Tuberculosis

Edited by
Giovanni Battista Migliori, Graham Bothamley,
Raquel Duarte and Adrian Rendon

Editor in Chief
Robert Bals

This book is one in a series of *ERS Monographs*. Each individual issue provides a comprehensive overview of one specific clinical area of respiratory health, communicating information about the most advanced techniques and systems required for its investigation. It provides factual and useful scientific detail, drawing on specific case studies and looking into the diagnosis and management of individual patients. Previously published titles in this series are listed at the back of this *Monograph*.

ERS Monographs are available online at www.books.ersjournals.com and print copies are available from www.ersbookshop.com

Editorial Board: Antonio Anzueto (San Antonio, TX, USA), Leif Bjermer (Lund, Sweden), John R. Hurst (London, UK) and Carlos Robalo Cordeiro (Coimbra, Portugal).

Managing Editor: Rachel Gozzard
European Respiratory Society, 442 Glossop Road, Sheffield, S10 2PX, UK
Tel: 44 114 2672860 | E-mail: monograph@ersnet.org

Production and editing: Caroline Ashford-Bentley, Alice Bartlett, Alyson Cann, Jonathan Hansen, Emma Jones, Claire Marchant, Catherine Pumphrey, Kay Sharpe and Ben Watson

Published by European Respiratory Society ©2018
December 2018
Print ISBN: 978-1-84984-099-6
Online ISBN: 978-1-84984-100-9
Print ISSN: 2312-508X
Online ISSN: 2312-5098
Typesetting by Nova Techset Private Limited
Printed by Charlesworth Press, Wakefield, UK

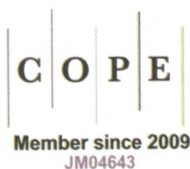

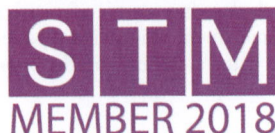

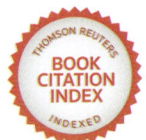

C|O|P|E
Member since 2009
JM04643

STM
MEMBER 2018

MIX
Paper from
responsible sources
FSC® C016379
www.fsc.org

THOMSON REUTERS
BOOK
CITATION
INDEX
INDEXED

ERS | monograph

Contents

Preface

Robert Bals

While most European chest physicians have little contact with TB patients, the disease is still of outstanding importance in our field, for a number of reasons.

1) TB was a major killer in Europe for hundreds of years, and phthisiology has helped develop many aspects of pulmonology.

2) TB is still a major cause of mortality and morbidity, and its prevalence in developing countries highlights the political dimensions of the disease.

3) TB is present in Europe and the clinical context of its presentation has changed in recent decades. Patients from a migratory background, those who are immunosuppressed and those with chronic lung diseases are now within the focus of care.

4) Diagnosis and treatment of TB is still a complicated issue. TB can mimic most other lung diseases and treatment has become a challenge in the age of multidrug resistancy.

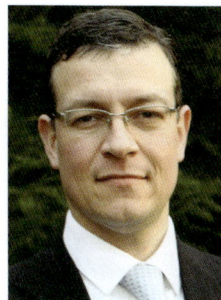

With these issues in mind, the United Nations General Assembly initiated concerted action and developed new guidelines. This *ERS Monograph* considers such guidelines, and provides a comprehensive and detailed overview of all aspects of TB. As such, it represents a unique source of information. The book covers the field's historical development, epidemiology, basic science and the clinical approach to the TB patient. It also includes chapters on drug therapy and special patient populations, as well as comorbidities.

The broad ranging and comprehensive topics covered in this book were selected by Guest Editors Giovanni Battista Migliori, Graham Bothamley, Raquel Duarte and Adrian Rendon. They worked to bring together expert authors in the field and in doing so, have successfully integrated different views on various aspects of TB. They have produced a *Monograph* that will not only be useful in the clinical practice of a broad range of respiratory physicians, but will be a trusted resource for many years to come.

Copyright ©ERS 2018. Print ISBN: 978-1-84984-099-6. Online ISBN: 978-1-84984-100-9. Print ISSN: 2312-508X. Online ISSN: 2312-5098.

https://doi.org/10.1183/2312508X.10032018

ERS | *monograph*

Guest Editors

Giovanni Battista Migliori

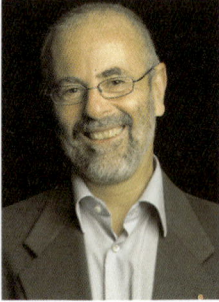

Giovanni Battista Migliori is a specialist in respiratory medicine and medical statistics, and an auditor of quality systems. He has over 20 years of experience in design, implementation, and monitoring and evaluation of TB and TB/HIV control programmes globally.

Giovanni Battista Migliori is Head of Clinical Epidemiology of the Respiratory Diseases Service and Director of the WHO Collaborating Centre for TB and Lung Diseases at Maugeri Care and Research Institute (Tradate, Italy).

Giovanni Battista Migliori is active in TB control, training and research activities at a global level. In 2012, he was elected a Fellow of the Royal College of Physicians, (London, UK) (honorary nomination, by-law 39b); and in 2014, he was elected Foundation Fellow of the European Respiratory Society (ERS).

Giovanni Battista Migliori has published more than 400 peer-reviewed papers on COPD, asthma, pulmonary rehabilitation and TB (h-index: 59). He was: one of the authors of the first ERS TB guidelines in 1999; an author/coordinator of several guidelines supporting ECDC/WHO development of a European Union TB control policy; an author on all of the guidelines belonging to the Wolfheze series (the European WHO/ International Union Against Tuberculosis and Lung Disease (IUATLD)/ECDC Consensus); a coordinator of the European Standards for Tuberculosis Care (ESTC); a promoter of the newly created Kosovo national TB Programme, in collaboration with the United States Agency for International Development (USAID), and of the implementation of TB control in countries experiencing war or mass migration; a coordinator of DST external quality assessment studies and drug-resistance surveys in several countries (Italy, Mozambique, Burkina, Kosovo, Russia and the Ukraine); a pioneer of the TB under-reporting evaluation with a series of important studies in different journals, which have been used by WHO to implement better surveillance

Copyright ©ERS 2018. Print ISBN: 978-1-84984-099-6. Online ISBN: 978-1-84984-100-9. Print ISSN: 2312-508X. Online ISSN: 2312-5098.

https://doi.org/10.1183/2312508X.10031218

guidance; a promoter of treatment-outcome evaluation as a surveillance and research tool; and an author on the 2013 WHO educational package supporting countries to develop national strategic plans and to apply to the Global Fund for funding. He demonstrated with experimental data the adequacy of the XDR-TB definition, the impossibility of using the TDR definition and the need to stratify outcomes beyond XDR-TB. He coordinated the USAID-funded project, which developed a tool that supported countries in the identification of gaps and in the proposal of solutions to prevent and manage MDR- and XDR-TB. This has become the standard tool used by the WHO Green Light Committee. He is the coordinator of the European TB Elimination movement, which involves the conceptualisation of TB elimination, the development of the first framework, creation of a feasibility white paper within the ERS Forum initiative, a European survey on preparedness and finalisation of the WHO framework resulting from the ERS/WHO event in Rome, Italy (2014).

Giovanni Battista Migliori has created and directed over 100 WHO training courses for consultants/managers of: TB and TB/HIV, the public–private mix, the laboratory, infection control and the Global Fund to Fight AIDS.

He is currently an Associate Editor of the *European Respiratory Journal* and the *International Journal of Tuberculosis and Lung Disease*. He was previously Secretary General of ERS.

Graham Bothamley

Graham Bothamley has been a respiratory physician for 35 years and has looked after >4000 patients with TB. He gained a PhD with the Medical Research Council (MRC) and Royal Postgraduate Medical School, Hammersmith Hospital (London, UK) in TB monoclonal antibodies, diagnostics and pathogenesis. He is currently a member of the TB Centre and Immunology and Infections Department at the London School of Hygiene and Tropical Medicine (London, UK) and at the Blizard Institute (Queen Mary University of London, London, UK).

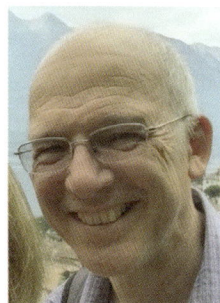

Graham Bothamley leads the British Thoracic Society (BTS) TB advisory group, is Head of the Respiratory Infections Assembly at the European Respiratory Society and is on the steering committee of TBnet as Past Chair.

Raquel Duarte

Raquel Duarte is a Portuguese pulmonologist, with a Masters in Public Health and Health Economics and a PhD in Public

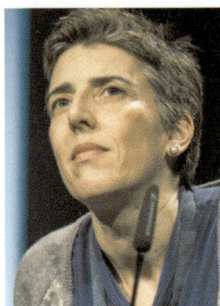

Health. She is the Coordinator of the National Reference Centre for MDR-TB, the Director of the National Programme for TB, and Associate Professor at the Medical School and at the Institute of Public Health of Porto University (Porto, Portugal).

In terms of international appointments, Raquel Duarte is Vice-President of the Europe Region Officers of the International Union Against Tuberculosis and Lung Disease, and Chair of the European Respiratory Society's Tuberculosis Group.

Raquel Duarte combines interests in public health with clinical, academic and research activities. Her main fields of interest are TB in vulnerable populations, the effects of social and economic determinants on TB incidence, LTBI, MDR-TB and XDR-TB, and NTM.

Adrian Rendon

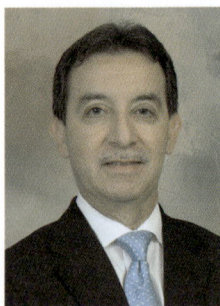

Adrian Rendon is a specialist in internal medicine and pulmonary and critical care medicine. He is Professor of Medicine at the School of Medicine and the University Hospital of Monterrey of the Universidad Autonoma de Nuevo Leon (Mexico), where he has run a busy TB clinic since 1994.

Adrian Rendon was trained in both Mexico and the USA. He graduated with honours as the first of his class, and later became Chief Resident of Internal Medicine and Chief Fellow of Pulmonary Medicine at the University Hospital of Monterrey.

For the last 15 years, Adrian Rendon has lead a TB Research, Prevention and Care Center in Monterrey (Mexico) that has become a referral centre for the Nuevo Leon State TB Program. The centre was something of a pioneer in Mexico and Latin America, as it was the first to routinely perform DST in all new TB cases, and has been doing so since 1994. In 2013, the Nuevo Leon State Public Health Society officially recognised his work in TB.

Adrian Rendon is the leading clinician involved in the local TB consilium and a consultant for the Mexican TB Consilium. He also is a founding member of the international European Respiratory Society (ERS)/WHO Tuberculosis Consilium.

Adrian Rendon's research focuses on several fields: basic, clinical and epidemiological TB topics, COPD, asthma, coccidioidomycosis and pneumonia, among others. He has published more than 50 peer-reviewed papers (h-index: 15), has participated in several COPD and TB guidelines and has collaborated with several international journals as a

https://doi.org/10.1183/2312508X.10031218

reviewer. He has also written several TB chapters in pulmonary medicine books.

Adrian Rendon is considered an opinion leader not only in Mexico but also in Latin America and has developed several collaborative projects with researchers and institutions in the USA and Europe. He is currently the Director of the TB Department of the Latin American Association of Thorax (ALAT) and the incoming President of the Mexican Society of Pulmonary Medicine and Thoracic Surgery (SMNYCT).

ERS | *monograph*

Introduction

Giovanni Battista Migliori[1], Graham Bothamley[2,3,4], Raquel Duarte[5,6,7] and Adrian Rendon[8]

🐦 @ERSpublications

Physicians feel TB is either very easy to treat with standard regimens or is too complex. This book: provides trainees with basic TB management knowledge; offers insight into addressing complexities in individual patients; is a useful resource for experts. http://ow.ly/zroQ30mipoT

On 26 September 2018, the United National General Assembly agreed to take concerted action on TB. With over 10 million new TB cases (90% in adults and 9% in HIV co-infected individuals) and 1.6 million deaths (300 000 in HIV coinfected persons) in 2017, TB is a global health priority [1]. Of particular concern for both clinicians and national TB programmes is MDR-TB: in 2017, WHO were notified of 558 000 new rifampicin-resistant cases and 460 000 confirmed MDR-TB cases [1]. Heads of state and government agreed to mobilise US$13 billion a year by 2022 in order to ensure that TB care is received by 40 million people and preventive treatment is given to 30 million people [2].

Although the "white plague" has historically been studied in an extensive manner (it was "the" respiratory disease in the pre-antibiotic era), there is still much to learn about its prevention, diagnosis and treatment. TB is therefore a hot topic in respiratory medicine, attracting an increasing amount of interest from clinicians, scientists, public health officers and the pharmaceutical industry, given that new drugs are finally available after more than 40 years of neglect. The High-Level Meeting on the Fight to End Tuberculosis also agreed to fund a US$2-billion research agenda [2].

With this *Monograph*, our aim is to provide an accessible resource that will help the young physician in training to recognise and treat TB in all its manifestations, as well as address a need for help with other mycobacterial diseases which might become apparent during the diagnostic process. Primarily providing clinical support, this book will also act as a reference resource for difficult TB. It will introduce topics of interest and scientific advances in TB that can be investigated by the interested reader at their leisure. Many of the chapters also indicate where TB management is going.

[1]Istituti Clinici Scientifici Maugeri IRCCS, Tradate, Italy. [2]Homerton University Hospital, London, UK. [3]Blizard Institute, Barts and The London School of Medicine and Dentistry, Queen Mary University of London, London, UK. [4]London School of Hygiene and Tropical Medicine, London, UK. [5]Departamento de Pneumologia, Centro Hospitalar Vila Nova de Gaia, Vila Nova de Gaia, Portugal. [6]Departamento de Ciências da Saúde Pública e Forenses e Educação Médica, Faculdade de Medicina, Universidade do Porto, Porto, Portugal. [7]ISPUP-EPIUnit, Faculdade de Medicina, Universidade do Porto, Porto, Portugal. [8]TB Dept, University Hospital of Monterrey, Monterrey, Mexico.

Correspondence: Giovanni Battista Migliori, Istituti Clinici Scientifici Maugeri IRCCS, Via Roncaccio 16, Tradate, Varese, 21049, Italy. E-mail: giovannibattista.migliori@icsmaugeri.it

Copyright ©ERS 2018. Print ISBN: 978-1-84984-099-6. Online ISBN: 978-1-84984-100-9. Print ISSN: 2312-508X. Online ISSN: 2312-5098.

https://doi.org/10.1183/2312508X.10031118

This *Monograph* will discuss the main issues related to TB, with an innovative approach, beginning with a patient's perspective [3]. The role of patients is very important, given the burden of the disease on healthcare systems globally.

A chapter on the history of TB discusses recent advances in human and TB genetics and presents historical vignettes that are relevant to the current introduction of new treatments [4]. Social determinants are included in the chapter on epidemiology, so that the measures to control and eventually eliminate TB are more holistic [5]. Molecular biology has made significant advances since the last *ERS Monograph* on TB was published in 2012 [6], and clinically relevant material has been included in a number of chapters [4, 7–12]. The diagnostic aspects (clinical diagnosis, laboratory diagnosis, imaging, bronchoscopy and other invasive procedures) are reiterated and updated so that they are accessible to the physician in training [5, 9, 13, 14]. The treatment of drug-susceptible and drug-resistant cases, new and repurposed drugs, adverse events and the role of surgery are discussed, together with broad principles, so that physicians can apply these to the likely rapid changes in this area [15–18]. Specific patient groups (children, pregnant women and the elderly) are addressed [19]. Comorbidities have become an increasing problem in the management of TB, and diabetes, chronic renal impairment, liver disease and transplantation are addressed, in addition to coinfection with HIV [20]. The modern TB physician has to work with a team to manage homelessness, alcohol and opiate addictions, poverty and malnutrition and the disruptions caused by migration and fleeing war zones and persecutions [21].

A later chapter includes both treatment and therapeutic drug monitoring, noting that the latter will become increasingly important in personalised treatments regimens [22]. Rehabilitation after TB has become an important topic and receives its own chapter [23]. NTM have been included, as they are frequently diagnosed when TB is considered their increasing importance may merit an entire *Monograph* in the not-too-distant future [24]! Preventive issues have come to the fore, especially with the End TB Strategy and there are chapters on vaccines [10], infection control [25] and latent TB infection management [11]. Looking to the future, there is a chapter on research priorities [12], and one addressing the needs of the physician training [26].

Lastly, to emphasise the realities of managing TB, there are some clinical cases drawn from the experience of early career members with expertise in managing MDR-TB [27].

The developments and challenges over the last 6 years, since the publication of the first TB *Monograph* [6], have exceeded our expectations. We expect the recent pledges of world leaders to defeat TB will be met by a mixture of attention to patients' needs and scientific advances, in addition to those we have outlined in this *Monograph*. We hope the *Monograph* will encourage TB physicians and basic scientists to see the gaps and fill these with their own excellent research for the next TB *Monograph*.

References

1. World Health Organization. Global Tuberculosis report 2018. WHO/CDS/TB/2018.20. Geneva, World Health Organization, 2018. http://apps.who.int/iris/bitstream/handle/10665/274453/9789241565646-eng.pdf?ua=1
2. UNGA High Level Meeting on Tuberculosis, 26 September 2018. https://www.un.org/pga/73/event-detail/fight-to-end-tuberculosis/.

3. Spita G, Clegg H, Dumitru M, *et al.* The patients' perspective. *In:* Migliori GB, Bothamley G, Duarte R, *et al.*, eds. Tuberculosis (ERS Monograph). Sheffield, European Respiratory Society, 2018; pp. 1–7.

4. Loddenkemper R, Murray JF, Gradmann C, *et al.* History of tuberculosis. *In:* Migliori GB, Bothamley G, Duarte R, *et al.*, eds. Tuberculosis (ERS Monograph). Sheffield, European Respiratory Society, 2018; pp. 8–27.

5. Duarte R, Santos JV, Santos Silva A, *et al.* Epidemiology and socioeconomic determinants. *In:* Migliori GB, Bothamley G, Duarte R, *et al.*, eds. Tuberculosis (ERS Monograph). Sheffield, European Respiratory Society, 2018; pp. 28–35.

6. Lange C, Migliori GB, eds. Tuberculosis. Sheffield, European Respiratory Society, 2012.

7. Barreira-Silva P, Torrado E, Nebenzahl-Guimaraes, *et al.* Aetiopathogenesis, immunology and microbiology. *In:* Migliori GB, Bothamley G, Duarte R, *et al.*, eds. Tuberculosis (ERS Monograph). Sheffield, European Respiratory Society, 2018; pp. 62–82.

8. Zellweger J-P, Sousa P, Heyckendorf J. Clinical diagnosis. *In:* Migliori GB, Bothamley G, Duarte R, *et al.*, eds. Tuberculosis (ERS Monograph). Sheffield, European Respiratory Society, 2018; pp. 83–98.

9. Tagliani E, Nikolayevskyy V, Tortoli E, *et al.* Laboratory diagnosis. *In:* Migliori GB, Bothamley G, Duarte R, *et al.*, eds. Tuberculosis (ERS Monograph). Sheffield, European Respiratory Society, 2018; pp. 99–115.

10. Ruhwald M, Andersen PL, Schrager L. Towards a new vaccine. *In:* Migliori GB, Bothamley G, Duarte R, *et al.*, eds. Tuberculosis (ERS Monograph). Sheffield, European Respiratory Society, 2018; pp. 343–363.

11. Rendon A, Goletti D, Matteelli A. Diagnosis and treatment of latent tuberculosis infection. *In:* Migliori GB, Bothamley G, Duarte R, *et al.*, eds. Tuberculosis (ERS Monograph). Sheffield, European Respiratory Society, 2018; pp. 381–398.

12. Bothamley G. What next? Basic research, new treatments and a patient-centred approach. *In:* Migliori GB, Bothamley G, Duarte R, *et al.*, eds. Tuberculosis (ERS Monograph). Sheffield, European Respiratory Society, 2018; pp. 414–429.

13. Chesov D, Botnaru V. Imaging for diagnosis and management. *In:* Migliori GB, Bothamley G, Duarte R, *et al.*, eds. Tuberculosis (ERS Monograph). Sheffield, European Respiratory Society, 2018; pp. 116–136.

14. Bhowmik A, Herth FJF. Bronchoscopy and other invasive procedures for diagnosis. *In:* Migliori GB, Bothamley G, Duarte R, *et al.*, eds. Tuberculosis (ERS Monograph). Sheffield, European Respiratory Society, 2018; pp. 137–151.

15. Caminero JA, Scardigli A, van der Werf T, *et al.* Treatment of drug-susceptible and drug-resistant tuberculosis. *In:* Migliori GB, Bothamley G, Duarte R, *et al.*, eds. Tuberculosis (ERS Monograph). Sheffield, European Respiratory Society, 2018; pp. 152–178.

16. Krutikov M, Bruchfeld J, Migliori GB, *et al.* New and repurposed drugs. *In:* Migliori GB, Bothamley G, Duarte R, *et al.*, eds. Tuberculosis (ERS Monograph). Sheffield, European Respiratory Society, 2018; pp. 179–204.

17. Caminero JA, Lasserra P, Piubello A, *et al.* Adverse anti-tuberculosis drug events and their management. *In:* Migliori GB, Bothamley G, Duarte R, *et al.*, eds. Tuberculosis (ERS Monograph). Sheffield, European Respiratory Society, 2018; pp. 205–227.

18. Olland A, Falcoz P-E, Guinard S, *et al.* Surgery as a treatment. *In:* Migliori GB, Bothamley G, Duarte R, *et al.*, eds. Tuberculosis (ERS Monograph). Sheffield, European Respiratory Society, 2018; pp. 228–233.

19. Repossi A, Bothamley G. Pregnancy and the elderly. *In:* Migliori GB, Bothamley G, Duarte R, *et al.*, eds. Tuberculosis (ERS Monograph). Sheffield, European Respiratory Society, 2018; pp. 263–275.

20. Magis-Escurra C, Carvalho ACC, Kritski AL, *et al.* Comorbidities. *In:* Migliori GB, Bothamley G, Duarte R, *et al.*, eds. Tuberculosis (ERS Monograph). Sheffield, European Respiratory Society, 2018; pp. 276–290.

21. Viney K, Wingfield T, Kuksa L, *et al.* Access and adherence to prevention and care for hard-to-reach groups. *In:* Migliori GB, Bothamley G, Duarte R, *et al.*, eds. Tuberculosis (ERS Monograph). Sheffield, European Respiratory Society, 2018; pp. 291–307.

22. Alffenaar J-WC, Akkerman OW, Bothamley G, *et al.* Monitoring during and after treatment. *In:* Migliori GB, Bothamley G, Duarte R, *et al.*, eds. Tuberculosis (ERS Monograph). Sheffield, European Respiratory Society, 2018; pp. 308–325.

23. Muñoz-Torrico M, Cid S, Galicia-Amor S, *et al.* Sequelae assessment and rehabilitation. *In:* Migliori GB, Bothamley G, Duarte R, *et al.*, eds. Tuberculosis (ERS Monograph). Sheffield, European Respiratory Society, 2018; pp. 326–342.

24. Zweijpfenning S, Hoefsloot W, van Ingen J, *et al.* Nontuberculous mycobacteria. *In:* Migliori GB, Bothamley G, Duarte R, *et al.*, eds. Tuberculosis (ERS Monograph). Sheffield, European Respiratory Society, 2018; pp. 399–413.

25. Nardell E, Volchenkov G. Transmission control: a refocused approach. *In:* Migliori GB, Bothamley G, Duarte R, *et al.*, eds. Tuberculosis (ERS Monograph). Sheffield, European Respiratory Society, 2018; pp. 364–380.

26. Casalini C, Matteelli A, Komba A, *et al.* Opportunities for training and learning. *In:* Migliori GB, Bothamley G, Duarte R, *et al.*, eds. Tuberculosis (ERS Monograph). Sheffield, European Respiratory Society, 2018; pp. 430–445.

27. Tiberi S, Payen MC, Manika K, *et al.* Clinical cases. *In:* Migliori GB, Bothamley G, Duarte R, *et al.*, eds. Tuberculosis (ERS Monograph). Sheffield, European Respiratory Society, 2018; pp. 446–460.

Disclosures: None declared.

https://doi.org/10.1183/2312508X.10031118

List of abbreviations

ART	antiretroviral therapy
BCG	bacille Calmette–Guérin
CDC	Centers for Disease Control and Prevention
COPD	chronic obstructive pulmonary disease
DILI	drug-induced liver injury
DM	diabetes mellitus
DOTS	directly observed therapy, short course
DR-TB	drug-resistant tuberculosis
DST	drug-susceptibility testing
EPTB	extrapulmonary tuberculosis
ETTB	extrathoracic tuberculosis
IFN	interferon
IGRA	interferon-γ release assay
IUATLD	International Union Against Tuberculosis and Lung Disease
LFT	liver function tests
LTBI	latent tuberculosis infection
MDR-TB	multidrug-resistant tuberculosis
MIC	minimum inhibitory concentration
MTBC	*Mycobacterium tuberculosis* complex
NGO	nongovernmental organisation
NTM	nontuberculous mycobacteria
PAS	para-aminosalicylic acid
PTB	pulmonary tuberculosis
RCT	randomised controlled clinical trial
RR-TB	rifampicin-resistant tuberculosis
SDGs	sustainable development goals
SLIDs	second-line injectable drugs
TB	tuberculosis
TDM	therapeutic drug monitoring
TST	tuberculin skin test
WHO	World Health Organization
XDR-TB	extensively drug-resistant tuberculosis

Chapter 1

The patients' perspective

Gabi Spita[1], Helen Clegg[2], Marius Dumitru[3], Paul Sommerfeld[4], Courtney Coleman[5] and Pippa Powell[5]

This chapter looks at TB and MDR-TB from the patients' perspective by posing three questions: how does TB and MDR-TB affect the daily lives of patients, how can the care of TB be improved, and where should we go with TB care in the next 10 years? The answers draw on the authors' experience and knowledge, and on published literature and case studies.

Cite as: Spita G, Clegg H, Dumitru M, *et al.* The patients' perspective. *In:* Migliori GB, Bothamley G, Duarte R, *et al.*, eds. Tuberculosis (ERS Monograph). Sheffield, European Respiratory Society, 2018; pp. 1–7 [https://doi.org/10.1183/2312508X.10020517].

🐦 @ERSpublications
To improve TB care from the patients' perspective, we need to learn from others, work together, improve education and understand the changing profile of the patient to diagnose quicker, keep patients out of hospital, improve awareness and provide support. http://ow.ly/cfVQ30lqCfE

This innovative chapter aims to set the scene for this timely *ERS Monograph* by looking at TB and MDR-TB from the patients' perspective – what are the big issues and where do we need to go in the next 10 years?

The European Lung Foundation (ELF) was asked to lead on the writing of this chapter, and to do so it worked with a selection of individuals and organisations from the ELF patient organisation network, including people who have lived with the condition and representatives of patient and advocacy organisations. The author group represents a number of European countries, which is important when thinking about the prevalence of the condition and the treatment options available in different regions.

The three questions presented here were asked by the Guest Editors of this *Monograph*, and these questions were posed to the authors. The points presented are based on their experience and knowledge, and on those of people linked to their organisations. In addition, the ELF performed a literature review to see what had been published about the patient experience in these areas. A total of 64000 papers were identified. The majority of

[1]Former TB Patient, Iasi, Romania. [2]TB Alert, Brighton, UK. [3]Romanian Association of TB Patients (ARB-TB), Bucharest, Romania. [4]TB Europe Coalition, Brussels, Belgium. [5]European Lung Foundation, Sheffield, UK.

Correspondence: Pippa Powell, European Lung Foundation, 442 Glossop Road, Sheffield S10 2PX, UK. E-mail: pippa.powell@europeanlung.org

This article has supplementary material available from books.ersjournals.com

the papers identified were from outside the Europe region but in some cases have been used to support points highlighted by the authors.

Finally, we have included quotes from case studies from different regions. These case studies highlight and bring to life some of the issues summarised in the chapter. The full collection of case studies is available in the online supplementary material. It is hoped that this mix of overarching messages and personal stories will set the tone for the rest of this *Monograph*.

How do tuberculosis and multidrug-resistant tuberculosis affect the daily lives of patients?

Stigma

> Friends reacted in different ways. Some people freaked out and didn't want to visit me, which I desperately needed.
>
> Jess, UK.

There remains a huge stigma around TB. All of the case studies collected for this chapter talk about the impact of stigma. People who are diagnosed with TB can often feel rejected by society, including by family and friends and people they trust. They often feel isolated, both because of the diagnosis and also due to their treatment regimes. There is a large risk that patients are not welcomed back into their old job and careers, especially if they are working in public-facing positions (*e.g.* doctors, teachers).

In a systematic review published by THOMAS *et al.* [1], stigma was identified as one of the main issues faced by MDR-TB patients from 282 published studies.

Self-image

> I found myself with the world crumbling around me. I thought of myself as a healthy person, to whom nothing could happen because I am young.
>
> Simona, Romania.
>
> I never thought something like that could happen to me. I had a healthy life style, have been pretty sporty and never smoked a cigarette in my life. I was not meant to have TB! But TB, like many other diseases, doesn't differentiate, it just hits!
>
> Cristina, Romania.

Many patients feel real shock when they find out they have TB. People who felt they were fit and healthy suddenly find out they have a disease that needs substantial long-term treatment. Individuals are often young and therefore find it hard to accept that they are seriously ill. This also can cause problems and delays with diagnosis, as people may ignore symptoms, or healthcare professionals may overlook the diagnosis of TB due to an individual's age or the fact that they are not in a high-risk group and are generally in good health.

Financial impact

TB has a huge impact on a person's entire life. It is not a condition that can sit in the background and be managed with little effect on daily living.

https://doi.org/10.1183/2312508X.10020517

The first financial impact can hit if a person has to travel to get a diagnosis. People have to stop working. They have to spend a lot of time interacting with the healthcare system, which incurs travel costs. They may also have to travel out of their own country for treatment. Patients with coinfections or other conditions, including HIV, may have to visit multiple locations to receive treatment for each condition.

There is a strong financial impact on every TB patient, which is often on top of the fact that the people most likely to get TB are from lower socioeconomic backgrounds. Often, there is no recourse to public funds, and this can impact on access to housing and benefits, all of which are important to support the patient.

In a study in Ethiopia, GETAHUN et al. [2] found that, despite the availability of free-of-charge anti-TB drugs, TB patients were making many out-of-pocket payments that they could not afford, which in turn were hampering the efforts to end TB. A report from the Regional Eastern Europe and Central Asian TB Project (TB-REP) and TB Europe Coalition noted that providing care in ambulatory rather than hospital settings can reduce the financial burden for both individual patients and healthcare systems. Related savings should be reinvested into good-quality people-centred care, such as offering patients incentives for treatment adherence [3]. Similarly, offering multiple health services at a single location would allow more integrated access and ease related financial challenges [4].

Fear for others

> After tests, it appeared I'd given TB to my brother, cousin and brother-in-law. I was so relieved my grandma was ok.
>
> Jess, UK.

> Eventually at the end of July, I was diagnosed with TB. In Switzerland, I was immediately put into isolation and was told if I didn't take my medicine I would end up in prison. Then my family, friends and class (I'm a teacher) were all tested. My family and friends were cleared, but three children in my class were diagnosed with TB. Consequently, their families were tested but no one else had it.
>
> Irene, Switzerland.

As TB is a contagious disease, and people may have been living with the condition for some time before being diagnosed, there is often a great deal of fear about having passed the condition on to others. This could be family, friends or work colleagues. This worry and fear, and often guilt, can also add to the stigma of TB.

Resilience

> Now I hope everything will be alright. I feel like I've been born again. This is the feeling I get. To the ones that are still under treatment, I wish them to be strong and to have the will to fight and to believe that everything will turn out fine.
>
> Bella, Romania.

> I was very lucky to have a loving and supportive family beside me, who gave me strength and courage; they supported me all the time and this is why I had a positive tone during the entire treatment.
>
> Gabi, Romania.

The overwhelming sense from the case studies received by ELF for the writing of this chapter was around the need for strength and resilience, the feeling that if a person can live through and recover from TB they can do anything. This is a real positive from the experiences of those living with the condition.

How can the care of tuberculosis be improved from the patients' perspective?

Quicker diagnosis

Diagnosis should be made as soon as possible. Diagnosis often takes 3–4 months, and this can be due to a number of factors, such as poor public awareness, people not thinking there is a serious problem and so not visiting their doctor soon enough, and poor understanding of the disease by healthcare professionals.

A study by BONADONNA *et al.* [5] carried out in Lima concluded that more human and material resources are required to promote TB case-finding initiatives, reduce TB-associated stigma and address the social determinants underlying diagnostic delay.

Keeping out of hospital

It is possible to be treated in the main from home rather than in hospital if you have TB, achieving similar or better treatment outcomes in most cases [3]. The advantages of maximising time at home are that it is more likely that a person will have a personal support network close at hand, helping to reduce stigma and discrimination, and allowing patients to better manage their treatment routine.

In a study in Uganda, home-based treatment and care was found to be acceptable to patients, families, communities and healthcare workers, and was seen as preferable to hospital-based care by most respondents [6]. Home-based care was perceived as safe, conducive to recovery, facilitating psychosocial support, and allowing more free time and earning potential for patients and care-givers.

Home-based care, however, is still not available throughout Eastern Europe and Central Asia as the default option for patients without complications. Challenges around healthcare system set-ups and misconceptions about the safety of home-based treatment among professionals and patients continue to prevent comprehensive uptake. A particular danger of overuse of hospitalisation is that patients who start with drug-sensitive TB may contract MDR-TB from fellow patients while in hospital [7]. There is a need to explain more clearly to healthcare staff, as well as to patients and their families, that, once started on a proper course of treatment, a TB patient, whether drug sensitive or multidrug resistant, becomes noninfectious within a matter of days [8].

Improved awareness and education

Awareness and education about TB is vital. It can help in early identification and diagnosis, and with stigma and adherence. In Romania and much of Eastern Europe, the majority of TB patients are in poorer socioeconomic groups [9]. However, there are patients from higher socioeconomic groups who could play more of a public role in education and dissemination. However, this is difficult in reality as not many patients are happy to talk about their TB experience and just want to forget about it.

Companies and businesses need to be educated on what TB is and how to treat employees fairly and equitably in the workplace, in line with the principles of dignity and security set out in *The Patients' Charter for Tuberculosis Care* [10].

https://doi.org/10.1183/2312508X.10020517

ZACHARIAH *et al.* [11], in their study about the language of TB, put out a plea to the healthcare community to change the terms used in TB care: terms such as "defaulter", "suspect" and "control" used in TB care are inappropriate, coercive and disempowering. They urge simple steps, such as replacing the term "defaulter" with "person lost to follow-up", "TB suspect" with "person with presumptive TB" or "person to be evaluated for TB", and "control" with "prevention and care". The language used around TB should be nonjudgemental and patient centred [10].

Peer support and counselling

More peer support and counselling are needed to ensure that people who live with TB are supported. In the UK, vulnerable patients get close support, directly observed treatment and social support (*e.g.* housing, travel, nutrition).

Peer support can also be given *via* tools such as HealthUnlocked (www.healthunlocked.com) and civil society organisations. However, peer support often lacks funding, meaning that it is unsustainable. An increase in the availability of funding for patient support grants by local authorities and governments would be a big step forward.

LEWIS AND NEWELL [12], in a study in Nepal, found that, in order to support people with TB more during their treatment, health policies and practice must appreciate that TB affects all aspects of TB patients' lives.

PAZ-SOLDÁN *et al.* [13], based in Peru, looked at the provision of social support. Here they found that psychosocial support was given to many patients by their families when they disclosed their diagnosis. High levels of depression were identified in patients, with many requesting psychological support. Patients who were involved in the programme locally advised that educational opportunities should be extended to patients' families and the wider community, increasing the existing amount of nutritional support and programmatic provision of vocational activities to increase economic opportunities.

In their assessment of efforts to tackle MDR- and XDR-TB in the European Region, the TB Europe Coalition highlighted a number of recommendations to improve treatment outcomes [14]. This included extending TB treatment beyond physical care to include access to social and psychological support. They recognised the role of civil society and patient organisations in the provision of psychosocial support, particularly in supporting socially vulnerable groups (including migrant communities, homeless people and people who inject drugs). One example of this is in the Azerbaijani penal system, where civil society organisations are involved in patient follow-up, treatment adherence and psychosocial support, allowing the country to achieve some of the best cure rates for MDR- and XDR-TB in prisons in the region. Loss to follow-up has also been reduced to almost zero, and the treatment success rate for new TB patients has increased to 88% [14].

Where should we go with tuberculosis care in the next 10 years?

Learn from others

Networking and learning from each other are vital to establish consistent levels of care across Europe [14].

The vast amount of knowledge and expertise that is available in Europe should be used in order to inspire confidence at a national level. Global expertise is important but should be combined with local expertise and context. Conversely, people working at a local level should always be conscious of sharing experiences and best practices that others can learn from. The 2014 assessment of efforts to tackle MDR- and XDR-TB in the European Region noted that local and national TB knowledge, attitude and practice studies provided crucial information to develop areas for priority action and to identify best practices [14].

One study, which compared the TB services across London in the UK, found significant variations, with best practices taking place in one area that were not transferred to others [15]. The authors highlighted that, even in London, what was needed was more consistent strategic planning/co-ordination and sharing of best practice. They also noted that these findings would be relevant to the development of TB services in other European cities.

Common standards of TB care should be developed and adapted to ensure fair and equitable treatment across Europe.

Work together

Patients and professionals should be ready to lobby together to try and get equal care for all TB patients across Europe. The patient–professional partnership is key to effecting policy change at national and international levels.

Develop strategies for migrant populations

In Europe, some of the biggest challenges in TB elimination are around migration and the need to manage TB care in people who are homeless or on the move. Patient-centred care models provide tools to facilitate tailored, high-quality care for individuals with multiple and complex needs [3].

Improve education

Public education is still needed to ensure that people understand TB, so that the stigma can be reduced further.

Professionals need to be better educated so that TB diagnosis is sped up. Education should also not be focused solely on doctors. Doctors often do not have enough time for a full discussion with patients. Therefore, key targets should be nurses, families and schools. Patient organisations can play an important role in delivering information and awareness-raising activities, and joint education efforts between advocacy, professional and patient organisations should be encouraged. For example, in Bulgaria, civil society organisations were contracted by the National TB Programme to expand community awareness and patient support activities, contributing to Bulgaria's significant drop in TB incidence, which has almost halved over a 5-year period [14].

Understanding the changing profile of patients

There needs to be a greater awareness of the changing profile of TB patients. There is a preconceived idea of what a TB patient looks like, which is no longer necessarily the case.

https://doi.org/10.1183/2312508X.10020517

The changing nature of TB means patients can get missed, and different organisations should be engaged in order to spread awareness as widely as possible. In the UK, work is being done with the Royal College of Midwives on TB in pregnancy, including BCG vaccine uptake in neonates.

Support in other aspects of a patient's life

Patients need support to rebuild their lives. This may go beyond what can be provided by their direct healthcare team, so there should be processes in place for referral to outside resources and assistance.

References

1. Thomas BE, Shanmugam P, Malaisamy M, *et al.* Psycho-socio-economic issues challenging multidrug resistant tuberculosis patients: a systematic review. *PLoS One* 2016; 11: e0147397.
2. Getahun B, Wubie M, Dejenu G, *et al.* Tuberculosis care strategies and their economic consequences for patients: the missing link to end tuberculosis. *Infect Dis Poverty* 2016; 5: 93.
3. Voitzwinkler F, Sommerfeld P, Stillo J, *et al.* Moving to people-centred care: achieving better TB outcomes. London, TB Europe Coalition, 2017. www.tbcoalition.eu/wp-content/uploads/2017/07/TBEC-brochure-on-PCC_EN_final.pdf
4. TB Europe Coalition. Transitioning From Donor Support for TB and HIV in Europe. Estonia: a Health System Approach to TB and HIV Response. London, TB Europe Coalition, 2017. www.tbcoalition.eu/wp-content/uploads/2018/03/FINAL-Estonia-case-study.pdf
5. Bonadonna LV, Saunders MJ, Zegarra R, *et al.* Why wait? The social determinants underlying tuberculosis diagnostic delay. *PLoS One* 2017; 12: e0185018.
6. Horter S, Stringer B, Reynolds L, *et al.* "Home is where the patient is": a qualitative analysis of a patient-centred model of care for multi-drug resistant tuberculosis. *BMC Health Serv Res* 2014; 14: 81.
7. Bantubani N, Kabera G, Connolly C, *et al.* High rates of potentially infectious tuberculosis and multidrug-resistant tuberculosis (MDR-TB) among hospital inpatients in KwaZulu Natal, South Africa indicate risk of nosocomial transmission. *PLoS One* 2014; 9: e90868.
8. Dharmadhikari S, Mphahlele M, Venter K, *et al.* Rapid impact of effective treatment on transmission of multidrug-resistant tuberculosis. *Int J Tuberc Lung Dis* 2014; 18: 1019–1025.
9. TB Europe Coalition/ACTION. Transitioning From Donor Support. HIV and TB Programmes in Eastern Europe and Central Asia: Challenges and Effective Solutions. London, TB Europe Coalition, 2016. www.tbcoalition.eu/wp-content/uploads/2016/05/TBEC-Position-Paper-Transitioning-from-donor-support-HIVTB-programmes-in-EECA.pdf
10. World Care Council/Conseil Mondial de Soins. The Patients' Charter for Tuberculosis Care: Parents' Rights and Responsibilities. Viols en Lava, World Care Council/Conseil Mondial de Soins, 2006. www.who.int/tb/publications/2006/istc_charter.pdf
11. Zachariah R, Harries AD, Srinath S, *et al.* Language in tuberculosis services: can we change to patient-centred terminology and stop the paradigm of blaming the patients? *Int J Tuberc Lung Dis* 2012; 6: 714–717.
12. Lewis CP, Newell JN. Improving tuberculosis care in low income countries – a qualitative study of patients' understanding of "patient support" in Nepal. *BMC Public Health* 2009; 9: 190.
13. Paz-Soldán VA, Alban RE, Jones CD, *et al.* The provision of and need for social support among adult and pediatric patients with tuberculosis in Lima, Peru: a qualitative study. *BMC Health Serv Res* 2013; 13: 290.
14. TB Europe Coalition/ACTION. Falling Short: a Civil Society Perspective of the Response to Multi and Extensively Drug Resistant Tuberculosis (M/XDR-TB) in the European Region. London, TB Europe Coalition, 2014. www.tbcoalition.eu/wp-content/uploads/2012/03/1410_report-falling-short-final.pdf
15. Belling R, McLaren S, Boudioni M, *et al.* Pan-London tuberculosis services: a service evaluation. *BMC Health Serv Res* 2012; 12: 203.

Disclosures: M. Dumitru works as a volunteer at the Romanian Association of Tuberculosis Patients. M. Dumitru is also a medical consultant and a qualified pharmacovigilance person (QPPV), and offers specialised consultancy to pharmaceutical companies in drug-registration procedures. C. Coleman is an employee of the ELF. P. Powell is an employee of the ELF.

| Chapter 2

History of tuberculosis

Robert Loddenkemper[1], John F. Murray[2], Christoph Gradmann[3], Philip C. Hopewell[4] and Midori Kato-Maeda[5]

This chapter begins with the supposition that *Mycobacterium tuberculosis* and humans co-evolved during their greater than 70000-year partnership, but how and where are still not fully understood. During the Neolithic revolution the size of the population and its farming and animal domestication activities contributed to the maintenance and transmission of *M. tuberculosis*. TB continued its increase beginning around 1750 owing to the deplorable conditions prevailing during the first half of the Industrial revolution (overcrowding, malnutrition and absent sanitation), but then began to decline. Even after Robert Koch's seminal discovery of *M. tuberculosis* in 1882, methods of diagnosis, treatment and prevention advanced slowly. But then TB mortality again increased sharply in many countries during world war I and II. In 1944, effective TB antibiotics first appeared and even better ones followed. Major impediments to TB eradication or elimination remain HIV infection and drug resistance. The WHO created the End TB Strategy in 2014, but achieving its goals appears unlikely by 2035. Possible solutions include widespread treatment for LTBI and an effective vaccine.

Cite as: Loddenkemper R, Murray JF, Gradmann C, *et al.* History of tuberculosis. *In:* Migliori GB, Bothamley G, Duarte R, *et al.*, eds. Tuberculosis (ERS Monograph). Sheffield, European Respiratory Society, 2018; pp. 8–27 [https://doi.org/10.1183/2312508X.10020617].

@ERSpublications
TB originated about 73000 years ago. It became the largest cause of adult deaths from any single infectious disease. Today it ranks among the top 10 causes of death worldwide. Drug resistance and HIV are the major impediments to TB elimination. http://ow.ly/cfVQ30lqCfE

Co-evolution of *Mycobacterium tuberculosis* and humans during the Neolithic period

The precise origins of TB are unknown. A study based on the genomic analysis of more than 250 strains of MTBC suggests that it originated approximately 73000 years ago in Africa [1]. MTBC is composed of both animal-adapted and human-adapted strains, the latter of which are composed of seven lineages (figure 1a) [2].

[1]German Central Committee against Tuberculosis, Berlin, Germany. [2]University of California San Francisco, San Francisco, CA, USA. [3]Institute for Health and Society, Section for Medical Anthropology and Medical History, University of Oslo, Oslo, Norway. [4]Division of Pulmonary and Critical Care Medicine, University of California San Francisco, San Francisco General Hospital, San Francisco, CA, USA. [5]Division of Pulmonary and Critical Care Medicine, University of California San Francisco, Zuckerberg San Francisco General Hospital, San Francisco, CA, USA.

Correspondence: Robert Loddenkemper, German Central Committee against Tuberculosis, Hertastr. 3, 14169 Berlin, Germany. E-mail: robert.loddenkemper@pneumologie.de

Copyright ©ERS 2018. Print ISBN: 978-1-84984-099-6. Online ISBN: 978-1-84984-100-9. Print ISSN: 2312-508X. Online ISSN: 2312-5098.

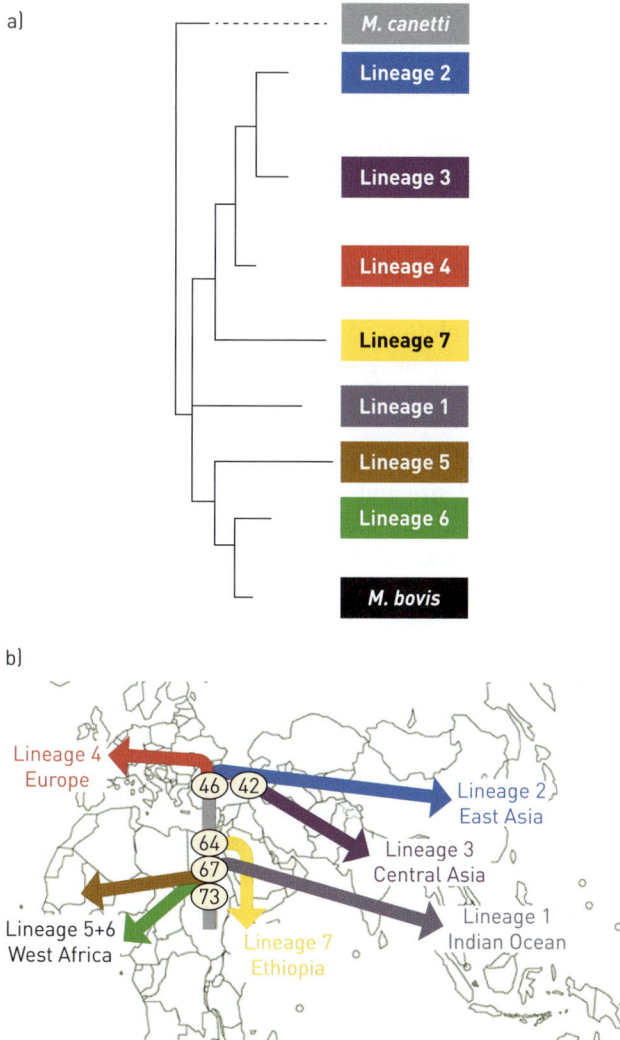

Figure 1. a) Phylogeny of the MTBC. The phylogeny is rooted with *Mycobacterium canettii*. The MTBC comprises seven human-adapted lineages and several lineages adapted to various wild and domestic animals, represented here only by *Mycobacterium bovis*. Reproduced and modified from [2] with permission. b) Out-of-Africa and Neolithic expansion of MTBC. The map summarises the results of the phylogeographic and dating analyses for MTBC. Colour coding of lineages is the same as in a. The major splits are annotated with the median value (in thousands of years) of the dating of the relevant node. Reproduced and modified from [1] with permission.

Until the 1990s it was thought that *M. tuberculosis* derived from *Mycobacterium bovis*, a pathogen mainly affecting cattle [3], which was then passed to humans through domesticated animals during the Neolithic period [4]. However, whole genome sequence-based studies in the late 1990s revealed that the animal-adapted strains were derived from human-adapted *M. tuberculosis*, specifically from the same ancestor of *M. tuberculosis* lineage 6 (figure 1a) [5]. Interestingly, the phylogeographic distribution and the shape and spacial relationships of the branches of the phylogenetic tree of the *M. tuberculosis* lineages, and the mitochondrial genomes of the major human haplogroups are similar, with early branching found only in Africa [1]. Moreover, the branching of *M. tuberculosis* into different lineages is estimated to have occurred between 73 000 and 42 000 years ago, which coincides with the estimated migration and dispersal of human populations out of Africa (figure 1b) [1]. These data, together with the fact that human-adapted *M. tuberculosis* mainly affects humans, suggests that both MTBC and humans have co-evolved for the last 70 000 years.

The Neolithic demographic revolution started roughly 10 000 years ago when hunter-gatherers began to settle down permanently and adopt a new life of agriculture and animal domestication [6]. This monumental change evolved at different times in different regions: 10 000 BC in Mesopotamia [7] and 7000 BC in Greece [8]. Significant benefits included an increase in birth rates, the evolution of novel forms of labour and production, and the development of unique administrative functions. Overall health declined, but the population grew and the world changed forever [9–11].

It is believed that the number of humans with TB increased during the Neolithic period, not only because of an increased size and density of the host populations but also because of changes in the virulence of *M. tuberculosis* [1, 12, 13]. Although there is no definitive proof of the increase in the number of TB cases, the study of skeletons from an ancient Egyptian necropolis dated between 3500 BC and 2600 BC showed that nine (11%) of the 83 mummies had morphological alterations characteristic of vertebral TB and six (7%) showed the presence of MTBC confirmed by molecular markers [1]. Studies in a later Egyptian necropolis dated between 2000 BC and 500 BC showed a similar frequency of morphological alterations suggestive of TB, indicating that the disease was prevalent in ancient Egypt [14].

Because *M. tuberculosis* is primarily a human pathogen, it requires survival of the host to be transmitted. How *M. tuberculosis* and humans co-evolved during the 70 000 year-partnership is still not fully understood. It is possible that the ability of *M. tuberculosis* to become dormant was, in early years, an adaptive mechanism. Reactivation after several years of being infected ensured the transmission of *M. tuberculosis* to new generations of susceptible population, avoiding extinction of the small hunter-gatherer populations and thereby avoiding elimination of the disease [15]. Later, the larger size of the settlements during the Neolithic period increased the size of the susceptible population, enabling the maintenance and transmission of *M. tuberculosis*. Ecology theory suggests that *M. tuberculosis* would become more virulent in a large vulnerable population by indirect selection, in which an increase in opportunities for *M. tuberculosis* transmission will select for virulence to maximise transmission to new hosts [16, 17]. Overall, the evidence suggests that the transition to urban living during the Neolithic period resulted in the increase in the number of individuals with TB, highlighting the impact of increasing population density on the evolution of the disease.

The European tuberculosis epidemic and industrialisation: 1750–1950

The European TB epidemic was already flourishing in 1750 at the beginning of the Industrial revolution. Although centred in England the Industrial revolution soon spread to neighbouring countries. In Western Europe during the 17th, 18th and 19th centuries, TB was by far the most important cause of death, and it remained the highest or one of the highest causes of mortality until the 1900s [18]. Today, TB remains the most common acute bacterial infection in the world [19].

https://doi.org/10.1183/2312508X.10020617

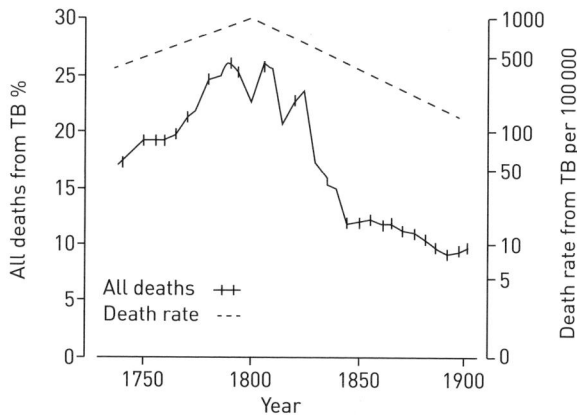

Figure 2. The percentage of deaths attributed to TB in the city of London (UK) compared with total deaths from all causes and a log-scale plot of mortality rates due to TB in England and neighbouring countries. Reproduced and modified from [18] and [20] with permission.

Industrial revolution

The Industrial revolution created one of the most consequential financial and social achievements of mankind. According to the data presented in figure 2, two distinct phases in the time-course of events occurred. First, there was a rise in both the percentage of deaths attributed to TB in the city of London (UK) and in the log plot of deaths from TB in England and neighbouring countries. Following this both time-plots show simultaneous peaks around 1800. Secondly, TB deaths in London decreased erratically, whereas those in Europe declined continuously [18, 20].

The early and late phases of the Industrial revolution were accompanied by strikingly different socioeconomic outcomes. During the first half of the Industrial revolution, TB rose because conditions in the mills and factories deteriorated to an unprecedented extent causing overcrowding, poor nutrition, absence of sanitation and medical care, and 12-hour-long hazardous shifts of children as young as 5 years of age. During the second half of the industrial revolution, owing to the prodigious population augmentation occurring in the 1800s, previously non-existent jobs became available (e.g. bankers, business men, storekeepers, doctors and lawyers), thereby creating a new and increasingly prosperous middle class. Although millions of workers continued to suffer in TB-enhancing mills and factories, millions of others benefitted from improved living circumstances and TB death rates declined [18].

Other important developments between 1882 and 1950 are described in the following paragraphs and additional achievements [21] are listed in table 1.

Sanatoria

Hermann Brehmer created the first TB sanatorium at Görbersdorf (then Germany, today Poland), in 1859 at an altitude of 500 m. His open-air facility featured bed rest, a rich diet and structured exercise. The idea caught on and spread widely throughout the affluent world [22]. In 1882, the year Robert Koch discovered tubercle bacilli, Carlo Forlanini

Table 1. Developments in TB between 1882 and 1950

Diagnostic steps
  1895: Discovery of radiographs: Wilhelm Conrad Röntgen
  1907: Introduction of the TST for diagnosis of LTBI: Clemens von Pirquet
Therapeutic steps
  1854: Creation of first TB sanatorium: Hermann Brehmer
  1882: Introduction of pneumothorax for collapse therapy: Carlo Forlanini
  1885: Thoracoplasty: Edouard de Cérenville
  1916: Completion of pneumothorax by thoracoscopy: Hans-Christian Jacobaeus
  1944: Discovery of first anti-TB antibiotics (PAS), Jorgen Lehmann, and streptomycin,
        Selman A. Waksman
Preventative steps
  1887: First TB dispensary (Edinburgh, UK): Robert W. Philip
  End of 19th century: First of TB organisations created and dispensaries established
  1921: BCG vaccination; Albert Calmette and Camille Guérin
  1948: WHO established

invented pneumothorax [23]. Later, in 1910, Hans-Christian Jacobaeus first used thoracoscopy, which in 1916 was augmented by pulmonary collapse procedures [24] and, sometimes, by heroic surgical interventions.

Radiographic techniques

The outstanding importance of radiographic techniques for diagnosing active PTB was acknowledged only a few years after Wilhelm Conrad Röntgen discovered the immense value of radiographs in 1895. But they were not used routinely until after world war II, either for individuals suspected of TB or for screening large populations. Photofluorography, which was better suited to screening, was initially extensively used in military services before world war I [25].

Vaccination for TB

BCG vaccination with the attenuated *M. bovis* strain was developed by the French researchers Albert Calmette and Camille Guérin and was first used for TB prevention in 1921 [26]. Initial acceptance was slow and then virtually stopped following the Lübeck disaster in 1930 [27]. After world war II, vaccination was vigorously promoted, particularly by the United Nations International Children's Emergency Fund (UNICEF). For decades, BCG was the most frequently used vaccination worldwide. It is especially valuable in preventing miliary TB and TB meningitis in infants and young children, but is much less effective in older persons and other forms of TB [25].

International participation

The WHO was officially established by the United Nations (UN) in 1948 when malaria, TB and venereal diseases were declared as the "three main scourges demanding prior and special attention", a statement which is still valid today. Exemplary international models that helped to eliminate famine after world war II were UN partnerships such as the UNRRA (UN Relief and Rehabilitation Administration), founded in 1943 to help displaced persons and, later, refugees; its successor organisation is the UN High Commissioner for

https://doi.org/10.1183/2312508X.10020617

Refugees (UNHCR). UNICEF was created by the UN General Assembly in 1946 to provide emergency food and healthcare to children in countries that had been devastated by world war II [25].

Robert Koch, Rudolf Virchow and tuberculin

It is thought that there was never more TB in Europe than during the Industrial revolution, and only towards the end of that period Robert Koch became famous for his discovery of the cause of TB (*M. tuberculosis*), which was presented on March 24, 1882 [28]. In his discussion that night, Robert Koch (figure 3) [29] commented that the tubercle bacillus accounted for roughly one-seventh of all deaths at the time and he shaped our modern view of the condition as a bacterial infection [30]. However, Koch's triumph has to be seen as the completion of work begun by others [31], and what he discovered was not quite what we think TB is today.

A century before Koch, few physicians thought of a whole set of clinical conditions such as phthisis, lupus and scrofula, today considered to be TB of the lungs, skin and glands, as clinical manifestations of a single disease. This idea was first suggested by Rene Théophile Laënnec who, in 1819, drawing on his information from pathological anatomy, suggested that these and several other manifestations were all one and the same disease [32].

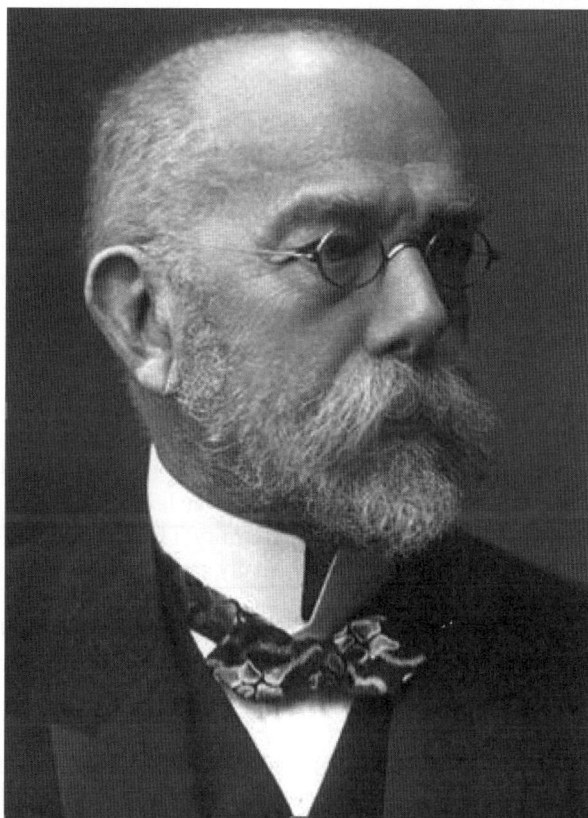

Figure 3. Robert Koch (1843–1910), who discovered *M. tuberculosis* in 1882. Nobel Laureate Physiology or Medicine, 1905. Reproduced and modified from [29] with permission.

As evidence, he pointed to a common structure, the tubercle, found in affected tissues. Later, in 1865, Jean Antoine Villemin demonstrated that infectious material from humans could be used to produce TB in animal experiments [33]. Koch knew about Villemin's work but the concept of infection was virtually unknown at the time. Instead, most physicians understood TB within the framework of Rudolf Virchow's cellular pathology. Virchow showed little concern with external causes of diseases, instead, focusing his research on internal pathophysiology [34]. Tubercular processes could be seen as transitional phases of other diseases such as when cancers turned tuberculous. The result was a highly artificial edifice in which the so-called caseous pneumonia of phthisis became separated from the other forms of the disease such as lupus.

Not only did Koch deliver a refutation of Virchow and a vindication of Laënnec, he was also innovative; he added a bacterium to Laënnec's concept of TB, thereby elevating what had been a description of a pathological anatomic finding to an analysis of causes, in this case bacteria [34]. Koch's presentation in March 1882 was a breakthrough, for the new science of medical bacteriology, vindicating an older concept of TB. The causal argument stood central and it is no coincidence that Koch's work on TB is the most important source of what became known as his postulates. Knowing the necessary causes facilitated intervention, and Koch's own ideas about pathogenic bacteria were far from modest: "in the future the fight against this dreadful scourge of human kind will no longer be against an indefinable something but against a tangible parasite" [28] was how he put it in 1882. He conceived medical bacteriology as the very basis of public health and clinical medicine. What had been elucidated for TB held for infectious diseases in general.

What is different in our modern understanding of TB is not so much its aetiology, which Koch had established, but the importance that he attributed to it: lacking an immunological framework, he saw TB as an exclusively bacterial activity. The shortcomings of this approach were exposed in 1890, when Koch presented tuberculin as a cure for the condition [35]. For Koch, who made no distinction between infection and disease, the idea that the strong reaction to tuberculin could indicate a previous infection was beyond imagination. Instead, even after it had failed as a medicine, he suggested using tuberculin for the diagnosis of acute conditions.

Decline in tuberculosis mortality before specific antibiotics

TB has been afflicting humans for millennia, but only in the past 300–400 years have there been attempts to quantify the disease [36–38]. From at least the 1700s through to the first quarter of the 1900s, the statistic presented to quantify TB in a population was the number of deaths (either absolute or per population, usually per 100 000) attributed to the disease, as shown in figure 4 [38, 39]. A fundamental principle in determining the incidence, prevalence or mortality of any disease is to establish an accurate case definition. Even many years after Koch's discovery of M. tuberculosis in 1882, the definition of TB was based largely on clinical features and, in a few instances, autopsy findings [40].

Based on data, presented in a variety of ways (table 2), it has been widely accepted that the decrease in TB deaths reported in western Europe, beginning in the early 1800s and later in the USA, reflected a decrease in incidence. Moreover, it has been stated that none of the control measures implemented prior to antimicrobial therapy had any impact on TB morbidity [41]. But this contention continues to be a matter of debate [38].

https://doi.org/10.1183/2312508X.10020617

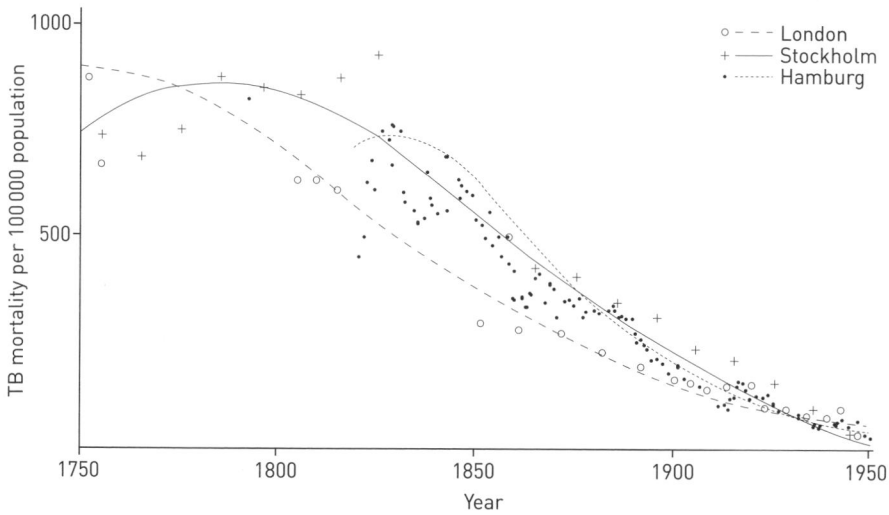

Figure 4. Biological phenomena exhibit cyclic patterns and TB, as a group disease, makes no exception as shown in the three TB mortality population curves. Mortality from TB probably reached its peak before 1750 in London, UK, around 1790 in Stockholm, Sweden, and around 1830 in Hamburg, Germany. Reproduced and modified from [3] with permission.

However, while it is reasonable to assume that TB morbidity and mortality were decreasing, it is likely that there were gross inaccuracies in the reported numbers of deaths and that the decline in TB deaths did not accurately reflect a decline in incidence, as shown in table 3. Given the frequency of comorbidities in persons with TB, death with TB is difficult to distinguish from death from TB [42]. This was even more likely to have been true in the pre-chemotherapy era.

The data are correct

It has been widely accepted that the decline in deaths was caused by improved living conditions and nutrition [40]. Better nutrition could result in a more robust immune response leading to a smaller proportion of those infected with tubercle bacilli progressing to TB. This reduced incidence of the disease would, in turn, decrease transmission. It is also possible that, at least in England, isolation of patients with TB in hospitals (and the many infirmaries located in workhouses for the poor) reduced transmission [38].

Deaths from any condition are determined by both its incidence and the proportion of those with the disease who die; thus, case fatality proportions could decrease for any of a number of reasons while the incidence could go up, go down or be unchanged. In the USA

Table 2. Death statistics for TB

Absolute number of deaths (usually per year)
Percentage of total deaths (usually per year)
Death rate (deaths per population, usually per 100 000 per year)
Case fatality proportion (percentage) of patients with TB who die (may be all-cause mortality or
    specific TB-caused death)

Table 3. Potential reasons for the decline in TB deaths, 1750–1950

The data are correct
TB incidence was declining
Case fatality proportion was decreasing
The data are incorrect
TB was over-diagnosed, but diagnoses became more accurate over time
Based on clinical assessment any wasting illness or chronic respiratory condition was likely to be diagnosed as TB
Over the decades diseases clinically mimicking TB were diagnosed more accurately, thereby progressively decreasing false-positive TB diagnoses
The population base (denominator) was inaccurate (applies when the data are expressed as a rate per population)

in the 1940s, death rates from TB fell from 45.8 per 100 000 in 1940 to 40 per 100 000 in 1945, a 15% decline, whereas the case rate increased from 76 per 100 000 to 89 per 100 000, a 17% increase.

The data are incorrect

There are many reasons why the data could be incorrect. First of all, it seems probable that the case definition was inaccurate. By-and-large during the course of the mortality decline, TB was commonly diagnosed when its clinical features were much more likely to be advanced than subtle. This difference creates an artefact by inflating the proportion of cases that died, because only the most severe cases would be included in the denominator of "established" cases.

It is also possible that there was increasing familiarity with TB and its clinical features, thus, increasing the accuracy of a clinical diagnosis. Moreover, at the same time the accuracy of identifying other conditions that could have mimicked TB could have increased. This would lead to less diagnostic confusion and fewer "false-positive" diagnoses of TB, thereby reducing the apparent deaths from TB.

The precise reasons for the declining TB deaths prior to chemotherapy will never be disentangled. All the factors described herein, as well as others [13], probably played a role. Such an interpretation should not, however, be used to minimise the importance of specific measures to prevent, treat and ultimately eradicate this still deadly disease.

Tuberculosis during world war I and world war II

TB is one of the most frequent and deadly diseases to complicate the special circumstances of warfare. When TB and war occur simultaneously, the inevitable consequences are disease, human misery, suffering and heightened mortality. This has been observed in particular in world war I and II [25].

World war I

Nearly all diagrams that depict death rates from TB in various Western European cities and countries from the mid-18th century through to the mid-19th century show similar

 https://doi.org/10.1183/2312508X.10020617

configurations. After reaching a particular summit of TB mortality in whatever city or country was being analysed, there followed a nearly consistent decline that lasted as long as 100 years, sometimes even longer. Suddenly, that monotonous pattern abruptly stopped and at nearly the same time in Western Europe, shortly after the beginning of world war I.

As illustrated in figure 5, the majority of the striking upsurge of TB mortality reached its peak in 1918 and was succeeded by equally precipitous decreases in fatalities. This may have been prolonged slightly to 1920 or even a year or two afterward because of the overlapping death toll triggered by the "Spanish Influenza pandemic", which erupted in March 1918 [44]. The lengthy well-established pre-war reductions of TB deaths had resumed their previous downward tracks around 1920; as if the war and its remarkable 6–7 year harvest of suffering and death hadn't actually happened.

Ordinary and war-related factors influencing the epidemiology of world war I
Although neutral, neighbouring countries such as Norway, Sweden and Denmark had the typical rise then fall in TB mortality observed in belligerent countries. Switzerland, however, had the expected increase but it failed to decrease as predicted. For unknown reasons, TB death rates in both France and the USA failed to show the world war I increase observed elsewhere; both countries, however, did experience the widely shared steep drop in post-wartime fatalities [45].

Figure 5 shows that in 1885 TB mortality was high, 200–300 per 100 000 population, but was continuously decreasing until the stunning and totally unforeseen sharp increase followed by an equally astounding decrease back to previously expected rates of decline. No one really knows the exact mechanism(s) that created the phenomenon. Possible culprits

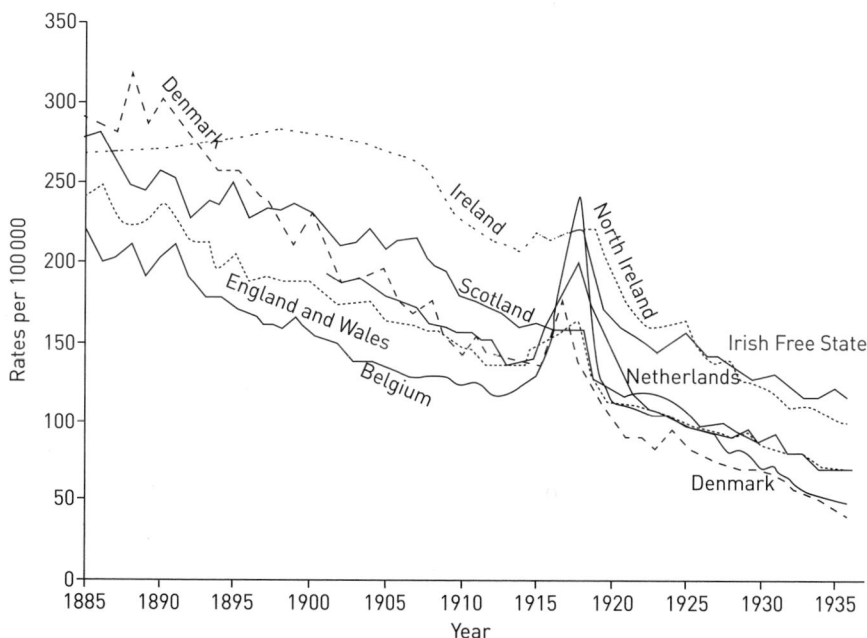

Figure 5. Mortality rates from TB per 100 000 population during the 50-year period 1885–1935. Reproduced and modified from [44] with permission.

Table 4. Major factors that contribute to the increase of TB mortality during wartime

Ordinary factors
1. Inadequate ventilation
2. Overcrowding
3. Malnutrition
4. Immune deficiency
5. Inadequate medical care

War-related factors
1. Shortage of healthcare personnel
2. Shortage of adequate medical supplies and hospital beds
3. Poison gas

are listed in table 4 and include both ordinary and war-related factors that promote the onset, spread, severity and death from TB.

During the early 1900s, the annual risk of TB infection was about 10%. According to RIEDER [46] this meant that during world war I roughly 80% of infants and children were infected by tubercle bacilli by 15 years of age, as indicated by a positive TST, and 88% by 20 years of age, when TB infections peak in adult life. Even though there wasn't much "room" for new infections to occur, many uninfected adults probably did become infected with tubercle bacilli, many of whom may have developed TB and some of whom died. But that doesn't account for the large majority who already harboured organisms. The detrimental effects of ongoing transmission through reinfection(s) of *M. tuberculosis* during wartime certainly played a pathogenic role, as did nutritional deficiencies and the logistic interferences that limited or prevented access to medical supplies and healthcare personnel. Poison gas played a minor role at best.

World war II

The data from several countries that participated in world war II have been summarised in an article by DANIELS [47]. Figure 6 shows conspicuously sharp rises in TB mortality in seven major European cities; Warsaw and Rome peaked in 1944 and Berlin, Budapest, Vienna, Hamburg and Amsterdam reached their peaks in 1945. After peaking, mortality declined strikingly in all affected cities except Berlin and Hamburg, which had less dramatic decreases. The remarkable similarity between the results of world war I and world war II strongly suggest a common war-related phenomenon, such as an aggregate of multiple factors and/or weakening of host resistance.

To date, world war II is by far the deadliest conflict in human history, with more than 60 million estimated fatalities, including about 20 million military personnel and 40 million civilians. Many of the civilians died because of deliberate genocide, massacres, mass bombings, disease, and starvation [25]. According to the British TB specialist M. Daniels, who analysed the TB outcome in several countries after the war, TB was the major health disaster of world war II [47].

Although the absolute rise in TB mortality that occurred during world war I was not reached in world war II, the increase over the global pre-war rate was proportionately even greater [48]. Although there were exceptions, TB mortality rose during world war II, as in world war I, in some countries soon after the start of the war, and in other countries gradually during the war or steeply after the war. Even some non-belligerent (neutral) countries observed an increase in TB, whereas a few belligerent countries saw a fall in

https://doi.org/10.1183/2312508X.10020617

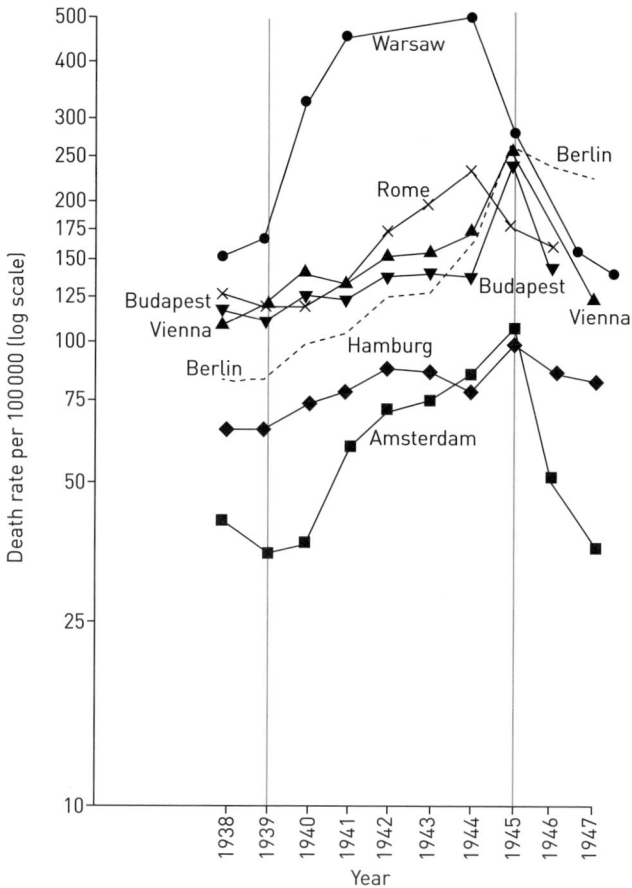

Figure 6. TB mortality in European cities, 1938–1947. Reproduced and modified from [47] with permission.

numbers of TB cases (Bulgaria, Denmark, England and Wales) [47]. As Daniels points out, there was a rise then a fall in TB mortality during world war II in England and Wales. The increase was highest in capital cities, as shown in figure 6 for seven European cities [47].

One has to bear in mind all the uncertainties and difficulties in the retrieval of reliable epidemiological data during wartime, problems include: the destruction of the public health infrastructure; the redeployment, transfer or elimination of health resources and personnel; the collapse of communication systems; the lack of diagnostic capabilities; and the presence of censorship, propaganda, and the intentional falsification of information [49]. But at least it is likely that the observed trends in most involved countries are germane and plausible.

Reducing the risk and burden of TB after world war II
Crowded living conditions in the ghettos and concentration camps, poor sanitation and near starvation diets contributed to the spread of TB [50]. Prisoner of war camps and the Nazi labour camps were also high-risk situations for TB, as observed in displaced persons after the war [51].

Solving the huge problem of providing sufficient quantities of food during famines, warfare, and other catastrophes, has historically been extremely difficult, but new organisations and technologies have lessened the burden to some extent. Exemplary international models that helped to eliminate famine after world war II are UN organisations such as the UNRRA, founded in 1943, essentially to organise help for displaced persons and, later, for refugees; its successor organisation is the UNHCR. UNICEF was created by the UN General Assembly in 1946 to provide emergency food and healthcare to children in countries that had been devastated by world war II. In 1947, the highly successful Marshall Plan was developed by the USA, with the purpose of aiding Western European countries in restoring their economies.

In addition, many non-governmental charitable organisations supported countries or certain populations (refugees, Jews, prisoners) suffering from hunger and in great need of food. In some countries, to ensure a fair supply of food to the general population, food ration cards were introduced.

Obviously, the black market for food, medications and other essentials flourished in many affected regions, and hoarding of food from agricultural sources was widespread.

Further post-war control measures aimed at: improving the housing situation; combating bovine TB; and stopping the use of mass radiography, tuberculin testing and BCG vaccination; plus other aspects of epidemiological research [52]. Among the recommendations of the Expert Committee to the WHO were the collection of data on TB morbidity and mortality rates, which were published for the first time in 1948 [53].

The health services, which had been severely disrupted during and after world war II in Europe, had to be reorganised [54]. Training programmes for TB had to be instituted for specialists and general practitioners as well as post-graduate courses for medical students. The lack of trained nurses was partially resolved by using domestic staff who became responsible for hospital duties that did not require special knowledge. There were also shortages of specialised instruments and equipment, including microscopes, fluoroscopes, and other radiographic apparatus, as well as analysers for chemical and microbiological measurements.

5 months before the end of the war in Europe the first effective anti-TB agents were discovered, which signalled the onset of curative chemotherapy [55].

The history of tuberculosis chemotherapy

It would be a simplification to view the history of TB chemotherapy as one of pills and injections. Commencing, as it did shortly after the end of world war II, it was a component of other major changes taking place. The decline of TB in industrial societies was well underway by that time and had been achieved through powerful public health interventions. TB had been framed as a social disease and addressing its social causes had been the road to control [31]. Suddenly, in 1944, not one but two effective TB-antimicrobials appeared, PAS and streptomycin; combined usage of both agents helped delay drug resistance. Later, the sought after, crucial anti-TB agent proved to be isoniazid. By 1952, "triple therapy" had become standard treatment for all forms of TB [56].

In subsequent decades, the promises of triple therapy and its replacements for PAS and streptomycin had steadily improved, but the challenges that they posed were immense: within less than two decades almost all the important effective "first-line" antimicrobial TB agents had been invented, including ethambutol, rifampicin and other rifamycins, and

https://doi.org/10.1183/2312508X.10020617

pyrazinamide. The bonanza ended after the discovery of rifampicin in 1965; to date, the last major anti-TB drug invented. New "second-line" agents for the treatment of drug resistance initially received scanty attention, but availability has much improved in recent years [57]. The main reason for this void is that drug development of TB antimicrobials was abandoned by big pharmaceutical companies around 1970, when TB had become a condition almost exclusively found in low-income countries, thereby holding little commercial promise [58].

A therapeutic challenge, virtually from the start, was TB drug resistance [59], which was hard to avoid in days when treatment took 18 or even 24 months. The hazards of resistance inspired research into combination therapies, starting from the simple combination of PAS, streptomycin and isoniazid in the 1950s. Later, increasingly refined compounds using modern antimicrobials were designed, particularly to shorten the length of therapy. Developing countries, and East Africa in particular, became centres for such work from the late 1950s and contributed substantially to the development of RCTs in the decades following world war II. The practical consequences, however, were limited, as the trials failed to improve TB control in the countries where they were hosted. As Brandon Lush wrote in 1962, "I cannot help making the point that the trials are not directly making any real impact on the incidence of TB in East Africa" [60]. What Africa saw instead was the spread of drug resistance originating from simplistic regimens and regimens that were too short. In the absence of a working health system, TB drugs had become "a definite public health menace" [61], as the head of Kenya's TB programme commented.

The field trials in three African countries conducted by the International Union Against Tuberculosis (IUATLD) from 1977 finally gave combination therapies traction in local health systems. Instead of seeking sophisticated regimens, the IUATLD focused on building up national TB programmes, putting the emphasis on operations research: training of personnel; provision of drugs; transport of patients; and engendering political commitment. When it came to drugs, the IUATLD used off-the-shelf Medical Research Council regimens, ultimately employing a 1970s short-course combination regimen that facilitated treatment completion in 8 months [62]. In particular, the hugely successful Tanzanian trials from 1977 to 1987, which were led by the memorable Karel Styblo (figure 7) [63, 64]. These trials became the prime inspiration for the global TB control strategy recommended by the WHO known as DOTS [65].

Ongoing progress, however, was considerably threatened and then reversed by the rise of HIV/AIDS in the 1980s which resulted in a worldwide explosion of TB, especially in Asia and Africa. Then, beginning in the early 2000s, TB workers have had to deal with the steadily increasing numbers of patients with MDR-TB [66].

Moving toward tuberculosis elimination

"Disease eradication provides global health equity, the highest aspiration of public health" [67]. The lofty humanitarian goal of eradication, however, is not easily accomplished. The eradication of smallpox required a huge worldwide effort [68], which in addition to its impact on global health, provided many lessons for current and future eradication or elimination initiatives [69, 70]. Important lessons also have been gleaned from earlier failed eradication efforts, particularly of malaria, a campaign that failed disastrously. An important lesson learned from all these campaigns is that eradication or elimination campaigns should not be undertaken lightly and may have serious unintended negative consequences, if unsuccessful.

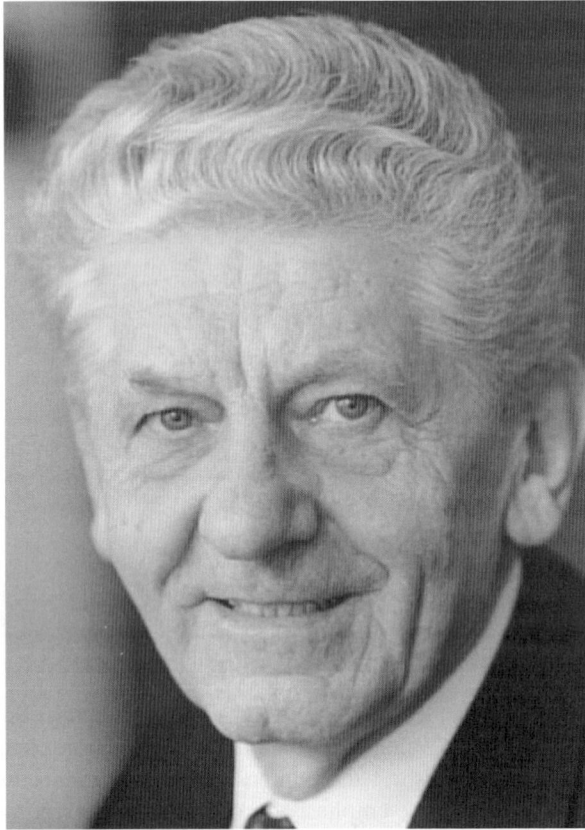

Figure 7. Karel Styblo (1921–1998). Reproduced and modified from [10] with permission.

Disease eradication is most commonly defined as a permanent reduction to zero of the worldwide incidence of infection caused by a specific agent as a result of deliberate efforts: intervention measures are no longer needed. Elimination differs in that worldwide it is not specified and that continued measures to prevent re-establishment of transmission are required [67, 71]. When applied to TB, elimination is generally defined as no more than one case per million population. In addition, the qualifier "as a disease of public health concern," is often appended to elimination.

Calls for the eradication (or elimination) of TB in the USA began in 1958 when Carroll Palmer, an influential US Public Health Service epidemiologist, stated that global public health authorities had an "obligation" to move from TB control to eradication [72]. This call was echoed in the same year by James Perkins, Director of the National Tuberculosis Association [73]. In 1959, the epidemiological background for an eradication programme in Denmark was presented, but no campaign was mounted [74]. Parenthetically, as of 2016, Denmark's TB case rate was 5.7per 100 000, which is far from elimination [75].

In 1963 the Chief of the US Public Health Service Tuberculosis Program, Edward Bloomquist, presented a framework for TB elimination in the USA [76]. However, it was not until 1989 that the Division of Tuberculosis Control at the CDC developed a strategic plan for tuberculosis elimination and changed its name to the Division of Tuberculosis

https://doi.org/10.1183/2312508X.10020617

Table 5. Milestones and targets for the WHO End TB Strategy

Indicators with baseline values for 2015	Milestones			Targets 2035
	2020	2025	2030	
Percentage reduction in deaths due to TB (projected 2015 baseline: 1.3 million deaths)	35%	75%	90%	95%
Percentage and absolute reduction in TB incidence rate (projected 2015 baseline: 110/100000)	20% (<85/ 100000)	50% (<55/ 100000)	80% (<20/ 100000)	90% (<10/ 100000)
Percentage of affected families facing catastrophic costs due to TB (projected 2015 baseline: not yet available)	Zero	Zero	Zero	Zero

Reproduced and modified from [80] with permission.

Elimination [77]. The strategic plan with updated recommendations was reaffirmed in 1999 [78]. The goal of reaching a case rate of 3.5 per 100000 by the year 2000 was delayed until 2010–2011; the ultimate goal of elimination, 1 per 1000000 by 2010, has receded well into the future with the current rate (in 2016) being 2.9 per 100000 [79].

In 2014, the WHO created the End TB Strategy [80], whose goal is "to end the global TB epidemic." While the "end" is not quantified, milestones and targets are specified and are highly ambitious (table 5).

Although the strategy is directed mainly toward high-incidence countries, because TB remains a global disease, strategies and elimination plans in low-incidence countries will not be successful until and unless high-incidence countries succeed in meeting the WHO targets.

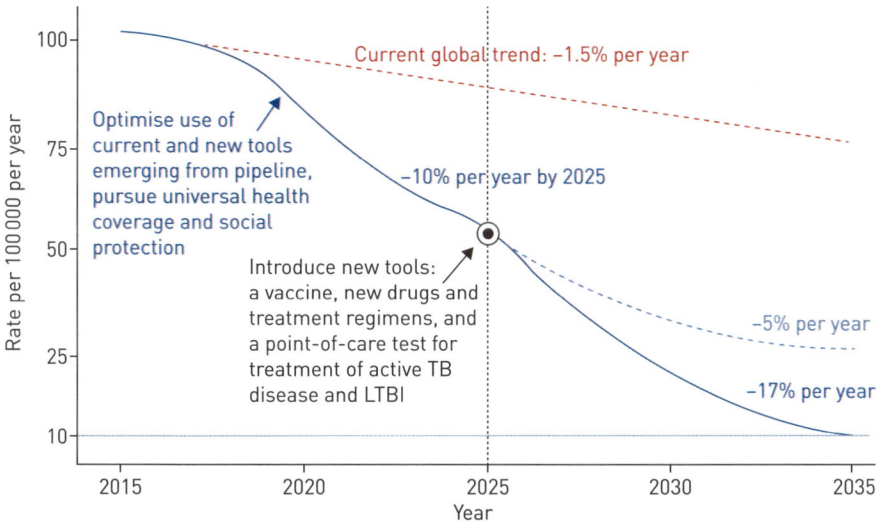

Figure 8. Rates of decline in TB incidence to reach 2035 targets. Reproduced and modified from [80] with permission.

https://doi.org/10.1183/2312508X.10020617

The natural history of TB is often marked by lengthy latent phases during which asymptomatic infection persists. Currently, thousands upon thousands of emigrants and refugees seeking better lives in industrialised countries has led to the maintenance of reservoirs of LTBI in low-incidence areas. This is clearly evident in the USA where foreign-born persons who have settled in America now comprise about 70% of newly reported cases of TB [79]. In the European Union, 33% of new cases of TB in 2016 were foreign-born [75].

Achieving the End TB Strategy goals by 2035 will be very difficult. Figure 8 shows the rate of decline in TB incidence (17% per year) that will be necessary to reach the 2035 target.

This is a greater decline than has ever been recorded except, perhaps, in very limited areas. Clearly, to reach this target either wide-spread preventive treatment for LTBI or an effective vaccine (or both) will be needed, together with intensified efforts in implementation of current measures, namely the eight core action areas for the WHO TB End Strategy: 1) ensure political commitment, funding and stewardship for planning and essential services of high quality; 2) address the most vulnerable and hard-to-reach groups; 3) address special needs of migrants and cross-border issues; 4) undertake screening for active TB and LTBI in TB contacts and selected high-risk groups and provide appropriate treatment; 5) optimise the prevention and care of DR-TB; 6) ensure continued surveillance, programme monitoring and evaluation and case-based data management; 7) invest in research and new tools; and 8) support global TB prevention, care and control [81].

Conclusion

TB remains the largest cause of adult deaths from any single infectious disease and ranks among the top 10 causes of death worldwide. Multiple factors are responsible for the increases and decreases in TB during the course of history. This chapter describes the various measures taken to combat TB, but they have not always been successful. The elimination of TB by the WHO is programmed to occur in 2035 but it is unlikely to occur on schedule. The increasing use of preventive diagnosis and treatment of LTBI and the invention of a potent vaccine should contribute to TB elimination.

References

1. Comas I, Coscolla M, Luo T, *et al.* Out-of-Africa migration and Neolithic coexpansion of *Mycobacterium tuberculosis* with modern humans. *Nat Genet* 2013; 45: 1176–1182.
2. Coscolla M, Gagneux S. Consequences of genomic diversity in *Mycobacterium tuberculosis*. *Semin Immunol* 2014; 26: 431–444.
3. Stead WW, Eisenach KD, Cave MD, *et al.* When did *Mycobacterium tuberculosis* infection first occur in the New World? An important question with public health implications. *Am J Respir Crit Care Med* 1995; 151: 1267–1268.
4. Manchester K. Tuberculosis and leprosy in antiquity: an interpretation. *Med History* 1984; 28: 162–173.
5. Brosch R, Gordon SV, Marmiesse M, *et al.* A new evolutionary scenario for the *Mycobacterium tuberculosis* complex. *Proc Natl Acad Sci USA* 2002; 99: 3684–3689.
6. Diamond J. Evolution, consequences and future of plant and animal domestication. *Nature* 2001; 418: 700–707.
7. Moore AMT, Hillman GC, Legge AJ. Village on the Euphrates: from foraging to farming at Abu Hureyra. 1st Edn. New York, Oxford University Press, 2000.
8. Paschou P, Drineas P, Yannaki E, *et al.* Maritime route of colonization of Europe. *Proc Natl Acad Sci USA* 2014; 111: 9211–9216.
9. Smith BD. The Emergence of Agriculture (Scientific American Library). 1st Edn. New York, W.H. Freeman & Co, 1994.

https://doi.org/10.1183/2312508X.10020617

10. Latham KJ. Human health and the Neolithic revolution: an overview of impacts of the agricultural transition on oral health, epidemiology, and the human body. *Nebraska Anthropologist* 2013; 28: 895–1002.

11. Smith BD. Documenting plant domestication: the consilience of biological and archaeological approaches. *Proc Natl Acad Sci USA* 2001; 98: 1324–1326.

12. Brites D, Gagneux S. Co-evolution of *Mycobacterium tuberculosis* and *Homo sapiens. Immunol Rev* 2015; 264: 6–24.

13. Barnes I, Duda A, Pybus OG, *et al.* Ancient urbanization predicts genetic resistance to tuberculosis. *Evolution* 2011; 65: 842–848.

14. Zink AR, Grabner W, Reischl U, *et al.* Molecular study on human tuberculosis in three geographically distinct and time delineated populations from ancient Egypt. *Epidemiol Infect* 2003; 130: 239–249.

15. Zheng N, Whalen CC, Handel A. Modeling the potential impact of host population survival on the evolution of *M. tuberculosis* latency. *PLoS One* 2014; 9: e105721.

16. Ebert D, Bull JJ. Challenging the trade-off model for the evolution of virulence: is virulence management feasible? *Trends Microbiol* 2003; 11: 15–20.

17. Gagneux S. Ecology and evolution of *Mycobacterium tuberculosis. Nat Rev Microbiol* 2018; 16: 202–213.

18. Murray JF. The Industrial revolution and the decline in death rates from tuberculosis. *Int J Tuberc Lung Dis* 2015; 19: 502–503.

19. World Health Organization. Global Tuberculosis Report 2017. World Health Organization, Geneva, Switzerland, 2017.

20. Murray JF. The white plague: down and out, or up and coming? *Am Rev Respir Dis* 1989; 140: 1788–1795.

21. Daniel TM. The history of tuberculosis. *Respir Med* 2006; 100: 1862–1870.

22. Davis AL. History of the sanatorium movement. *In:* Rom WN, Garay SM, eds. Tuberculosis. New York, Little, Brown and Company, 1996; pp. 35–54.

23. Hansson N, Polianski IJ. Therapeutic pneumothorax and the Nobel Prize. *Ann Thorac Surg* 2015; 100: 761–765.

24. Loddenkemper, R, Mathur PN, Noppen M, *et al.* Medical thoracoscopy/pleuroscopy: manual and atlas. Stuttgart, Thieme, 2011.

25. Loddenkemper R, Murray JF. Tuberculosis and war. Lessons learned from world war II. *In:* Murray JF, Loddenkemper R, eds. Tuberculosis and war. Lessons learned from world war II. Basel, Karger, 2018; pp. 214–228.

26. Calmette A. On preventive vaccination of the new-born against tuberculosis by B.C.G. *Br J Tuberc* 1928; 22: 161–165.

27. The Lubeck Disaster. *Science* 1930; 72: 198–199.

28. Koch R. Die Aetiologie der Tuberkulose. *Berlin klin Wschr* 1882; 19: 221–230.

29. Migliori GB, Loddenkemper R, Blasi F, *et al.* 125 years after Robert Koch's discovery of the tubercle bacillus: the new XDR-TB threat. Is "science" enough to tackle the epidemic? *Eur Respir J* 2007; 29: 423–427.

30. Murray J. *Mycobacterium tuberculosis* and the cause of consumption: from discovery to fact. *Am J Respir Dis Crit Care Med* 2004; 169: 1086–1088.

31. Dubos R, Dubos J. Tuberculosis, man, and society. New Brunswick, Rutgers University Press, 1952.

32. Duffin J. To see with a better eye. A life of R.T.H. Laennec. Princeton, Princeton University Press, 1998.

33. Daniel TM. Jean-Antoine villemin and the infectious nature of tuberculosis. *Int J Tuberc Lung Dis* 2015; 19: 267–268.

34. Faber K. Nosography: The Evolution of Clinical Medicine in Modern Times. New York, Paul B. Hoeber, 1930; pp. 76–81.

35. Gradmann C. Laboratory Disease: Robert Koch's medical bacteriology. Baltimore, Johns Hopkins University Press, 2009.

36. Roberts CA. Old World tuberculosis: evidence from human remains with a review of current research and future prospects. *Tuberculosis (Edinb)* 2015; 95: Suppl 1: S117–S121.

37. Frith J. History of Tuberculosis. Part 1 – Phthisis, consumption and the White Plague. *J Military and Veterans' Health* 2014; 22: 29–35.

38. Grigg ER. The arcana of tuberculosis with a brief epidemiologic history of the disease in the U.S.A. *Am Rev Tuberc Pul Dis* 1958; 78: 151–172.

39. Wilson LD. Commentary: medicine, population, and tuberculosis. *Int J Epidem* 2005; 34: 521–524.

40. Daniel TM. René Théophile Hyacinthe Laënnec and the founding of pulmonary medicine. *Int J Tuberc Lung Dis* 2004; 8: 517–518.

41. McKeown T, Record RG. Reasons for the decline of mortality in England and Wales during the nineteenth century. *Popul Stud* 1962; 16: 94–122.

42. Beavers SF, Pascopella L, Davidow AL, *et al.* Tuberculosis mortality in the United States: epidemiology and prevention opportunities. *Ann Am Thoracic Soc* 2018; in press https://doi.org/10.1513/AnnalsATS.201705-405OC.

43. Hopewell PC. Tuberculosis in the United States before, during, and after world war II. *In:* Murray JF, Loddenkemper R, eds. Tuberculosis and war. Lessons learned from world war II. Basel, Karger, 2018; pp. 179–187.

44. Drolet GL. World War I and tuberculosis: a statistical summary and review. *Am J Public Health* 1945; 35: 689–697.

45. Murray JF. Tuberculosis and World War I. *Am J Respir Crit Care Med* 2015; 192: 411–414.
46. Rieder HL. Methodological issues in the estimation of the tuberculosis problem from tuberculin surveys. *Tuber Lung Dis* 1995; 76: 114–121.
47. Daniels M. Tuberculosis in Europe during and after the Second World War. *Br Med J* 1949; 2: 1065–1072.
48. Sartwell PE, Moseley CH, Long ER. Tuberculosis in the German population, United States Zone of Germany. *Am Rev Tuberc* 1949; 59: 481–493.
49. Smallman-Raynor M, Cliff AD. War and disease: some perspectives on the spatial and temporal occurrence of tuberculosis in wartime. *In:* Gandy M, Zumla A, eds. The Return of the White Plague: Global Poverty and the "New" Tuberculosis. New York, Verso, 2003; pp. 70–92.
50. Lipscomb FM. Medical aspects of Belsen concentration camp. *Lancet* 1945; 246: 313–315.
51. Wyman M. DPs: Europe's displaced persons, 1945–1951 (reprinted). New York, Cornell University Press, 1998.
52. Expert Committee on Tuberculosis Report of the Expert Committee on Tuberculosis. *Bull World Health Organ* 1948; 1: 205–212
53. World Health Organization. Monthly supplement to the weekly epidemiological record. *Epidemiol Vital Statistics Rep* 1948; 1: 223–227.
54. Daniels M. Tuberculosis in Europe during and after the Second World War. *Br Med J* 1949; 2: 1135–1140.
55. Murray JF, Schraufnagel DE, Hopewell PC. Treatment of tuberculosis. A historical perspective. *Ann Am Thorac Soc* 2015; 12: 1749–1759.
56. Murray JF. A century of tuberculosis. *Am J Respir Crit Care Med* 2004; 169: 1181–1186.
57. Horsburgh CR Jr, Haxaire-Theeuwes M, Lienhardt C, *et al.* Compassionate use of and expanded access to new drugs for drug-resistant tuberculosis. *Int J Tuberc Lung Dis* 2013; 17: 146–152.
58. Greenwood D. Antimicrobial Drugs. Chronicle of a Twentieth Century Triumph. Oxford, Oxford University Press, 2008.
59. Gradmann C. Re-inventing infectious disease: antibiotic resistance and drug development at the Bayer company 1945–1980. *Med History* 2016; 59: 155–180.
60. Lush B. Memoradum of 20.2.1962, Medical Research Council 1962, Public Records Office, PRO FD 12/552, Tuberculosis Research Unit, 11.1.1962–1.3.63. www.nationalarchives.gov.uk/
61. McMillen CW. Discovering Tuberculosis: A Global History, 1900 to Present. New Haven, Yale University Press, 2015.
62. Arnadottir T. Tuberculosis and Public Health: Policy and Princples in Tuberculosis Control. Paris, IUATLD, 2009.
63. Styblo K. Overview and epidemiologic assessment of the current global tuberculosis situation with an emphasis on control in developing countries. *Rev Infect Dis* 1989; 11: Suppl. 2, S339–S346.
64. Broekmans JF. In memoriam Dr. K. Styblo. *Ned Tijdschr Geneeskd* 1998; 142: 1636–1637.
65. Ogden J, Walt G, Lush L. The politics of 'branding' in policy transfer: the case of DOTS for tuberculosis control. *Soc Sci Med* 2003; 57: 179–188.
66. Dirlikov E, Raviglione M, Scano F. Global tuberculosis control: toward the 2015 targets and beyond. *Ann Intern Med* 2015; 163: 52–58.
67. Dowdle WR, Cochi SL. The principles and feasibility of disease eradication. *Vaccine* 2011; 29: Suppl. 4, D70–D73.
68. Henderson DA. Eradication: lessons from the past. *Bull WHO* 1988; 76: Suppl. 2, 7–21.
69. World Health Organization. Eradication of poliomyelitis. Report of the Director General. A71/26. 20 March 2018. http://apps.who.int/gb/ebwha/pdf_files/WHA71/A71_26-en.pdf
70. The Carter Center. Guinea worm eradication program www.cartercenter.org/health/guinea_worm/index.html Date last accessed: May 25, 2018.
71. Soper FL. Problems to be solved if eradication of tuberculosis is to be realized. *Am J Public Health Nations Health* 1962; 52: 734–745.
72. Palmer C. Tuberculosis: a decade in retrospect and in prospect. *Lancet* 1958; 78: 257–260.
73. Perkins J. Global tuberculosis eradication. *Am Rev Tuberc* 1959; 80: 138–139.
74. Groth-Petersen E, Knudsen J, Wilbek E. The epidemiological basis of tuberculosis eradication in an advanced country. *Bull World Health Organ* 1959; 21: 5–49.
75. European Centre for Disease Prevention and Control, World Health Organization. Tuberculosis surveillance and monitoring in Europe 2018: 2016 data. https://ecdc.europa.eu/sites/portal/files/documents/ecdc-tuberculosis-surveillance-monitoring-Europe-2018-19mar2018.pdf
76. Bloomquist ET. Program aimed at eradication of tuberculosis. *Pub Health Reports* 1963; 78: 897–904.
77. Center for Disease Control. A strategic plan for the elimination of tuberculosis in the United States. *MMWR Suppl* 1989; 38: 1–25.
78. Centers for Disease Control and Prevention. Tuberculosis elimination revisited: obstacles, opportunities, and a renewed commitment. Advisory Council for the Elimination of Tuberculosis (ACET). *MMWR Morb Mortal Wkly Rep* 1999; 48: 1–12.
79. Centers for Disease Control and Prevention (CDC). Reported Tuberculosis in the United States, 2016. Atlanta, GA, US Department of Health and Human Services, CDC, 2017.

https://doi.org/10.1183/2312508X.10020617

80. World Health Organization. The End TB Strategy. Geneva, WHO, 2014.

81. Lönnroth K, Migliori GB, Abubakar I, *et al.* Towards tuberculosis elimination: a framework for low incidence countries. *Eur Respir J* 2015; 45: 928–952.

Disclosures: None declared.

Acknowledgements: The authorship of this chapter is as follows. Co-evolution of *Mycobacterium tuberculosis* and humans during the Neolithic period: M. Kato-Maeda. The European tuberculosis epidemic and industrialisation: 1750–1950: J.F. Murray and R. Loddenkemper. Robert Koch, Rudolf Virchow and tuberculin: C. Gradmann. Decline in tuberculosis mortality before specific antibiotics: P.C. Hopewell. Tuberculosis during world war I and world war II: J.F. Murray and R. Loddenkemper. The history of tuberculosis chemotherapy: C. Gradmann. Moving toward tuberculosis elimination: P.C. Hopewell.

Chapter 3

Epidemiology and socioeconomic determinants

Raquel Duarte[1,2,3], João V. Santos[4,5,6], André Santos Silva[7,8] and Giovanni Sotgiu[9]

The incidence rate of TB has declined worldwide but remains unacceptably high. TB is currently the ninth leading cause of death and the leading cause of death among infectious diseases worldwide. Several behavioural and biological factors are associated with TB, such as HIV infection, tobacco smoking, DM, alcohol abuse and poor nutrition. Socioeconomic factors, such as poor housing, crowded living conditions, migration, low income and advanced age, are also associated with TB. There is an established link between poverty and TB, and increasing evidence suggests that actions or policies that target the socioeconomic determinants of TB can reduce its incidence. In addition, the costs of treatment faced by patients, which can be significant in countries without universal health coverage, must be assessed so that interventions can be implemented at the clinical, public health and socioeconomic levels to reduce the burden of TB.

Cite as: Duarte R, Santos JV, Santos Silva A, *et al.* Epidemiology and socioeconomic determinants. *In:* Migliori GB, Bothamley G, Duarte R, *et al.*, eds. Tuberculosis [ERS Monograph]. Sheffield, European Respiratory Society, 2018; pp. 28–35 [https://doi.org/10.1183/2312508X.10020717].

@ERSpublications
The worldwide incidence of TB is unacceptably high. Increasing evidence shows that addressing the socioeconomic determinants of TB may help to achieve the WHO goal of TB elimination. http://ow.ly/cfVQ30lqCfE

The burden of TB remains high, and the rate of progress appears insufficient to achieve the WHO targets [1]. Despite our current knowledge of the biology of *Mycobacterium tuberculosis* and its epidemiology, a holistic approach is needed to improve clinical management and to identify factors associated with infection [2].

[1]Departamento de Pneumologia, Centro Hospitalar Vila Nova de Gaia, Vila Nova de Gaia, Portugal. [2]Departamento de Ciências da Saúde Pública e Forenses e Educação Médica, Faculdade de Medicina, Universidade do Porto, Porto, Portugal. [3]ISPUP-EPIUnit, Faculdade de Medicina, Universidade do Porto, Porto, Portugal. [4]Dept of Community Medicine, Information and Health Decision Sciences (MEDCIDS), Faculty of Medicine, University of Porto, Porto, Portugal. [5]CINTESIS – Center for Health Technology and Services Research, Porto, Portugal. [6]Public Health Unit, ACeS Grande Porto VIII, Espinho-Gaia, Portugal. [7]Departamento de Doenças Infeciosas, Centro Hospitalar de São João, Porto, Portugal. [8]Departamento de Medicina, Faculdade de Medicina da Universidade do Porto, Porto, Portugal. [9]Dept of Medical, Surgical and Experimental Sciences, University of Sassari, Sassari, Italy.

Correspondence: Raquel Duarte, ISPUP-EPIUnit, Faculdade de Medicina, Universidade do Porto, Rua das Taipas No. 135, 4050-600 Porto, Portugal. E-mail: rdmelo@med.up.pt

Copyright ©ERS 2018. Print ISBN: 978-1-84984-099-6. Online ISBN: 978-1-84984-100-9. Print ISSN: 2312-508X. Online ISSN: 2312-5098.

https://doi.org/10.1183/2312508X.10020717

Overview of the epidemiology of tuberculosis

Almost 90% of the incident cases of TB in 2016 were in the WHO Southeast Asia Region, the WHO African Region and the WHO Western Pacific Region [3]. There were lower incidences in the WHO Eastern Mediterranean Region (7%), the WHO European Region (3%) and the WHO Region of the Americas (3%) [3].

The latest WHO report estimated an incidence of 10.4 million TB cases in 2016, with most cases in India, Indonesia, China, The Philippines and Pakistan [4]. Among the 10 countries with the highest incidence of TB, five are in the WHO African Region, including South Africa and Lesotho (table 1) [3]. Individuals in these counties have also high rates of co-infection with HIV [4].

TB was responsible for more than 1.7 million deaths in 2016, and is now the ninth leading cause of death worldwide and the leading cause of death among infectious diseases [3]. TB-related mortality is especially significant in the WHO African and Southeast Asian Regions. Poor therapeutic adherence, infection with drug-resistant strains and immunodepression are significantly associated with increased mortality from TB.

HIV co-infection, RR-TB and MDR-TB are the main reasons for the ongoing global epidemic [4]. Annually, >600 000 TB cases are RR-TB, and >80% of these cases are MDR-TB. Among the 10 countries with the highest incidence rates of MDR-TB, nine are in the WHO European Region (table 2) [3]. In former Soviet Union nations (Belarus, Moldova, Kazakhstan and the Russian Federation), the rate of MDR-TB is >50% among cases requiring retreatment [5].

In comparison with drug-susceptible TB (DS-TB), MDR- and XDR-TB have higher rates of mortality and relapse, and lower rates of treatment success [4]. In particular, the treatment success rate of DS-TB is ~85–90%, but is <60% for MDR-TB and <30% for XDR-TB [6].

Overall, the incidence of TB worldwide has decreased at an estimated rate of 4% year^{-1}, and the fastest decline was in the WHO European Region [4]. There have also been

Table 1. Countries with the highest incidence rates of TB according to the WHO

Country	Incidence rate per 100 000 inhabitants per year
South Africa	781
Lesotho	724
Kiribati	566
The Philippines	554
Mozambique	551
Democratic People's Republic of Korea	513
East Timor	498
Gabon	485
Namibia	446
Papua New Guinea	432

Information from [3].

Table 2. Countries with the highest percentages of MDR-TB among all TB cases according to the WHO

Country	MDR-TB cases %
Belarus	38–72
Russian Federation	27–65
Uzbekistan	24–63
Kyrgyzstan	27–60
Moldova	26–56
Ukraine	27–47
Kazakhstan	26–44
Tajikistan	22–45
Bahamas	11–50
Lithuania	12–47

Information from [3].

declining rates in several counties with high TB burdens, including Ethiopia, Kenya, Lesotho, Namibia, the Russian Federation, Tanzania, Zambia and Zimbabwe. Globally, the TB mortality rate declined by 37% between 2000 and 2016 [4]. Regionally, the fastest declines since 2010 were in the WHO European Region (6.0% year^{-1}) and the WHO Western Pacific Region (4.6% year^{-1}) [4]. During the last decade, the incidence and prevalence of TB have declined significantly in low-income countries, particularly in Central and Eastern Europe and sub-Saharan Africa [7]. However, these improvements have not been fast enough to reach the WHO targets, and a high burden of disease remains [3].

Effect of alcohol, tobacco and intravenous drugs

Immunodepression is the major predisposing factor for TB [8], and patients with HIV infections have the highest relative risk for TB [8]. Several studies have shown that low CD4$^+$ counts and high viral load are surrogate risk factors for the occurrence of TB, whereas initiation of ART is associated with a significantly reduced risk [9, 10]. At the population level, an increased HIV notification rate is associated with an increased TB notification rate [11, 12].

However, other behavioural and biological determinants (such as smoking, DM, alcohol use and malnutrition) can also increase the risk of TB infection and contribute to the pathogenesis of TB. Socioeconomic determinants, such as poor housing, crowded living conditions, migration, low income and advanced age, are also important [13].

Use of tobacco, alcohol and *i.v.* drugs is frequently associated with poverty, overcrowding, HIV infection and viral hepatitis [14]. A case–control study in 1961 first reported an association of alcohol and tobacco use with TB [15]. Other studies confirmed these initial findings, and also reported correlations of these same factors with more contagious and severe disease (*e.g.* cavitary TB) [16–18]. Data on active TB cases from 22 countries with high TB burdens indicated that 21% of cases were attributable to smoking, 13.4% to alcohol abuse and 16% to HIV infection [19].

https://doi.org/10.1183/2312508X.10020717

The most frequently reported risk factor for TB is being an active or former tobacco smoker, and up to one-third of all TB cases are attributable to smoking [20]. The association of tobacco smoking with TB is weaker if adjusted for confounding by alcohol use, even in prolonged and heavy tobacco users. Moreover, an analysis of never-smokers, former smokers and active smokers indicated a progressive increase in the rate of LTBI. There is also an increased risk of LTBI and active TB in children exposed to second-hand smoke [21] and in nonsmoking adults who have close household contact with heavy smokers [22].

Smokers with TB have an ~9-fold greater mortality rate than never-smokers with TB, although the risk to smokers decreases significantly after cessation of smoking. Therefore, medical counselling on smoking cessation is highly recommended to reduce the burden of TB, and national programmes should include strategies to reduce the number of individuals exposed to tobacco smoke [23].

Several previous studies have reported a relationship between heavy alcohol use and TB, but only recently has there been an estimate of the TB burden attributable to alcohol use. Worldwide, ~10% of TB patients are alcohol abusers, and avoidance of heavy alcohol use could reduce the number of TB cases by 17% and the number of TB deaths by 15% [14]. Excessive alcohol consumption (>40 g·day^{-1}) is associated with a 3-fold increased risk of sputum smear-positive cavitary disease, with a longer time to sputum smear conversion and with an increased risk of adverse events to anti-TB medication [18, 24]. Alcoholism is also linked to other determinants of poor clinical and treatment outcomes, such as low socioeconomic status, homelessness and malnutrition [25].

Treatment of alcohol abuse may be even harder than treatment of smoking, because psychosocial factors linked to heavy drinking may play a stronger role. The lack of adequate human resources, the high cost of drugs used to treat alcoholism and the severity of alcohol addiction limit the efficacy of counselling and other medical interventions [14].

Another global risk factor for TB is *i.v.* drug use, especially in Eastern Europe and the Americas [26]. According to the United Nations Office on Drugs and Crime, almost 12 million people use *i.v.* drugs, and one in eight (1.6 million) of these individuals is HIV positive [26]. Drug use is frequently associated with homelessness, incarceration and HIV infection.

There are frequently barriers to the care and treatment of *i.v.* drug users. These individuals also typically have poor treatment adherence, due to the social stigma and criminalisation of drug use [27]. Furthermore, the delayed diagnosis of TB in these individuals may contribute to a higher rate of transmission and the presence of more severe disease [28]. Former *i.v.* drug users exposed to opiate substitution therapy may also experience drug toxicities following the administration of potentially hepatotoxic TB drugs or rifampicin, due to the accelerated metabolism of methadone, and this could increase the risk of abstinence syndrome.

Socioeconomic determinants

The socioeconomic determinants of health include the social, political and economic conditions to which all population groups are exposed [29], as well as their health status [30, 31]. These determinants can affect living conditions, behaviours and access to healthcare.

People in low socioeconomic groups have a higher risk of contact with persons with active TB, of living in crowded and poorly ventilated settings, and of engaging in unhealthy behaviours, such as having a poor diet, not exercising and having poor hygiene [32].

Recent modelling studies estimated that, by 2035, the incidence of TB will decline by 33.5% if appropriate actions are taken against extreme poverty, and by 76.1% if there are expansions of social protection [33]. Both interventions together could achieve a reduction of 84.3% by 2035, with an annual decrease of ~9.1% [33].

Effect of diabetes mellitus and employment in healthcare

Researchers have increasingly recognised DM, whose worldwide prevalence is expected to double by 2030 [34], as a risk factor for TB. Several population studies, systematic reviews and a meta-analysis point to a link between poor glycaemic control or overt DM with TB [35–38]. In particular, these individuals have an overall 3-fold increased risk of active PTB, regardless of background or underlying medical conditions [35]. DM is also associated with more severe TB, delayed sputum conversion, increased risk of treatment failure [39], and higher rates of relapse and recurrence. In 2008, LÖNNROTH AND RAVIGLIONE [8] calculated that the population attributable fraction (PAF) of TB cases due to DM was 6% worldwide, but more recent estimates are that this PAF is 11–15%, comparable to the PAF of HIV/AIDS [36].

TB was recognised as an occupational hazard for healthcare workers in the 1950s [40]. Healthcare workers have a greater risk of LTBI and active TB, most probably due to their exposure to patients with unrecognised or inappropriately treated TB. A recent meta-analysis, which updated the estimates of the occupational risks for latent and active TB, identified a 2-fold increased risk of LTBI and a 3-fold increased risk of active TB among healthcare workers, although these vary among different healthcare settings [41–43] and usually mirror the TB incidence in the general population. Overall, at least one-third of healthcare workers may have LTBI, and their risk of developing active TB can be 2–3-fold higher than that of the general population. However, because healthcare workers typically account for a small fraction of the total population, the PAF of healthcare workers does not exceed 5%, and is comparable among different countries [41].

Costs of tuberculosis control and elimination

The Global Plan to End TB 2016–2020, established by the Stop TB Partnership, estimated that US$58 billion is needed to implement TB programmes, and up to US$9 billion to develop new tools to achieve the 90-(90)-90 targets ("reach 90% of all people who need TB treatment, including 90% of people in key populations, and achieve at least 90% treatment success") [44]. This could lead to a return of US$27 for each dollar spent [44]. However, low- and middle-income countries had yearly funding gaps of nearly US$2 billion in 2016 and 2017, according to the Global Plan [4, 45]. Furthermore, international donors are still the main source of funding in low-income countries, mainly by the Global Fund to Fight AIDS, Tuberculosis and Malaria, whose largest donor is the USA [4].

The Global TB Caucus projected that 28 million people will die from TB between 2015 and 2030, assuming the current rate of decline in the annual incidence, and the associated global economic costs will be US$983 billion [46]. A delay of investments in research and development could dramatically increase future costs [44].

https://doi.org/10.1183/2312508X.10020717

In the European Union (EU), the costs associated with TB treatment and loss of productivity was more than €0.5 billion during 2011 [47]. This is less than the EU costs associated with other respiratory diseases, such as obstructive sleep apnoea syndrome (by a factor of ~13), asthma (by a factor of ~63) and COPD (by a factor of ~90) [48].

Although the incidence rate of TB decreased between 2005 and 2015 in Europe and globally [49], drug-resistant forms became more common [50]. Relative to DS-TB, the estimated cost for treatment of MDR-TB is ~5.6–7.6-fold greater, and the cost of treatment for XDR-TB is ~16.6-fold greater [4, 47, 51]. Furthermore, the high price for these TB regimens could significantly increase costs for clinical and public healthcare [52].

Another important consideration when attempting to eliminate TB is the costs faced by patients, which can be catastrophic in poor countries and countries without universal health coverage. Thus, additional funds are needed to reduce the prevalence and incidence of TB to achieve the WHO's SDGs and End TB Strategy targets. The Millennium Development Goals previously described the steps required to achieve these targets [53]. Addressing the socioeconomic determinants of health and improving the socioeconomic status of affected households can help to achieve these goals.

Conclusion

The worldwide incidence of TB is unacceptably high. Increasing evidence shows that addressing the socioeconomic determinants of TB may help to achieve the WHO goal of TB elimination.

References

1. WHO. Global Strategy and Targets for Tuberculosis Prevention, Care and Control after 2015. Document EB134/12. Geneva, WHO, 2013. http://apps.who.int/gb/ebwha/pdf_files/EB134/B134_12-en.pdf
2. Wingfield T, Tovar MA, Huff D, *et al.* Beyond pills and tests: addressing the social determinants of tuberculosis. *Clin Med* 2016; 16: s79–s91.
3. Frieden TR, Brudney KF, Harries AD. Global tuberculosis: perspectives, prospects, and priorities. JAMA 2014; 312: 1393–1994.
4. WHO. Global Tuberculosis Report 2017. Geneva, WHO, 2017. www.who.int/tb/publications/global_report/en/
5. WHO. Roadmap to Implement the Tuberculosis Action Plan for the WHO European Region 2016–2020. Geneva, WHO, 2016. www.euro.who.int/__data/assets/pdf_file/0020/318233/50148-WHO-TB-Plan_May17_web.pdf
6. Matteelli A, Roggi A, Carvalho ACC. Extensively drug-resistant tuberculosis: epidemiology and management. *Clin Epidemiol* 2014; 6: 111–118.
7. Dye C, Lönnroth K, Jaramillo E, *et al.* Trends in tuberculosis incidence and their determinants in 134 countries. *Bull World Health Organ* 2009; 87: 683–691.
8. Lönnroth K, Raviglione M. Global epidemiology of tuberculosis: prospect for control. *Sem Respir Crit Care Med* 2008; 29: 481–491.
9. Lange C, van Leth F, Sester M. Viral load and risk of tuberculosis in HIV infection. *J Acquir Immune Defic Syndr* 2016; 71: e51–e53.
10. Badri M, Wilson D, Wood R. Effect of highly active antiretroviral therapy on incidence of tuberculosis in South Africa: a cohort study. *Lancet* 2002; 359: 2059–2064.
11. Harries A, Dye C. Tuberculosis. *Ann Trop Med Parasitol* 2006; 100: 415–431.
12. Sousa P, Oliveira A, Gomes M, *et al.* Longitudinal clustering of tuberculosis incidence and predictors for the time profiles: the impact of HIV. *Int J Tuberc Lung Dis* 2016; 20: 1027–1032.
13. Murray M, Oxlade O, Lin HH. Modeling social, environmental and biological determinants of tuberculosis. *Int J Tuberc Lung Dis* 2011; 15: 64–70.
14. Rehm J, Samokhvalov AV, Neuman MG, *et al.* The association between alcohol use, alcohol use disorders and tuberculosis (TB). A systematic review. *BMC Public Health* 2009; 9: 450.

15. Brown KE, Campbell AH. Tobacco, alcohol and tuberculosis. *Br J Dis Chest* 1961; 55: 150–158.

16. Yen YF, Yen MY, Lin YS, *et al.* Smoking increases risk of recurrence after successful anti-tuberculosis treatment: a population-based study. *Int J Tuberc Lung Dis* 2014; 18: 492–498.

17. Patra J, Jha P, Rehm J, *et al.* Tobacco smoking, alcohol drinking, diabetes, low body mass index and the risk of self-reported symptoms of active tuberculosis: Individual Participant Data (IPD) meta-analyses of 72,684 individuals in 14 high tuberculosis burden countries. *PLoS One* 2014; 9: e96433.

18. Lönnroth K, Castro KG, Chakaya JM, *et al.* Tuberculosis control and elimination 2010–50: cure, care, and social development. *Lancet* 2010; 375: 1814–1829.

19. Hutahaean LM. Effects of smoking habit on the development of tuberculosis disease. *IOSR J Nurs Health Sci* 2013; 2: 2320–1940.

20. Zellweger JP, Cattamanchi A, Sotgiu G. Tobacco and tuberculosis: could we improve tuberculosis outcomes by helping patients to stop smoking? *Eur Respir J* 2015; 45: 583–585.

21. Lin HH, Ezzati M, Murray M. Tobacco smoke, indoor air pollution and tuberculosis: a systematic review and meta-analysis. *PLoS Med* 2007; 4: e20.

22. Santos-Silva AF, Migliori GB, Duarte R. Tuberculosis, alcohol and tobacco: dangerous liaisons. *Rev Port Pneumol* 2017; 23: 177–178.

23. Francisco J, Oliveira O, Felgueiras Ó, *et al.* How much is too much alcohol in tuberculosis? *Eur Respir J* 2017; 49: 1601468.

24. Lönnroth K, Williams BG, Stadlin S, *et al.* Alcohol use as a risk factor for tuberculosis – a systematic review. *BMC Public Health* 2008; 8: 289.

25. Duarte R, Lönnroth K, Carvalho C, *et al.* Tuberculosis, social determinants and co-morbidities (including HIV). *Rev Port Pneumol* 2017; 24: 115–119.

26. United Nations Office on Drugs and Crime (UNODC). Executive Summary. Conclusion and Policy Implications of the World Drug Report 2017. Vienna, UNODC, 2017. www.unodc.org/wdr2017/field/Booklet_1_EXSUM.pdf

27. Getahun H, Baddeley A, Raviglioni M. Managing tuberculosis in people who use and inject illicit drugs. *Bull World Health Organ* 2013; 91: 154–156.

28. Deiss RG, Rodwell TC, Garfein RS. Tuberculosis and illicit drug use: review and update. *Clin Infect Dis* 2009; 48: 72–82.

29. WHO. World Conference on Social Determinants of Health. Geneva, WHO, 2011. www.who.int/social_determinants/sdhconference/declaration/en/

30. Braveman P, Gottlieb L. The social determinants of health: it's time to consider the causes of the causes. *Public Health Rep* 2014; 129: 19–31.

31. Epstein D, Jiménez-Rubio D, Smith PC, *et al.* Social determinants of health: an economic perspective. *Health Econ* 2009; 18: 495–502.

32. Lönnroth K, Jaramillo E, Williams BG, *et al.* Drivers of tuberculosis epidemics: the role of risk factors and social determinants. *Soc Sci Med* 2009; 68: 2240–2246.

33. Carter DJ, Glaziou P, Lönnroth K, *et al.* The impact of social protection and poverty elimination on global tuberculosis incidence: a statistical modelling analysis of Sustainable Development Goal 1. *Lancet Glob Heal* 2018; 6: e514–e522.

34. WHO. Global Report on Diabetes. Geneva, WHO, 2016. www.who.int/diabetes/publications/grd-2016/en/

35. Jiménez-Corona ME, Cruz-Hervert LP, García-García L, *et al.* Association of diabetes and tuberculosis: impact on treatment and post-treatment outcomes. *Thorax* 2013; 68: 214–220.

36. Stevenson CR, Forouhi NG, Roglic G, *et al.* Diabetes and tuberculosis: the impact of the diabetes epidemic on tuberculosis incidence. *BMC Public Health* 2007; 7: 1–8.

37. Alisjahbana B, van Crevel R, Sahiratmadja E, *et al.* Diabetes mellitus is strongly associated with tuberculosis in Indonesia. *Int J Tuberc Lung Dis.* 2006; 10: 696–700.

38. Jeon CY, Murray MB. Diabetes mellitus increases the risk of active tuberculosis: a systematic review of 13 observational studies. *PLoS Med* 2008; 5: 1091–1101.

39. Da Costa JC, Oliveira O, Baía L, *et al.* Prevalence and factors associated with diabetes mellitus among tuberculosis patients: a nationwide cohort. *Eur Respir J* 2016; 48: 264–268.

40. Sepkowitz K. Tuberculosis and the health care worker: a historical perspective. *Ann Intern Med* 1994; 120: 71–79.

41. Baussano I, Nunn P, Williams B, *et al.* Tuberculosis among health care workers. *Emerging Infect Dis* 2011; 17: 488–494.

42. Uden L, Barber E, Ford N, *et al.* Risk of tuberculosis infection and disease for health care workers: an updated meta-analysis. *Open Forum Infect Dis* 2017; 4: 1–7.

43. Meireles JM, Gaio R, Duarte R. Factors influencing tuberculosis screening in healthcare workers in Portugal. *Eur Respir J* 2015; 45: 834–838.

44. Stop TB Partnership. The Paradigm Shift 2016–2020: Global Plan to End TB. Geneva, Stop TB Partnership, UNOPS, 2015. www.stoptb.org/assets/documents/global/plan/globalplantoendtb_theparadigmshift_2016-2020_stoptbpartnership.pdf

https://doi.org/10.1183/2312508X.10020717

45. WHO. Global Tuberculosis Report 2016. Geneva, WHO, 2016. http://apps.who.int/iris/bitstream/handle/10665/250441/9789241565394-eng.pdf?sequence=1

46. Global TB Caucus. The Price of a Pandemic 2017. Global TB Caucus, 2017. https://docs.wixstatic.com/ugd/309c93_56d4ef0e87d24667b1d3edae55f6eeb5.pdf

47. Diel R, Vandeputte J, De Vries G, *et al.* Costs of tuberculosis disease in the European Union: a systematic analysis and cost calculation. *Eur Respir J* 2014; 43: 554–565.

48. The economic burden of lung disease. *In:* Gibson J, Loddenkemper R, Sibille Y, *et al.* eds. European Lung White Book. 2nd Edn. Sheffield, European Respiratory Society, 2013; pp. 16–27.

49. Kyu HH, Maddison ER, Henry NJ, *et al.* The global burden of tuberculosis: results from the Global Burden of Disease Study 2015. *Lancet Infect Dis* 2018; 18: 261–284.

50. van der Werf MJ, Kodmon C, Hollo V, *et al.* Drug resistance among tuberculosis cases in the European Union and European Economic Area, 2007 to 2012. *Euro Surveill* 2014; 19: 1–13.

51. Laurence YV, Griffiths UK, Vassall A. Costs to health services and the patient of treating tuberculosis: a systematic literature review. *Pharmacoeconomics* 2015; 33: 939–955.

52. Günther G, Gomez GB, Lange C, *et al.* Availability, price and affordability of anti-tuberculosis drugs in Europe: a TBNET survey. *Eur Respir J* 2015; 45: 1081–1088.

53. Floyd K, Pantoja A. Financial resources required for tuberculosis control to achieve global targets set for 2015. *Bull World Health Organ* 2008; 86: 568–576.

Disclosures: **None declared.**

| Chapter 4

Evolution of the strategies for control and elimination

Mario C. Raviglione

TB still affects millions of people every year, causing 1.6 million deaths annually. Attempts to control this disease intensified after the discovery of its infectious nature over the past century, when both diagnosis and treatment became widely available. After a period of neglect, linked with the conviction that TB was declining, new information about global burden and major outbreaks in rich countries in the early 1990s prompted a renewed effort. The first WHO global strategy, DOTS, was widely implemented in countries from the mid-1990s and contributed towards standardising control activities and reverting TB incidence. However, emerging challenges, including HIV-associated TB, MDR-TB, how to engage the private sector and communities, and the need for new tools, have required a revisiting of the strategy in the form of the new WHO Stop TB Strategy launched in 2006. Lately, multiple actors have become prominent in the global fight against TB, and the new framework of the SDGs has prompted innovations in the global approach, with more emphasis placed on patient-centred care, policies addressing the social and economic determinants of TB, and the role of research. The new WHO End TB Strategy is currently the approach universally recommended in the SDG era, while TB enjoys growing political attention thanks to two unprecedented events in 2017–2018 that should transform the global struggle against this disease.

Cite as: Raviglione MC. Evolution of the strategies for control and elimination. *In:* Migliori GB, Bothamley G, Duarte R, *et al.*, eds. Tuberculosis (ERS Monograph). Sheffield, European Respiratory Society, 2018; pp. 36–61 [https://doi.org/10.1183/2312508X.10020817].

🐦 @ERSpublications
Approaches to TB control have evolved from DOTS to the End TB Strategy 2016–2035. While TB incidence and mortality are slowly declining, political commitment and proper financing are necessary to end TB. http://ow.ly/cfVQ30lqCfE

With 1.3 million people dying every year, TB is currently the top cause of infectious death from a single pathogen worldwide, ranking in 10th position after mainly noncommunicable and noncontagious conditions [1]. Over the past two decades, TB control activities have intensified in most countries, and the resources available have increased substantially leading to better practices [1]. An estimated 54 million lives have been saved since 2000 compared with the number of predicted deaths. International standards have been promoted since 1995 by the WHO through its global strategies. In addition, after the

---

Global Health Centre, University of Milan, Milan, Italy.

Correspondence: Mario C. Raviglione, 415F Route des Alpes, 01280 Prévessin-Moëns, France. E-mail: mario.raviglione@unimi.it

Copyright ©ERS 2018. Print ISBN: 978-1-84984-099-6. Online ISBN: 978-1-84984-100-9. Print ISSN: 2312-508X. Online ISSN: 2312-5098.

https://doi.org/10.1183/2312508X.10020817

persistent increases in TB during the 1990s, linked to the HIV/AIDS epidemic in Africa and the collapse of the public health infrastructure in the former Soviet Union, the global incidence of TB and death rates have begun to decline since the early 2000s, although as slowly as 1–2% per year and 3–4% per year, respectively [2, 3].

Despite these achievements, the availability of sound strategies, good scientific knowledge and life-saving tools for diagnosis, treatment and prevention, some of which have been used for decades, efforts to fully control TB and eventually eliminate this millennia-old scourge of humanity have not been sufficient to guarantee a faster decline of the disease burden [4]. Many national TB control programmes lack capacity, resources or just clear objectives to face TB in an optimal way. As a result, over one-third of TB cases estimated to emerge annually (3.6 million out of 10 million) are not officially reported by surveillance systems. A high proportion of these are "hidden" in the private for-profit sector where case-management practices are unknown or inappropriate [5]. MDR-TB is rampant in some parts of the world, and most patients are not detected due to a lack of systematic, universal DST [2]. For those detected, treatment is often poorly effective due to difficulties in accessing second-line drugs, the toxicity of these drugs and the long duration of treatment [6]. HIV-associated TB, with three-quarters of its burden concentrated in sub-Saharan Africa, is often not addressed properly due to limited collaboration between dedicated TB and HIV/AIDS programmes, preventing implementation of the full package of care available for coinfected persons [7]. Resources, both human and financial, are not growing at the appropriate speed to face the epidemic. Financial gaps, estimated to be over US$3.5 billion for implementation efforts and at least US$1.3 billion for research, are a testimony of the lukewarm commitment by most governments and stakeholders to confront the challenge. Finally, "epidemics" of noncommunicable conditions, including DM, tobacco smoking and alcohol abuse, are factors increasing the risk of TB in the population and opposing control efforts [8].

Apart from inadequacies within the health systems, often due to a lack of policies promoting universal health coverage (UHC), many other factors, social and economic in nature and linked with the general development of people and societies at large, are responsible for the current status of the TB epidemic. Poverty, lack of social protection, malnutrition, poor living conditions (especially in slums), indoor air pollution due to toxic fuels, inequities, gender inequality, instability and wars in many countries are determining the fate of the TB epidemic [9, 10]. In this situation, political engagement, such as that derived from momentous events including those held recently in Moscow in November 2017 and at the United Nations (UN) General Assembly High Level Meeting in September 2018, is essential to pursue a stronger response in all sectors.

Methods of research

The literature has been searched extensively for coverage of the various topics presented in this chapter. The chapter draws mainly on a narrative scientific literature review. However, given the policy-oriented structure, "grey papers", reports from key international meetings and conferences, and, where necessary, nonscientific journals and magazines have also been used to provide additional information. Among others, PubMed was searched. Information from countries presented in this chapter relies largely on reported programme implementation and policy data.

Historical overview of tuberculosis control in the 19th and first half of the 20th century

The modern era of the global fight against TB began at the time of the discovery of the TB bacillus, *Mycobacterium tuberculosis,* by the German Nobel Prize winner Robert Koch in 1882 [11]. This revolutionary event prompted scientists to focus on control and care approaches directed at detecting a micro-organism after centuries of debates on the aetiology of the disease, and at identifying means to combat it effectively. Following the discovery of the agent of TB, Ehrlich, Ziehl and Neelsen perfected the staining technique. This resulted in wide-scale implementation of sputum smear microscopy, thus opening the way towards accurate bacteriological diagnosis [12].

This was a major advance against a disease that, as in Koch's own statement, caused one out of seven deaths in Europe. In this pre-antibiotic era, the solution that was sought was a vaccine. Koch developed a glycerine extract of tubercle bacilli (known as "old tuberculin") in the hope that it would be curative. However, this was in fact risky and could be fatal. It took three decades for the development in 1921 of the BCG vaccine, the only vaccine for TB with some efficacy still available today. Calmette and Guerin at the Pasteur Institute in Lille, France, discovered that inactivating *Mycobacterium bovis* bacilli through multiple passages on a glycerine–potato medium to render them less virulent provided protection in humans. Several trials were undertaken between the 1930s and 1960s in an attempt to demonstrate the efficacy of the BCG vaccine. The results were controversial, with an efficacy ranging from −70% to +70% depending on the population and location, with more favourable outcomes in the north of the world, where a vaccine is less important [13–15]. Today, the BCG vaccine is recognised as effective in preventing the severe, disseminated forms of childhood TB. The WHO recommends that it should be used as soon as possible in life in children from high-incidence settings or in selected risk groups [16].

Throughout the first half of the 20th century, the main measures to control TB were therefore a good standard of living, adequate nutrition and isolation of infectious individuals in sanatoria. Sanatoria were facilities where TB patients could be provided with the best possible care, and with rest, food and continued assistance [17]. These measures, applied with intensity in Europe and North America, resulted in a progressive reduction in TB incidence and deaths, with annual declines in countries with good surveillance capacity such as the Netherlands, Norway, Denmark, the UK and the USA that reached >3% per year. In Denmark, for instance, the incidence fell by 53% between 1921 and 1940 [18]. Overall societal development, better living conditions, improved nutrition and general poverty reduction contributed in a major way to the decline of TB in the western world. However, in the absence of a curative intervention, mortality remained high and some 65% of TB patients had a fatal outcome at 5 years, with the remainder either becoming chronic cases with bouts of disease alternating with remissions and a long course that also meant continuous transmission, or self-curing with often serious fibrotic changes in their lung tissue and sequelae [19, 20]. Moreover, the situation in other parts of the world was not well known, and in fact in most developing countries TB remained a threat to individuals and communities.

The antibiotic era of tuberculosis control: the second half of the 20th century

What eventually revolutionised the management of TB was the discovery of the first effective anti-TB drugs during the 1940s and their wide-scale introduction into treatment in

 https://doi.org/10.1183/2312508X.10020817

the years immediately after. The first effective drug, discovered in 1943 by Schatz, Bugie and Waksman, was the aminoglycoside streptomycin [21, 22]. Just like Robert Koch for his discovery of the cause of TB more than half a century before, Waksman received the Nobel Prize in 1955. However, the discovery should also be attributed to Schatz, a young PhD student who first isolated streptomycin in Waksman's laboratory from the products of *Streptomyces griseus*. The molecule was very effective against *M. tuberculosis*. The developing company, Merck & Co., purified it and started massive production. Almost simultaneously with the discovery of streptomycin, the Swedish physician Lehmann discovered PAS, another effective drug [23]. More discoveries of new anti-TB drugs followed rapidly over the next two decades, and the introduction of isoniazid, ethambutol, pyrazinamide and thiacetazone allowed the first combination regimens, as it soon became clear that the use of a single agent would facilitate the emergence of drug-resistant strains [24]. Thus, by the late 1950s, the best regimen to treat TB had become a combination of streptomycin, isoniazid and a third drug. With this approach, a much higher cure rate and lower relapse rate were achieved. The discovery and introduction of rifampicin, still the most potent agent available, in the early 1970s allowed the first large clinical trials to define the most effective drug combinations [25]. These trials, mostly run by the British Medical Research Council (BMRC), are often cited as pioneering examples of systematic, statistically sound controlled trials in the history of medicine [26]. The results showed clearly that the best regimen needed to include isoniazid, rifampicin and pyrazinamide with the addition of ethambutol to "protect" against drug resistance. By the early 1980s, therefore, the treatment strategy against TB was well defined. However, despite this promising situation and three to four decades of fruitful intensive research efforts, TB control was far from being reached and the feeling of failing elimination became widespread, especially in poor countries [27].

Meanwhile, the WHO had initiated campaigns to eliminate TB through massive BCG vaccination [28]. Later, it introduced new case-management practices that relied mainly on experiences in Madras and Bangalore, India, and focused on integrated primary care approaches rather than specialised vertical delivery. These included ambulatory treatment instead of prolonged hospitalisation, intermittent regimens, the adoption of direct observation of drug intake to ensure adherence to months-long treatment, and the possibility of relying on sputum smear microscopy for diagnosis [29–32]. To make policy recommendations, the WHO established Expert Committees that met regularly between 1947 and 1973. The 1964 Eighth Committee incorporated these innovations into WHO policies [33]. In 1974, the Ninth and last Expert Committee promoted a full package of interventions beyond treatment, such as standard definitions and cohort-based reporting, thus creating the basis of the future DOTS strategy [34]. This last Expert Committee was led by Wallace Fox, a major authority in the TB field, who had run the BMRC clinical trials that established the best-regimen options.

Despite the existence of sound recommendations, implementation in countries was minimal and without any accountability or reliable monitoring systems. Meanwhile, a major turmoil in international health was brought by the Alma-Ata Declaration in 1978 [35], which underemphasised vertical, disease-specific efforts in favour of primary care services and community engagement. The extreme interpretation of the new "philosophy" resulted in a hot debate between those favouring horizontal, holistic, primary care approaches and those who were instead pursuing "vertical", disease-specific approaches [36]. The debate did not help the global fight against TB. TB programmes in countries were minimised or dismantled without proper, well-thought-out compensatory measures. The end result was that TB was left unchecked for more than a decade during which awareness of what was happening in poor countries was limited. During the 1980s, the WHO itself, with two or three TB specialists at its headquarters in Geneva, did not have a dedicated TB programme under the false impression that more horizontal efforts would automatically address what is indeed a complex public health intervention requiring good coordination and essential measures to be successful.

Fortunately, piloting and operational research did not stop, despite WHO neglect and lack of global direction in policies and innovations. The IUATLD, an international federation of national NGOs devoted to the care and control of TB, and the Dutch NGO Royal Netherlands Tuberculosis Association (KNCV) kept assisting countries in their efforts. Mainly thanks to the work of Karel Styblo, recognised as the "father" of modern TB control, the essential elements of the TB response were piloted starting in the late 1970s [37]. These large-scale implementation pilots were conducted in countries such as Tanzania, Malawi and Nicaragua through a pragmatic operationalisation of the principles described by the 1974 WHO Expert Committee. Styblo could demonstrate what TB control needed to succeed. This included a standardised bacteriological approach to diagnosis and treatment, a proper drug supply system, and a strict monitoring and evaluation approach that utilised quarterly reports on a few key indicators, as well as six standard definitions of treatment results in any given cohort of patients. The latter was a truly fundamental shift in assessing results as it pursued simple evidence from the field to evaluate and correct poor performance. It was indeed a key part of a new monitoring system starting at the clinics and ending at the Ministry of Health, through the district and intermediate levels. The KNCV also followed this approach when becoming active in countries such as Indonesia and Vietnam. China, which received a major World Bank loan in the early 1990s, was another model for implementation of sound practices [38].

The World Health Organization gets back to the global fight against tuberculosis

In 1989, after a decade of neglect, the WHO was made acutely aware of the unfavourable situation of TB control in the world. What prompted this change of direction towards a more proactive effort were several factors. Probably the most important was the realisation in the USA that TB had again become a public health issue. After decades of decline, a "U-shaped curve of concern" showed that, starting in 1985, TB incidence was increasing again, reaching a peak in 1992 [39]. This resulted in what the CDC estimated to be an excess of 63 800 cases from the previously observed declining trends [40]. In addition, to complicate things further, major outbreaks of MDR-TB were detected in New York and Miami, affecting high-risk individuals such as people with HIV infection and the homeless [41, 42]. These facts engendered a worldwide reaction and alarm, with the media, especially in the USA, paying finally attention to TB. The US Government reacted by reshaping a national TB control effort led by the CDC through allocation of new financial resources. Simultaneously, similar reversing trends were noted in most countries in western Europe, also resulting in renewed attention to TB [43]. In Africa, the HIV epidemic was uncontrolled, and reports started to acknowledge the strong association between the TB and HIV epidemics and the major burden imposed on poorly developed health systems and services with growing suffering and increasing numbers of deaths [44, 45]. Finally, the collapse of the former Soviet Union and of its public health infrastructure was responsible, together with the social and economic struggle of its people, for a reversal of the previous incidence decline and a steep increase in the TB burden in all new former Soviet republics [46]. All these events

https://doi.org/10.1183/2312508X.10020817

called for a revisiting of the WHO approach. New estimates of the global situation became available [47, 48]. They revealed a massive TB burden, estimated to be in the range of 9–10 million new cases and 3 million deaths per year, making TB a top priority again to be addressed internationally. In 1991, this new information was presented and discussed at the World Health Assembly (WHA) [49]. The resolution proposed new targets to be reached everywhere: ensuring a case detection rate of 70% of all sputum smear-positive cases and a cure rate of 85%. These figures were not random but were based on models predicting that reaching these levels of case detection and cure would result in a regular 8–12% annual decline in TB incidence and an even faster reduction in TB mortality [50]. The 1991 WHA and the global awareness of the TB threat were followed by an increase in resources. The small WHO TB unit embedded anonymously within a general communicable disease department became a full department in itself in 1993 called the Global TB Programme (GTB), directed by Dr Arata Kochi. Kochi and his collaborators (Mr Bumgarner, Dr Spinaci and Dr Nunn) contributed greatly to make TB a visible priority at the WHO after more than a decade of silence. Funding was made available to establish surveillance, for research and policy making, to create regional teams, and to facilitate operations in the highest-burden countries. Importantly, in the middle of a conservative environment that was not very conversant with effective technical communication, advocacy was strengthened to target politicians and stakeholders, and to make them commit resources to global and national TB responses. Thanks to assertive communication led by Mr Klaudt, an innovator in advocacy, the Director-General of the WHO, Dr Hiroshi Nakajima, was prompted to declare TB a global health emergency in 1993 [51]. That declaration, which was no more than a press release, remained in the decades to come as a key advocacy tool to convince politicians of the importance of TB. Well-illustrated WHO reports, complementing the first scientific reports, were published to inform donors and partners about the burden and the progress. Some of these media-friendly documents created a sense of the WHO becoming an advocacy rather than a technical agency. However, being simple and communicative, they were fundamental in spreading information about the poor status of TB control in the world and the response to the disease. In 1994, after assessing the results of programmes in Africa that had adopted the basic elements of the strategy to control TB developed by Dr Styblo, the WHO published the *Framework for Effective Tuberculosis Control* [52]. This was the first attempt to standardise and simplify the approach to an otherwise complex health issue. The framework was based on five elements: 1) government commitment to a nationwide programme, 2) case detection through predominantly passive case findings, 3) administration of standardised short-course chemotherapy to at least all smear-positive cases under proper case-management conditions, 4) establishment of a system of regular drug supply and 5) establishment and maintenance of a monitoring system. These elements aimed to put order into the chaotic control efforts that predominated worldwide at the time. The treatment regimens, in particular, despite scientific proof by the BMRC of the highly effective four-drug regimen, were left to decisions made by individual and often poorly trained physicians, a situation that P. Chaulet defined "anarchie thérapeutique". The end results were catastrophic with, for instance, 80 different regimens often of unknown efficacy being used by 100 prescribers in the private sector in India [53]. This situation was not just ineffective but also dangerous in terms of the potential creation of drug-resistant strains. The WHO's new framework promoted instead a proven regimen for new cases to be used universally. More complex was the issue of DR-TB, on which data were lacking in the mid-1990s and for which there was no proven regimen that could be promoted universally [54]. The framework also established rules for surveillance and monitoring of control efforts, starting with definitions of cases and treatment outcomes that were disseminated to all countries in 1995 when a global monitoring system was developed.

In the rich and advanced Europe, the situation was equally chaotic, and key efforts by the KNCV and WHO addressed surveillance, treatment outcome data and other components of TB control through annual all-Europe meetings in Wolfheze, the Netherlands [55]. They generated common standards in Europe, although adoption of new norms in the former Soviet Union countries remained mostly on paper for a long time.

The first global strategy: the DOTS era begins

In 1995, at a meeting in New York, the GTB launched the "DOTS strategy". Originally, this was an acronym standing for "directly observed treatment, short-course". The acronym was created to incorporate what US experts considered crucial in case management: directly observed therapy (DOT). DOTS soon became a brand for the comprehensive approach detailed in the 1994 framework. This prevented further misinterpretation of the strategy that was well beyond DOT [56]. In fact, the WHO had to face attacks from academicians who were questioning DOT, interpreting it not as a support approach, but as a quasi-military instrument that humiliated TB patients. In addition, the claim was that DOT was promoted in the absence of clinical trial evidence. The debate was polemic and resulted in scientific journal articles and rebuttals [57–60]. In reality, due to acronym similarities, DOT was often confused with the DOTS strategy as a whole, and was interpreted as the sole focus of a comprehensive five-element approach of which DOT was a subelement. This shows how careful one must be when branding an intervention. Fortunately, implementers in countries pursued implementation of DOTS, regardless of well-published academic polemics.

As a result, the DOTS package was adopted almost everywhere, although it was put into practice in its entirety in only a small number of countries. The World Bank assessment of the high cost-effectiveness of TB control compared with most other public health interventions, which had been published in 1993 in a World Development Report devoted to health, served as a catalyst to facilitate wide implementation in countries such China and later India [61]. However, delays were obvious, and by the second half of the 1990s, it became clear that the international targets set by the WHA in 1991 could not be reached by the year 2000 [62].

A better understanding of the global situation was made possible thanks to two projects established in the mid-1990s that have been informing the world ever since. The first was the global Drug Resistance Surveillance project, set up in 1994 [63]. Until then, the prevalence of MDR-TB was unknown. Only scattered studies were available, and they were for the most part nonrepresentative of the national situation, nor were they following correct standards in laboratory procedures and definitions. The new project allowed standardisation of procedures, making data from a country comparable with those originating in other settings. This required establishment of a supranational reference laboratory network sharing strains for quality assurance [64], the promotion of common epidemiological definitions and the conduct of sound surveys that were statistically representative of the territory under study. The first global report was published in September 1997 in Washington to attract attention from the US Government, until then poorly engaged in the global fight against TB [65]. Subsequent reports progressively added information that some regions, especially the former Soviet Union, suffered from an overwhelming epidemic of highly resistant TB [66–70].

The second project was the establishment of a global surveillance and monitoring system that prompted countries to report information in a comparable standard format. This system became necessary after a meeting of a committee of stakeholders and donors (the Coordination, Advisory and Review Group (CARG)) in September 1995 in Oslo. At that meeting, a key decision point was on the need to monitor progress towards the achievement of the 2000 global targets set by the WHA in 1991. At the time, no standardised global monitoring system existed. While clear definitions of TB cases and treatment outcomes were key components of DOTS, the only available information had come from epidemiological bulletins from better-off countries and occasional ad-hoc reports from low-income countries following reviews and monitoring missions. Given that global targets had been set in 1991, it is surprising that the need for precise data was felt only 4 years later, but at the time most programmes did not have information systems in place. The GTB was a pioneer in this endeavour. A new database and a new standard data collection form (in both paper and digital formats) were distributed to all member states with the aim of "globalising" the local recording and reporting system [71] recommended within DOTS and derived from the experience of Dr Styblo in several countries. By mid-1996, most countries had provided information to the WHO using the same definitions. For the first time, global progress towards the 2000 targets could be assessed reliably. The results showed that <20% of all cases estimated worldwide were detected in programmes that had adopted the DOTS strategy, and that the cure rate in those countries was <80% [72]. In the following years, the global TB monitoring and evaluation system evolved further with the inclusion of additional information and more sophisticated analyses, including on financial data. Better estimates of the burden of disease using impact indicators (incidence, prevalence and mortality) and new ways of measuring them, including through national TB prevalence surveys and vital registration systems, substantially improved the understanding of the TB epidemic over the following two decades.

The consideration that the targets for 2000 could not be reached prompted a new assessment of the TB situation. The WHO convened a milestone meeting of an Ad-hoc Committee on the TB Epidemic in London, in March 1998 [73]. The committee was also composed of several public health and political authorities from outside the TB community and was aimed at conceiving new approaches to accelerate adoption and implementation of DOTS. A few innovative ideas were put on the table. The first addressed the frequent drug stock-outs, a clear weakness of national programmes at the time. The response was the call for a "global TB drug facility" that would buffer stock-outs everywhere in the world, aiming to provide quality medicines at affordable price. The second was the notion of making TB a political issue, as was the case for HIV/AIDS. The third was the call for the establishment of a "coordinated partnership". However, these visionary recommendations of the Ad-hoc Committee were not all implemented immediately. The WHO underwent a major reform under the new Director-General, Dr G.H. Brundlandt, that resulted in the dismantling of the GTB and dilution of WHO efforts against TB. This was a time of confusion within and outside the WHO caused by the sudden disappearance of the global guidance function that the GTB had provided, although at times with controversy, for nearly a decade. During the first 2 years of the Brundlandt administration, while at WHO headquarters there was no longer a TB department, following the Ad-hoc Committee recommendations, partners organised themselves in the Stop TB Initiative (hosted by the WHO and composed of WHO staff and some seconded staff) to promote the TB cause. Later, in 2001, it became the Stop TB Partnership, "built to widen engagement of all forces available, from WHO to the World Bank, bilateral development assistance agencies, NGOs and the global research community" [74, 75].

A ministerial-level conference with the 22 highest-burden countries was organised in March 2000 in Amsterdam on the occasion of World TB Day: the resulting declaration committed all to increase efforts [76]. Meanwhile, the failed 2000 targets were postponed to 2005. Following the Amsterdam political declaration, little happened until the WHO got its act together again. By the end of 2000, three large working groups were created by the WHO and actively started to convene high-burden country governments and stakeholders. They reflected the top priorities: DOTS expansion, HIV-associated TB and MDR-TB. The global movement against TB began once again. The WHO finally established a new TB department under the direction of Dr J.W. Lee, who later became Director-General of the WHO. It was called the Stop TB Department and consisted of two teams: a technical team responsible for the main functions of the WHO, and a Stop TB Partnership team that placed itself in the position of a facilitator of collaboration among partners. Immediately, action accelerated. The Stop TB Partnership governance was finally agreed upon after 2 years of inconclusive debates at an historical meeting hosted by the Rockefeller Foundation in Bellagio in February 2001. The Global Drug Facility (GDF), inspired by the London Ad-hoc Committee 3 years earlier, was launched thanks to a major grant by the Canadian development agency. It delivered its first free drugs to Moldova in late 2001 [77]. The existing working groups created by the WHO and three new ones devoted to research for new diagnostics, drugs and vaccines became an integral part of the Stop TB Partnership structure. Funds were rapidly mobilised to address the major issues, and a new partnership trust fund was established, first at the World Bank and later, after long negotiations, at the WHO at a reduced overhead cost.

The Stop TB Partnership is born

The Stop TB Partnership was born in an era during which "public–private" partnerships flourished rapidly as mechanisms that could complement the WHO and government work through smooth engagement of all stakeholders. They mobilised attention and funds, and perhaps due to some loss of trust in official institutions, aimed to influence policies by sitting at the table with both WHO and its Member States. The hosting of some of them at the WHO, however, was not without major challenges, since partnerships were focused on their specific issue and aimed to enjoy special rights that normal WHO programmes could not afford. This resulted at times in a competition for both funding and visibility, besides, on a wider scale, recreating the old debate between vertical and horizontal approaches to solutions [78]. The Stop TB Partnership, in its first decade and until 2010, under the able and diplomatic leadership of Dr M. Espinal, was long considered the best model of a WHO-hosted partnership. Being embedded within the same department as the other WHO TB technical teams was key to close collaboration. The Partnership reported in principle both to the WHO through the usual hierarchical lines and to its own coordinating board, in which the WHO had a permanent seat; however, this board was fully responsible for setting strategic direction. During its first decade, the work of the Partnership was fully complementary to that of the WHO. Where the WHO could not operate, the Partnership could. This guaranteed the engagement of many partners who felt influential in determining strategies to promote the cause against TB. As the Partnership was an advocacy-driven entity, three major Partners Fora attended by ministers of health were held in the first decade of the new century: Washington in 2001, Delhi in 2004 and Rio de Janeiro in 2009. One of these events, that in Delhi, went down in history for being very fruitful, as it produced a healthy level of competition among the highest-burden countries: it appears that the Chinese Government decided to act and reach the 2005 international targets after realising at the Delhi event what India had achieved. The Stop TB Partnership kept administering the GDF and releasing, thanks to grants from Canada

https://doi.org/10.1183/2312508X.10020817

and the US Agency for International Development (USAID), free drugs to millions of patients worldwide. It also administered other major initiatives such as those addressing the case detection gap, the engagement of communities and civil society, and the collaboration with nongovernmental partners. The success of the Stop TB Partnership during the first decade of its life was not necessarily paralleled by that of some other hosted partnerships that in fact ended up competing for visibility and resources, or suffering from the administrative rules and regulations of WHO. This was eventually also the case for the Stop TB Partnership. Through a decision of its board, it formally separated from the WHO in 2014.

A changing global health environment and new challenges in the era of Millennium Development Goals, 2000–2015

With the new millennium, global health became an integral part of the UN Millennium Development Goals (MDGs): three out of eight MDGs were fully devoted to health issues and one of them (MDG-6) called for "combating HIV, malaria and other diseases", with indicators and targets on HIV, malaria and TB [79, 80]. The reasons why TB was not mentioned in the title of MDG-6 remain unclear but reflect its lack of visibility compared with the other two major epidemics. Nevertheless, the inclusion of TB indicators under MDG-6 allowed intensive advocacy efforts worldwide and helped increase the sense of urgency. Meanwhile, a few major challenges received attention and became popular among policy makers, donors and communities: the coepidemic of TB and HIV/AIDS, especially in Africa, and the emerging of DR-TB as a major public health threat.

HIV/AIDS and drug resistance as threats to tuberculosis control and care

Initially, addressing HIV-associated TB proved difficult, with little engagement of the HIV community and old concerns by the TB community. In many countries, these two epidemics were managed by separate programmes not interacting with each other [81]. The WHO proposed policy recommendations through a new framework on HIV-associated TB collaborative activities in 2004 (revised in 2012 [82]). This document outlined measures that were common to the two programmes such as the establishment of a coordinating body, joint planning and monitoring and surveillance activities, interventions that are the responsibility of HIV/AIDS health workers – including the so-called "3Is" (intensified case finding among people living with HIV infection, isoniazid preventative therapy, and infection control in healthcare facilities and congregate settings [83, 84]) – and interventions to be implemented by TB care providers such as HIV testing in all TB patients, co-trimoxazole prophylaxis and provision of antiretroviral drugs. While norms are clear, progress in implementation has not always been fast, given the resistance towards some of these measures by overconcerned programme managers on both sides.

More complex was the challenge of MDR-TB. As late as 1997, there was no knowledge of the true extent of DR-TB in the world. It was the first WHO global report published in 1997 that started revealing the reality: MDR-TB was at unprecedented high prevalence in some countries, especially those of the former Soviet Union [65, 85]. This provoked a reaction by NGOs, such as Médecins sans Frontière (MSF) and Partners in Health (PIH), that had been working on highly resistant cases in small projects. In 1998, a meeting was held at Harvard University during which "DOTS-Plus", described as a "strategy to manage MDR-TB with the use of second-line drugs within the DOTS strategy", was defined [86]. The main concern was how to provide access to expensive, rare and toxic second-line drugs while at the same time ensuring that their use was appropriate, so that additional drug resistance was not created, especially in the absence of well-funded research efforts to develop new drugs. The WHO, supported by partners, established the "Green Light Committee" (GLC) with the aim of providing access and ensuring proper use [87, 88]. For a decade, the GLC reviewed proposals from countries, technically assisted the programmes and provided access to second-line drugs through negotiations with pharmaceutical companies, so that the lowest possible price was achieved and drugs could reach those in need. The GLC operated effectively although slowly, given the lack of resources in countries to buy even heavily discounted drugs. It was the establishment of the Global Fund against AIDS, TB and Malaria, a new financial mechanism to provide support to low- and middle-income countries against these three diseases, that facilitated access through unprecedented millionaire grants [89]. Later, some activist groups criticised the GLC as an impediment to quicker access, not realising in fact that slowness depended on the countries themselves not implementing MDR-TB care and control measures, rather than on a central mechanism created to facilitate access to drugs. This polemic grew fast and resulted in a reform of the GLC mechanism in an era of new resources available compared with a decade before. Despite new funding, even in recent years the progress in enrolment of MDR-TB cases on treatment has been slow and disappointing due to the lack of universal DST and insufficient commitment by many governments to adopt new diagnostics and provide proper MDR-TB care. This suggests that the GLC mechanism was not the reason for the slow response, which depended instead on systematic issues and political neglect of the problem in most of the high-burden countries [90].

System challenges and opportunities

Another challenge in an era where health rapidly became an issue transcending governmental and public health institutions and expanding towards other nongovernmental actors was that of the private for-profit sector [91]. In some large Asian countries, such as India and Indonesia, and in many other settings, the role of nonstate practitioners grew in importance and became a challenge and an opportunity at the same time. Solutions were complex and ranged from complete exclusion *via* regulations of private practitioners to proactive attempts to engage them. Many pilot projects have been conducted on how to involve nonstate practitioners in programme activities, although replicable and large-scale models have rarely been successful. The results are that, in some high-burden countries where privately provided care is rampant, standards may not be followed, reporting is not done and risks of creation of drug resistance exist. However, some successful models of engagement of the for-profit practitioners were piloted and are in need of scaling up through commitment by national programmes [92].

The engagement of affected communities for both public mobilisation and care contribution was an additional issue to be faced. During the 1990s, the HIV/AIDS epidemic had shown how civil society awareness and strong advocacy were fundamental in the response of governments and stakeholders. It also showed that communities could be fully engaged and self-activated to become not only advocates *vis-à-vis* their own politicians but also to contribute to home- and community-based care in settings that governmental facilities could not reach. Based on the HIV/AIDS model, earlier operational research conducted by the WHO had already shown in the late 1990s that TB care too could benefit from deeper engagement of communities [93, 94]. However, pilot studies in Africa and elsewhere, due to a lack of interest by programmes, did not reach the scale necessary to

https://doi.org/10.1183/2312508X.10020817

become an integral part of the response. A new attempt was therefore made to promote activism in the TB community, mainly through engagement of HIV activists, especially in the African continent. There were mixed results. Some successful engagement in Africa was due to community and civil society organisations able to address the needs of local communities. At the same time, the perception that what was done for HIV/AIDS could easily be replicated in TB proved wrong. In fact, the HIV/AIDS epidemic enjoyed unprecedented "exceptionalism" at all levels and attracted political attention by heads of state and celebrities [95]. In high-income countries, this was the result of an epidemic also affecting well-resourced segments of population, such as the gay community in San Francisco and New York. In some low-income countries, it was the result of major awareness campaigns led by NGOs and local celebrities that managed to activate governments to address AIDS in their heavily affected communities [96]. It was a revolution in health and a model of how far one can go when people take their health as a priority to be addressed. It was the demonstration that the Alma-Ata principles of community participation and self-determination may work under certain circumstances. It was not the same for TB. First, in all settings, TB affects the poorest, the voiceless and marginalised people; there is stigma and discrimination that persist; and TB, after all, is curable and not for life. In those early years, activism in TB frequently failed to become sustainable and was not necessarily seen as an opportunity to make the case and obtain support. The result at the international level was sterile polemics against international actors, rather than a focused and outcome-oriented effort in countries. In the attempt to support local communities, the Stop TB Partnership in the mid-2000s established a small grant mechanism for local organisations willing to embark on activities in both the care and social mobilisation spheres. However, sustainability remained an issue, partly alleviated through new funding to finance local projects by international donors. Later, the WHO also embarked on a project to engage existing African NGOs that are operating in fields such as maternal and child health or general primary care. The results were promising and showed that deeply rooted NGOs could contribute effectively to TB care [97].

The era of the MDGs raised other challenges for those engaged in TB control at the policy level. The "horizontal/vertical pendulum" was debated again. After the post-Alma-Ata emphasis on primary care and the consequent dismantling or weakening of national TB programmes, interpreted as examples of verticalism, the re-emergence of TB as a major health issue in the early 1990s eventually resurrected the old debate. At the WHO, the Nakajima administration prioritised TB and a strong programme was established. Under Brundlandt's administration, the programme was dismantled, TB experts were distributed in "function-oriented" departments, and external partners organised themselves into the Stop TB Partnership, hosted at the WHO, to sustain the global fight against TB, trying to buffer the lack of WHO leadership. When, by early 2001, the WHO administration felt threatened by the growing complaints of partners and the call to focus attention on TB control, a specific programme was re-established. Meanwhile, work began to create new, powerful financial mechanisms such as the Global Fund and Unitaid. Unprecedented large amounts of funds for TB control became soon available in the poorest settings. This situation resulted in more focus by the global health community on TB along with HIV/AIDS and malaria. At the same time, it generated the sense that these three diseases persisted in a vertical approach, rather than favouring strengthening of health systems on a more "horizontal" axis [98]. The ideological debate came to the point of interpreting well-funded programmes as distortion to health systems. While there was some truth in this sentiment, global experts raised the criticism that verticality in health was no longer an option. Harsh debates ensued, generating a strong dualism between system development and focused disease-oriented approaches. Instead, it would have been more constructive to understand that "diagonal" approaches can help both general system strengthening and disease control. It was a matter of finding the right balance under the leadership of ministries of health in all countries. This debate is not yet fully resolved and is likely to continue in the future. What international and national policy decision makers often fail to realise is that any premature attempt to dismantle TB programmes when systems and services are not yet fully operational may result in additional deaths. Even in some well-resourced countries, the re-establishment of focused programmes was necessary, regardless of the wide availability of clinical services, as proven by the response of the USA to the MDR-TB threat in the 1990s [99].

The lack of new tools becomes a recognised issue

Finally, a major issue as we entered the MDG era was the lack of new tools to fight TB more effectively. TB care and control were still based mainly on diagnostics such as sputum smear microscopy and solid media cultures, regimens with drugs developed half a century before and a weak 80-year-old vaccine. Technology, apart from liquid cultures, did not evolve over the previous several decades. Research was badly underfunded, including in rich, high-income countries. A resurrection of research efforts against TB was necessary. Thanks to efforts by agencies such as the Rockefeller Foundation and new philanthropic foundations, such as the Bill & Melinda Gates Foundation (BMGF), TB research received a new impulse [100]. Investments grew rapidly in the decade after 2000. The US National Institutes of Health (NIH) started investing more in TB research. A few product-development partnerships were created to facilitate prioritisation and develop links with the industry: the TB Alliance (TBA) in New York for new TB drugs and the Foundation for Innovative New Diagnostics (FIND) in Geneva. Vaccine development enjoyed important investments: the nonprofit organisation Aeras received hundreds of millions of US$ from the BMGF, while the European Commission funded a new TB Vaccine Initiative (TBVI). As a result of these efforts and increased awareness, new rapid diagnostics such as the Xpert MTB/RIF nucleic acid amplification test (Cepheid, Sunnyvale, CA, USA) and line probe assays became available. Two new drugs active against MDR-TB were developed by the pharmaceutical industry: bedaquiline, approved in 2012, and delamanid, approved in 2013. The TBA, after developing pretomanid, started testing it as part of promising novel regimens including new or repurposed drugs. In the vaccine field, a new vaccine, MVA25A, was tested but failed to demonstrate benefits, showing how complex the development of a new vaccine against *M. tuberculosis* is when the full understanding of the immunopathogenesis of the disease is not complete. A dozen candidates, however, are under testing as a result of investments [101].

The new WHO Stop TB Strategy, 2006–2015

All of the challenges that emerged in the first few years of the MDG era were taken into consideration at the time of formulating a new global strategy, which was necessary when the 2001 international targets came to their final deadline in 2005. By then, the case detection rate was about 50%, 20% short of the target, and the treatment success was 84%, a near miss. A new approach was necessary to rapidly improve case detection. Together with the challenges highlighted above, finding cases soon became the main target to be pursued when the new strategy was formulated and branded as the WHO Stop TB Strategy, in line with the need to revert the increasing incidence trend observed during the previous years and as part of the MDG targets [102]. The new WHO Stop TB Strategy was backed by the second Global Plan to Stop TB 2006–2015 [103, 104]. This budgeted plan succeeded the previous one, which was developed mainly on the request of US investors in 2000. The new one required a broader exercise of estimation and projection, with engagement of many stakeholders.

The WHO Stop TB Strategy, summarised in table 1, reflects in its six elements the agreed priorities. Clearly, this approach acknowledged that the epidemic needed more than the essential DOTS elements to achieve TB control. It was more complex, as it addressed system issues well beyond what national programme managers had been trained to do until then. There was some apprehension about the feasibility of implementing a new, broader strategy that required adoption of different, innovative interventions. For instance, engaging the nonstate sector was a challenge in most countries, empowering affected communities was difficult in the absence of new resources, and working within the context of health system reforms and strengthening was not easy, especially in countries that ideologically kept looking at TB programmes as a different, almost parallel system instead of taking a more visionary direction and seriously thinking how categorical disease-control programmes could be constructively supported within general systems and services. There were some good examples of programmes that used primary services to deliver care while maintaining the desirable level of managerial specificity that is necessary for complex public health problems.

The global efforts against TB progressed intensively during the MDG era. The target of reverting the epidemic, called by some an "unambitious" target, was reached in the early to mid-2000s, due to a combination of investments in TB control and achievements in reducing the incidence of the HIV/AIDS epidemic in Africa, which was the main factor responsible for the previous rapidly increasing TB incidence worldwide. Starting in the mid-2000s, the appearance of the Global Fund on the international scene was a crucial determinant of the highly increased financing for TB control in most low- and middle-income countries. Large amounts of funds arriving in poor countries allowed implementation of new interventions promoted by the WHO Stop TB Strategy. At the same time, two important commissions established by the WHO published their reports. In 2001, the Commission of Macroeconomics and Health emphasised that "ill health undermines economic development and efforts to reduce poverty. Investments in health are essential for economic growth and should be a key component of national development strategies. The greatest achievements can be made by focusing on the health of the poor and on the least developed countries." It added that "a few diseases and conditions account for most of the avoidable deaths in low- and middle-income countries. Efforts to scale up access to existing interventions against infectious diseases, to address reproductive and child health, and to confront malnutrition will prevent millions of deaths in poor countries and considerably improve health" [107]. Among infectious diseases, TB was prominent in a report that backed the MDG framework as a whole and called for increased investments to accelerate the development of nations.

In 2008, the Commission on Social Determinants of Health published another landmark report, which, building on the concepts of social justice and equity, pursued universal access to health [108]. Health was seen as a result of holistic approaches and the impact of multiple sectors on improving health. Opposing poverty and inequalities was recognised as a new means to achieve better health for the world. Three main recommendations emerged from the report: first, improve the conditions of daily life, *i.e.* the circumstances in which people are born, grow, live, work and age; second, tackle the inequitable distribution of power, money and resources, and address the structural drivers of inequities in daily life,

Table 1. The WHO Stop TB Strategy (2006–2015) at a glance

Vision	A TB-free world
Goal	To dramatically reduce the global burden of TB by 2015 in line with the MDGs and the Stop TB Partnership targets
Objectives	To achieve universal access to quality diagnosis and patient-centred treatment
	To reduce the human suffering and socioeconomic burden associated with TB
	To protect vulnerable populations from TB, HIV-associated TB and DR-TB
	To support development of new tools and enable their timely and effective use
Targets	MDG 6, Target 8: halt and begin to reverse the incidence of TB by 2015
Targets endorsed by the Stop TB Partnership	2005: detect at least 70% of infectious TB cases and cure at least 85% of them
	2015: reduce prevalence of and deaths due to TB by 50%
	2050: eliminate TB as a public health problem
Components	1) Pursue quality DOTS expansion and enhancement
	Political commitment with increased and sustained financing
	Case detection through quality-assured bacteriology
	Standardised treatment, with supervision and patient support
	Effective drug supply and management system
	Monitoring and evaluation system, and impact measurement
	2) Address HIV-associated TB, MDR-TB and other challenges
	HIV-associated TB collaborative activities
	Prevention and control of MDR-TB
	Addressing prisoners, refugees, other risk groups and special situations
	3) Contribute to health system strengthening
	Active participation in efforts to improve system-wide policy, human resources, financing, management, service delivery and information systems
	Sharing innovations that strengthen systems, including the WHO Practical Approach to Lung Health
	Adapting innovations from other fields
	4) Engage all care providers
	Public–public and public–private mix approaches
	WHO International Standards for TB Care
	5) Empower people with TB and communities
	Advocacy, communication and social mobilisation
	Community participation in TB care
	6) Enable and promote research
	Programme-based operational research
	Research to develop new diagnostics, drugs and vaccines

Reproduced and modified from [105] and [106] with permission.

https://doi.org/10.1183/2312508X.10020817

globally, nationally and locally; third, measure the problem, evaluate action, expand the knowledge base, develop a workforce that is trained in the social determinants of health and raise public awareness about the social determinants of health. This report prompted a deeper assessment of the importance of economic and social determinants of TB, probably the best model of a disease of poverty, with a view to addressing them to reach elimination. Through this assessment, which was among the side products of the Commission, a new vision, eventually inspiring the future WHO End TB Strategy 2016–2035, began to look at UHC and social protection as essential in strategic approaches towards controlling TB [109, 110].

Thanks to advances in financing, commitment and policies, the era of the MDGs was characterised by progress in implementation and research, although this was slow. On the implementation side, new investments resulted in a regular increase in case notifications, which reached 6.4 million in 2017, and a better understanding of the TB epidemic overall thanks to the availability of funds to conduct prevalence surveys and additional measurement methods and capacity. It also resulted in better treatment success (~85% among new cases), wider implementation of HIV-associated TB collaborative interventions, and ultimately a continuous annual decline in both TB incidence (1.5–2%) and mortality (3%) [2].

However, progress in addressing MDR-TB and other drug-resistant forms of TB remained disappointing, largely due to the lack of universal DST and of second-line drugs and regimens. As of today, less than one-quarter of all estimated MDR-TB and RR-TB cases are detected, reported and treated appropriately [2]. The Ministerial Conference called by the WHO and the Chinese Government in Beijing in 2009, influential meetings such as the Pacific Health Summit in Seattle in 2009, resolutions at the WHA, and innumerable scientific articles and advocacy events have not succeeded in raising sufficient commitment and resources to tackle MDR-TB effectively. Likewise, the one-third general case detection gap persisted.

Between 2005 and 2009, TB research investments almost doubled, reaching figures of US$600–700 million per year. However, the curve flattened after 2009, with just a small increase in 2017 to over US$700 million per year [111]. Half of this funding has come from two agencies: the US NIH and the BMGF. The concrete outcomes of the investments have been relatively important but small in number. Probably the most transformational new tool is the rapid molecular diagnostic Xpert MTB/RIF, which allows, in 2 h, the detection of TB and rifampicin resistance and, as a result, immediate decisions on treatment options [112]. Other new rapid diagnostics, such as line probe assays, have also been introduced. Two new drugs, bedaquiline and delamanid, have been developed and were approved by stringent regulatory authorities in 2012 and 2013, respectively, after phase IIB clinical trials, given the potential to save lives [113, 114]. Promising regimens, containing a new drug (pretomanid), bedaquiline, and a repurposed drug (linezolid) or the four drugs pretomanid, bedaquiline, moxifloxacin and pyrazinamide are in advanced phases of clinical trials conducted by TBA [115, 116]. Some 12 vaccine candidates have entered the pipeline. Overall, TB research was resurrected in the MDG era but revolutionary new tools are not yet on the horizon. The amount of investment in TB research today is still a small fraction of what it should be for the top infectious disease killer worldwide. The desired amount of US$2 billion, as proposed in the Global Plan to Stop TB 2016–2020, is far from being achieved, but even if it were, it would be insufficient if one looks at the rapid results obtained in the case of other diseases that have benefitted from hugely larger sums.

In conclusion, the MDG era allowed progress on many fronts: investments (both external and domestic), degree of implementation of new strategies, engagement of new actors, establishment of new financial mechanisms, political visibility, some new tools out of the research pipelines, and, above all, some measurable impact on the burden with the MDG-6 target of reverting the epidemic achieved and a slow but regular decline in incidence and mortality. Nevertheless, in 2018, TB is the top infectious killer with an annual 1.6 million deaths, including 300 000 among people with HIV infection, more than 10 million new cases every year, an insufficiently addressed problem of drug resistance, and gaps in funding for both implementation and research [2].

The era of sustainable development goals, 2016–2030, and the WHO End TB Strategy

Facing these staggering figures and recognising the urgency of intensifying efforts, the WHA in May 2014 approved a new strategy for the post-2015 SDGs era. This new era, building on concepts of sustainable development, universality of challenges and multisectoriality differs substantially from the previous global development framework, and emphasises equity and, in addressing health, UHC and social protection (figure 1). This meant the need to rethink the global strategy against TB, taking full advantage of the new concepts within the new UN SDG framework [117]. The establishment of an SDG devoted to health (SDG-3) where UHC becomes a means to "ensure healthy lives and promote well-being for all at all ages" is a significant step forward that can allow TB control and care to progress in a faster way. This sentiment guided the formulation of a new strategy, which began in 2012 following the request by WHO member states during the WHA to develop an ambitious approach and a set of impact-focused international targets. During 2 years of intensive consultations with country governments, NGOs and civil society, the GTB/WHO produced a document outlining a new strategy (branded the WHO End TB Strategy, to conform with the language of SDG-3 calling to "end the epidemics of…TB") that was discussed and endorsed through a formal resolution by the 67th WHA on May 21, 2014 [118]. The document described three pillars and four basic principles underpinning the strategy, as well as highly ambitious, aspirational targets with 5-year milestones. The 2030 milestone became the targets to be reached during the SDG era ending in 2030: a 90% reduction in TB deaths and 80% reduction in TB incidence compared with 2015, and zero catastrophic costs to TB-affected people and families. Table 2 illustrates in detail all components of the WHO End TB Strategy. The discussion about the targets was intense, given the resolute position by the civil society during a public

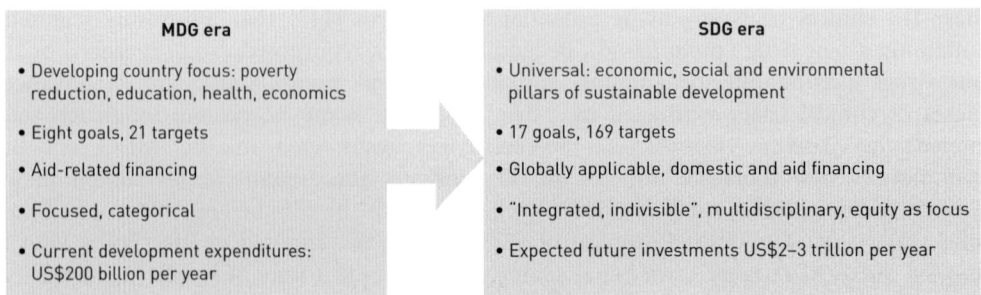

MDG era	SDG era
• Developing country focus: poverty reduction, education, health, economics	• Universal: economic, social and environmental pillars of sustainable development
• Eight goals, 21 targets	• 17 goals, 169 targets
• Aid-related financing	• Globally applicable, domestic and aid financing
• Focused, categorical	• "Integrated, indivisible", multidisciplinary, equity as focus
• Current development expenditures: US$200 billion per year	• Expected future investments US$2–3 trillion per year

Figure 1. Conceptual differences between the Millennium Development Goals (MDG) and SDG eras.

https://doi.org/10.1183/2312508X.10020817

Table 2. The WHO End TB Strategy at a glance, with targets for 2030 (SDG-3) and 2035

Vision	A world free of TB: zero deaths, disease and suffering due to TB
Goal	End the global TB epidemic
SDG targets for 2030	90% reduction in TB deaths (compared with 2015)
	80% reduction in TB incidence rate
	No affected families facing catastrophic costs due to TB
Targets for 2035	95% reduction in TB deaths (compared with 2015)
	90% reduction in TB incidence rate (less than 10 TB cases per 100 000 population)
	No affected families facing catastrophic costs due to TB
Principles	1) Government stewardship and accountability, with monitoring and evaluation
	2) Strong coalition with civil society organisations and communities
	3) Protection and promotion of human rights, ethics and equity
	4) Adaptation of the strategy and targets at country level, with global collaboration
Pillars and components	1) Integrated, patient-centred care and prevention
	• Early diagnosis of TB including universal DST, and systematic screening of contacts and high-risk groups
	• Treatment of all people with TB including DR-TB and patient support
	• Collaborative HIV-associated TB activities, and management of comorbidities
	• Preventative treatment of persons at high risk, and vaccination against TB
	2) Bold policies and supportive systems
	• Political commitment with adequate resources for TB care and prevention
	• Engagement of communities, civil society organisations, and public and private care providers
	• Universal health coverage policy, and regulatory frameworks for case notification, vital registration, quality and rational use of medicines, and infection control
	• Social protection, poverty alleviation and actions on other determinants of TB
	3) Intensified research and innovation
	• Discovery, development and rapid uptake of new tools, interventions and strategies
	• Research to optimise implementation and impact, and promote innovations

Reproduced and modified from [119] with permission.

discussion in Kuala Lumpur in November 2012. This prompted the WHO to convene a meeting to specifically revisit the formulation of targets [120]. Contrary to expectations, no government delegates at the WHA opposed the ambitions expressed in the targets by the civil society. In addition, the slogan of "Zero deaths, disease and suffering due to TB", proposed by activists and inspired by the Joint United Nations Programme on HIV/AIDS (UNAIDS) advocacy against HIV/AIDS, was accepted as an expression of the vision endorsed by the WHA. The way to face the TB problem evolved in the same direction as the decade-long political advocacy against HIV/AIDS and its powerful slogans and communication approaches. Concerning the four basic principles, they reiterate in clear language the prominence of governments in providing stewardship and being responsible and accountable; the importance of engaging with civil society; the protection of human rights, ethics and equity; and the need to adapt the strategy at the country level. These principles are all well aligned with the sustainable development framework.

The three pillars introduce several innovations in policies. The emphasis in the pillar devoted to care is that of placing the patient at the centre, which means considering the needs of individuals affected by TB in their globality, and adapting the care model to the circumstances surrounding each person. This translates into universal DST, screening of all potential contacts to offer chemoprophylaxis, equal consideration for all types of TB and management of comorbidities. The pillar devoted to general health policies emphasises the need for sound and supportive systems to face TB. There must be political commitment (already recognised as key since the time of DOTS) backed by adequate financing, facilitation of engagement of the nonstate sector, broad health policies on information systems, rational use of medicines, infection control measures in health facilities and, crucially, UHC and social protection mechanisms. Finally, the third pillar on research strongly underlines the need for new tools and their rapid introduction in the field. This also means interpreting research as a continuum from basic to development and operational research to influence choices and directions, as well as the need by all countries to contribute with their own institutions in the piloting and implementation phase.

These innovative elements comprising the WHO End TB Strategy clearly call for a multisectorial response to TB that goes beyond traditional areas of action and responsibilities of the national TB programme and Ministry of Health. In particular, broad policies to ensure access by all and financial protection through poverty alleviation mechanisms are today an essential component of a sound and comprehensive response to TB. With respect to the universality of the SDG framework, the WHO End TB Strategy, however, is not limited to high-burden countries but must be adapted to the needs of the low-burden countries that are aiming to eliminating TB. For this reason, the WHO in partnership with the European Respiratory Society (ERS), low-incidence country representatives and other agencies worked to adapt the new strategy to low-incidence countries, publishing a framework document [121]. The document highlights eight main priorities to be addressed, emphasising the major challenges faced by high-income countries, including the focus on high-risk groups and migrants, the importance of active screening and treatment of LTBI, and the relevance of research and innovations (figure 2).

The largest ever advocacy movement to "end tuberculosis"

The principles expressed in the WHO End TB Strategy were the inspiration for two historical events in the 2017–2018 biennium [4]: the "First WHO Global Ministerial Conference on Ending TB in the Sustainable Development Era: a Multisectoral Response", co-organised by the WHO and the Ministry of Health of the Russian Federation in Moscow, Russia, on December 16–17, 2017; and the High-Level Meeting on ending TB at the UN General Assembly in September 2018. The Moscow conference aimed to accelerate

https://doi.org/10.1183/2312508X.10020817

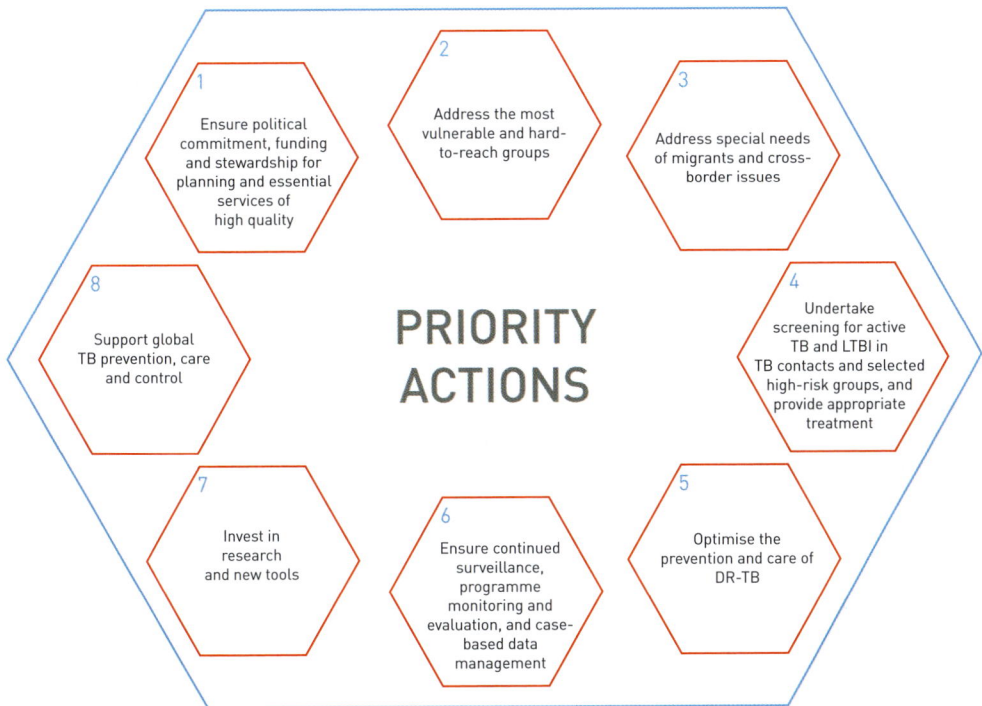

PRIORITY ACTIONS

1 Ensure political commitment, funding and stewardship for planning and essential services of high quality

2 Address the most vulnerable and hard-to-reach groups

3 Address special needs of migrants and cross-border issues

4 Undertake screening for active TB and LTBI in TB contacts and selected high-risk groups, and provide appropriate treatment

5 Optimise the prevention and care of DR-TB

6 Ensure continued surveillance, programme monitoring and evaluation, and case-based data management

7 Invest in research and new tools

8 Support global TB prevention, care and control

Figure 2. Action framework for TB elimination in low-incidence countries. Reproduced and modified from [122] with permission.

implementation of the WHO End TB Strategy and address gaps in access to care. Its goal was to reach the End TB targets set by the WHA and UN SDGs through national and global commitments towards clear deliverables and accountability, eventually to be endorsed at the UN General Assembly High-Level Meeting on TB in 2018. The event, opened by the Russian President and with delegations from 125 WHO Member States and more than 70 ministers (mainly of health but also from other sectors) concluded that there were three top priorities to accelerate the reduction of incidence and mortality proposed by the WHA in 2014. They were described in the Moscow Declaration document: 1) advancing the TB response within the SDG agenda, 2) ensuring sufficient and sustainable financing and 3) pursuing science, research and innovation. A fourth strong recommendation was that of developing a Multisectoral Accountability Framework [123].

Under the recommendation of advancing the TB response, ministers committed to scale up interventions for diagnosis, treatment and care, and to work towards the goal of UHC through all providers to achieve ambitious targets of 90% diagnostic coverage and 90% cure. Rapid molecular diagnostics, the WHO standards of care and the introduction of digital health innovations were specifically mentioned as means to achieve the new targets. The ministers also committed to engage civil society and focus on high-risk groups and populations in vulnerable situations, including indigenous people, migrants and refugees, prisoners and people living with HIV/AIDS. National emergency responses were identified as an option to accelerate care of MDR-TB patients, and emphasis was placed on the association between TB and HIV and other comorbidities. Patient-centred care was reiterated as a primary goal jointly with abolition of discrimination and stigma. The second recommendation of ensuring sufficient and sustainable financing was underpinned by the commitment to work with heads of state and other ministries and sectors "to mobilize the domestic financing needed for health systems strengthening with the ultimate goal of reaching universal health coverage, in keeping with national legislative frameworks, and with the Addis Ababa Action Agenda of the Third International Conference on Financing for Development" [123]. Among the commitments made by ministers was the development of well-funded plans inclusive of measures to address catastrophic costs to patients such as social protection mechanisms. The third recommendation, to pursue science, research and innovation, proposed expansion of multidisciplinary TB research and innovation, and the establishment of national TB research networks cooperating internationally towards the development of transformational new tools. One request to the WHO was to work on a new strategic and prioritised global research agenda.

However, apart from these outcomes, which addressed the main policy issues and needs, the recommendation to develop a Multisectoral Accountability Framework (MAF) was the most important political decision. It created intense debate in the preparation of the conference declaration, as some Member States had strong ideas about the MAF, who should develop it and what it should contain. The WHO was eventually asked to work on it and ensure that a framework monitoring the commitments made and allowing measures to accelerate implementation of the recommended interventions would be ready by the time of the next political event, the 2018 UN General Assembly High-level Meeting on Ending TB. Some initial suggestions were made on the aims of the MAF that would be multisectoral in nature, thus implying reporting beyond the WHA if other sectors were equally accountable for ending TB. The Moscow Declaration also proposed that ministries of health in partnership with civil society convene national inter-ministerial commissions on TB with the direct engagement of the Heads of State. The signatory ministers ultimately committed "to act immediately on this Declaration in coordination with the WHO, and to engage with leaders and all relevant sectors of Government, UN agencies, bilateral and multilateral funding agencies and donors, academia, research organisations, scientific community, civil society and the private sector to prepare for and follow-up on the UN General Assembly High-Level Meeting on Tuberculosis in 2018 in New York" [123].

The future towards ending tuberculosis: finally, a high-level political issue

The Moscow event promoted wide attention towards TB. It coincided with the beginning of a new administration at the WHO and at the Global Fund against AIDS, TB and Malaria, the most important international financial mechanism supporting the global fight against TB. This increased the visibility of the TB problem, after decades of fairly lukewarm commitment by virtually all multilateral agencies, and obliged the new administration of the WHO to take a stand, especially in view of the first-ever UN General Assembly High-level Meeting on Tuberculosis held in September 2018 in New York [124]. Despite perplexities by some UN Member States that are not keen to hold health-related discussions at the UN General Assembly, if one believes that the ultimate solutions to TB and other poverty-related health conditions are multisectoral, it is inevitable to rely on international mechanisms going beyond ministries of health and their assemblies.

After Moscow, the WHO Secretariat prepared an MAF proposal to be discussed at the Executive Board of the WHO in January 2018 and at the WHA in May 2018 [125]. This document described accountability as being responsible for commitments made or actions

https://doi.org/10.1183/2312508X.10020817

taken at national or international and regional levels, and proposed that the SDG-3 targets relevant to TB, the WHO End TB Strategy targets, the implementation of the three pillars of the new strategy and its four principles, and the political declarations made at the UN General Assembly on HIV in 2016 and on TB in 2018 be the key indicators for the MAF. The document also proposed examples of actions: preparation of plans, financial commitments and existence of norms, as well as monitoring and review systems. In the end, what will count is a clear description: of who is accountable, on what actions one is accountable for, of whom one responds to in accountability terms, of how accountability is monitored and of which measures are in place for lack of compliance. Accountability should first be with governments, as they are responsible for public health issues. However, currently there are many actors with powerful influential means in global health and TB response. Therefore, a comprehensive framework must include the UN family of agencies, donors, philanthropic foundations, partnerships, NGOs, academic institutions, research institutions and civil society at large. Facing a complex multifactorial issue such as TB requires that all work in collaboration and towards the same aims. While accountability is clear for governmental entities and UN agencies, it is much less so for the others who do not respond to citizens. The key is in identification of means to ensure that all are part of the framework and feel responsible to act in a responsible manner. Actions to be monitored should clearly be placed in the context of established international and national targets. In addition, given the multisectoral nature of the TB response, beyond the operational indicators developed over the years specifically for TB, additional indicators related to SDG-3 health targets as well as those in SDGs other than SDG-3 need to be monitored at national and global levels. The WHO has identified seven SDG-3 indicators relevant to TB and seven other indicators within SDG-1, -7, -8, -10 and -11 that are crucial for TB elimination [2]. Therefore, a new monitoring and evaluation system needs to be put in place in all countries that allows a comprehensive multisectoral assessment. More difficult to establish is to whom one is accountable for actions undertaken or neglected. While the WHA is the logical place to report and evaluate progress or lack thereof, the awareness that the response to TB, and to most other complex health issues, goes beyond ministries of health makes it unquestionable that one needs to target a higher level of decision-making to seek solutions and ensure success. Therefore, the most appropriate setting for monitoring of the TB response needs to be the UN General Assembly, which could periodically review the progress made by governments and nonstate actors alike. This will require strong advocacy and resisting the push-back by some Member States who believe that all health issues should be handled at the WHA, ignoring the fact that solutions are more often not technical but political. TB is a good example, given its multisectoral nature, its links with development in general, its dependence on better living and nutritional conditions, and its need for innovation and research. Only through an expanded approach that engages decision makers responsible for financing and for broad policies with social and economic implications will TB be faced effectively.

References

1. WHO. World Health Statistics 2018: Monitoring Health for the SDGs. Geneva, WHO, 2018. www.who.int/gho/publications/world_health_statistics/2018/en/
2. WHO. Global Tuberculosis Report 2018. Geneva, WHO, 2018. www.who.int/tb/publications/global_report/en/
3. Floyd K, Glaziou P, Zumla A, et al. The global tuberculosis epidemic and progress in care, prevention and research: an overview in year 3 of the End TB era. Lancet Respir Med 2018; 6: 299–314.
4. Raviglione M, Uplekar M, Weil D, et al. Tuberculosis makes it onto the international political agenda for health…finally. Lancet Glob Health 2017; 6: e20–e21.

5. WHO. Engaging all care providers in TB control: Guidance on Implementing Public–Private Mix Approaches. Geneva, WHO, 2006. www.who.int/tb/publications/who_htm_tb_2006_360/en/

6. Daley CL, Caminero JA. Management of multidrug resistant tuberculosis. *Semin Respir Crit Care Med* 2013; 34: 44–59.

7. Harries AD, Zachariah R, Lawn SD. Providing HIV care for co-infected tuberculosis patients: a perspective from sub-Saharan Africa. *Int J Tuberc Lung Dis* 2009; 13: 6–16.

8. Creswell J, Raviglione M, Ottmani S, *et al.* Tuberculosis and non-communicable diseases: neglected links and missed opportunities. *Eur Respir J* 2011; 37: 1269–1282.

9. Lönnroth K, Castro GK, Chakaya JM, *et al.* Tuberculosis control and elimination 2010–50: cure, care, and social development. *Lancet* 2010; 375: 1814–1829.

10. Lönnroth K, Raviglione M. Global epidemiology of tuberculosis: prospects for control. *Semin Respir Crit Care Med* 2008; 29: 481–491.

11. Koch R. Die Atiologie der Tuberkulose. [The aetiology of tuberculosis.] *Berl Klin Wochenschr* 1882; 19: 221–230.

12. Bulloch W. The History of Bacteriology. New York, Oxford University Press, 1938.

13. Mangtani P, Abubakar I Ariti C, *et al.* Protection by BCG vaccine against tuberculosis: a systematic review of randomized controlled trials. *Clin Infect Dis* 2014; 58: 470–480.

14. Trunz BB, Fine P, Dye C. Effect of BCG vaccination on childhood tuberculous meningitis and miliary tuberculosis worldwide: a meta-analysis and assessment of cost-effectiveness. *Lancet* 2006; 367: 1173–1180.

15. Roy A, Eisenhut M, Harris RJ, *et al.* Effect of BCG vaccination against *Mycobacterium tuberculosis* infection in children: systematic review and meta-analysis. *BMJ* 2014; 349: g4643.

16. WHO. BCG vaccines: WHO position paper – February 2018. *Wkly Epidemiol Rec* 2018; 93: 73–96.

17. Dubos R, Dubos J. The White Plague: Tuberculosis, Man, and Society. New Brunswick/London, Rutgers University Press, 1987.

18. Styblo K. Epidemiology of Tuberculosis. The Hague, Royal Netherlands Tuberculosis Association (KNCV), 1991.

19. Rutledge CJA, Crouch JB. The ultimate results in 1694 cases of tuberculosis treated at the Modern Woodmen of America Sanatorium. *Am Rev Tuberc* 1919; 2: 755–763.

20. Springett VH. Ten-year results during the introduction of chemotherapy for tuberculosis. *Tubercle* 1971; 52: 73–87.

21. Schatz A, Bugie E, Waksman S. Streptomycin, a substance exhibiting antibiotic activity against Gran-positive and Gran-negative bacteria. *Proc Soc Exp Biol Med* 1944; 55: 66–69.

22. Schatz A, Waksman SA. Effects of streptomycin and other antibiotic substances upon *Mycobacterium tuberculosis* and related organisms. *Proc Soc Expt Biol Med* 1944; 57: 244–248.

23. Lehmann J. Para-aminosalicylic acid in the treatment of tuberculosis. *Lancet* 1946; 1: 15–16.

24. Crofton J, Mitchison DA. Streptomycin resistance in pulmonary tuberculosis. *Br Med J* 1948; 2: 1009–1015.

25. Sensi P. History of the development of rifampin. *Rev Infect Dis* 1983; 5: Suppl. 3, S402–S406.

26. Fox W, Ellard GA, Mitchison DA. Studies on the treatment of tuberculosis undertaken by the British Medical Research Council Tuberculosis Units, 1946–1986, with relevant subsequent publications. *Int J Tuberc Lung Dis* 1999; 10: Suppl. 2, S231–S279.

27. Canetti G. The eradication of tuberculosis: theoretical problems and practical solutions. *Tubercle* 1962; 43: 301–321.

28. Raviglione MC, Pio A. Evolution of WHO policies for tuberculosis control, 1948–2001. *Lancet* 2002; 359: 775–780.

29. Mahler H. The tuberculosis programme in the developing countries. *Bull Int Union Tuberc* 1966; 37: 77–82.

30. Fox W. The problem of self-administration of drugs, with particular reference to pulmonary tuberculosis. *Tubercle* 1958; 39: 269–274.

31. Fox W. Self-administration of medicaments: a review of published work and a study of the problem. *Bull Int Union Tuberc* 1962; 32: 307–331.

32. Banerji D. Tuberculosis: a problem of social planning in developing countries. *Med Care* 1965; 3: 151–161.

33. WHO. WHO Expert Committee on Tuberculosis: Eighth Report. WHO Technical Report Series No. 290. Geneva, WHO, 1964. www.who.int/iris/handle/10665/40606

34. WHO. Expert Committee on Tuberculosis: Ninth report. WHO Technical Reports Series No. 552. Geneva, WHO, 1974. www.who.int/iris/handle/10665/41095

35. WHO. Alma-Ata 1978. Primary Health Care. Geneva, WHO, 1978. Health for All Series No. 1. www.unicef.org/about/history/files/Alma_Ata_conference_1978_report.pdf

36. Uplekar M, Raviglione MC. The "vertical–horizontal" debates: time for the pendulum to rest (in peace)? *Bull World Health Organ* 2007; 85: 413–414.

37. Styblo K. Overview and epidemiological assessment of the current global tuberculosis situation with an emphasis on control in developing countries. *Rev Infect Dis* 1989; 11: Suppl. 2, S339–S346.

38. Wang LD, Liu JJ, Chin DP. Progress in tuberculosis control and the evolving public-health system in China. *Lancet* 2007; 369: 691–696.

39. Reichman LB. The U-shaped curve of concern. *Am Rev Respir Dis* 1991; 144: 741–742.

40. CDC. Epidemiologic notes and reports – expanded tuberculosis surveillance and tuberculosis morbidity – United States, 1993. *MMWR Morb Mortal Wkly Rep* 1994; 43: 361–366.

https://doi.org/10.1183/2312508X.10020817

41. CDC. Epidemiologic notes and reports nosocomial transmission of multidrug-resistant tuberculosis among hiv-infected persons – Florida and New York, 1988–1991. *MMWR Morb Mortal Wkly Rep* 1991; 40: 585–591.

42. Pablos-Mendez A, Raviglione MC, Battan R, *et al.* Drug-resistant tuberculosis among the homeless in New York City. *NY State J Med* 1990; 90: 351–355.

43. Raviglione MC, Sudre P, Rieder HL, *et al.* Secular trends of tuberculosis in Western Europe. *Bull World Health Organ* 1993; 71: 297–306.

44. Harries AD. Tuberculosis and human immunodeficiency virus infection in developing countries. *Lancet* 1990; 335: 387–390.

45. Narain JP, Raviglione MC, Kochi A. HIV-associated tuberculosis in developing countries: epidemiology and strategies for prevention. *Tuberc Lung Dis* 1992; 73: 311–321.

46. Raviglione MC, Rieder HL, Styblo K, *et al.* Tuberculosis trends in Eastern Europe and the former USSR. *Tuberc Lung Dis* 1994; 75: 400–416.

47. Sudre P, ten Dam HG, Kochi A. Tuberculosis: a global overview of the situation today. *Bull World Health Organ* 1992; 70: 149–159.

48. Dolin JP, Raviglione MC, Kochi A. Estimates of future global tuberculosis morbidity and mortality. *MMWR Morb Mortal Wkly Rep* 1993; 42: 961–964.

49. WHO. Forty-fourth World Health Assembly. Resolutions and Decisions. Resolution WHA 44.8. Document WHA44/1991/REC/1.WHO, Geneva, 1991. www.who.int/iris/handle/10665/173858

50. Styblo K, Bumgarner R. Tuberculosis can be controlled with existing technologies: evidence. *In:* Tuberculosis Surveillance Research Unit, Progress Report. The Hague, Tuberculosis Surveillance Unit, 1991, pp. 60–72.

51. WHO. WHO declares tuberculosis a global emergency. Press release WHO/31, April 23, 1993. Geneva, WHO, 1993.

52. WHO. Global Tuberculosis Programme. Framework for Effective Tuberculosis Control. Document WHO/TB/94.179. Geneva, WHO, 1994. www.who.int/iris/handle/10665/58717

53. Uplekar MW, Shepard DS. Treatment of tuberculosis by private general practitioners in India. *Tubercle* 1991; 72: 284–290.

54. Chaulet P, Raviglione M, Bustreo F. Epidemiology, control and treatment of multidrug-resistant tuberculosis. *Drugs* 1996; 52: Suppl. 2, 103–108.

55. Veen J, Migliori GB, Raviglione M, *et al.* Harmonisation of TB control in the WHO European region: the history of the Wolfheze Workshops. *Eur Respir J* 2011; 37: 950–959.

56. Maher D, Raviglione M. The history of the DOTS strategy: achievements and perspectives. *In:* Schaaf S, Zumla A, eds. Tuberculosis – a Comprehesive Clinical Reference. London, Elsevier Publishers, 2008, pp. 930–939.

57. Zwarenstein M, Schoeman J, Vundule C, *et al.* Randomised controlled trial of self-supervised and directly observed treatment of tuberculosis. *Lancet* 1998; 352: 1340–1343.

58. Volmink J, Garner P. Systematic review of randomised controlled trials of strategies to promote adherence to tuberculosis treatment. *BMJ* 1997; 315: 1403–1406.

59. Walley JD, Khan MA, Newell JN, *et al.* Effectiveness of the direct observation component of DOTS for tuberculosis: a randomised controlled trial in Pakistan. *Lancet* 2001; 357: 664–669.

60. Maher D, Raviglione M, Lee JW. Direct observation for tuberculosis treatment. *Lancet* 2001; 358: 421.

61. World Bank. World Development Report 1993. Investing in Health. New York, Oxford University Press, 1993. Available from: https://openknowledge.worldbank.org/handle/10986/5976

62. WHO. Fifty-third World Health Assembly. Resolutions and Decisions. Resolution WHA 53.1. Geneva, WHO, 2000. www.who.int/iris/handle/10665/260181

63. Cohn DL, Bustreo F, Raviglione MC. Drug resistance in tuberculosis: review of the worldwide situation and WHO/IUATLD's Global Surveillance Project. *Clin Infect Dis* 1997; 24: Suppl. 1, S121–S130.

64. Laszlo A, Rahman M, Raviglione M, *et al.* Quality assurance programme for drug susceptibility testing of *Mycobacterium tuberculosis* in the WHO/IUATLD Supranational Laboratory Network: first round of proficiency testing. *Int J Tuberc Lung Dis* 1997; 1: 231–238.

65. Pablos-Méndez A, Raviglione MC, Laszlo A, *et al.* Global surveillance for antituberculosis-drug resistance: 1994–1997. *N Engl J Med* 1998; 338: 1641–1649.

66. Espinal MA, Laszlo A, Simonsen L, *et al.* Global trends in resistance to antituberculosis drugs. *N Engl J Med* 2001; 344: 1294–1303.

67. Aziz MA, Wright A, Laszlo A, *et al.* Epidemiology of antituberculosis drug resistance (the Global Project on Anti-tuberculosis Drug Resistance Surveillance): an updated analysis. *Lancet* 2006; 368: 2142–2154.

68. Wright A, Zignol M, Van Deun A, *et al.* Epidemiology of antituberculosis drug resistance 2002–2007: an updated analysis of the Global Project on Anti-Tuberculosis Drug Resistance Surveillance. *Lancet* 2009; 373: 1861–1873.

69. Zignol M, Van Gemert W, Falzon D, *et al.* Surveillance of anti-tuberculosis drug resistance in the world: an updated analysis, 2007–2010. *Bull World Health Organ* 2012; 90: 111–119D.

70. Zignol M, Dean AS, Falzon D, *et al.* Twenty years of global surveillance of anti-tuberculosis drug resistance. *N Eng J Med* 2016; 375: 1081–1089.

71.   Raviglione MC, Dye C, Schmidt S, *et al.* Assessment of worldwide tuberculosis control. *Lancet* 1997; 350: 624–629.
72.   WHO. Global Tuberculosis Control: WHO Report 1997. Document WHO/TB/97.225. Geneva, WHO, 1997. http://apps.who.int/iris/bitstream/handle/10665/63354/WHO_TB_97.225_(part1).pdf?sequence=1
73.   WHO. Report of the ad hoc Committee on the Tuberculosis Epidemic. London 17–19 March 1998. Document WHO/TB/98.245. Geneva, WHO, 1998. www.who.int/iris/handle/10665/63941
74.   Heitkamp PI, Espinal Fuentes MA. Advancing and advocating tuberculosis control globally through the Stop Tuberculosis Partnership. *In:* Raviglione MC, ed. Tuberculosis. A Comprehensive International Approach. 3rd Edn. New York, Informa Health Care USA, 2006, pp. 685–704.
75.   Kumaresan J, Heitkamp P, Smith I, *et al.* Global Partnership to Stop TB: a model of an effective public health partnership. *Int J Tuberc Lung Dis* 2004; 8: 120–129.
76.   WHO. Tuberculosis and Sustainable Development. Stop TB Initiative and Ministerial Conference on Tuberculosis and Sustainable Development. Document WHO/CDS/STB/2000.6. Geneva, WHO, 2000. www.who.int/iris/handle/10665/66473
77.   Arnold VC, Smith IM. The Global Drug Facility: a revolution in tuberculosis control. *In:* Raviglione MC, ed. Tuberculosis. A Comprehensive International Approach. 3rd Edn. New York, Informa Health Care USA, 2006, pp. 705–715.
78.   Lorenz N. Effectiveness of global health partnerships: will the past repeat itself? *Bull World Health Organ* 2007; 85: 567–568.
79.   United Nations. United Nations Millennium Declaration. United Nations General Assembly Resolution 55/2. New York, United Nations, 2000. www.un.org/millennium/declaration/ares552e.htm
80.   Haines A, Cassels A. Can the millennium development goals be attained? *BMJ* 2004; 329: 394–397.
81.   Reid A, Scano F, Getahun H, *et al.* Towards universal access to HIV prevention, treatment, care and support: the role of tuberculosis/HIV collaboration. *Lancet Infect Dis* 2006; 6: 483–495.
82.   WHO. WHO Policy on Collaborative TB/HIV Activities: Guidelines for National Programmes and Other Stakeholders. Documents WHO/HTM/TB/2012.1 and WHO/HIV/2012.1. Geneva, WHO, 2012. www.who.int/tb/publications/2012/tb_hiv_policy_9789241503006/en/
83.   Getahun H, Raviglione M. Active case finding for tuberculosis in the community: time to act. *Lancet* 2010; 376: 1205–1206.
84.   Getahun H, Granich R, Sculier D, *et al.* Implementation of isoniazid preventive therapy for people living with HIV worldwide: barriers and solutions. *AIDS* 2010; 24: Suppl. 5, S57–S65.
85.   WHO. Anti-tuberculosis Drug Resistance in the World/the WHO/IUATLD Global Project on Anti-tuberculosis Drug Resistance Surveillance 1994–1997. Document WHO/TB/97.229. Geneva, WHO, 1997. www.who.int/iris/handle/10665/64090
86.   Espinal M, Dye C, Raviglione M, *et al.* Rational 'DOTS Plus' for the control of MDR-TB. *Int J Tuberc Lung Dis* 1999; 3: 561–563.
87.   Gupta R, Kim JY, Espinal MA, *et al.* Responding to market failure in tuberculosis control. *Science* 2001; 293: 1049–1051.
88.   Gupta R, Cegielski JP, Espinal MA, *et al.* Increasing transparency in partnership for health – introducing the Green Light Committee. *Trop Med Intern Health* 2002; 7: 970–976.
89.   Brugha R, Donohue M, Starling M, *et al.* The Global Fund: managing great expectations. *Lancet* 2004; 364: 95–10.
90.   Nathanson E, Nunn P, Uplekar M, *et al.* MDR tuberculosis – critical steps for prevention and control. *N Engl J Med* 2010; 363: 1050–1058.
91.   Uplekar M, Pathania V, Raviglione M. Private practitioners and public health: weak links in tuberculosis control. *Lancet* 2001; 358: 912–916.
92.   Dewan PK, Lal SS, Lonnroth K, *et al.* Improving tuberculosis control through public–private collaboration in India: literature review. *BMJ* 2006; 332: 574–578.
93.   Maher D, Hausler HP, Raviglione MC, *et al.* Tuberculosis care in community care organizations in sub-Saharan Africa: practice and potential. *Int J Tuberc Lung Dis* 1997; 1: 276–283.
94.   Maher D, Gorkom Jv, Gondrie PCFM, *et al.* Community contribution to tuberculosis care in high tuberculosis prevalence countries: past, present and future. *Int J Tuberc Lung Dis* 1999; 3: 762–768.
95.   Smith JH, Whiteside A. The history of AIDS exceptionalism. *J Int AIDS Soc* 2010; 13: 47.
96.   Mbali M. South African AIDS Activism and Global Health Politics. London, Palgrave Macmillan, 2013.
97.   Getahun H, Raviglione M. Transforming the global tuberculosis response through effective engagement of civil society organizations: the role of the WHO. *Bull World Health Organ* 2011; 89: 616–618.
98.   Travis P, Bennett S, Haines A, *et al.* Overcoming health-systems constraints to achieve the Millennium Development Goals. *Lancet* 2004; 364: 900–906.
99.   Iademarco MF, Castro KG. Tuberculosis in the United States. *In:* Raviglione MC, ed. Tuberculosis. A Comprehensive International Approach. 3rd Edn. New York, Informa Health Care USA, 2006, pp. 767–792.
100.   Lienhardt C, Glaziou P, Uplekar M, *et al.* Successes and challenges of global tuberculosis control. *Nat Rev Microbiol* 2012; 10: 407–416.

https://doi.org/10.1183/2312508X.10020817

101. Pai M, Behr MA, Dowdy D, *et al*. Tuberculosis. *Nat Rev Dis Primers* 2016; 2: 16076.

102. Uplekar M, Weil D, Lönnroth K, *et al*. WHO's End TB Strategy. *Lancet* 2015; 385: 1799–1801.

103. Maher D, Dye C, Floyd K, *et al*. Planning to improve global health: the next decade of tuberculosis control. *Bull World Health Organ* 2007; 85: 341–347.

104. Raviglione MC. The new Stop TB Strategy and the Global Plan to Stop TB, 2006–2015. *Bull World Health Organ* 2007; 85: 327.

105. WHO. The Stop TB Strategy. Geneva, WHO, 2006. http://apps.who.int/iris/bitstream/handle/10665/69241/WHO_HTM_STB_2006.368_eng.pdf;jsessionid=C3CB9DE2D4FA2B6C65FFB85C9A7A6E06?sequence=12

106. Raviglione MC, Uplekar M. WHO's new StopTB Strategy. *Lancet* 2006; 367: 952–955.

107. WHO. Macroeconomics and Health: Investing in Health for Economic Development: Executive Summary/Report of the Commission on Macroeconomics and Health. Geneva, WHO, 2001. www.who.int/iris/handle/10665/42463

108. WHO/Commission on Social Determinants of Health. Closing the Gap in a Generation – Health Equity Through Action on the Social Determinants of Health. Geneva, WHO, 2008. www.who.int/social_determinants/thecommission/finalreport/en/

109. Lönnroth K, Jaramillo E, Williams B, *et al*. Tuberculosis: the role of risk factors and social determinants. *In:* Blas E, Sivasankara Kurup A, eds. Equity, Social Determinants and Public Health Programmes. Geneva, WHO, 2010, pp. 219–241.

110. Lönnroth K, Jaramillo E, Williams BG, *et al*. Drivers of tuberculosis epidemics: the role of risk factors and social determinants. *Soc Sci Med* 2009; 68: 2240–2246.

111. Treatment Action Group. The Ascent Begins: Tuberculosis Research Funding Trends, 2005–2016. New York, Treatment Action Group, 2017.

112. Boehme CD, Nabeta P, Hillemann D, *et al*. Rapid molecular detection of tuberculosis and rifampin resistance. *N Engl J Med* 2010; 363: 1005–1015.

113. Diacon AH, Pym A, Grobusch M, *et al*. The diarylquinoline TMC207 for multidrug-resistant tuberculosis. *N Engl J Med* 2009; 360: 2397–2405.

114. Gler MT, Skripconoka V, Sanchez-Garavito E, *et al*. Delamanid for multidrug-resistant pulmonary tuberculosis. *N Engl J Med* 2012; 366: 2151–2160.

115. Lienhardt C, Lönnroth K, Menzies D, *et al*. Translational research for tuberculosis elimination: priorities, challenges, and action. *PLOS Med* 2016; 13: e1001965.

116. Zumla AI, Gillespie SH, Hoelscher M, *et al*. New antituberculosis drugs, regimens, and adjunct therapies: needs, advances, and future prospects. *Lancet Infect Dis* 2014; 14: 327–340.

117. United Nations General Assembly. Resolution A/RES/70/1. Transforming Our World: the 2030 Agenda for Sustainable Development. New York, United Nations, 2015. https://undocs.org/A/RES/70/1

118. WHO. Agenda item 12.1, 21 May 2014. Global Strategy and Targets for Tuberculosis Prevention, Care and Control after 2015. Sixty-seventh World Health Assembly WHA67.1. Resolutions and Decisions. Geneva, WHO, 2014. Available from: http://apps.who.int/gb/e/e_wha67.html

119. WHO. Global Tuberculosis Report 2014. Geneva, WHO, 2014. www.who.int/iris/handle/10665/137094

120. Raviglione MC. Setting new targets in the fight against tuberculosis. *Nat Med* 2013; 19: 263.

121. Lönnroth K, Migliori GB, Abubakar I, *et al*. Towards tuberculosis elimination: an action framework for low-incidence countries. *Eur Respir J* 2015; 45: 928–952.

122. WHO. Framework Towards Tuberculosis Elimination in Low-incidence Countries. Geneva, WHO, 2014. www.who.int/tb/publications/elimination_framework/en/

123. WHO. First WHO Global Ministerial Conference. Ending TB in the Sustainable Development Era: a Multisectoral Response, November 16–17, 2017, Moscow, Russian Federation. Geneva, WHO, 2017. www.who.int/tb/features_archive/Moscow_Declaration_to_End_TB_final_ENGLISH.pdf?ua=1

124. United Nations General Assembly. Seventy-first Session. Resolution adopted by the General Assembly on 15 December 2016. Global Health and Foreign Policy: Health Employment and Economic Growth. Document A/RES/71.159. New York, United Nations, 2017. www.un.org/ga/search/view_doc.asp?symbol=A/RES/71/159

125. WHO. Seventy-First World Health Assembly. Preparation for a High-level Meeting of the General Assembly on Ending Tuberculosis. Development Process for a Draft Multisectoral Accountability Framework to Accelerate Progress to End Tuberculosis. Document A71/16. Geneva, WHO, 2018. http://apps.who.int/gb/ebwha/pdf_files/WHA71/A71_16-en.pdf

---

Disclosures: None declared.

| | Chapter 5 |

Aetiopathogenesis, immunology and microbiology

Palmira Barreira-Silva[1,2], Egídio Torrado[1,2],
Hanna Nebenzahl-Guimaraes[1,2], Gunilla Kallenius[3] and
Margarida Correia-Neves[1,2,3]

The interaction of *Mycobacterium tuberculosis* with a host may result in a number of distinct outcomes: the host can either eliminate the micro-organisms immediately or allow the establishment of an infection, which in turn can progress to active TB or remain as LTBI. The nature of this outcome depends on a number of factors, most of which are related to the immune response developed by the host and the particularities of the bacterial genetics. Here, we summarise the major concepts and unanswered questions on the host response to infection and *M. tuberculosis* strain-related differences associated with distinct outcomes. In addition, detection of infection before individuals develop clear signs of active disease is challenging, as is the recognition of those who are at a higher risk of progressing towards active TB. Thus, new biomarkers for active and latent TB are presented.

Cite as: Barreira-Silva P, Torrado E, Nebenzahl-Guimaraes H, *et al.* Aetiopathogenesis, immunology and microbiology. *In:* Migliori GB, Bothamley G, Duarte R, *et al.*, eds. Tuberculosis (ERS Monograph). Sheffield, European Respiratory Society, 2018; pp. 62–82 [https://doi.org/10.1183/2312508X.10020917].

🐦 @ERSpublications
Following infection with *Mycobacterium tuberculosis*, individuals develop distinct outcomes from cure to latent or active TB. The mediators of these differences, as well as new biomarkers to identify distinct forms of the disease, are discussed. http://ow.ly/cfVQ30lqCfE

Immune response to *Mycobacterium tuberculosis*

The immune response to *M. tuberculosis* is an intricate mechanism involving both innate and adaptive immune cell populations. Studies with human subjects and, to a greater extent, animal models have shown that macrophages play a key role in orchestrating this immune response, given their ability to engulf bacteria, present antigens and produce cytokines that activate T-cells. The central role of activated T-cells has also been unravelled, in particular the cytokines produced by CD4[+] T-cells and their ability to activate the antimicrobial mechanisms of macrophages. As will be discussed in this chapter, while

[1]Life and Health Sciences Research Institute (ICVS), School of Medicine, University of Minho, Braga, Portugal. [2]ICVS/3B's, PT Government Associate Laboratory, Braga/Guimarães, Portugal. [3]Dept of Medicine Solna Enheten för Infektionssjukdomar MEDS, Division of Infectious Diseases, Karolinska Institutet, Stockholm, Sweden.

Correspondence: Margarida Correia-Neves, Life and Health Sciences Research Institute (ICVS), University of Minho, Campus of Gualtar, 4710-057 Braga, Portugal. E-mail: mcorreianeves@med.uminho.pt

Copyright ©ERS 2018. Print ISBN: 978-1-84984-099-6. Online ISBN: 978-1-84984-100-9. Print ISSN: 2312-508X. Online ISSN: 2312-5098.

https://doi.org/10.1183/2312508X.10020917

several key aspects of the *M. tuberculosis*–host interaction have been unveiled, including the recruitment of particular immune cell populations, secretion of certain cytokines, and the formation and organisation of granulomas, the precise nature of a fully protective immunity remains to be elucidated.

Innate immune response to *Mycobacterium tuberculosis*

Recognition and engulfment

Following *M. tuberculosis* infection, pattern recognition receptors (PRRs) present in antigen-presenting cells (*e.g.* macrophages, dendritic cells (DCs) and neutrophils) recognise the mycobacterial pathogen-associated molecular patterns (PAMPs) and phagocytose the invading bacilli [1–3]. Most *M. tuberculosis* infections are air-borne and occur after the inhalation of *M. tuberculosis*-containing droplets [4]: in these cases, the bacteria are taken up initially by the alveolar macrophages and the resident DCs. The particularities of this initial *M. tuberculosis* recognition, including which *M. tuberculosis* PAMPs bind to the PRRs in macrophages and DCs, are key to the outcome of the infection. Table 1 summarises the main PRRs known to recognise *M. tuberculosis* PAMPs and their interaction outcomes [5–16].

Mycobacterium tuberculosis evasion of innate mechanisms

After engulfment, *M. tuberculosis* may evade the killing mechanisms of phagocytes by preventing fusion between the lysosome and the phagosome and by blocking maturation of the phagolysosome: the bacilli can then escape to the cytosol and proliferate within the infected cell [17–20]. Moreover, certain *M. tuberculosis* strains are able to prevent apoptosis of infected macrophages, which is thought to be a protective host response [21]. In fact, some highly virulent *M. tuberculosis* strains clearly favour macrophage necrosis, as opposed to apoptosis, facilitating the infection of surrounding cells [22, 23]. Additionally, some *M. tuberculosis* strains can limit the apoptosis process of neutrophils, delaying the priming and initiation of the adaptive immune response [24] and probably the migration of DCs to the draining lymph nodes [25]. Recently, it has been shown that the differentiation of foamy macrophages (macrophages with a high lipid content) after *M. tuberculosis* infection may be favourable to the growth of these bacteria, as these cells present immunosuppressive properties [26].

Adaptive immune response to *Mycobacterium tuberculosis*

From priming to activation of T-cells

When the innate immune response is unable to successfully clear bacteria, antigen-presenting cells carrying antigen and/or bacteria migrate to the draining lymph nodes and mediate T-cell priming. Studies using a mouse model of low-dose aerosol infection have shown that T-cell priming occurs only ∼8 days after infection [27–29]. During this process, T-cells with receptors specific for *M. tuberculosis* antigen expand and migrate to the site of infection, initiating the adaptive immune response [29]. Primed T-cells need three main distinct signals to become fully activated: 1) direct interaction of the T-cell receptors with the infected cell's peptide–major histocompatibility complex (MHC) proteins, 2) interaction between T-cell costimulatory surface molecules (*e.g.* CD28) and their antigen-presenting cell receptors (*e.g.* CD80 or CD86), and 3) cytokines secreted by infected cells (*e.g.* interleukin (IL)-12) [30–35]. Thus, individuals carrying a genetic deficiency in the IL-12p40 subunit are particularly prone to develop active TB [36], and mice lacking

Table 1. Pattern recognition receptors (PRRs) known to recognise *Mycobacterium tuberculosis* pathogen-associated molecular patterns (PAMPs) and the resulting outcome

PRR	PAMP	Outcome	First author [ref.]
TLR family			
TLR2	Liposaccharides and lipopeptides	Inhibits cytokine synthesis Represses MHC type II transactivator expression in macrophages	Doz [5]; Gupta [6] Harding [7]
		Induces the loss of peptide-loaded MHC type II molecules on macrophages	Harding [7]
		Cooperates with TLR9, which is essential for resistance	Bafica [8]
TLR4	Undetermined	Single missense mutation results in inability to control bacterial load	Jo [9]
TLR9	GC-rich genome	Regulates the granulomatous response	Ito [10]
		Regulates IL-12 synthesis by dendritic cells	Pompei [11]
		Essential for regulation of the Th1 response	Bafica [8]
NOD family			
NOD2	*N*-glycolyl muramyl dipeptide	Promotes the production of pro-inflammatory cytokines and nitric oxide	Coulombe [12]; Jo [13]
C-type lectins			
DC-SIGN	Mannose-capped lipoarabinomannan	Induces expression of IL-10 *via* crosstalk with TLRs	Jo [13]
Dectin-1	Undetermined	Activates the expression of several cytokines (such as TNF, IL-6, IL-1β, IL-12, IL-23 and IL-17A) Cooperates with TLRs	Yadav [14]; Zenaro [15]
Mincle	Trehalose-6,6′-dimycolate	Induces the expression of pro-inflammatory cytokines	Ishikawa [16]

TLR: Toll-like receptor; MHC: major histocompatibility complex; IL: interleukin; Th1: T-helper type 1 cell; NOD: nucleotide-binding oligomerisation domain-like receptor; DC-SIGN: dendritic cell-specific intercellular adhesion molecule-3-grabbing nonintegrin; TNF: tumour necrosis factor; Mincle: macrophage inducible Ca^{2+}-dependent lectin receptor.

IL-12p40 are highly susceptible to *M. tuberculosis* infection [37, 38]. Following activation, T-cells secrete pro-inflammatory molecules, namely IFN-γ and tumour necrosis factor (TNF), which further activate the microbicidal mechanisms of macrophages. One of these mechanisms includes the production of nitric oxide (NO) by the inducible NO synthase (iNOS). IFN-γ, TNF and NO play a crucial role in the host defence against *M. tuberculosis*. In fact, individuals with genetic alterations in the IFN-γ pathway are highly susceptible to developing active TB [39]. Moreover, the use of TNF-targeted therapies, in the context of autoimmune diseases, promotes the progression from LTBI to active TB [40]. Additionally, mice lacking IFN-γ (or its receptor), TNF (or its receptor) or iNOS die prematurely following *M. tuberculosis* infection [41–44]. Of note is that, as well as the type of T-cells

https://doi.org/10.1183/2312508X.10020917

and related cytokines present in the lung, their quantity and localisation (vasculature *versus* parenchyma, and within the different zones of the granuloma) are crucial in determining infection outcome [45, 46]. This fact may potentially explain contradictory results regarding the role of different types of T-cells during *M. tuberculosis* infection, as will be described.

Among the different T-cells, CD4[+] T-cells play a crucial role in the *M. tuberculosis*-induced immune response. Thus, HIV-infected individuals with low CD4[+] T-cell counts have a markedly high susceptibility towards developing active TB [47]. In agreement, mice depleted of CD4[+] T-cells or lacking MHC class II succumb to the infection much earlier than their wild-type counterparts [48]. The role played by the different subsets of CD4[+] T-cells (and the cytokines produced by each) in the immune response against *M. tuberculosis* has been extensively addressed. T-helper type 1 (Th1) cells, in particular, have been broadly studied, as well as the role of IFN-γ (produced by these cells) in activation of the microbicidal mechanisms of macrophages. As with Th17 cells, and the corresponding IL-17, they play an important role in Th1 cell recruitment to the site of infection, as well as in the establishment of protection after vaccination [49, 50]. Despite this role, IL-17 has also been associated with the inhibition of apoptosis in infected macrophages, and with the promotion of *M. tuberculosis* intracellular growth [51]. T-follicular-helper cells constitute another subset of CD4[+] T-cells known to play a role in granuloma formation [52]. Moreover, IL-21, which is produced mainly by these cells, has been shown to be elevated in paediatric TB and reduced in adults with active TB (when compared with individuals with LTBI) [53, 54]. In the mouse model, production of IL-21 increases following *M. tuberculosis* infection [55], and IL-21 signalling has been shown to play a crucial role in the T-cell-mediated immune response [56]. Finally, CD4[+] T-regulatory (Treg) cells constrain the inflammatory response and reduce immune-mediated tissue damage [57]. However, elevated levels of Treg cells in TB patients have been associated with an increased bacterial load [58–60]. Accordingly, inhibition of the function of Treg cells in mice results in a decreased *M. tuberculosis* burden [61, 62].

In addition to CD4[+] T-cells, CD8[+] T-cells are also able to produce a set of relevant cytokines in the context of *M. tuberculosis* infection, namely IFN-γ and TNF [63–65]. Determining the precise role of CD8[+] T-cells is hampered by the fact that their regulation may be dependent on the action of CD4[+] T-cells. Accordingly, the absence of CD4[+] T-cells during an *M. tuberculosis* infection has been associated with the impaired generation of cytotoxic CD8[+] T-cells, as well as with decreased production of IFN-γ by CD8[+] T-cells [66–68]. However, several indicators suggest that CD8[+] T-cells play an important role in the generation of a protective immune response to *M. tuberculosis*. In fact, CD8[+] T-cells can eliminate *M. tuberculosis*-infected cells using mechanisms such as Fas- and TNF-mediated killing and granule exocytosis, involving the release of perforin and granzyme (in humans and mice) and granulysin (in humans) [69, 70]. *M. tuberculosis*-specific CD8[+] T-cells are present in granulomas and in the pleural fluid of patients with active TB or LTBI, as well as in those who have been BCG vaccinated [71–77]. Mice lacking CD8[+] T-cell responses exhibit a shorter survival period after infection when compared with their wild-type counterparts [78–84]. In addition, the depletion of CD8[+] T-cells in mice already lacking CD4[+] T-cells further decreases their survival period [48]. Interestingly, it has recently been shown that CD8[+] T-cells specific to the immunodominant *M. tuberculosis* epitope TB10.4 are unable to recognise infected macrophages, which may indicate a possible evasion method [85]. Nevertheless, considerable efforts in the investigation of CD8[+] T-cell-mediated immunity are still needed to clarify its relevance in TB resistance/susceptibility.

B-cell-mediated response

The first studies concerning the role of B-lymphocytes in the immune response against *M. tuberculosis* were centred on the production of anti-*M. tuberculosis* antibodies. However, the contribution of humoral immunity to the host defence against *M. tuberculosis* was controversial [86]. More recently, B-cells regained relevance in TB, as several investigators have explored both antibody-dependent and antibody-independent B-cell responses in this scenario [86, 87]. One particular study showed that IgGs produced by LTBI individuals are more effective than those produced by patients with active TB in terms of promoting inflammasome activation, phagolysosome fusion and macrophage killing activity of phagocytosed mycobacteria [88]. Another study found that anti-*M. tuberculosis* IgA inhibits the infection of human epithelial cells, whereas anti-*M. tuberculosis* IgG promotes it [89]. Several studies have suggested that B-cells may play a role in neutrophil mobility, CD4$^+$ T-cell-mediated responses and macrophage polarisation during *M. tuberculosis* infection [52, 86, 90, 91].

Question marks over the protective immune response to *Mycobacterium tuberculosis*

Although the majority of *M. tuberculosis*-infected individuals are able to mount an immune response against the pathogen, triggering key features such as activation of T-cells and the production of cytokines such as IL-12, IFN-γ and TNF, many still develop either active TB or LTBI. Additionally, vaccination-induced IFN-γ production does not correlate with protection against *M. tuberculosis* [39, 92]. Furthermore, the immune response to *M. tuberculosis* in the mouse model includes the production of IFN-γ and NO but is ultimately unable to clear the bacteria, whose population grows until achieving a plateau (at ~4 weeks post-infection) [93]. Accordingly, IFN-γ-independent CD4$^+$ T-cell-mediated mechanisms of protection are known to occur during *M. tuberculosis* infection, as the transfer of effector cells unable to produce IFN-γ to infected mice is as protective as that of wild-type effector cells [94, 95]. These are a few of the remaining unclear aspects concerning the *M. tuberculosis* immune response, illustrating our incomplete understanding of what constitutes an adequate and fully protective immunity against this bacterium.

Latent tuberculosis infection and progression to active disease

M. tuberculosis latency can be maintained throughout the life of an infected individual or may progress to active TB at a certain time (most frequently within 2 years after infection) [96, 97]. The WHO classifies LTBI as a state of persistent immune response to stimulation by *M. tuberculosis* antigen without clinical manifestations of active TB [98]. From a practical point of view, this means that LTBI patients have a positive reaction to the TST and the IGRA, while their sputum and radiographic examination are negative for the presence of bacilli and TB-related lesions, respectively. The development of reliable LTBI diagnosis tools is essential to understand the differences between the immune response during LTBI and active disease, as well as to determine which host and/or bacterial variables can predict the progression from one to the other.

The most important risk factors for progression from LTBI to active TB characterised so far include Mendelian susceptibility to mycobacteria [99], HIV/AIDS coinfection [100], uncontrolled type 2 DM [101, 102], anti-TNF therapy [40, 103], organ transplantation [104], cancer chemotherapy [105], smoking and pulmonary comorbidities [106]. Moreover,

https://doi.org/10.1183/2312508X.10020917

older individuals have been shown to be more susceptible to developing active TB and to dying from the disease [107–109]. Importantly, a large proportion of patients with active TB present none of the major risk factors identified so far, which underscores the need to investigate this topic further.

Recent developments using mouse models include the acknowledgement of a bidirectional relationship between the gut microbiome and M. tuberculosis infection: not only is the gut microbiome able to have an impact on control of the M. tuberculosis infection, but M. tuberculosis infection itself is able to alter the gut microbiome [110, 111]. The lung microbiome is also altered in TB patients and after TB chemotherapy [112], although this area of knowledge needs further investigation [113]. The role of metabolism as a factor mediating progression to active TB has been gaining attention. In fact, there is metabolic variation within each granuloma (from the centre to the periphery), which has been shown to be associated with the eicosanoid pathway both in humans and in the rabbit model [114]. Additionally, the production of glucocorticoids modulates the maintenance of latency versus progression to active TB [115, 116]. Patients with active TB are also known to have alterations in their glucose and cholesterol levels, a deregulation that may facilitate disease progression [117, 118]. So far, and regardless of all the effort invested in understanding the mechanisms that trigger progression from LTBI to active TB, we are still far from knowing which individuals with LTBI are at higher risk of progressing to the active form of the disease.

Tuberculosis granulomas

Granulomas are the pathological hallmark and most distinctive histological feature of human TB [119]. During the initial stages of infection, granulomas comprise aggregates of innate immune cells (including macrophages, monocytes, DCs and neutrophils) that are recruited to the site of infection. It is only after the onset of the acquired immune response that granulomas acquire their characteristic structure, composed of a macrophage-rich centre surrounded by a lymphocyte cuff of $CD4^+$ and $CD8^+$ T- and B-cells [119–123]. As infection progresses, granulomas undergo extensive remodelling, and in some cases develop a central necrotic core known as caseous necrosis. The caseum can then liquefy and fuse with the adjacent airways, a process known as cavitation [124]. While this is the basic architecture of a "typical" human granuloma, it is important to note that TB granulomas have a wide morphological heterogeneity, even within the same patient [125, 126]. Indeed, and in addition to caseous granulomas, other types of granuloma may occur, including nonnecrotising, neutrophilic rich, mineralised, and completely fibrotic or cavitary ones [127, 128].

Granuloma function

A TB granuloma is a local outcome of the interaction between the host immune cells and M. tuberculosis. The classical view is that granulomas result from an efficient host response to the pathogen while preserving the function of neighbouring tissue. This view is supported by the observation that fibrotic and calcified human granulomas only seldom contain live bacteria [129]. Additionally, several immunocompromising risk factors that lead to the development of defective granulomas also result in hypersusceptibility to M. tuberculosis infection [130, 131]. However, and as has been highlighted earlier, is important to note that M. tuberculosis is an exquisite manipulator of the macrophage response [131]. As such, the hypersusceptibility to *M. tuberculosis* underlying the aforementioned immunosuppressive conditions may not simply be the result of poorly formed granulomas but rather a combination with a decreased microbicidal capacity of macrophages. Furthermore, the granuloma does not fully prevent dissemination of the bacteria to other tissues. Indeed, the initiation of acquired immunity requires shuttling of the bacteria to the draining lymph nodes [28, 29]. Therefore, it is possible that the immune response in the periphery is more efficient at controlling bacterial growth than the one that occurs in the lungs [131]. Accordingly, control of an *M. tuberculosis* infection in mice after a systemic challenge has been shown to be more efficient than after an aerosol challenge [132]. Finally, recent data support the hypothesis that the early recruitment of permissive macrophages to the forming granuloma may facilitate the early proliferation and dissemination of an *M. tuberculosis* infection [130, 133, 134]. Moreover, and while the granuloma may indeed serve to "wall off" the pathogen initially, it may later facilitate its transmission to other individuals. In fact, caseation followed by liquefaction of the granuloma can lead to rupture of the lesion and to the release of infectious material into the airways. This material can then be aerosolised in cough droplets, thus promoting bacterial transmission to other individuals.

Impact of granuloma heterogeneity on disease outcome

As discussed above, TB granulomas display a high morphological variability associated with distinct outcomes, even within the same host [125, 126]. Defining these micro-environments might provide important clues as to what constitutes protective immunity to TB.

Owing to the limited availability of human samples, animal models have been used to understand the development of granulomas. The use of nonhuman primates has been particularly useful, confirming the diversity of granulomas within each individual and their independence in terms of the total number of cells, proportion of T-cells, pattern of cytokine response and bacterial burden [126]. Granulomas containing T-cells producing both pro- and anti-inflammatory cytokines are more often related to bacterial sterilisation [126]. These results suggest that the balance between pro- and anti-inflammatory responses is critical for control of *M. tuberculosis* infection, as will be discussed further. Another intriguing observation of this study was that only a relatively small proportion of T-cells within the granuloma actually produced cytokines [126]. While some of these cells may be recruited to the granuloma because of the ongoing inflammatory response, it is possible that most of them do not interact with *M. tuberculosis* antigen. In this regard, a recent study on nonhuman primates infected with *M. tuberculosis* reported that the majority of antigen-specific CD4$^+$ T-cells that crossed the vascular endothelium into the lung parenchyma were located in the outer cuffs of the granuloma, and only a few were found in the myeloid cell core (where the *M. tuberculosis*-infected macrophages are located) [46]. This is important because direct recognition of infected macrophages by CD4$^+$ T-cells is required for the control of intracellular *M. tuberculosis* growth [135]. When taken together, these data suggest that the defective positioning of CD4$^+$ T-cells may be an important hurdle to T-cell-mediated immunity during TB. Although the expression of specific chemokine receptors is now recognised to be essential for the correct positioning of CD4$^+$ T-cells [52], the inflammatory environment that T-cells encounter in the granuloma alters their differentiation state, phenotype and survival [131, 136, 137]. Therefore, the T-cell response drives and is driven by the inflammatory environment. Further research is crucial to define the mechanism that prevents the correct positioning of T-cells.

https://doi.org/10.1183/2312508X.10020917

Compartmentalisation of granuloma inflammation

A robust pro-inflammatory environment promotes extensive granuloma remodelling and results in liquefaction of the caseum, a process that enables the transmission of *M. tuberculosis* [138]. In contrast, an anti-inflammatory milieu is associated with a better outcome of infection and a reduced risk of progression from LTBI to active TB [138, 139]. A recent study has shown that the balance between pro- and anti-inflammatory programmes is spatially compartmentalised and occurs at the level of individual granulomas [114]. Examination of different areas of intact, caseous and cavitary human granulomas has shown that the centre of more advanced lesions (caseous and cavitary) are enriched in pro-inflammatory pathways (with the presence of anti-microbial peptides, reactive oxygen species and pro-inflammatory eicosanoids), while the most exterior layers display an anti-inflammatory, tissue-preserving signature [114]. The spatial compartmentalisation of inflammatory programmes is consistent with the organisation of pro- and anti-inflammatory macrophage subsets in granulomas from humans and nonhuman primates [140]. However, the impact of this compartmentalisation of T-cell responses is yet to be understood. Future research focused on the accumulation and organisation of T-cells within TB granulomas is likely to provide important clues to define T-cell correlates of protection.

Potential new biomarkers for tuberculosis diagnosis

Currently available markers/tests for TB diagnosis exhibit serious limitations, and none is a point-of-care diagnostic test. Moreover, none of the available tests can fully differentiate between LTBI and past TB, or predict disease progression in LTBI patients [141–143]. Therefore, there is an ongoing intensive search for diagnostic and prognostic TB biomarkers [144–148].

Detection of mycobacterial antigens

The utilisation of *M. tuberculosis* antigen for TB diagnosis has obvious advantages over the utilisation of immune-response biomarkers, as the latter might reflect a past and fully resolved infection [149]. The *M. tuberculosis* antigen lipoarabinomannan (LAM), which is a mycobacterial cell wall glycolipid, represents one of the most promising antigens for the development of new diagnostic tests. In active TB patients, LAM has been found in serum and urine [150, 151]. Tests for urinary LAM have generated great enthusiasm and numerous publications but have also met several difficulties [152–155]. The current consensus is that these tests are not yet sensitive enough for detection of LTBI or for the detection of active TB in HIV-negative patients [152–155], but that this strategy merits further investment.

Immune responses to *Mycobacterium tuberculosis* antigens used as tuberculosis biomarkers

M. tuberculosis-activated T-cells incubated with *M. tuberculosis* antigen respond by secreting cytokines. In fact, the currently available IGRA tests, the QuantiFERON-TB Gold (Qiagen, Hilden, Germany), the T-Spot.*TB* (Oxford Immunotec, Abingdon, UK) and the more recent QuantiFERON-TB Gold Plus (Qiagen), rely on the fact that *M. tuberculosis*-specific T-cells release IFN-γ when exposed to the *M. tuberculosis* antigens ESAT-6 and CFP-10. Although very useful, these tests nevertheless present several limitations [141–143, 156, 157], and their use is not endorsed by the WHO in countries with a high TB burden [158].

The identification of *M. tuberculosis* antigen other than ESAT-6 and CFP-10, as well as of their corresponding T-cell markers and/or induced cytokines/chemokines, is a promising strategy to develop alternative diagnostic tools [159]. Ultimately, these diagnostic tools aim to differentiate between LTBI and active TB, and to identify LTBI patients who are at a high risk of progressing to active TB [160–162]. In this regard, heparin-binding haemagglutinin and DosR regulon-encoded antigen, for example, have been associated with LTBI [147]. Moreover, several other cytokines and chemokines besides IFN-γ are expressed by activated T-cells, some at much higher levels [159]. IFN-γ-induced protein 10 (IP-10), macrophage inflammatory protein (MIP)-1α/β, monocyte chemotactic protein-1 (MCP-1), and monokine induced by IFN-γ (MIG) are particularly promising in the context of immunodiagnostic tests [159].

Antibody responses are prominent during active TB [163, 164], and antibody levels against particular *M. tuberculosis* antigens may increase even before the appearance of symptoms [163]. Stemming from these findings, a number of commercial tests based on antibody detection were developed [165]. However, none reached the required thresholds of specificity and sensitivity, and the WHO has therefore recommended against utilisation in their current form [166]. Nevertheless, and as described earlier, B-cells have been attracting increasing interest in the TB field [86, 167, 168]. Accordingly, the design of diagnostic strategies based on new findings concerning TB-related B-cell responses and antibody production is a promising route.

Host marker signatures

Another potential approach to identify patients with TB at different stages involves the detection of host marker signatures, as opposed to individual biomarkers. In fact, a whole-blood transcriptomic mRNA expression signature was identified following a prospective analysis of a large cohort of South African adolescents with LTBI [169]. This study resulted in the definition of a correlate of risk signature composed of the transcription pattern of 16 genes, which was able to establish the risk of progression from LTBI to active TB. Additionally, a four-gene blood signature was found to be able to predict the progression towards active TB in exposed household contacts up to 2 years preceding actual disease development [170]. Table 2 summarises the host marker signatures presented in these two studies. Finally, the results of a few small studies have highlighted the potential of differentially expressed patient cell microRNAs as TB biomarker candidates [148].

Mycobacterium tuberculosis strain-related differences

Although differences in the immune response and their possible roles in *M. tuberculosis* infection outcomes have been explored for decades, the role of *M. tuberculosis* strain differences in these dynamics has only recently been addressed. This late assessment can be attributed to the lack of obvious virulence factors and reduced genetic diversity in *M. tuberculosis*, as revealed by whole-genome sequencing. Unlike other bacterial pathogens, where genetic diversity arises as a result of recombination, duplication, insertion and deletion events, *M. tuberculosis* presents a markedly clonal evolution due to the lack of gene exchange [180]. There are three widely used genotyping tools to differentiate *M. tuberculosis* strains, namely IS*6110* restriction fragment length polymorphism (RFLP), spacer oligotyping (spoligotyping) and mycobacterial interspersed repeat units/variable number of tandem repeats (MIRU-VNTR), the last of which, due to its comparable

https://doi.org/10.1183/2312508X.10020917

Table 2. Host marker signatures as an approach towards predicting progression to active TB

Reporting study	Gene	Described/potential relationship to TB	First author [ref.]
ZAK [169]	ANKRD22	Undetermined	
	APOL1	Undetermined	
	BATF2	Promotes inflammatory response	ROY [171]
	ETV7	Undetermined	
	FCGR1A	Undetermined	
	FCGR1B	Undetermined	
	GBP1	Cell-autonomous immunity to TB	KIM [172]
	GBP2	Undetermined	
	GBP4	Undetermined	
	GBP5	Inflammasome activation	SHENOY [173]
	SCARF1	Undetermined	
	SEPT4	Undetermined	
	SERPING1	Undetermined	
	STAT1	Its absence increases susceptibility to TB in mice	SUGAWARA [174]
	TAP1	Important for TB antigen presentation	BEHAR [79]
	TRAFD1	Undetermined	
SULIMAN [170]	GAS6	Inhibition of TNF, IL-6 and IL-1 expression on macrophages	ALCIATO [175]
	SEPT4	Undetermined	
	CD1C	Lipid presentation and recognition by T-cells	MOODY [176]; MATSUNAGA [177]; ROY [178]; ROURA-MIR [179]
	BLK	Undetermined	

TNF: tumour necrosis factor; IL: interleukin. Reproduced and modified from [169] with permission.

specificity to IS6110 RFLP and its faster as well as cheaper performance [181, 182], has become the new standard in public health applications of *M. tuberculosis* in the USA, Europe and other parts of the world. Spoligotyping, a rapid, PCR-based method, is also widely used and is highly reproducible [183].

Analysis of large sequence polymorphisms has allowed the identification of seven distinct *M. tuberculosis* lineages, categorised as either "ancient" or "modern" according to the presence or absence of the TbD1 sequence [184]. The "ancient" lineages 1, 5, 6 and 7 are geographically restricted [185–187], while the "modern" lineages 2, 3 and 4 form a monophyletic group [184], with lineages 2 and 4 frequently being isolated from patients with diverse locations [188, 189]. Table 3 summarises the genetic markers that characterise the major *M. tuberculosis* lineages described to date.

Mycobacterium tuberculosis genetic diversity and virulence/immune response/transmission

Many experimental studies have found evidence suggesting that different *M. tuberculosis* lineages have distinct virulence profiles, reflected by differences in the uptake of bacteria by host cells, intracellular growth, pathology progression and cytokine induction. This variability may mirror the ability of strains to undermine the innate and/or adaptive

Table 3. Major *Mycobacterium tuberculosis* lineages and their genetic markers

Genetic markers and corresponding classification	*M. tuberculosis* lineage						
	Lineage 1	Lineage 2	Lineage 3	Lineage 4	Lineage 5	Lineage 6	Lineage 7
TbD1	Ancestral	Modern	Modern	Modern	Ancestral	Ancestral	Intermediate
LSP-based classification	Indo-Oceanic	East Asian	East African–Indian	Euro-American	West African 1	West African 2	Ethiopian
Spoligotype	East African–Indian	Beijing	Central Asian	Haarlem, LAM, S, T, X, etc.	AFRI2, AFRI3	AFRI1	Ethiopian
Regional association	East Africa, South Asia, South India [190]	East Asia, former USSR, South Africa [191]	East Africa, North India, Central Asia [186]	Americas, Europe, North Africa [192]	West Africa [193]	West Africa [193]	The Horn of Africa [194]

LSP: large sequence polymorphisms; USSR: Union of Soviet Socialist Republics; LAM: Latin-American Mediterranean. Reproduced and modified from [195] with permission.

https://doi.org/10.1183/2312508X.10020917

immunity, or their capacity to exploit the host immune system through the induction of a detrimental inflammatory response, which leads to tissue damage and culminates in the formation of cavities that promote disease transmission [196, 197]. More specifically, studies modelling infection with different *M. tuberculosis* lineages have shown that the modern lineages induce a lower and more delayed pro-inflammatory response following infection when compared with the others [198]. Modern lineages also have an enhanced ability to grow, reflected by faster replication in human macrophages *in vitro* and in the aerosol-infected mouse model [199]. Moreover, and within lineage 2, the Beijing sublineage strains are usually associated with highly virulent phenotypes, including an exacerbated cytotoxicity that leads to a worse pathology in the mouse model [200].

Among *M. tuberculosis* strains known for displaying a specific virulence phenotype, the W/Beijing HN878 strain stands out: immunocompetent mice infected with this strain die more rapidly than those infected with the clinical strain CDC-1551 or the standard laboratory strain H37Rv. Moreover, HN878 is also known to be associated with an increased rate of relapse from the latent state [201, 202]. The Beijing/K strain, in turn, is characterised by a severe pathology following infection and by a high-level of re-activation [203].

The growing body of experimental data associating *M. tuberculosis* genotypes with particular virulence phenotypes has a number of limitations: evidence gleaned from *in vitro* conditions may not always be extrapolated to the *in vivo* scenario, while the course of disease in animal models, such as the frequently used mouse model, is very different from that in humans. However, molecular epidemiological studies working with data on human transmission require the control of several host risk factors [204]. After doing so, these studies have identified associations between particular phylogenetic lineages and the ability to cause pulmonary disease [205], their proclivity to infect contacts [206, 207] and their likelihood of causing secondary cases [208, 209].

Mycobacterium tuberculosis genetic diversity and BCG vaccine efficacy

The efficacy of the BCG vaccine varies geographically, ranging from sites where it confers no protection to others where it accounts for a decrease of 80% in TB incidence. Among other factors (which include BCG vaccine–host interaction, host nutritional status and environmental status), differences in the genetic characteristics of the *M. tuberculosis* infecting strains might explain part of this variation [210, 211]. Furthermore, several epidemiological studies have suggested that extensive BCG vaccination might actually be one of the driving causes behind the emergence of the Beijing family [212], as it has been reported that isolates from this family were identified more regularly from BCG-immunised patients and from areas where the BCG vaccine was administered [210, 213]. The Beijing family is characterised by its ability to avoid BCG-induced immune responses: for instance, BCG-immunised mice die rapidly and at a higher rate following infection with a Beijing strain when compared with mice infected with *Mycobacterium canettii* or a lineage 1 strain [198, 210]. In addition, the insignificant prevention attained by the new-generation booster vaccine MVA85A has been attributed to a possible underestimation of *M. tuberculosis* genetic diversity [214].

Genetic diversity and drug resistance

The development of drug resistance through mutations in individual resistance genes was initially thought to have a cost in terms of bacterial infectivity [215]. However, recent studies have shown that DR-TB strains may develop compensatory mutations, thus remaining equally able to spread [198, 216]. Although DR-TB strains are found on a global scale, certain lineages and even particular clones, such as *M. tuberculosis* lineage 2 and KwaZulu-Natal, respectively, are particularly prone to developing drug-resistance mutations [217, 218]. The phylogenetic background has recently been shown to influence positive epistasis of major low-cost drug-resistance-conferring mutations, as these were found to increase transmission ability in MDR-TB strains of the modern (but not the ancient) Beijing sublineage [219].

Further prospective clinical studies are needed to determine the clinical significance of the associations found to date between phylogenetic lineages and drug-resistance profiles, including whether the prompt genotyping of isolates at the outset of treatment may be beneficial for patient management.

Conclusion

Notwithstanding the major efforts that have been made to understand the specificities of *M. tuberculosis* infection and characterise the associated immune response, our knowledge in this field remains very incomplete. One of the major unanswered questions pertains to the progression to active disease in patients with no obvious defects in their immune response. The characterisation of what constitutes a protective immune response against *M. tuberculosis* is thus a priority, as is the identification of biomarkers able to diagnose patients with LTBI or active TB, as well as to pinpoint those with LTBI who are at a high risk of progressing to active disease. Along with the decreasing cost of whole-genome sequencing analysis, identification of infecting strains and/or major lineage-specific single nucleotide polymorphisms may become a routine practise in certain settings [220, 221]. This is likely to improve TB control, namely in terms of the efficiency of contact tracing, the decision-making process regarding therapy initiation and the adaptation of vaccination programmes to different geographical regions.

References

1. Eum SY, Kong JH, Hong MS, *et al.* Neutrophils are the predominant infected phagocytic cells in the airways of patients with active pulmonary TB. *Chest* 2010; 137: 122–128.
2. Wolf AJ, Linas B, Trevejo-Nunez GJ, *et al.* Mycobacterium tuberculosis infects dendritic cells with high frequency and impairs their function *in vivo. J Immunol* 2007; 179: 2509–2519.
3. Eruslanov EB, Lyadova IV, Kondratieva TK, *et al.* Neutrophil responses to *Mycobacterium tuberculosis* infection in genetically susceptible and resistant mice. *Infect Immun* 2005; 73: 1744–1753.
4. Schlesinger LS. Entry of *Mycobacterium tuberculosis* into mononuclear phagocytes. *Curr Top Microbiol Immunol* 1996; 215: 71–96.
5. Doz E, Rose S, Court N, *et al.* Mycobacterial phosphatidylinositol mannosides negatively regulate host Toll-like receptor 4, MyD88-dependent proinflammatory cytokines, and TRIF-dependent co-stimulatory molecule expression. *J Biol Chem* 2009; 284: 23187–23196.
6. Gupta D, Sharma S, Singhal J, *et al.* Suppression of TLR2-induced IL-12, reactive oxygen species, and inducible nitric oxide synthase expression by *Mycobacterium tuberculosis* antigens expressed inside macrophages during the course of infection. *J Immunol* 2010; 184: 5444–5455.
7. Harding CV, Boom WH. Regulation of antigen presentation by *Mycobacterium tuberculosis*: a role for Toll-like receptors. *Nat Rev Microbiol* 2010; 8: 296–307.
8. Bafica A, Scanga CA, Feng CG, *et al.* TLR9 regulates Th1 responses and cooperates with TLR2 in mediating optimal resistance to *Mycobacterium tuberculosis. J Exp Med* 2005; 202: 1715–1724.
9. Jo EK, Yang CS, Choi CH, *et al.* Intracellular signalling cascades regulating innate immune responses to mycobacteria: branching out from Toll-like receptors. *Cell Microbiol* 2007; 9: 1087–1098.

https://doi.org/10.1183/2312508X.10020917

10. Ito T, Schaller M, Hogaboam CM, *et al.* TLR9 activation is a key event for the maintenance of a mycobacterial antigen-elicited pulmonary granulomatous response. *Eur J Immunol* 2007; 37: 2847–2855.

11. Pompei L, Jang S, Zamlynny B, *et al.* Disparity in IL-12 release in dendritic cells and macrophages in response to *Mycobacterium tuberculosis* is due to use of distinct TLRs. *J Immunol* 2007; 178: 5192–5199.

12. Coulombe F, Divangahi M, Veyrier F, *et al.* Increased NOD2-mediated recognition of *N*-glycolyl muramyl dipeptide. *J Exp Med* 2009; 206: 1709–1716.

13. Jo EK. Mycobacterial interaction with innate receptors: TLRs, C-type lectins, and NLRs. *Curr Opin Infect Dis* 2008; 21: 279–286.

14. Yadav M, Schorey JS. The β-glucan receptor dectin-1 functions together with TLR2 to mediate macrophage activation by mycobacteria. *Blood* 2006; 108: 3168–3175.

15. Zenaro E, Donini M, Dusi S. Induction of Th1/Th17 immune response by *Mycobacterium tuberculosis*: role of dectin-1, mannose receptor, and DC-SIGN. *J Leukoc Biol* 2009; 86: 1393–1401.

16. Ishikawa E, Ishikawa T, Morita YS, *et al.* Direct recognition of the mycobacterial glycolipid, trehalose dimycolate, by C-type lectin Mincle. *J Exp Med* 2009; 206: 2879–2888.

17. Armstrong JA, Hart PD. Phagosome–lysosome interactions in cultured macrophages infected with virulent tubercle bacilli. Reversal of the usual nonfusion pattern and observations on bacterial survival. *J Exp Med* 1975; 142: 1–16.

18. Frehel C, Rastogi N. *Mycobacterium leprae* surface components intervene in the early phagosome–lysosome fusion inhibition event. *Infect Immun* 1987; 55: 2916–2921.

19. Clemens DL, Horwitz MA. Characterization of the *Mycobacterium tuberculosis* phagosome and evidence that phagosomal maturation is inhibited. *J Exp Med* 1995; 181: 257–270.

20. van der Wel N, Hava D, Houben D, *et al. M. tuberculosis* and *M. leprae* translocate from the phagolysosome to the cytosol in myeloid cells. *Cell* 2007; 129: 1287–1298.

21. Balcewicz-Sablinska MK, Keane J, Kornfeld H, *et al.* Pathogenic *Mycobacterium tuberculosis* evades apoptosis of host macrophages by release of TNF-R2, resulting in inactivation of TNF-α. *J Immunol* 1998; 161: 2636–2641.

22. Woodworth JS, Shin D, Volman M, *et al. Mycobacterium tuberculosis* directs immunofocusing of CD8[+] T cell responses despite vaccination. *J Immunol* 2011; 186: 1627–1637.

23. Martin CJ, Booty MG, Rosebrock TR, *et al.* Efferocytosis is an innate antibacterial mechanism. *Cell Host Microbe* 2012; 12: 289–300.

24. Blomgran R, Desvignes L, Briken V, *et al. Mycobacterium tuberculosis* inhibits neutrophil apoptosis, leading to delayed activation of naive CD4 T cells. *Cell Host Microbe* 2012; 11: 81–90.

25. Blomgran R, Ernst JD. Lung neutrophils facilitate activation of naive antigen-specific CD4[+] T cells during *Mycobacterium tuberculosis* infection. *J Immunol* 2011; 186: 7110–7119.

26. Genoula M, Marin Franco JL, Dupont M, *et al.* Formation of foamy macrophages by tuberculous pleural effusions is triggered by the interleukin-10/signal transducer and activator of transcription 3 axis through ACAT upregulation. *Front Immunol* 2018; 9: 459.

27. Chackerian AA, Alt JM, Perera TV, *et al.* Dissemination of *Mycobacterium tuberculosis* is influenced by host factors and precedes the initiation of T-cell immunity. *Infect Immun* 2002; 70: 4501–4509.

28. Wolf AJ, Desvignes L, Linas B, *et al.* Initiation of the adaptive immune response to *Mycobacterium tuberculosis* depends on antigen production in the local lymph node, not the lungs. *J Exp Med* 2008; 205: 105–115.

29. Reiley WW, Calayag MD, Wittmer ST, *et al.* ESAT-6-specific CD4 T cell responses to aerosol *Mycobacterium tuberculosis* infection are initiated in the mediastinal lymph nodes. *Proc Natl Acad Sci USA* 2008; 105: 10961–10966.

30. Burnt FM. The Clonal Selection Theory of Acquired Immunity. Nashville, Vanderbilt University Press, 1959.

31. Zinkernagel RM, Doherty PC. Immunological surveillance against altered self components by sensitised T lymphocytes in lymphocytic choriomeningitis. *Nature* 1974; 251: 547–548.

32. Cunningham AJ, Lafferty KJ. A simple conservative explanation of the H-2 restriction of interactions between lymphocytes. *Scand J Immunol* 1977; 6: 1–6.

33. Linsley PS, Clark EA, Ledbetter JA. T-cell antigen CD28 mediates adhesion with B cells by interacting with activation antigen B7/BB-1. *Proc Natl Acad Sci USA* 1990; 87: 5031–5035.

34. Scott P. IL-12: initiation cytokine for cell-mediated immunity. *Science* 1993; 260: 496–497.

35. Booty MG, Nunes-Alves C, Carpenter SM, *et al.* Multiple inflammatory cytokines converge to regulate CD8[+] T cell expansion and function during tuberculosis. *J Immunol* 2016; 196: 1822–1831.

36. Casanova JL, Abel L. Genetic dissection of immunity to mycobacteria: the human model. *Annu Rev Immunol* 2002; 20: 581–620.

37. Cooper AM, Magram J, Ferrante J, *et al.* Interleukin 12 (IL-12) is crucial to the development of protective immunity in mice intravenously infected with *Mycobacterium tuberculosis*. *J Exp Med* 1997; 186: 39–45.

38. Cooper AM, Kipnis A, Turner J, *et al.* Mice lacking bioactive IL-12 can generate protective, antigen-specific cellular responses to mycobacterial infection only if the IL-12 p40 subunit is present. *J Immunol* 2002; 168: 1322–1327.

39. Alcais A, Fieschi C, Abel L, et al. Tuberculosis in children and adults: two distinct genetic diseases. J Exp Med 2005; 202: 1617–1621.

40. Keane J, Gershon S, Wise RP, et al. Tuberculosis associated with infliximab, a tumor necrosis factor α-neutralizing agent. N Engl J Med 2001; 345: 1098–1104.

41. Cooper AM, Dalton DK, Stewart TA, et al. Disseminated tuberculosis in interferon gamma gene-disrupted mice. J Exp Med 1993; 178: 2243–2247.

42. Flynn JL, Chan J, Triebold KJ, et al. An essential role for interferon gamma in resistance to Mycobacterium tuberculosis infection. J Exp Med 1993; 178: 2249–2254.

43. MacMicking JD, North RJ, LaCourse R, et al. Identification of nitric oxide synthase as a protective locus against tuberculosis. Proc Natl Acad Sci USA 1997; 94: 5243–5248.

44. Flynn JL, Goldstein MM, Chan J, et al. Tumor necrosis factor-α is required in the protective immune response against Mycobacterium tuberculosis in mice. Immunity 1995; 2: 561–572.

45. Sallin MA, Sakai S, Kauffman KD, et al. Th1 differentiation drives the accumulation of intravascular, non-protective CD4 T cells during tuberculosis. Cell Rep 2017; 18: 3091–3104.

46. Kauffman KD, Sallin MA, Sakai S, et al. Defective positioning in granulomas but not lung-homing limits CD4 T-cell interactions with Mycobacterium tuberculosis-infected macrophages in rhesus macaques. Mucosal Immunol 2018; 11: 462–473.

47. Jones BE, Young SM, Antoniskis D, et al. Relationship of the manifestations of tuberculosis to CD4 cell counts in patients with human immunodeficiency virus infection. Am Rev Respir Dis 1993; 148: 1292–1297.

48. Mogues T, Goodrich ME, Ryan L, et al. The relative importance of T cell subsets in immunity and immunopathology of airborne Mycobacterium tuberculosis infection in mice. J Exp Med 2001; 193: 271–280.

49. Khader SA, Bell GK, Pearl JE, et al. IL-23 and IL-17 in the establishment of protective pulmonary CD4+ T cell responses after vaccination and during Mycobacterium tuberculosis challenge. Nat Immunol 2007; 8: 369–377.

50. Khader SA, Cooper AM. IL-23 and IL-17 in tuberculosis. Cytokine 2008; 41: 79–83.

51. Cruz A, Ludovico P, Torrado E, et al. IL-17A promotes intracellular growth of Mycobacterium by inhibiting apoptosis of infected macrophages. Front Immunol 2015; 6: 498.

52. Slight SR, Rangel-Moreno J, Gopal R, et al. CXCR5+ T helper cells mediate protective immunity against tuberculosis. J Clin Invest 2013; 123: 712–726.

53. Pavan Kumar N, Anuradha R, Andrade BB, et al. Circulating biomarkers of pulmonary and extrapulmonary tuberculosis in children. Clin Vaccine Immunol 2013; 20: 704–711.

54. Kumar NP, Sridhar R, Hanna LE, et al. Decreased frequencies of circulating CD4+ T follicular helper cells associated with diminished plasma IL-21 in active pulmonary tuberculosis. PLoS One 2014; 9: e111098.

55. Li L, Jiang Y, Lao S, et al. Mycobacterium tuberculosis-specific IL-21+IFN-γ+CD4+ T cells are regulated by IL-12. PLoS One 2016; 11: e0147356.

56. Booty MG, Barreira-Silva P, Carpenter SM, et al. IL-21 signaling is essential for optimal host resistance against Mycobacterium tuberculosis infection. Sci Rep 2016; 6: 36720.

57. Parkash O, Agrawal S, Madhan Kumar M. T regulatory cells: Achilles' heel of Mycobacterium tuberculosis infection? Immunol Res 2015; 62: 386–398.

58. Pang H, Yu Q, Guo B, et al. Frequency of regulatory T-cells in the peripheral blood of patients with pulmonary tuberculosis from Shanxi Province, China. PLoS One 2013; 8: e65496.

59. Singh A, Dey AB, Mohan A, et al. Foxp3+ regulatory T cells among tuberculosis patients: impact on prognosis and restoration of antigen specific IFN-γ producing T cells. PLoS One 2012; 7: e44728.

60. Guyot-Revol V, Innes JA, Hackforth S, et al. Regulatory T cells are expanded in blood and disease sites in patients with tuberculosis. Am J Respir Crit Care Med 2006; 173: 803–810.

61. Bhattacharya D, Dwivedi VP, Maiga M, et al. Small molecule-directed immunotherapy against recurrent infection by Mycobacterium tuberculosis. J Biol Chem 2014; 289: 16508–16515.

62. Scott-Browne JP, Shafiani S, Tucker-Heard G, et al. Expansion and function of Foxp3-expressing T regulatory cells during tuberculosis. J Exp Med 2007; 204: 2159–2169.

63. Woodworth JS, Behar SM. Mycobacterium tuberculosis-specific CD8+ T cells and their role in immunity. Crit Rev Immunol 2006; 26: 317–352.

64. Lewinsohn DM, Zhu L, Madison VJ, et al. Classically restricted human CD8+ T lymphocytes derived from Mycobacterium tuberculosis-infected cells: definition of antigenic specificity. J Immunol 2001; 166: 439–446.

65. Tully G, Kortsik C, Hohn H, et al. Highly focused T cell responses in latent human pulmonary Mycobacterium tuberculosis infection. J Immunol 2005; 174: 2174–2184.

66. Serbina NV, Lazarevic V, Flynn JL. CD4+ T cells are required for the development of cytotoxic CD8+ T cells during Mycobacterium tuberculosis infection. J Immunol 2001; 167: 6991–7000.

67. Green AM, Difazio R, Flynn JL. IFN-γ from CD4 T cells is essential for host survival and enhances CD8 T cell function during Mycobacterium tuberculosis infection. J Immunol 2013; 190: 270–277.

68. Bold TD, Ernst JD. CD4+ T cell-dependent IFN-γ production by CD8+ effector T cells in Mycobacterium tuberculosis infection. J Immunol 2012; 189: 2530–2536.

https://doi.org/10.1183/2312508X.10020917

69. Woodworth JS, Wu Y, Behar SM. *Mycobacterium tuberculosis*-specific CD8$^+$ T cells require perforin to kill target cells and provide protection *in vivo*. *J Immunol* 2008; 181: 8595–8603.

70. Stenger S, Hanson DA, Teitelbaum R, *et al*. An antimicrobial activity of cytolytic T cells mediated by granulysin. *Science* 1998; 282: 121–125.

71. Randhawa PS. Lymphocyte subsets in granulomas of human tuberculosis: an *in situ* immunofluorescence study using monoclonal antibodies. *Pathology* 1990; 22: 153–155.

72. Guzman J, Bross KJ, Wurtemberger G, *et al*. Tuberculous pleural effusions: lymphocyte phenotypes in comparison with other lymphocyte-rich effusions. *Diagn Cytopathol* 1989; 5: 139–144.

73. Manca F, Habeshaw J, Dalgleish A. The naive repertoire of human T helper cells specific for gp120, the envelope glycoprotein of HIV. *J Immunol* 1991; 146: 1964–1971.

74. Rees A, Scoging A, Mehlert A, *et al*. Specificity of proliferative response of human CD8 clones to mycobacterial antigens. *Eur J Immunol* 1988; 18: 1881–1887.

75. Smith SM, Malin AS, Pauline T, *et al*. Characterization of human *Mycobacterium bovis* bacille Calmette–Guerin-reactive CD8$^+$ T cells. *Infect Immun* 1999; 67: 5223–5230.

76. Lewinsohn DM, Alderson MR, Briden AL, *et al*. Characterization of human CD8$^+$ T cells reactive with *Mycobacterium tuberculosis*-infected antigen-presenting cells. *J Exp Med* 1998; 187: 1633–1640.

77. Stenger S, Mazzaccaro RJ, Uyemura K, *et al*. Differential effects of cytolytic T cell subsets on intracellular infection. *Science* 1997; 276: 1684–1687.

78. Flynn JL, Goldstein MM, Triebold KJ, *et al*. Major histocompatibility complex class I-restricted T cells are required for resistance to *Mycobacterium tuberculosis* infection. *Proc Natl Acad Sci USA* 1992; 89: 12013–12017.

79. Behar SM, Dascher CC, Grusby MJ, *et al*. Susceptibility of mice deficient in CD1D or TAP1 to infection with *Mycobacterium tuberculosis*. *J Exp Med* 1999; 189: 1973–1980.

80. D'Souza CD, Cooper AM, Frank AA, *et al*. A novel nonclassic β$_2$-microglobulin-restricted mechanism influencing early lymphocyte accumulation and subsequent resistance to tuberculosis in the lung. *Am J Respir Cell Mol Biol* 2000; 23: 188–193.

81. Sousa AO, Mazzaccaro RJ, Russell RG, *et al*. Relative contributions of distinct MHC class I-dependent cell populations in protection to tuberculosis infection in mice. *Proc Natl Acad Sci USA* 2000; 97: 4204–4208.

82. Rolph MS, Raupach B, Kobernick HH, *et al*. MHC class Ia-restricted T cells partially account for β$_2$-microglobulin-dependent resistance to *Mycobacterium tuberculosis*. *Eur J Immunol* 2001; 31: 1944–1949.

83. Turner J, D'Souza CD, Pearl JE, *et al*. CD8- and CD95/95L-dependent mechanisms of resistance in mice with chronic pulmonary tuberculosis. *Am J Respir Cell Mol Biol* 2001; 24: 203–209.

84. Urdahl KB, Liggitt D, Bevan MJ. CD8$^+$ T cells accumulate in the lungs of *Mycobacterium tuberculosis*-infected Kb$^-$/$^-$Db$^-$/$^-$ mice, but provide minimal protection. *J Immunol* 2003; 170: 1987–1994.

85. Yang JD, Mott D, Sutiwisesak R, *et al*. *Mycobacterium tuberculosis*-specific CD4$^+$ and CD8$^+$ T cells differ in their capacity to recognize infected macrophages. *PLoS Pathog* 2018; 14: e1007060.

86. Achkar JM, Chan J, Casadevall A. B cells and antibodies in the defense against *Mycobacterium tuberculosis* infection. *Immunol Rev* 2015; 264: 167–181.

87. Casadevall A. Antibodies to *Mycobacterium tuberculosis*. *N Engl J Med* 2017; 376: 283–285.

88. Lu LL, Chung AW, Rosebrock TR, *et al*. A functional role for antibodies in tuberculosis. *Cell* 2016; 167: 433–443e414.

89. Zimmermann N, Thormann V, Hu B, *et al*. Human isotype-dependent inhibitory antibody responses against *Mycobacterium tuberculosis*. *EMBO Mol Med* 2016; 8: 1325–1339.

90. Kondratieva TK, Rubakova EI, Linge IA, *et al*. B cells delay neutrophil migration toward the site of stimulus: tardiness critical for effective bacillus Calmette–Guerin vaccination against tuberculosis infection in mice. *J Immunol* 2010; 184: 1227–1234.

91. Maglione PJ, Chan J. How B cells shape the immune response against *Mycobacterium tuberculosis*. *Eur J Immunol* 2009; 39: 676–686.

92. Majlessi L, Simsova M, Jarvis Z, *et al*. An increase in antimycobacterial Th1-cell responses by prime-boost protocols of immunization does not enhance protection against tuberculosis. *Infect Immun* 2006; 74: 2128–2137.

93. Rhoades ER, Frank AA, Orme IM. Progression of chronic pulmonary tuberculosis in mice aerogenically infected with virulent *Mycobacterium tuberculosis*. *Tuber Lung Dis* 1997; 78: 57–66.

94. Cowley SC, Elkins KL. CD4$^+$ T cells mediate IFN-γ-independent control of *Mycobacterium tuberculosis* infection both *in vitro* and *in vivo*. *J Immunol* 2003; 171: 4689–4699.

95. Gallegos AM, van Heijst JW, Samstein M, *et al*. A gamma interferon independent mechanism of CD4 T cell mediated control of *M. tuberculosis* infection *in vivo*. *PLoS Pathog* 2011; 7: e1002052.

96. Getahun H, Matteelli A, Chaisson RE, *et al*. Latent *Mycobacterium tuberculosis* infection. *N Engl J Med* 2015; 372: 2127–2135.

97. Trauer JM, Moyo N, Tay EL, *et al*. Risk of active tuberculosis in the five years following infection…15%? *Chest* 2016; 149: 516–525.

98.   WHO. Latent TB Infection: Updated and Consolidated Guidelines for Programmatic Management. Geneva, WHO, 2018. www.who.int/tb/publications/2018/latent-tuberculosis-infection/en/

99.   Bustamante J, Boisson-Dupuis S, Abel L, *et al.* Mendelian susceptibility to mycobacterial disease: genetic, immunological, and clinical features of inborn errors of IFN-γ immunity. *Semin Immunol* 2014; 26: 454–470.

100. Bruchfeld J, Correia-Neves M, Kallenius G. Tuberculosis and HIV coinfection. *Cold Spring Harb Perspect Med* 2015; 5: a017871.

101. Critchley JA, Restrepo BI, Ronacher K, *et al.* Defining a research agenda to address the converging epidemics of tuberculosis and diabetes: part 1: epidemiology and clinical management. *Chest* 2017; 152: 165–173.

102. Ronacher K, van Crevel R, Critchley JA, *et al.* Defining a research agenda to address the converging epidemics of tuberculosis and diabetes: part 2: underlying biologic mechanisms. *Chest* 2017; 152: 174–180.

103. Bruns H, Meinken C, Schauenberg P, *et al.* Anti-TNF immunotherapy reduces CD8$^+$ T cell-mediated antimicrobial activity against *Mycobacterium tuberculosis* in humans. *J Clin Invest* 2009; 119: 1167–1177.

104. Meije Y, Piersimoni C, Torre-Cisneros J, *et al.* Mycobacterial infections in solid organ transplant recipients. *Clin Microbiol Infect* 2014; 20: Suppl. 7, 89–101.

105. Jacobs RE, Gu P, Chachoua A. Reactivation of pulmonary tuberculosis during cancer treatment. *Int J Mycobacteriol* 2015; 4: 337–340.

106. Inghammar M, Ekbom A, Engstrom G, *et al.* COPD and the risk of tuberculosis – a population-based cohort study. *PLoS One* 2010; 5: e10138.

107. WHO. Global Tuberculosis Report 2017. Geneva, WHO, 2017. www.who.int/tb/publications/global_report/en/

108. Zevallos M, Justman JE. Tuberculosis in the elderly. *Clin Geriatr Med* 2003; 19: 121–138.

109. Negin J, Abimbola S, Marais BJ. Tuberculosis among older adults – time to take notice. *Int J Infect Dis* 2015; 32: 135–137.

110. Winglee K, Eloe-Fadrosh E, Gupta S, *et al.* Aerosol *Mycobacterium tuberculosis* infection causes rapid loss of diversity in gut microbiota. *PLoS One* 2014; 9: e97048.

111. Khan D, Ansar Ahmed S. The immune system is a natural target for estrogen action: opposing effects of estrogen in two prototypical autoimmune diseases. *Front Immunol* 2015; 6: 635.

112. Hong BY, Maulen NP, Adami AJ, *et al.* Microbiome changes during tuberculosis and antituberculous therapy. *Clin Microbiol Rev* 2016; 29: 915–926.

113. Adami AJ, Cervantes JL. The microbiome at the pulmonary alveolar niche and its role in *Mycobacterium tuberculosis* infection. *Tuberculosis* 2015; 95: 651–658.

114. Marakalala MJ, Raju RM, Sharma K, *et al.* Inflammatory signaling in human tuberculosis granulomas is spatially organized. *Nat Med* 2016; 22: 531–538.

115. Rook G, Baker R, Walker B, *et al.* Local regulation of glucocorticoid activity in sites of inflammation. Insights from the study of tuberculosis. *Ann N Y Acad Sci* 2000; 917: 913–922.

116. Rey AD, Mahuad CV, Bozza VV, *et al.* Endocrine and cytokine responses in humans with pulmonary tuberculosis. *Brain Behav Immun* 2007; 21: 171–179.

117. Lin Y, Yuan Y, Zhao X, *et al.* The change in blood glucose levels in tuberculosis patients before and during anti-tuberculosis treatment in China. *Glob Health Action* 2017; 10: 1289737.

118. Gebremicael G, Amare Y, Challa F, *et al.* Lipid profile in tuberculosis patients with and without human immunodeficiency virus infection. *Int J Chronic Dis* 2017; 2017: 3843291.

119. Orme IM, Basaraba RJ. The formation of the granuloma in tuberculosis infection. *Semin Immunol* 2014; 26: 601–609.

120. Gonzalez-Juarrero M, Turner OC, Turner J, *et al.* Temporal and spatial arrangement of lymphocytes within lung granulomas induced by aerosol infection with *Mycobacterium tuberculosis*. *Infect Immun* 2001; 69: 1722–1728.

121. Ulrichs T, Kosmiadi GA, Trusov V, *et al.* Human tuberculous granulomas induce peripheral lymphoid follicle-like structures to orchestrate local host defence in the lung. *J Pathol* 2004; 204: 217–228.

122. Silva Miranda M, Breiman A, Allain S, *et al.* The tuberculous granuloma: an unsuccessful host defence mechanism providing a safety shelter for the bacteria? *Clin Dev Immunol* 2012; 2012: 139127.

123. Ndlovu H, Marakalala MJ. Granulomas and inflammation: host-directed therapies for tuberculosis. *Front Immunol* 2016; 7: 434.

124. Russell DG, Cardona PJ, Kim MJ, *et al.* Foamy macrophages and the progression of the human tuberculosis granuloma. *Nat Immunol* 2009; 10: 943–948.

125. Lin PL, Ford CB, Coleman MT, *et al.* Sterilization of granulomas is common in active and latent tuberculosis despite within-host variability in bacterial killing. *Nat Med* 2014; 20: 75–79.

126. Gideon HP, Phuah J, Myers AJ, *et al.* Variability in tuberculosis granuloma T cell responses exists, but a balance of pro- and anti-inflammatory cytokines is associated with sterilization. *PLoS Pathog* 2015; 11: e1004603.

127. Cadena AM, Fortune SM, Flynn JL. Heterogeneity in tuberculosis. *Nat Rev Immunol* 2017; 17: 691–702.

128. Flynn JL, Chan J, Lin PL. Macrophages and control of granulomatous inflammation in tuberculosis. *Mucosal Immunol* 2011; 4: 271–278.

https://doi.org/10.1183/2312508X.10020917

129. Cosma CL, Sherman DR, Ramakrishnan L. The secret lives of the pathogenic mycobacteria. *Annu Rev Microbiol* 2003; 57: 641–676.
130. Ramakrishnan L. Revisiting the role of the granuloma in tuberculosis. *Nat Rev Immunol* 2012; 12: 352–366.
131. Fraga AG, Barbosa AM, Ferreira CM, *et al.* Immune-evasion strategies of mycobacteria and their implications for the protective immune response. *Curr Issues Mol Biol* 2018; 25: 169–198.
132. Cooper AM, Callahan JE, Keen M, *et al.* Expression of memory immunity in the lung following re-exposure to *Mycobacterium tuberculosis*. *Tuber Lung Dis* 1997; 78: 67–73.
133. Davis JM, Ramakrishnan L. The role of the granuloma in expansion and dissemination of early tuberculous infection. *Cell* 2009; 136: 37–49.
134. Cambier CJ, Takaki KK, Larson RP, *et al.* Mycobacteria manipulate macrophage recruitment through coordinated use of membrane lipids. *Nature* 2014; 505: 218–222.
135. Srivastava S, Ernst JD. Cutting edge: direct recognition of infected cells by CD4 T cells is required for control of intracellular *Mycobacterium tuberculosis* in vivo. *J Immunol* 2013; 191: 1016–1020.
136. Torrado E, Fountain JJ, Liao M, *et al.* Interleukin 27R regulates CD4$^+$ T cell phenotype and impacts protective immunity during *Mycobacterium tuberculosis* infection. *J Exp Med* 2015; 212: 1449–1463.
137. Pearl JE, Torrado E, Tighe M, *et al.* Nitric oxide inhibits the accumulation of CD4$^+$CD44^{hi}Tbet$^+$CD69^{lo} T cells in mycobacterial infection. *Eur J Immunol* 2012; 42: 3267–3279.
138. Kaplan G, Post FA, Moreira AL, *et al.* *Mycobacterium tuberculosis* growth at the cavity surface: a microenvironment with failed immunity. *Infect Immun* 2003; 71: 7099–7108.
139. Lin PL, Maiello P, Gideon HP, *et al.* PET CT identifies reactivation risk in cynomolgus macaques with latent *M. tuberculosis*. *PLoS Pathog* 2016; 12: e1005739.
140. Mattila JT, Ojo OO, Kepka-Lenhart D, *et al.* Microenvironments in tuberculous granulomas are delineated by distinct populations of macrophage subsets and expression of nitric oxide synthase and arginase isoforms. *J Immunol* 2013; 191: 773–784.
141. Pai M, Denkinger CM, Kik SV, *et al.* Gamma interferon release assays for detection of *Mycobacterium tuberculosis* infection. *Clin Microbiol Rev* 2014; 27: 3–20.
142. Auguste P, Tsertsvadze A, Pink J, *et al.* Comparing interferon-gamma release assays with tuberculin skin test for identifying latent tuberculosis infection that progresses to active tuberculosis: systematic review and meta-analysis. *BMC Infect Dis* 2017; 17: 200.
143. Nemes E, Rozot V, Geldenhuys H, *et al.* Optimization and interpretation of serial QuantiFERON testing to measure acquisition of *Mycobacterium tuberculosis* infection. *Am J Respir Crit Care Med* 2017; 196: 638–648.
144. Weiner J, Kaufmann SH. High-throughput and computational approaches for diagnostic and prognostic host tuberculosis biomarkers. *Int J Infect Dis* 2017; 56: 258–262.
145. Goletti D, Petruccioli E, Joosten SA, *et al.* Tuberculosis biomarkers: from diagnosis to protection. *Infect Dis Rep* 2016; 8: 6568.
146. Wallis RS, Doherty TM, Onyebujoh P, *et al.* Biomarkers for tuberculosis disease activity, cure, and relapse. *Lancet Infect Dis* 2009; 9: 162–172.
147. Petruccioli E, Scriba TJ, Petrone L, *et al.* Correlates of tuberculosis risk: predictive biomarkers for progression to active tuberculosis. *Eur Respir J* 2016; 48: 1751–1763.
148. Walzl G, McNerney R, du Plessis N, *et al.* Tuberculosis: advances and challenges in development of new diagnostics and biomarkers. *Lancet Infect Dis* 2018.
149. Flores LL, Steingart KR, Dendukuri N, *et al.* Systematic review and meta-analysis of antigen detection tests for the diagnosis of tuberculosis. *Clin Vaccine Immunol* 2011; 18: 1616–1627.
150. Sada E, Aguilar D, Torres M, *et al.* Detection of lipoarabinomannan as a diagnostic test for tuberculosis. *J Clin Microbiol* 1992; 30: 2415–2418.
151. Hamasur B, Bruchfeld J, Haile M, *et al.* Rapid diagnosis of tuberculosis by detection of mycobacterial lipoarabinomannan in urine. *J Microbiol Methods* 2001; 45: 41–52.
152. Sahle SN, Asress DT, Tullu KD, *et al.* Performance of point-of-care urine test in diagnosing tuberculosis suspects with and without HIV infection in selected peripheral health settings of Addis Ababa, Ethiopia. *BMC Res Notes* 2017; 10: 74.
153. Suwanpimolkul G, Kawkitinarong K, Manosuthi W, *et al.* Utility of urine lipoarabinomannan (LAM) in diagnosing tuberculosis and predicting mortality with and without HIV: prospective TB cohort from the Thailand Big City TB Research Network. *Int J Infect Dis* 2017; 59: 96–102.
154. Nicol MP, Allen V, Workman L, *et al.* Urine lipoarabinomannan testing for diagnosis of pulmonary tuberculosis in children: a prospective study. *Lancet Glob Health* 2014; 2: e278–e284.
155. Kroidl I, Clowes P, Reither K, *et al.* Performance of urine lipoarabinomannan assays for paediatric tuberculosis in Tanzania. *Eur Respir J* 2015; 46: 761–770.
156. Mahomed H, Hawkridge T, Verver S, *et al.* The tuberculin skin test *versus* QuantiFERON TB Gold in predicting tuberculosis disease in an adolescent cohort study in South Africa. *PLoS One* 2011; 6: e17984.

157. Banaei N, Pai M. Detecting new *Mycobacterium tuberculosis* infection. Time for a more nuanced interpretation of QuantiFERON conversions. *Am J Respir Crit Care Med* 2017; 196: 546–547.

158. WHO. Strategic and Technical Advisory Group for Tuberculosis. Report of 10th Meeting. Geneva, WHO, 2010. www.who.int/tb/advisory_bodies/stag_tb_report_2010.pdf

159. Chegou NN, Heyckendorf J, Walzl G, *et al.* Beyond the IFN-γ horizon: biomarkers for immunodiagnosis of infection with *Mycobacterium tuberculosis*. *Eur Respir J* 2014; 43: 1472–1486.

160. Frahm M, Goswami ND, Owzar K, *et al.* Discriminating between latent and active tuberculosis with multiple biomarker responses. *Tuberculosis* 2011; 91: 250–256.

161. Jeong YH, Hur YG, Lee H, *et al.* Discrimination between active and latent tuberculosis based on ratio of antigen-specific to mitogen-induced IP-10 production. *J Clin Microbiol* 2015; 53: 504–510.

162. Nonghanphithak D, Reechaipichitkul W, Namwat W, *et al.* Chemokines additional to IFN-γ can be used to differentiate among *Mycobacterium tuberculosis* infection possibilities and provide evidence of an early clearance phenotype. *Tuberculosis* 2017; 105: 28–34.

163. Gennaro ML, Affouf M, Kanaujia GV, *et al.* Antibody markers of incident tuberculosis among HIV-infected adults in the USA: a historical prospective study. *Int J Tuberc Lung Dis* 2007; 11: 624–631.

164. Laal S, Samanich KM, Sonnenberg MG, *et al.* Human humoral responses to antigens of *Mycobacterium tuberculosis*: immunodominance of high-molecular-mass antigens. *Clin Diagn Lab Immunol* 1997; 4: 49–56.

165. Steingart KR, Flores LL, Dendukuri N, *et al.* Commercial serological tests for the diagnosis of active pulmonary and extrapulmonary tuberculosis: an updated systematic review and meta-analysis. *PLoS Med* 2011; 8: e1001062.

166. WHO. Commercial Serodiagnostic Tests for Diagnosis of Tuberculosis: Policy Statement. Geneva, WHO, 2011. www.who.int/tb/publications/tb-serodiagnostic-policy/en/

167. Kozakiewicz L, Phuah J, Flynn J, *et al.* The role of B cells and humoral immunity in *Mycobacterium tuberculosis* infection. *Adv Exp Med Biol* 2013; 783: 225–250.

168. Jacobs AJ, Mongkolsapaya J, Screaton GR, *et al.* Antibodies and tuberculosis. *Tuberculosis* 2016; 101: 102–113.

169. Zak DE, Penn-Nicholson A, Scriba TJ, *et al.* A blood RNA signature for tuberculosis disease risk: a prospective cohort study. *Lancet* 2016; 387: 2312–2322.

170. Suliman S, Thompson E, Sutherland J, *et al.* Four-gene pan-African blood signature predicts progression to tuberculosis. *Am J Respir Crit Care Med* 2018; in press [DOI: https://doi.org/10.1164/rccm.201711-2340OC].

171. Roy S, Guler R, Parihar SP, *et al.* Batf2/Irf1 induces inflammatory responses in classically activated macrophages, lipopolysaccharides, and mycobacterial infection. *J Immunol* 2015; 194: 6035–6044.

172. Kim BH, Shenoy AR, Kumar P, *et al.* A family of IFN-γ-inducible 65-kD GTPases protects against bacterial infection. *Science* 2011; 332: 717–721.

173. Shenoy AR, Wellington DA, Kumar P, *et al.* GBP5 promotes NLRP3 inflammasome assembly and immunity in mammals. *Science* 2012; 336: 481–485.

174. Sugawara I, Yamada H, Mizuno S. STAT1 knockout mice are highly susceptible to pulmonary mycobacterial infection. *Tohoku J Exp Med* 2004; 202: 41–50.

175. Alciato F, Sainaghi PP, Sola D, *et al.* TNF-α, IL-6, and IL-1 expression is inhibited by GAS6 in monocytes/macrophages. *J Leukoc Biol* 2010; 87: 869–875.

176. Moody DB, Ulrichs T, Muhlecker W, *et al.* CD1c-mediated T-cell recognition of isoprenoid glycolipids in *Mycobacterium tuberculosis* infection. *Nature* 2000; 404: 884–888.

177. Matsunaga I, Sugita M. Mycoketide: a CD1c-presented antigen with important implications in mycobacterial infection. *Clin Dev Immunol* 2012; 2012: 981821.

178. Roy S, Ly D, Li NS, *et al.* Molecular basis of mycobacterial lipid antigen presentation by CD1c and its recognition by αβ T cells. *Proc Natl Acad Sci USA* 2014; 111: E4648–E4657.

179. Roura-Mir C, Wang L, Cheng TY, *et al.* *Mycobacterium tuberculosis* regulates CD1 antigen presentation pathways through TLR-2. *J Immunol* 2005; 175: 1758–1766.

180. Nicol MP, Wilkinson RJ. The clinical consequences of strain diversity in *Mycobacterium tuberculosis*. *Trans R Soc Trop Med Hyg* 2008; 102: 955–965.

181. de Beer JL, van Ingen J, de Vries G, *et al.* Comparative study of IS6110 restriction fragment length polymorphism and variable-number tandem-repeat typing of *Mycobacterium tuberculosis* isolates in the Netherlands, based on a 5-year nationwide survey. *J Clin Microbiol* 2013; 51: 1193–1198.

182. Allix-Beguec C, Harmsen D, Weniger T, *et al.* Evaluation and strategy for use of MIRU-VNTR*plus*, a multifunctional database for online analysis of genotyping data and phylogenetic identification of *Mycobacterium tuberculosis* complex isolates. *J Clin Microbiol* 2008; 46: 2692–2699.

183. Driscoll JR. Spoligotyping for molecular epidemiology of the *Mycobacterium tuberculosis* complex. *Methods Mol Biol* 2009; 551: 117–128.

184. Coll F, McNerney R, Guerra-Assuncao JA, *et al.* A robust SNP barcode for typing *Mycobacterium tuberculosis* complex strains. *Nat Commun* 2014; 5: 4812.

185. Hirsh AE, Tsolaki AG, DeRiemer K, *et al.* Stable association between strains of *Mycobacterium tuberculosis* and their human host populations. *Proc Natl Acad Sci USA* 2004; 101: 4871–4876.

https://doi.org/10.1183/2312508X.10020917

186. Gagneux S, DeRiemer K, Van T, *et al.* Variable host–pathogen compatibility in *Mycobacterium tuberculosis. Proc Natl Acad Sci USA* 2006; 103: 2869–2873.

187. Smith NH, Kremer K, Inwald J, *et al.* Ecotypes of the *Mycobacterium tuberculosis* complex. *J Theor Biol* 2006; 239: 220–225.

188. Gagneux S. Genetic diversity in *Mycobacterium tuberculosis. Curr Top Microbiol Immunol* 2013; 374: 1–25.

189. Galagan JE. Genomic insights into tuberculosis. *Nat Rev Genet* 2014; 15: 307–320.

190. Fenner L, Egger M, Bodmer T, *et al.* HIV infection disrupts the sympatric host–pathogen relationship in human tuberculosis. *PLoS Genet* 2013; 9: e1003318.

191. Mokrousov I, Ly HM, Otten T, *et al.* Origin and primary dispersal of the *Mycobacterium tuberculosis* Beijing genotype: clues from human phylogeography. *Genome Res* 2005; 15: 1357–1364.

192. Stucki D, Brites D, Jeljeli L, *et al. Mycobacterium tuberculosis* lineage 4 comprises globally distributed and geographically restricted sublineages. *Nat Genet* 2016; 48: 1535–1543.

193. Chihota VN, Niehaus A, Streicher EM, *et al.* Geospatial distribution of *Mycobacterium tuberculosis* genotypes in Africa. *PLoS One* 2018; 13: e0200632.

194. Nebenzahl-Guimaraes H, Yimer SA, Holm-Hansen C, *et al.* Genomic characterization of *Mycobacterium tuberculosis* lineage 7 and a proposed name: 'Aethiops vetus'. *Microb Genom* 2016; 2: e000063.

195. Chae H, Shin SJ. Importance of differential identification of *Mycobacterium tuberculosis* strains for understanding differences in their prevalence, treatment efficacy, and vaccine development. *J Microbiol* 2018; 56: 300–311.

196. Romero MM, Balboa L, Basile JI, *et al.* Clinical isolates of *Mycobacterium tuberculosis* differ in their ability to induce respiratory burst and apoptosis in neutrophils as a possible mechanism of immune escape. *Clin Dev Immunol* 2012; 2012: 152546.

197. Wang C, Peyron P, Mestre O, *et al.* Innate immune response to *Mycobacterium tuberculosis* Beijing and other genotypes. *PLoS One* 2010; 5: e13594.

198. Coscolla M, Gagneux S. Consequences of genomic diversity in *Mycobacterium tuberculosis. Semin Immunol* 2014; 26: 431–444.

199. Reiling N, Homolka S, Walter K, *et al.* Clade-specific virulence patterns of *Mycobacterium tuberculosis* complex strains in human primary macrophages and aerogenically infected mice. *MBio* 2013; 4: e00250-13.

200. Ribeiro SC, Gomes LL, Amaral EP, *et al. Mycobacterium tuberculosis* strains of the modern sublineage of the Beijing family are more likely to display increased virulence than strains of the ancient sublineage. *J Clin Microbiol* 2014; 52: 2615–2624.

201. Barczak AK, Domenech P, Boshoff HI, *et al. In vivo* phenotypic dominance in mouse mixed infections with *Mycobacterium tuberculosis* clinical isolates. *J Infect Dis* 2005; 192: 600–606.

202. Thwaites G, Caws M, Chau TT, *et al.* Relationship between *Mycobacterium tuberculosis* genotype and the clinical phenotype of pulmonary and meningeal tuberculosis. *J Clin Microbiol* 2008; 46: 1363–1368.

203. Jeon BY, Kwak J, Hahn MY, *et al. In vivo* characteristics of Korean Beijing *Mycobacterium tuberculosis* strain K1 in an aerosol challenge model and in the Cornell latent tuberculosis model. *J Med Microbiol* 2012; 61: 1373–1379.

204. Nebenzahl-Guimaraes H, Borgdorff MW, Murray MB, *et al.* A novel approach – the propensity to propagate (PTP) method for controlling for host factors in studying the transmission of *Mycobacterium tuberculosis. PLoS One* 2014; 9: e97816.

205. Aguilar D, Hanekom M, Mata D, *et al. Mycobacterium tuberculosis* strains with the Beijing genotype demonstrate variability in virulence associated with transmission. *Tuberculosis* 2010; 90: 319–325.

206. Jones-Lopez EC, Kim S, Fregona G, *et al.* Importance of cough and *M. tuberculosis* strain type as risks for increased transmission within households. *PLoS One* 2014; 9: e100984.

207. Albanna AS, Reed MB, Kotar KV, *et al.* Reduced transmissibility of East African Indian strains of *Mycobacterium tuberculosis. PLoS One* 2011; 6: e25075.

208. Kato-Maeda M, Kim EY, Flores L, *et al.* Differences among sublineages of the East-Asian lineage of *Mycobacterium tuberculosis* in genotypic clustering. *Int J Tuberc Lung Dis* 2010; 14: 538–544.

209. de Jong BC, Hill PC, Aiken A, *et al.* Progression to active tuberculosis, but not transmission, varies by *Mycobacterium tuberculosis* lineage in The Gambia. *J Infect Dis* 2008; 198: 1037–1043.

210. Abebe F, Bjune G. The emergence of Beijing family genotypes of *Mycobacterium tuberculosis* and low-level protection by bacille Calmette–Guerin (BCG) vaccines: is there a link? *Clin Exp Immunol* 2006; 145: 389–397.

211. Zhang L, Ru HW, Chen FZ, *et al.* Variable virulence and efficacy of BCG vaccine strains in mice and correlation with genome polymorphisms. *Mol Ther* 2016; 24: 398–405.

212. Jeon BY, Derrick SC, Lim J, *et al. Mycobacterium bovis* BCG immunization induces protective immunity against nine different *Mycobacterium tuberculosis* strains in mice. *Infect Immun* 2008; 76: 5173–5180.

213. Rook GA, Bahr GM, Stanford JL. The effect of two distinct forms of cell-mediated response to mycobacteria on the protective efficacy of BCG. *Tubercle* 1981; 62: 63–68.

214. McShane H, Williams A. A review of preclinical animal models utilised for TB vaccine evaluation in the context of recent human efficacy data. *Tuberculosis* 2014; 94: 105–110.

215. Lanzas F, Karakousis PC, Sacchettini JC, *et al.* Multidrug-resistant tuberculosis in panama is driven by clonal expansion of a multidrug-resistant *Mycobacterium tuberculosis* strain related to the KZN extensively drug-resistant *M. tuberculosis* strain from South Africa. *J Clin Microbiol* 2013; 51: 3277–3285.

216. Ford CB, Shah RR, Maeda MK, *et al.* *Mycobacterium tuberculosis* mutation rate estimates from different lineages predict substantial differences in the emergence of drug-resistant tuberculosis. *Nat Genet* 2013; 45: 784–790.

217. Buu TN, van Soolingen D, Huyen MN, *et al.* Increased transmission of *Mycobacterium tuberculosis* Beijing genotype strains associated with resistance to streptomycin: a population-based study. *PLoS One* 2012; 7: e42323.

218. Merker M, Blin C, Mona S, *et al.* Evolutionary history and global spread of the *Mycobacterium tuberculosis* Beijing lineage. *Nat Genet* 2015; 47: 242–249.

219. Li QJ, Jiao WW, Yin QQ, *et al.* Positive epistasis of major low-cost drug resistance mutations *rpoB*531-TTG and *katG*315-ACC depends on the phylogenetic background of *Mycobacterium tuberculosis* strains. *Int J Antimicrob Agents* 2017; 49: 757–762.

220. Dou HY, Lin CH, Chen YY, *et al.* Lineage-specific SNPs for genotyping of *Mycobacterium tuberculosis* clinical isolates. *Sci Rep* 2017; 7: 1425.

221. Stucki D, Malla B, Hostettler S, *et al.* Two new rapid SNP-typing methods for classifying *Mycobacterium tuberculosis* complex into the main phylogenetic lineages. *PLoS One* 2012; 7: e41253.

Disclosures: None declared.

Support statement: This work has been funded by FEDER funds, through the Competitiveness Factors Operational Programme (COMPETE), and by national funds, through the Foundation for Science and Technology (FCT), under the scope of project POCI-01-0145-FEDER-007038, and by project NORTE-01-0145-FEDER-000013, supported by the Northern Portugal Regional Operational Programme (NORTE 2020), under the Portugal 2020 Partnership Agreement, through the European Regional Development Fund (FEDER), as well as national funds, through the Foundation for Science and Technology (FCT) by IF/01390/2014 and by FEDER, through the Competitiveness Internationalization Operational Programme (POCI), and by national funds, through the Foundation for Science and Technology (FCT), under the scope of project POCI-01-0145-FEDER-029521.

Acknowledgements: The authors wish to acknowledge Catarina L. Santos for medical writing and editorial services.

https://doi.org/10.1183/2312508X.10020917

Chapter 6

Clinical diagnosis

Jean-Pierre Zellweger[1], Pedro Sousa[2] and Jan Heyckendorf [ID][3,4,5]

Clinical symptoms and signs of TB are very diverse, and depend on the localisation and extent of the disease as well as the age and immunological status of the affected patient. For each localisation, a differential diagnosis has to be considered. Symptoms are generally not specific enough to allow a diagnosis; however, they are indicators of the necessity to perform further diagnostic tests, usually radiographic and bacteriological examinations, in order to obtain a definitive diagnosis and start treatment. Due to the slowly progressive nature of TB, the nonspecific character of symptoms, the difficulty in access to healthcare in many settings or the lack of experience of primary healthcare clinicians, there may be a long delay between the onset of symptoms and the implementation of an appropriate treatment. During this interval, some patients with transmissible forms of TB may infect their contacts and caregivers. Reduction of the diagnostic delay may contribute to the decrease in transmission of TB in the population.

Cite as: Zellweger J-P, Sousa P, Heyckendorf J. Clinical diagnosis. *In:* Migliori GB, Bothamley G, Duarte R, *et al.*, eds. Tuberculosis (ERS Monograph). Sheffield, European Respiratory Society, 2018; pp. 83–98 [https://doi.org/10.1183/2312508X.10021017].

@ERSpublications
TB presents with various nonspecific localisation and symptoms. TB is evolving slowly and may change its presentation over time. In patients with unclear signs/symptoms, TB should be part of the differential diagnosis and appropriate diagnostic tests done. http://ow.ly/cfVQ30lqCfE

The most common symptoms of TB are related to the affected organ and to the presence of an infection. For PTB, the disease usually starts with cough with scanty sputum production, haemoptysis in advanced cases, dyspnoea and chest pain. The general symptoms the consequence of the reaction of the immune system to the infection, mostly in the form of low-grade intermittent fever, sweating (particularly during the night), fatigue and weight loss [1, 2]. For EPTB, the symptoms are very variable, depending on the localisation and extent of the infection [3]. Pain is common in pleural, abdominal and vertebral TB, but may be absent in lymphadenitis and in urogenital and osteoarticular TB. Meningeal TB is evidenced by progressive neurological

[1]Swiss Lung Association, Berne, Switzerland. [2]Family Health Unit Saúde em Família, Porto, Portugal. [3]Division of Clinical Infectious Diseases, Research Center Borstel, Borstel, Germany. [4]German Center for Infection Research (DZIF), TTU TB, Borstel, Germany. [5]International Health/Infectious Diseases, University of Lübeck, Lübeck, Germany.

Correspondence: Jean-Pierre Zellweger, Swiss Lung Association, Chutzenstrasse 10, 3007 Berne, Switzerland. E-mail zellwegerjp@swissonline.ch

Copyright ©ERS 2018. Print ISBN: 978-1-84984-099-6. Online ISBN: 978-1-84984-100-9. Print ISSN: 2312-508X. Online ISSN: 2312-5098.

signs, from headache to blurred vision, with impaired consciousness and coma in the ultimate phase.

The nature and severity of symptoms depend on the age and general immunological state of the patient. In children with PTB, cough is frequent but general symptoms such as failure to thrive and reduced activity are the most prominent signs [4, 5]. Even in children aged <3 years, the combination of persistent cough and failure to thrive has a fair diagnostic sensitivity [6]. In adolescents, the clinical picture and prevalence of symptoms are similar to adults [7]. In elderly patients, the symptoms may be very discrete, with cough, weight loss and fever being less prominent than in young patients [8]. Moreover, elderly patients may have comorbidities that interact with TB and the clinical picture may be a combination of simultaneous diseases. This is also the case in smokers, who may regard coughing as a normal phenomenon.

As TB is a slowly progressive disease, the symptoms are usually very discrete at the beginning, become more prominent with time and depend on the site of disease manifestation. In TB cases discovered by systematic screening (e.g. in migrants or during contact investigations), the prevalence of symptoms may be much lower than in patients spontaneously visiting a health institution because of illness [9]. Depending on the sensitivity of the patient, access to healthcare and experience of the clinician, the diagnosis may be made at an early stage or be delayed until the disease has progressed to large territories [10].

In 2016, 64.6% of cases of TB notified in the WHO European Region were PTB only, 11.7% were PTB and EPTB, and 22.8% were EPTB only, but some countries reported much higher proportions of EPTB (45.3% in the UK and 46% in the Netherlands) [11]. EPTB cases notified in the European Union (EU)/European Economic Area (EEA) were pleural (36.7%), lymphatic (30.5%), skeletal (9.0%), urogenital (6.9%), central nervous system (3.4%), gastrointestinal (2.7%), disseminated (1.5%) and other TB (9.4%) [12].

A TB case can be confirmed bacteriologically or diagnosed clinically [13]. Every effort should be undertaken to collect adequate samples for bacteriological examination, which will enable a definite diagnosis together with determining the identity and drug sensitivity of the strain. Clinical diagnosis is made in the absence of bacteriological confirmation, based on signs and symptoms suggestive of TB, and histological and/or radiological findings, sometimes supported by immune tests (e.g. IGRAs), by a physician or other medical practitioner who has decided to treat the patient with a full course of anti-TB therapy [13]. Clinical diagnosis without bacteriological confirmation should only be accepted in cases where no biological sample can be collected.

This chapter focuses on clinical aspects of TB, i.e. typical and atypical signs and symptoms, differential diagnosis, and delayed diagnosis.

Pulmonary tuberculosis

Typical and atypical signs and symptoms

Classic symptoms of PTB include persistent cough, haemoptysis, fever, night sweats and weight loss [14]. Cough, the most common symptom of PTB, may be nonproductive early

https://doi.org/10.1183/2312508X.10021017

in the course of the illness, but sputum is usually produced as inflammation continues [15]. Currently, there is no strong evidence concerning the minimal cough duration for when to screen for TB [16]. Coughing for $\geqslant 2$ weeks is the most common temporal criterion to consider the possible presence of TB [17, 18]. For high TB prevalence countries or settings it is suggested to initiate the evaluation for TB regardless of cough duration [16]. Additional to cough of any duration, the presence of fever, night sweats or weight loss has a particular relevance in increasing the diagnostic sensitivity in individuals with increased susceptibility, such as people with HIV infection [16, 17]. Haemoptysis is mostly self-limited, but can be massive and fatal [19]. TB-associated haemoptysis may result from bronchiectasis, rupture of Rasmussen's aneurysm, bacterial or fungal infection in a residual cavity, or erosion of broncholithiasis [15, 20]. Pleuritic pain can also occur due to inflammation of the lung parenchyma adjacent to a pleural surface [14]. Dyspnoea is unusual unless there is extensive disease with severe lung destruction [15]. The prevalence of clinical symptoms in smear-positive TB patients from four clinics in The Gambia is reported in table 1 [1].

Physical signs, which can be elicited during the clinical examination, are usually absent, except if the pulmonary lesions are extensive and give rise to a consolidation of a large territory, liable to be identified by percussion of the thorax. Crackles, wheezing and bronchial breath sounds may be heard, and these signs were used as diagnostic criteria for TB prior to the identification of *Mycobacterium tuberculosis* as the infectious agent [2, 14]. Clubbing occurs in up to one-third of patients with PTB [21, 22]. Uveitis, erythema nodosum and other skin conditions may be the first signs of PTB, which are thought to be caused by a hypersensitivity response to a variety of *M. tuberculosis* antigens [14, 23–25]. The prevalence of physical signs in smear-positive TB patients from four clinics in The Gambia is reported in table 1 [1].

Table 1. Prevalence of clinical symptoms and signs in 340 adult patients with smear-positive TB from four clinics in The Gambia

Symptoms	
Cough	100.0
Productive cough	97.1
Chest pain	78.8
Dyspnoea	53.8
Haemoptysis	35.9
Side pain	84.7
Night sweats	77.9
Fever	94.4
Weight loss	97.4
Anorexia	82.1
Other symptoms	14.4
Signs	
Pallor	37.1
Wasting	68.5
Clubbing	15.3
Lymphadenopathy	15.3
Hepatomegaly	2.9
Splenomegaly	2.1
Oedema	0.6

Data are presented as %. Reproduced from [1] with permission.

The classical symptoms of PTB, albeit not specific, may be the reason for a patient's visit to a healthcare institution or be used as a screening method for population surveys. In any case, the symptoms alone will not be sufficient to make a diagnosis of TB, but will be a first indicator of the necessity to perform further investigations, in most cases radiography of the thorax and, if this is abnormal, a bacteriological examination of sputum. In a prospective study conducted in South Africa among patients with cough and/or difficult breathing, a clinical evaluation by a nurse using a guideline in the form of an algorithm identified TB patients with a sensitivity of 76% and a specificity of 77%, and missed only four out of 40 patients with bacteriologically documented TB [26]. In that study, weight loss, pleuritic pain and night sweats were independently associated with bacteriologically confirmed TB. In another study, a clinical score integrating symptoms (cough, haemoptysis, dyspnoea and chest pain) and signs (fever, anaemia, tachycardia, abnormal findings at auscultation, low body mass index and wasting) was strongly correlated with clinical outcome and mortality [27]. A study comparing the relative contribution of symptoms and chest radiography in a TB prevalence survey demonstrated that the sensitivity of individual symptoms was low, ranging from 0.1 for fever to 0.54 for cough $\geqslant 2$ weeks, with a global specificity of 0.67, and that the sensitivity was lower than the sensitivity of chest radiography, but the specificity of both was similar (table 2) [28].

Children who have been in contact with a case of TB have an increased risk of infection and disease, and should be examined for potential signs of infection or disease. Efforts should be made to obtain biological samples (e.g. by induced sputum, gastric tubing or

Table 2. Sensitivity and specificity of classical TB symptoms and chest radiography in a population survey in South Africa[#]

	Smear-positive n (%)	Sensitivity (95% CI)	Specificity (95% CI)
Cough		0.67 (0.43–0.90)	0.82 (0.79–0.84)
No or <2 weeks	6 (0.7)		
$\geqslant$2 weeks	12 (5.7)		
Unknown	2 (2.9)		
Haemoptysis		0.30 (0.10–0.50)	0.92 (0.88–0.96)
No	14 (1.2)		
Yes	6 (15.0)		
Night sweats		0.60 (0.36–0.84)	0.85 (0.83–0.88)
No	8 (0.8)		
Yes	12 (6.7)		
Fever		0.10 (0.00–0.23)	0.96 (0.94–0.97)
No	18 (1.6)		
Yes	2 (3.8)		
Weight loss		0.50 (0.29–0.71)	0.83 (0.81–0.86)
No	10 (1.0)		
Yes	10 (4.9)		
Symptoms		0.75 (0.55–0.95)	0.67 (0.64–0.70)
No symptoms	5 (0.6)		
Any symptom	15 (3.9)		
Chest radiograph		0.95 (0.85–1.00)	0.66 (0.63–0.69)
Normal	1 (0.1)		
Abnormal	19 (4.7)		

[#]: 20 smear-positive TB cases among 1170 patients. Reproduced from [28] with permission.

https://doi.org/10.1183/2312508X.10021017

stool examination) for bacteriological tests. A symptom-based screening approach may help to identify those who need further evaluation and preventive or curative treatment [29]. A systematic approach based on the assessment of risk factors for infection and disease has been proposed for low-resource settings [30].

Differential diagnosis

No symptom is unique to TB and all of the symptoms may be observed in other pulmonary infections and diseases, *e.g.* COPD exacerbations, bronchiectasis, pneumonia, fungal lung disease, lung cancer and some immune disorders. Therefore, symptoms alone do not allow a diagnosis, but do point to the necessity to perform further diagnostic tests, usually chest radiography or computed tomography and bacteriological examination of sputum, bronchial fluid, gastric fluid or laryngeal swabs.

In elderly patients, the symptoms are usually less prominent than in young patients and may overlap with common symptoms (*e.g.* dyspnoea, fatigue, chest pain and cough) due to other frequent diseases in this age category, such as chronic pulmonary or cardiac disorders.

In children and in patients who are unable to produce sputum samples, the diagnosis often has to rely on a probability, integrating the symptoms and other information, such as recent TB contact, origin of the patient and probability of prior exposure to TB, results of biological tests (*e.g.* IGRAs), and radiology, but a final diagnosis of TB should not be made before all possible options for obtaining samples for bacteriological examination have been exhausted. A scoring system including the history of TB contact, incidence in the country of origin and classical symptoms has been used for the screening of migrants for active TB at the Swiss border, and has demonstrated a sensitivity comparable to systematic screening by chest radiography, albeit with a longer delay until the initiation of treatment [31].

Extrapulmonary tuberculosis

Pleural tuberculosis

Typical and atypical signs and symptoms
Pleural TB usually presents with fever, nonproductive cough and pleuritic chest pain [32, 33]. Other symptoms include breathlessness as the effusion increases, night sweats, weight loss and malaise. Tuberculous pleural effusion is typically unilateral, small to moderate in size and characterised by a lymphocytic differential, predominantly exudative with increased adenosine deaminase [33–35]. Neutrophil-predominant pleural effusions can occur at an early stage during the course of the disease [33, 34]. Pleural thickening, empyema and trapped lung are possible complications at later stages [36].

Physical examination of the thorax may reveal asymmetric expansion, decreased tactile fremitus on palpation, dullness to percussion, reduced or absent breath sounds over the pleural effusion, decreased vocal resonance, crackles and audible pleural rub [37].

Differential diagnosis
Malignancy (*e.g.* metastatic lung cancer, mesothelioma and lymphoma), bacterial and fungal infections, autoimmune diseases, pulmonary embolism, post-coronary artery bypass

graft, post-myocardial infarction pancreatitis, benign asbestos effusion, and yellow nail syndrome are some examples of exudative pleural effusions [35].

Lymph node tuberculosis

Typical and atypical signs and symptoms

Extrathoracic and intrathoracic lymph node TB accounts for 20.1% and 10.4%, respectively, of the EPTB cases notified in the EU/EEA [12]. Lymphatic intrathoracic TB occurs predominantly in children aged 0–14 years (40.9%) [12], usually in association with primary PTB [14]. Extrathoracic lymphatic TB mostly affects young adults aged 25–44 years (38.8%) [12].

The cervical region is the most commonly involved in nearly two-thirds of the cases, followed by mediastinal and axillary regions [38]. Historically, tuberculous cervical lymphadenitis is also known as scrofula or the "King's Evil", from when royal touch was believed to cure the disease (a belief based on the observation that some forms of cervical lymphadenitis tend to resolve spontaneously!) [39].

JONES and CAMPBELL [40] classified peripheral tuberculous lymphadenitis into five stages. Stage I (hyperplasia): enlarged, firm, mobile, discrete and slightly tender lymph nodes. Stage II (periadenitis): the lymph nodes become larger, rubbery in consistency and fixed to surrounding tissues with consequent loss of mobility. Stage III (abscess formation): an abscess may appear as a fluctuant swelling with little or no tenderness. Stage IV ("collar-stud" abscess): a purplish thin skin covers a fluctuant swelling and a deeper induration is palpable beneath the deep fascia. Stage V (sinus formation): nonhealing fistulas to the skin. Patients with ETTB lymphadenitis may also present with cough and/or systemic symptoms, such as weight loss, fever and night sweats [41, 42].

With regard to intrathoracic lymphatic TB, the most frequent symptoms are fever, weight loss, chest pain and cough [43]. Infrequently, dysphagia may occur related to a tracheo-oesophageal fistula or extrinsic compression of the gastrointestinal tract [44]. Chylothorax due to thoracic duct obstruction [45], pyopericardium and cardiac tamponade have also been described [46].

Differential diagnosis

Essential considerations in lymphadenopathy evaluation include the age of the patient, location and time duration of the lymphadenopathy, and presence of splenomegaly, fever, or other associated signs or symptoms [47]. Clinical diagnosis is often difficult as several diseases can follow the same course as lymphadenopathy. The acronym "CHICAGO" was proposed to group the extensive differential diagnoses: Cancers, Hypersensitivity syndromes, Infections, Connective tissue diseases, Atypical lymphoproliferative disorders, Granulomatous diseases, and Other unusual causes of lymphadenopathy [47].

Bone and joint tuberculosis

Typical and atypical signs and symptoms

Bone and joint TB account for 9.0% of the EPTB cases notified in the EU/EEA. In particular, the spine is involved in 3.9%, while other bones/joints are involved in 5.1% of

https://doi.org/10.1183/2312508X.10021017

skeletal TB cases [12]. In developed countries, the disease usually affects natives aged >55 years and immigrants aged 20–35 years [48].

The spine is the most commonly affected site (Pott's disease), followed by arthritis in weight-bearing joints and extraspinal tuberculous osteomyelitis [48, 49]. Thoracic and lumbar vertebrae are the most frequently affected levels [48, 50, 51]. The onset of symptoms is usually insidious and the disease progresses slowly [52]. Back pain is the most common symptom, followed by night sweats and fever [51]. At physical examination, restricted motion is the most common feature, followed by painful percussion and kyphosis [51]. Neurological deficits, cold abscesses and draining skin sinus tracts can also be found in patients with spinal TB [48, 49, 51]. Hip flexion may cause pain in the groin when a paraspinal abscess develops within the psoas muscle [14].

Articular TB mostly occurs in weight-bearing joints, such as the hips and knees, usually as monoarthritis [48]. The earliest symptom is pain, which may precede swelling and other signs of inflammation, for weeks or months. Systemic symptoms are usually absent [48]. The presence of cold abscesses, sinus tracts and cartilage destruction may be helpful in making the diagnosis [48, 53].

Extraspinal tuberculous osteomyelitis can affect virtually any bone. The onset is often insidious, and usually presents as a cold abscess with swelling and mild erythema and pain. Similar to articular TB and tuberculous spondylodiscitis, sinus tracts may also be observed [48].

Differential diagnosis
Bone TB infection may mimic several diseases, including primary and metastatic neoplastic disease (*e.g.* multiple myeloma and metastatic carcinoma), traumatic injury, osteoporosis, eosinophilic granuloma, sarcoidosis, cystic angiomatosis, bacterial and fungal infections, brucellosis, Paget's disease, and Scheuermann's disease [14, 48, 54, 55]. The differential diagnoses for joint TB include pyogenic and rheumatoid arthritis, tumours, gout, regional osteoporosis, idiopathic chondrolysis, brucellar arthritis, and pigmented villonodular synovitis [48, 55].

Urogenital tuberculosis

Typical and atypical signs and symptoms
Urogenital TB includes kidney TB, urinary tract TB, and both male and female genital TB [56]. The disease mainly affects adults aged 45–64 years (37.0%) and ⩾65 years (35.7%) [12]. Young children are rarely affected due to the long latency period after the primary TB infection [57–59].

The kidney is the most commonly affected organ of the urogenital system [59]. Renal infection usually develops slowly and without symptoms, but it can be highly destructive with cases of unilateral renal exclusion and renal failure [59–61]. Bladder TB usually manifests with urinary symptoms of frequency, urgency and haematuria [56]. Sterile pyuria, with or without haematuria, is a classic finding [61, 62]. Urinary TB is frequently misdiagnosed as chronic infection until bacteriological examination reveals the diagnosis. Other clinical features of urinary tract TB include back, flank and suprapubic pain [63]. Systemic symptoms are unusual [64].

The fallopian tubes are the most common site involved in female genital TB [65]. Female genital TB usually presents with infertility, pelvic pain and abnormal uterine bleeding [65]. Physical examination may reveal a pelvic mass, uterine enlargement, fistulas, and ulcerative and hypertrophic lesions in the cervix, vagina or vulva [65].

The epididymis is the commonest site affected in male genital TB [57]. Patients with male genital TB may present with complaints of scrotal mass (usually painless, but can be painful), urinary frequency, nocturia, dysuria, haematuria, haemospermia and infertility [57]. Physical examination may reveal prostatic indurations and nodules on rectal examination, hydrocele, sinus tracts discharging pus, ulcerative penile lesions, and a nodular enlargement of the epididymis [57].

Differential diagnosis
The differential diagnoses of urogenital TB include benign and malignant tumours, nephrolithiasis, cystic kidney, pyelonephritis, xanthogranulomatous pyelonephritis, and urinary malakoplakia [55, 64].

Central nervous system tuberculosis

Typical and atypical signs and symptoms
Diagnosing tuberculous meningitis is a clinical challenge due to the nonspecific characteristics of the signs and symptoms. In adults, the disease usually begins with malaise, weight loss, low-grade fever and gradual onset of headache over 1–2 weeks. In 2–3 weeks, the patient experiences worsening headache, vomiting and confusion, which at this stage may quickly evolve into stupor, coma and death if untreated [66, 67]. Clinical signs include neck stiffness, cranial nerve palsies, plegia/paresis, movement disorders and seizures [66, 67]. The most frequent symptom at hospital admission is headache, followed by fever and nausea or vomiting. The most frequent sign is neck stiffness. Cranial nerve palsy can be detected in 24% of tuberculous meningitis cases, most commonly the abducens nerve followed by the oculomotor nerve [68]. Atypical presentations include slowly progressive dementia, acute meningitis similar to pyogenic bacterial infection and TB encephalopathy [67, 69]. Young children and immunosuppressed adults have the highest risk to develop tuberculous meningitis [66, 70, 71]. In children, clinical features include apathy, irritability, decreased level of consciousness, anorexia, poor weight gain, headache, fever, vomiting (without diarrhoea), malaise, signs of increased intracranial pressure such as bulging fontanelle, cranial nerve palsy, and focal neurological signs and seizures [66, 67].

Cerebral tuberculomas without meningitis are often asymptomatic, but may either present signs and symptoms of focal brain lesions or increased intracranial pressure [72, 73]. The most common clinical manifestations are cranial nerve deficits, altered mental status, hemiparesis, seizures and headache [72].

Spinal cord TB is mostly related to the progression of vertebral tuberculous osteomyelitis (Pott's disease). Signs and symptoms are variable according to localisation, and include radicular pain, bladder dysfunction and plegia/paresis [71].

Differential diagnosis
The differential diagnoses that should be considered include bacterial, fungal, viral and parasitic infections, sarcoidosis, endocarditis, and collagen vascular disorders (*e.g.* systemic lupus erythematosus and polyarteritis) [55, 74, 75].

https://doi.org/10.1183/2312508X.10021017

Disseminated tuberculosis

Typical and atypical signs and symptoms

TB may develop in several organs simultaneously, usually by haematogenous dissemination (miliary TB, characterised by the presence of small nodular lesions with similar size) or sequentially (disseminated TB, characterised by the development of lesions of different size and stage in several organs one after the other, by continuity or lymphatic dissemination). The clinical manifestations of miliary TB depend on the organs involved. Fever, weakness, night sweats, anorexia, weight loss and cough are frequent presenting symptoms [76, 77]. Prolonged fever with daily morning spikes is also described to be characteristic of miliary TB [78]. Physical examination may reveal lymphadenopathy, splenomegaly, hepatomegaly, jaundice, cutaneous lesions and other findings related to the involved organs [76, 79]. Ophthalmoscopic examination may reveal choroidal tubercles, which are suggestive of disease [76, 77]. Atypical presentations include cryptic miliary TB and fulminant disease with acute respiratory distress syndrome and shock [76, 77, 80–82].

The clinical manifestations of disseminated TB are usually the addition of symptoms related to the organs involved. Constitutional symptoms are usually severe.

Differential diagnosis

The differential diagnoses include various infections (*e.g.* due to NTM or fungi), disseminated tumours, granulomatosis diseases and systemic diseases [55].

Abdominal tuberculosis

Typical and atypical signs and symptoms

Gastrointestinal TB most commonly affects the ileocaecal region followed by the jejunum and colon [83]. Regardless of the gastrointestinal portion involved, abdominal pain and systemic symptoms, such as weight loss, fever and anorexia, are frequent [84].

Additional to these symptoms, oesophageal TB may present with retrosternal pain, dysphagia and odynophagia [83, 84]. Cough while eating or massive haematemesis may represent the presence of complications associated with oesophageal TB such as tracheo-oesophageal or aorto-oesophageal fistulas. Gastric TB may present with vague epigastric discomfort or pain, features of gastric outlet obstruction, or a palpable mass [83, 84]. Small intestinal TB usually manifests features of obstruction, most frequently at the ileocaecal valve, such as colicky abdominal pain, nausea, vomiting and abdominal distension [83, 84]. Fistulas from the small intestine to vascular structures, skin and other gastrointestinal sites have been described [84]. Additional to abdominal pain and systemic features, colorectal TB may follow the same course as with diarrhoea, altered bowel habits and haematochezia [84]. When colonic TB involves the appendix, the presentation can be similar to classical appendicitis [84].

Peritoneal TB generally develops over a period of several weeks to months [85]. Abdominal pain is the commonest symptom and ascites the most frequent clinical sign [85]. Other clinical features include fever, weight loss, diarrhoea, constipation, abdominal tenderness, abdominal distension, hepatomegaly and splenomegaly [85, 86]. A large proportion of patients with abdominal TB have concomitant involvement of the lungs or pleura [87].

Differential diagnosis

Abdominal TB can imitate several other diseases such as Crohn's disease, malignancy (*e.g.* carcinoma, lymphoma, peritoneal carcinomatosis and gastrointestinal stromal tumour), NTM peritonitis, pseudo-membranous and ischaemic colitis, cirrhosis with spontaneous bacterial peritonitis, peptic ulcer disease, and amoebic colitis [55, 86].

Diagnostic delay

One of the greatest challenges in practice is the fact that a long time period may exist between the onset of symptoms and the final diagnosis of TB. This may be due to the slowly progressive nature of the disease, the apparent banality of symptoms (*e.g.* for most smokers cough is just normal and not a symptom of disease), the obstacles to access to healthcare, particularly for patients who belong to an underserved population such as undocumented migrants or persons without insurance coverage, and the experience and knowledge of the physician who receives the patient.

Total diagnosis delay is defined as the time between the onset of symptoms and initiation of treatment. Patient delay comprises the period from the debut of symptoms to the patient's first contact with a medical provider. Healthcare system delay is defined as the time from the patient's first medical consultation until initiation of treatment. Total diagnosis delay includes the sum of diagnosis delay by the patient and diagnosis delay by the healthcare system [88].

Several studies have analysed the duration and causes of delays in the management of patients with TB [89–91]. Most studies report an average duration of the total delay of 2–3 months [91, 92]. In some studies, the patient's delay is longer than the health system's delay, *e.g.* in undocumented migrants, whereas the health system's delay may be longer for patients belonging to the resident population, for whom the *a priori* likelihood of TB is considered as very low. A study in the USA demonstrated that undocumented migrants had a higher frequency of cough and haemoptysis and a longer duration of symptoms compared with US-born persons before having a medical evaluation for PTB [93]. In a meta-analysis, the main factors associated with delay were immunodeficiency, presence of chronic cough, low access to healthcare, repeated visits to the same healthcare facility or referral to several health institutions, reflecting the perplexity of medical doctors facing a disease they do not understand and do not recognise [89].

In countries where the TB incidence is high and most medical doctors have experience with the detection of TB, the delay may be shorter than in countries with a low incidence [94], but a large proportion of patients may wait for prolonged periods or the occurrence of several symptoms before visiting a health institution, or visit health institutions where no diagnostic facilities for TB are available [95]. Furthermore, the management of patients in the private sector may be less efficient than in health institutions depending on the national TB programme [96, 97]. Meeting with physicians and nurses with a broad experience in the diagnosis and management of TB, and knowledge of the history and origin of the patients, increases the diagnostic accuracy [98]. In countries with a low prevalence of TB, several studies report a progressive increase in the proportion of advanced (and transmissible) forms of TB, probably associated with the decrease in experience and awareness of TB by the health professionals, with increasing delays in diagnosis [10, 99].

https://doi.org/10.1183/2312508X.10021017

During the period between the first manifestation of symptoms and diagnosis, a patient with active TB may infect several other susceptible individuals and thus contribute to the transmission in the community. The infectiousness is low for an individual who has only recently become infectious and increases over time, tending to a saturation value [100]. To stop the spread of TB, the duration of infectiousness has to be kept to a minimum through an early diagnosis and treatment [101]. At the individual level, delay in treatment was associated with more severe clinical presentation [102] and mortality [103–105]. House-to-house screening activities and the availability of diagnostic clinics near the place of residence and work increase the TB case detection rate, whereas health promotion activities do not seem to increase the TB case detection rate [106].

Conclusion

No symptom or sign is specific for TB and any symptom frequently seen in TB may be caused by other diseases. The diagnosis of TB should not be made solely on the basis of clinical symptoms and signs, but symptoms are usually the first reason for a patient to seek medical attention and care, and thus should prompt further examination. Whenever possible, the final diagnosis should be documented by a bacteriological test, but in special instances (*e.g.* young children and EPTB) the diagnosis may have to be made on the basis of a simultaneous occurrence of several symptoms or signs and radiological features suggestive of TB.

The diagnostic delay is a problem in clinical practice as the patients may continue to actively transmit TB to their close contacts and caregivers during the period before the initiation of adequate therapy. Even in low-incidence regions, due attention to suspect symptoms must be maintained.

Case report
A young healthy Swiss bank employee, occasional smoker, developed left-sided chest pain, fever, unusual fatigue and cough in January 2006. Chest radiography demonstrated a left-sided pleural collection. A computed tomography (CT) scan revealed an infiltrate at the apex of the left lung (figure 1). The pleural fluid contained a lymphocytic exudative effusion, but smear and culture for TB remained negative. Over the following years, the patient suffered from repeated episodes of cough and fever, all apparently attributed to smoking and viral infections. Further chest radiography confirmed the presence of an infiltrate in the left upper lobe, with the progressive development of a cavity, which was overlooked by the family physician over the next months. Chest radiography (figure 2) and a new CT scan (figure 3) in April 2012 confirmed the extent of the infiltrate and the presence of a large cavity. A sputum examination was finally performed (during a visit to another medical doctor) and revealed the presence of mycobacteria, confirmed by culture and PCR as being *Mycobacterium tuberculosis*. In the meantime, the patient had infected his sister and two colleagues.

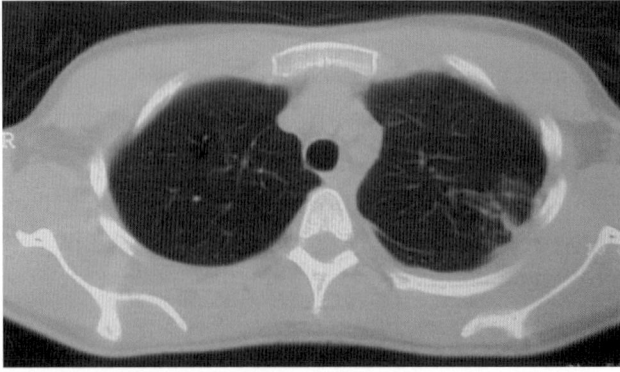

Figure 1. Computed tomography scan: January 2006.

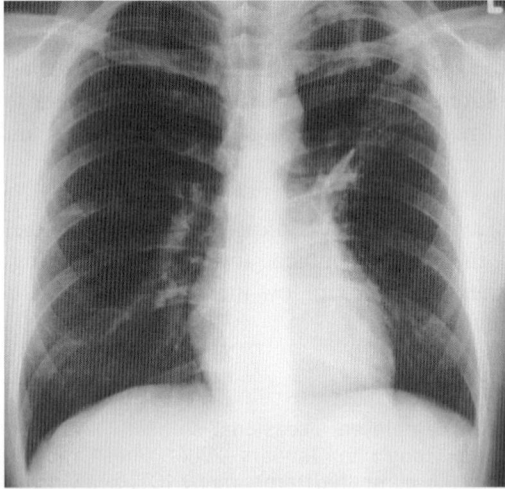

Figure 2. Chest radiograph: April 2012.

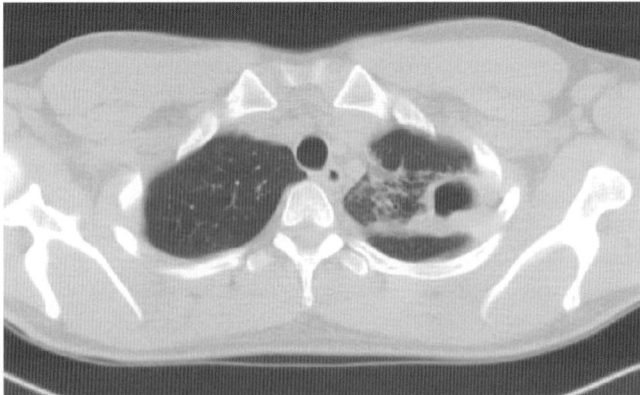

Figure 3. Computed tomography scan: April 2012.

https://doi.org/10.1183/2312508X.10021017

References

1. Rathman G, Sillah J, Hill PC, *et al.* Clinical and radiological presentation of 340 adults with smear-positive tuberculosis in The Gambia. *Int J Tuberc Lung Dis* 2003; 7: 942–947.
2. Laennec RTH. Traite de l'auscultation mediate et des maladies des poumons et du coeur. [A Treatise on Mediate Auscultation and on Diseases of the Lungs and Heart.] Paris, J.S. Chaude, 1826.
3. Norbis L, Alagna R, Tortoli E, *et al.* Challenges and perspectives in the diagnosis of extrapulmonary tuberculosis. *Expert Rev Anti Infect Ther* 2014; 12: 633–647.
4. Perez-Velez CM, Marais BJ. Tuberculosis in children. *N Engl J Med* 2012; 367: 348–361.
5. World Health Organization. Guidance for National Tuberculosis Programmes in the Management of Tuberculosis in Children. 2nd Edn. Geneva, WHO, 2014.
6. Marais BJ, Gie RP, Hesseling AC, *et al.* A refined symptom-based approach to diagnose pulmonary tuberculosis in children. *Pediatrics* 2006; 118: e1350–e1359.
7. Wong KS, Huang YC, Lai SH, *et al.* Validity of symptoms and radiographic features in predicting positive AFB smears in adolescents with tuberculosis. *Int J Tuberc Lung Dis* 2010; 14: 155–159.
8. Cruz-Hervert LP, Garcia-Garcia L, Ferreyra-Reyes L, *et al.* Tuberculosis in ageing: high rates, complex diagnosis and poor clinical outcomes. *Age Ageing* 2012; 41: 488–495.
9. Ravessoud M, Zellweger JP. Presentation clinique de la tuberculose chez les immigrants vus au Dispensaire antituberculeux de Lausanne. [Clinical presentation of tuberculosis among immigrants seen at the antituberculosis outpatient clinic in Lausanne.] *Schweiz Med Wochenschr* 1992; 122: 1037–1043.
10. Wallace RM, Kammerer JS, Iademarco MF, *et al.* Increasing proportions of advanced pulmonary tuberculosis reported in the united states: are delays in diagnosis on the rise? *Am J Respir Crit Care Med* 2009; 180: 1016–1022.
11. European Centre for Disease Prevention and Control/WHO Regional Office for Europe. Tuberculosis Surveillance and Monitoring in Europe 2018 – 2016 Data. Stockholm, European Centre for Disease Prevention and Control, 2018.
12. Sandgren A, Hollo V, van der Werf MJ. Extrapulmonary tuberculosis in the European Union and European Economic Area, 2002 to 2011. *Euro Surveill* 2013; 18 (12): 20431.
13. World Health Organization. Definitions and Reporting Framework for Tuberculosis – 2013 Revision. Geneva, WHO, 2013.
14. Loddenkemper R, Lipman M, Zumla A. Clinical aspects of adult tuberculosis. *Cold Spring Harb Perspect Med* 2015; 6: a017848.
15. American Thoracic Society, Centers for Disease Control and Prevention. Diagnostic standards and classification of tuberculosis in adults and children. *Am J Respir Crit Care Med* 2000; 161: 1376–1395.
16. Field SK, Escalante P, Fisher DA, *et al.* Cough due to TB and other chronic infections: CHEST Guideline and Expert Panel Report. *Chest* 2018; 153: 467–497.
17. TB CARE I. International Standards for Tuberculosis Care. 3rd Edn. The Hague, TB CARE I, 2014.
18. Bastos LG, Fonseca LS, Mello FC, *et al.* Prevalence of pulmonary tuberculosis among respiratory symptomatic subjects in an out-patient primary health unit. *Int J Tuberc Lung Dis* 2007; 11: 156–160.
19. Giraldo-Montoya AM, Rodriguez-Morales AJ, Hernandez-Hurtado JD, *et al.* Rasmussen aneurysm: a rare but not gone complication of tuberculosis. *Int J Infect Dis* 2018; 69: 8–10.
20. Seo JB, Song KS, Lee JS, *et al.* Broncholithiasis: review of the causes with radiologic–pathologic correlation. *Radiographics* 2002; 22: S199–S213.
21. Reeve PA, Harries AD, Nkhoma WA, *et al.* Clubbing in African patients with pulmonary tuberculosis. *Thorax* 1987; 42: 986–987.
22. Ddungu H, Johnson JL, Smieja M, *et al.* Digital clubbing in tuberculosis – relationship to HIV infection, extent of disease and hypoalbuminemia. *BMC Infect Dis* 2006; 6: 45.
23. Schwartz RA, Nervi SJ. Erythema nodosum: a sign of systemic disease. *Am Fam Physician* 2007; 75: 695–700.
24. Requena L, Yus ES. Erythema nodosum. *Dermatol Clin* 2008; 26: 425–438.
25. Shakarchi FI. Ocular tuberculosis: current perspectives. *Clin Ophthalmol* 2015; 9: 2223–2227.
26. English RG, Bachmann MO, Bateman ED, *et al.* Diagnostic accuracy of an integrated respiratory guideline in identifying patients with respiratory symptoms requiring screening for pulmonary tuberculosis: a cross-sectional study. *BMC Pulm Med* 2006; 6: 22.
27. Wejse C, Gustafson P, Nielsen J, *et al.* TBscore: signs and symptoms from tuberculosis patients in a low-resource setting have predictive value and may be used to assess clinical course. *Scand J Infect Dis* 2008; 40: 111–120.
28. den Boon S, White NW, van Lill SW, *et al.* An evaluation of symptom and chest radiographic screening in tuberculosis prevalence surveys. *Int J Tuberc Lung Dis* 2006; 10: 876–882.
29. Triasih R, Robertson CF, Duke T, *et al.* A prospective evaluation of the symptom-based screening approach to the management of children who are contacts of tuberculosis cases. *Clin Infect Dis* 2015; 60: 12–18.
30. Perez-Velez CM, Roya-Pabon CL, Marais BJ. A systematic approach to diagnosing intra-thoracic tuberculosis in children. *J Infect* 2017; 74: Suppl. 1, S74–S83.

31. Schneeberger Geisler S, Helbling P, Zellweger JP, *et al.* Screening for tuberculosis in asylum seekers: comparison of chest radiography with an interview-based system. *Int J Tuberc Lung Dis* 2010; 14: 1388–1394.

32. Jeon D. Tuberculous pleurisy: an update. *Tuberc Respir Dis* 2014; 76: 153–159.

33. Porcel JM. Tuberculous pleural effusion. *Lung* 2009; 187: 263–270.

34. Hooper C, Lee YCG, Maskell N. Investigation of a unilateral pleural effusion in adults: British Thoracic Society pleural disease guideline 2010. *Thorax* 2010; 65: Suppl. 2, ii4–ii17.

35. Valdes L, Alvarez D, San Jose E, *et al.* Tuberculous pleurisy: a study of 254 patients. *Arch Intern Med* 1998; 158: 2017–2021.

36. Sahn SA. Pleural thickening, trapped lung, and chronic empyema as sequelae of tuberculous pleural effusion: don't sweat the pleural thickening. *Int J Tuberc Lung Dis* 2002; 6: 461–464.

37. Wong CL, Holroyd-Leduc J, Straus SE. Does this patient have a pleural effusion? *JAMA* 2009; 301: 309–317.

38. Geldmacher H, Taube C, Kroeger C, *et al.* Assessment of lymph node tuberculosis in northern Germany: a clinical review. *Chest* 2002; 121: 1177–1182.

39. Bray FN, Alsaidan M, Simmons BJ, *et al.* Scrofula and the divine right of royalty: the King's Touch. *JAMA Dermatol* 2015; 151: 702.

40. Jones PG, Campbell PE. Tuberculous lymphadenitis in childhood: the significance of anonymous mycobacteria. *Br J Surg* 1962; 50: 302–314.

41. Dandapat MC, Mishra BM, Dash SP, *et al.* Peripheral lymph node tuberculosis: a review of 80 cases. *Br J Surg* 1990; 77: 911–912.

42. Prasad KC, Sreedharan S, Chakravarthy Y, *et al.* Tuberculosis in the head and neck: experience in India. *J Laryngol Otol* 2007; 121: 979–985.

43. Dhand S, Fisher M, Fewell JW. Intrathoracic tuberculous lymphadenopathy in adults. *JAMA* 1979; 241: 505–507.

44. Rathinam S, Kanagavel M, Tiruvadanan BS, *et al.* Dysphagia due to tuberculosis. *Eur J Cardiothorac Surg* 2006; 30: 833–836.

45. Kutlu O, Demirbas S, Sakin A. Chylothorax due to tuberculosis lymphadenitis. *North Clin Istanb* 2016; 3: 225–228.

46. Kasilingam SK, Sinha N, Kambar V, *et al.* Mediastinal tubercular lymph node eroding into pericardium causing acute pyopericardium and cardiac tamponade. *Trop Doct* 2014; 44: 114–115.

47. Habermann TM, Steensma DP. Lymphadenopathy. *Mayo Clin Proc* 2000; 75: 723–732.

48. Pigrau-Serrallach C, Rodríguez-Pardo D. Bone and joint tuberculosis. *Eur Spine J* 2013; 22: Suppl. 4, 556–566.

49. Garg RK, Somvanshi DS. Spinal tuberculosis: a review. *J Spinal Cord Med* 2011; 34: 440–454.

50. Gehlot PS, Chaturvedi S, Kashyap R, *et al.* Pott's spine: retrospective analysis of MRI scans of 70 cases. *J Clin Diagn Res* 2012; 6: 1534–1538.

51. Shi T, Zhang Z, Dai F, *et al.* Retrospective study of 967 patients with spinal tuberculosis. *Orthopedics* 2016; 39: e838–e843.

52. Pertuiset E, Beaudreuil J, Liote F, *et al.* Spinal tuberculosis in adults. A study of 103 cases in a developed country, 1980–1994. *Medicine* 1999; 78: 309–320.

53. Pattamapaspong N, Muttarak M, Sivasomboon C. Tuberculosis arthritis and tenosynovitis. *Semin Musculoskelet Radiol* 2011; 15: 459–469.

54. Kelley MA, El-Najjar MY. Natural variation and differential diagnosis of skeletal changes in tuberculosis. *Am J Phys Anthropol* 1980; 52: 153–167.

55. Lange C, Mori T. Advances in the diagnosis of tuberculosis. *Respirology* 2010; 15: 220–240.

56. Kulchavenya E, Naber K, Bjerklund Johansen TE. Urogenital tuberculosis: classification, diagnosis, and treatment. *Eur Urology Suppl* 2016; 15: 112–121.

57. Yadav S, Singh P, Hemal A, *et al.* Genital tuberculosis: current status of diagnosis and management. *Transl Androl Urol* 2017; 6: 222–233.

58. Cek M, Lenk S, Naber KG, *et al.* EAU guidelines for the management of genitourinary tuberculosis. *Eur Urol* 2005; 48: 353–362.

59. Figueiredo AA, Lucon AM. Urogenital tuberculosis: update and review of 8961 cases from the world literature. *Rev Urol* 2008; 10: 207–217.

60. Kerr WK, Gale GL, Peterson KS. Reconstructive surgery for genitourinary tuberculosis. *J Urol* 1969; 101: 254–266.

61. Kapoor R, Ansari MS, Mandhani A, *et al.* Clinical presentation and diagnostic approach in cases of genitourinary tuberculosis. *Indian J Urol* 2008; 24: 401–405.

62. Issack MI, Jinerdeb D. Sterile pyuria. *N Engl J Med* 2015; 372: 2373.

63. Eastwood JB, Corbishley CM, Grange JM. Tuberculosis and the kidney. *J Am Soc Nephrol* 2001; 12: 1307–1314.

64. Simon HB, Weinstein AJ, Pasternak MS, *et al.* Genitourinary tuberculosis. Clinical features in a general hospital population. *Am J Med* 1977; 63: 410–420.

65. Sharma JB. Current diagnosis and management of female genital tuberculosis. *J Obstet Gynaecol India* 2015; 65: 362–371.

https://doi.org/10.1183/2312508X.10021017

66. Thwaites GE, van Toorn R, Schoeman J. Tuberculous meningitis: more questions, still too few answers. *Lancet Neurol* 2013; 12: 999–1010.

67. Leonard JM. Central nervous system tuberculosis. *Microbiol Spectr* 2017; 5: TNMI7-0044-2017.

68. Pehlivanoglu F, Kart Yasar K, Sengoz G. Tuberculous meningitis in adults: a review of 160 cases. *Sci World J* 2012; 2012: 169028.

69. Kim HJ, Shim KW, Lee MK, *et al.* Tuberculous encephalopathy without meningitis: pathology and brain MRI findings. *Eur Neurol* 2011; 65: 156–159.

70. Berenguer J, Moreno S, Laguna F, *et al.* Tuberculous meningitis in patients infected with the human immunodeficiency virus. *N Engl J Med* 1992; 326: 668–672.

71. Thwaites G, Fisher M, Hemingway C, *et al.* British Infection Society guidelines for the diagnosis and treatment of tuberculosis of the central nervous system in adults and children. *J Infect* 2009; 59: 167–187.

72. Nicolls DJ, King M, Holland D, *et al.* Intracranial tuberculomas developing while on therapy for pulmonary tuberculosis. *Lancet Infect Dis* 2005; 5: 795–801.

73. Labhard N, Nicod L, Zellweger JP. Cerebral tuberculosis in the immunocompetent host: 8 cases observed in Switzerland. *Tuber Lung Dis* 1994; 75: 454–459.

74. Erdem H, Senbayrak S, Gencer S, *et al.* Tuberculous and brucellosis meningitis differential diagnosis. *Travel Med Infect Dis* 2015; 13: 185–191.

75. Ginsberg L, Kidd D. Chronic and recurrent meningitis. *Pract Neurol* 2008; 8: 348–361.

76. Sharma SK, Mohan A, Sharma A. Diagnosis and management of miliary tuberculosis: current state and future perspectives. *Indian J Med Res* 2012; 135: 703–730.

77. Sharma SK, Mohan A, Sharma A, *et al.* Miliary tuberculosis: new insights into an old disease. *Lancet Infect Dis* 2005; 5: 415–430.

78. Cunha BA, Krakakis J, McDermott BP. Fever of unknown origin (FUO) caused by miliary tuberculosis: diagnostic significance of morning temperature spikes. *Heart Lung* 2009; 38: 77–82.

79. Proudfoot AT, Akhtar AJ, Douglas AC, *et al.* Miliary tuberculosis in adults. *Br Med J* 1969; 2: 273–276.

80. Lee K, Kim JH, Lee JH, *et al.* Acute respiratory distress syndrome caused by miliary tuberculosis: a multicentre survey in South Korea. *Int J Tuberc Lung Dis* 2011; 15: 1099–1103.

81. Vasankari T, Liippo K, Tala E. Overt and cryptic miliary tuberculosis misdiagnosed until autopsy. *Scand J Infect Dis* 2003; 35: 794–796.

82. Singh K, Hyatali S, Giddings S, *et al.* Miliary tuberculosis presenting with ARDS and shock: a case report and challenges in current management and diagnosis. *Case Rep Crit Care* 2017; 2017: 9287021.

83. Debi U, Ravisankar V, Prasad KK, *et al.* Abdominal tuberculosis of the gastrointestinal tract: revisited. *World J Gastroenterol* 2014; 20: 14831–14840.

84. Choi EH, Coyle WJ. Gastrointestinal tuberculosis. *Microbiol Spectr* 2016; 4: TNMI7-0014-2016.

85. Sanai FM, Bzeizi KI. Systematic review: tuberculous peritonitis – presenting features, diagnostic strategies and treatment. *Aliment Pharmacol Ther* 2005; 22: 685–700.

86. Guirat A, Koubaa M, Mzali R, *et al.* Peritoneal tuberculosis. *Clin Res Hepatol Gastroenterol* 2011; 35: 60–69.

87. Chien K, Seemangal J, Batt J, *et al.* Abdominal tuberculosis: a descriptive case series of the experience in a Canadian tuberculosis clinic. *Int J Tuberc Lung Dis* 2918; 22: 681–685.

88. Yimer S, Bjune G, Alene G. Diagnostic and treatment delay among pulmonary tuberculosis patients in Ethiopia: a cross sectional study. *BMC Infect Dis* 2005; 5: 112.

89. Storla DG, Yimer S, Bjune GA. A systematic review of delay in the diagnosis and treatment of tuberculosis. *BMC Public Health* 2008; 8: 15.

90. Sreeramareddy CT, Panduru KV, Menten J, *et al.* Time delays in diagnosis of pulmonary tuberculosis: a systematic review of literature. *BMC Infect Dis* 2009; 9: 91.

91. Tattevin P, Che D, Fraisse P, *et al.* Factors associated with patient and health care system delay in the diagnosis of tuberculosis in France. *Int J Tuberc Lung Dis* 2012; 16: 510–515.

92. Kherad O, Herrmann FR, Zellweger JP, *et al.* Clinical presentation, demographics and outcome of tuberculosis (TB) in a low incidence area: a 4-year study in Geneva, Switzerland. *BMC Infect Dis* 2009; 9: 217.

93. Achkar JM, Sherpa T, Cohen HW, *et al.* Differences in clinical presentation among persons with pulmonary tuberculosis: a comparison of documented and undocumented foreign-born *versus* US-born persons. *Clin Infect Dis* 2008; 47: 1277–1283.

94. Yimer SA, Bjune GA, Holm-Hansen C. Time to first consultation, diagnosis and treatment of TB among patients attending a referral hospital in Northwest, Ethiopia. *BMC Infect Dis* 2014; 14: 19.

95. Senkoro M, Hinderaker SG, Mfinanga SG, *et al.* Health care-seeking behaviour among people with cough in Tanzania: findings from a tuberculosis prevalence survey. *Int J Tuberc Lung Dis* 2015; 19: 640–646.

96. Sulis G, Pai M. Missing tuberculosis patients in the private sector: business as usual will not deliver results. *Public Health Action* 2017; 7: 80–81.

97. Claassens MM, Jacobs E, Cyster E, *et al.* Tuberculosis cases missed in primary health care facilities: should we redefine case finding? *Int J Tuberc Lung Dis* 2013; 17: 608–614.

98.   Lam PK, Lobue PA, Catanzaro A. Clinical diagnosis of tuberculosis by specialists and non-specialists. *Int J Tuberc Lung Dis* 2009; 13: 659–661.

99.   Yang Z-H, Gorden T, Liu D-P, *et al.* Increased likelihood of advanced pulmonary tuberculosis at initial diagnosis in a low-incidence US state. *Int J Tuberc Lung Dis* 2018; 22: 628–636.

100. Uys PW, Warren RM, van Helden PD. A threshold value for the time delay to TB diagnosis. *PLoS One* 2007; 2: e757.

101. Lonnroth K, Castro KG, Chakaya JM, *et al.* Tuberculosis control and elimination 2010–50: cure, care, and social development. *Lancet* 2010; 375: 1814–1829.

102. Virenfeldt J, Rudolf F, Camara C, *et al.* Treatment delay affects clinical severity of tuberculosis: a longitudinal cohort study. *BMJ Open* 2014; 4: e004818.

103. Pablos-Mendez A, Sterling TR, Frieden TR. The relationship between delayed or incomplete treatment and all-cause mortality in patients with tuberculosis. *JAMA* 1996; 276: 1223–1228.

104. Liu YC, Lin HH, Chen YS, *et al.* Reduced health provider delay and tuberculosis mortality due to an improved hospital programme. *Int J Tuberc Lung Dis* 2010; 14: 72–78.

105. Bustamante-Montes LP, Escobar-Mesa A, Borja-Aburto VH, *et al.* Predictors of death from pulmonary tuberculosis: the case of Veracruz, Mexico. *Int J Tuberc Lung Dis* 2000; 4: 208–215.

106. Mhimbira FA, Cuevas LE, Dacombe R, *et al.* Interventions to increase tuberculosis case detection at primary healthcare or community-level services. *Cochrane Database Syst Rev* 2017; 11: CD011432.

Disclosures: J-P. Zellweger reports receiving speaker's honoraria from Qiagen, outside the submitted work. J. Heyckendorf reports receiving sponsorship for independent lectures performed at sponsored symposia from the following, outside the submitted work: Chiesi, Janssen and Lucane.

https://doi.org/10.1183/2312508X.10021017

Chapter 7

Laboratory diagnosis

Elisa Tagliani[1], Vlad Nikolayevskyy[2,3], Enrico Tortoli[1] and
Daniela Maria Cirillo[1]

Laboratory diagnosis of TB needs to be accurate, rapid and able to provide sufficient data to start patients on proper treatment. While culture and phenotypic DST remain pillars in the diagnostic process, molecular methods have the advantage of providing key data in a very short time. Worldwide roll-out of automated platforms able to detect TB and rifampicin resistance have substantially contributed to the increase of detection and treatment of MDR-TB cases. New, more comprehensive platforms are under development or have just started commercialisation, where the main advantage will be the capacity to detect resistance to isoniazid in addition to rifampicin. Some of the platforms are designed to be placed at a more centralised and high workload level. Whole-genome sequencing (WGS) and WGS-based technologies are the promise for the future. These tests will provide a very comprehensive range of information, from extensive resistance prediction to data on transmission in the population.

Cite as: Tagliani E, Nikolayevskyy V, Tortoli E, *et al.* Laboratory diagnosis. *In:* Migliori GB, Bothamley G, Duarte R, *et al.*, eds. Tuberculosis (ERS Monograph). Sheffield, European Respiratory Society, 2018; pp. 99–115 [https://doi.org/10.1183/2312508X.10021318].

@ERSpublications
The availability of more sensitive, accurate and affordable diagnostics for TB and DR-TB, including new point-of care tests, is one of the key pre-requisites to reach the 2035 targets of the End TB Strategy http://ow.ly/cfVQ30lqCfE

Rapid and accurate diagnosis of TB is key to avert death and to prevent further transmission of the disease. However, of the 10.4 million estimated new TB cases that occurred in 2016, 40% remained undiagnosed or underreported, including 450 000 cases (>75%) of RR-TB and MDR-TB [1]. Finding these 4 million missing cases will require 1) the development of improved diagnostics and to ensure their accessibility in low- and middle-income countries, and 2) the correct implementation and most efficient use of the existing tools.

The past few years have seen an increased interest in new technologies and progress in the field of TB diagnostics. The list of the TB diagnostic tools currently under development and validation is shown in table 1 [2]. The WHO has recently endorsed and issued policy

[1]Emerging Bacterial Pathogens Unit, Division of Immunology, Transplantation and Infectious Diseases, IRCCS San Raffaele Scientific Institute, Milan, Italy. [2]National Mycobacterium Reference Service South, Public Health England, London, UK. [3]Dept of Medicine, Imperial College London, London, UK.

Correspondence: Daniela Maria Cirillo, Emerging Bacterial Pathogens Unit, Division of Immunology, Transplantation and Infectious Diseases, IRCCS San Raffaele Scientific Institute, via Olgettina 58, 20132 Milan, Italy. E-mail: cirillo.daniela@hsr.it

Table 1. TB diagnostic landscape

	Development	Validation	Regulatory	WHO evaluation	Country transition
Rapid biomarker-based non-sputum-based test for detecting TB		Sensitive lipoarabinomannan assay (Fujifilm, Tokyo, Japan)			Determine TB LAM Ag (Alere, Waltham, MA, USA)
Rapid sputum-based test for detecting TB at the microscopy centre level of the healthcare system		ID-FISH assay (ID-FISH Technology, Palo Alto, CA, USA)	Truenat MTB (Molbio Diagnostics, Goa, India)		Loopamp MTBC assay (Eiken Chemical, Tokyo, Japan)
Next-generation DST at microscopy centres	TruArray MDR-TB and XDR-TB (Akonni Biosystems, Frederick, MD, USA) PoC (Bioneer, Daejon, South Korea) Xpert XDR (Cepheid, Sunnyvale, CA, USA) Omni (Cepheid) Q-POC TB/MDR-TB (QuantuMDx, Newcastle upon Tyne, UK) TB MultiTest (SelfDiagnostic, Leipzig, Germany) Stool testing with molecular tools (various)		Truenat MTB RIF Dx (Molbio Diagnostics)		Xpert MTB/RIF Ultra (Cepheid)
Centralised DST	FluoroType MTBXDR version 1.0 (Hain Lifescience, Nehren, Germany) LabChip-based rapid POCT (MicoBiomed,	INFINITI MDR-TB (AutoGenomics, Carlsbad, CA, USA) AccuPower XDR-TB real-time PCR (Bioneer)	TB resistance module series (Autoimmun Diagnostika, Strassberg, Germany) AccuPower TB&MDR real-time PCR (Bioneer)	RealTime MTB RIF/INH (Abbott Laboratories, Des Plaines, IL, USA)	

Continued

https://doi.org/10.1183/2312508X.10021318

Table 1. Continued

Development	Validation	Regulatory	WHO evaluation	Country transition
Geumcheon-gu, Seoul, Korea)		TB drug resistance detection array kit (CapitalBio Technology, Beijing, China)	BD MAX MDR-TB (BD, Franklin Lakes, NJ, USA)	
UltraFast LabChip real-time PCR MDR-TB kit (MicoBiomed)	INNO-LiPA Rif.TB (Fujirebio Europe, Gent, Belgium)		MGIT bedaquiline and delamanid (Becton Dickinson)	
	AdvanSure MDR-TB GenoBlot assay (LG Life Sciences, Seoul, South Korea)	MTB drug-resistant mutation test kits (QuanDx, San Jose, CA, USA)	FluoroType MTBDR version 1.0 (Hain Lifescience)	
	PrimeSuite TB (Longhorn Vaccines and Diagnostics, San Antonio, TX, USA)	Mycolor TK platform (Salubris, Shenzhen, China)	Cobas MTB-RIF/INH (Roche, Basel, Switzerland)	
	QMAC DST (QuantaMatrix, Seoul, South Korea)	Anyplex assays for MDR/XDR (Seegene, Seoul, South Korea)		
	VereMTB detection kit (Veredus Laboratories, Singapore)	VersaTREK (Thermo Fisher, Waltham, MA, USA)		
		Sensititre MYCOTB MIC plate (Thermo Fisher)		
		MolecuTech REBA MDR/XDR assays (YD Diagnostics, Gyeonggi-do, South Korea)		
		MeltPro MTB (MDR-TB, XDR-TB) kits (Zeesan Biotech, Fujian, China)		

Reproduced and modified from [2] with permission.

guidelines on multiple tests, including Xpert MTB/RIF and Xpert MTB/RIF Ultra (Xpert Ultra) assays [3, 4], line probe assays (LPAs) for the detection of resistance to isoniazid and rifampicin and to second-line anti-TB drugs [5, 6], loop-mediated isothermal amplification (TB-LAMP) [7], the lateral flow urine lipoarabinomannan (LF-LAM) assay [8], and a policy framework to guide countries in the implementation of TB diagnostics [9]. Nonetheless, many challenges for active TB diagnosis remain, including the lack of a point-of-care test deployable at the most decentralised level of care and having minimal infrastructure and training requirements, the unavailability of sensitive tools for the diagnosis of EPTB and TB in children, and the lack of molecular tools for accurate DST to more anti-TB drugs and implementable in decentralised settings.

In this chapter we provide an overview of the current diagnostics for active TB endorsed by the WHO and of tools that are currently undergoing multicentre evaluation. In addition, we describe the current applications of whole-genome sequencing (WGS) as next-generation DST and the use of targeted next-generation sequencing (NGS) for drug susceptibility and resistance prediction starting from clinical specimens. Finally, we provide some considerations on the future perspectives of the TB diagnostic landscape.

Current methodologies for tuberculosis detection

Direct microscopy

Microscopy still plays a major role in TB diagnosis and follow-up. The high lipid content of the mycobacterial cell wall makes the uptake of dyes problematic; however, once the primary colour has penetrated, it forms stable complexes resistant to decolourisation with acid-alcohol solutions (acid-fast bacilli (AFB) microscopy). Classical methods, i.e. Ziehl–Neelsen and Kinyoun staining, use different carbol fuchsin concentrations requiring, or not requiring, heating for cell wall penetration [10–12]. A valid alternative is represented by the fluorescence-based methods using auramine O as the primary stain. Mycobacteria stained with fuchsin appear red; those stained with auramine are yellow-orange fluorescent. The need for an expensive fluorescence microscope has long hampered the spread of florescence microscopy, despite its higher sensitivity in comparison with classical staining; in recent years the availability of cheaper and more durable light-emitting diode microscopes has made the latter approach preferred worldwide [13]. The reading of fluorescent AFB microscopy requires lower magnification with a significant reduction of the reading time in comparison with fuchsin.

Although smear microscopy on concentrated sputum samples has an increased sensitivity compared with the direct method, the WHO does not recommend it because of the increased biosafety risk of centrifugation methods at the peripheral microscopy laboratory level and the feasibility and costs of implementing such methods on a large scale [14].

AFB microscopy provides important information of a patient's infectiousness and allows the response to therapy to be evaluated. Its major limit is the poor sensitivity, in particular with extrapulmonary specimens and in HIV-positive patients (2000–10 000 bacilli·mL^{-1} are needed for a positive result).

The use of fluorescein diacetate, a viability stain that fluoresces only when hydrolysed by esterases of viable bacteria, has been proposed since the 1980s for mycobacteria [15].

https://doi.org/10.1183/2312508X.10021318

The method revealed excellent correlation with quantitative culture and potentially represents an inexpensive tool for treatment monitoring [16].

Culture methods

Culture is at least 100 times more sensitive than microscopy in detecting mycobacteria. Due to the slow growth rate of *Mycobacterium tuberculosis*, the risk of overgrowth by the contaminating flora present in specimens from nonsterile sites needs to be minimised. Of the various methods developed for this purpose, the one using *N*-acetylcysteine-NaOH is recommended; *N*-acetylcysteine is mucolytic and 2% NaOH eliminates most of the contaminant flora. The objective is to keep the contamination rate of cultures between 3% and 5%. A contamination rate <3% may indicate a too harsh procedure detrimental for mycobacteria, while a rate >5% is at risk of missing positive cultures.

Different solid media are available for culture of mycobacteria, either egg- or agar-based. Liquid media were rarely used because of problems with frequent contamination; it was only following the introduction of supplements consisting of antimicrobial blends active against common bacteria and yeasts that they have become more widely used. Culture in liquid media is both more sensitive and rapid in comparison with solid media. At present, to get maximum yield, the international guidelines recommend culture to be performed in parallel on both solid and liquid media, with Löwenstein–Jensen medium and the Mycobacteria Growth Indicator Tube (MGIT) being the most used, respectively [10, 11, 17]. The MGIT is a commercial liquid medium consisting of Middlebrook 7H9 broth supplemented with an antibiotic mixture (PANTA) (BD, Franklin Lakes, NJ, USA). An indicator, embedded in a silicon film at the bottom of the tube, becomes fluorescent when the oxygen concentration decreases in the medium, consumed by mycobacterial metabolism. Despite the high costs, the BACTEC MGIT 960 System, consisting of a fully automated machine for incubation and detection of positivity in MGIT tubes, is nowadays used in many laboratories worldwide, including in low-income countries [18, 19].

Rapid molecular tools for active tuberculosis detection

Xpert MTB/RIF

Xpert MTB/RIF (Cepheid, Sunnyvale, CA, USA) is a cartridge-based real-time PCR assay for the simultaneous detection of MTBC and rifampicin resistance from clinical specimens [20]. The test is fully automated, and takes ~2 h for sample processing, DNA extraction, PCR amplification and data analysis. The WHO issued policy recommendations on using Xpert MTB/RIF in early 2011 [21] and a policy update in 2013 [3], stating that Xpert MTB/RIF may be used as the initial diagnostic test for all adults and children with signs and symptoms of TB, rather than microscopy and culture (conditional recommendation acknowledging resource implications). Xpert MTB/RIF can be performed directly on sputum, processed sputum sediment and selected extrapulmonary specimens from adults and children [3]. The Xpert MTB/RIF pooled estimates of sensitivity and specificity for PTB detection are 88% and 99%, respectively [22]. However, the test sensitivity remains suboptimal compared with culture in smear-negative TB patients, in patients with HIV infection and in children [22, 23]. For extrapulmonary samples, the sensitivity varies depending on the sample type, being higher for lymph node tissues and aspirates, cerebrospinal fluid [24], and gastric aspirates, but low for pleural fluid [25].

https://doi.org/10.1183/2312508X.10021318

Xpert MTB/RIF Ultra

The Xpert Ultra assay (Cepheid) was launched in 2017 as a next-generation more sensitive assay for TB and rifampicin resistance detection [26]. Xpert Ultra uses the same GeneXpert platform and sample processing procedures as the Xpert MTB/RIF assay, but targets additional genetic regions, *i.e.* the multicopy genes IS6110 and IS1081, to enhance its sensitivity for MTBC detection. In addition, Xpert Ultra is characterised by a larger DNA reaction chamber, more rapid thermal cycling, and improved fluidics and enzymes [4]. Xpert Ultra uses the same semiquantitative categories used in the Xpert MTB/RIF assay with an additional category "trace" to identify the paucibacillary samples positive to IS6110/IS1081 targets but negative to *rpoB* [26].

In January 2017, a WHO expert consultation found the Xpert Ultra cartridge noninferior to the original assay for TB and rifampicin resistance detection based on data from a multicentre study coordinated by the Foundation for Innovative New Diagnostics (FIND) [4]. The study showed that Xpert Ultra's overall sensitivity was 5% higher than that of Xpert MTB/RIF with a higher incremental sensitivity among paucibacillary forms of TB: 17% higher for smear-negative, culture-positive patients and 13% higher for HIV-positive patients [27]. In a study assessing the performance of Xpert Ultra for the diagnosis of tuberculous meningitis against uniform clinical case definition, the assay sensitivity was 70% compared with 43% for Xpert MTB/RIF and liquid culture [28]. In a recent study on the accuracy of Xpert Ultra for the diagnosis of PTB in children, the assay detected 73.7% of microbiologically confirmed TB cases compared with 63.2% for Xpert MTB/RIF and 82.9% for culture [29].

However, Xpert Ultra's increased sensitivity came at a trade-off of decreased specificity, with an overall reduction of 2.7% [27]. In patients with a history of TB, Xpert Ultra specificity was 93% compared with 98% for Xpert MTB/RIF, possibly due to the presence of *M. tuberculosis* DNA or intact *M. tuberculosis* bacilli in the participant's respiratory system [27]. Based on these results, the WHO Technical Expert Group agreed that an Xpert Ultra "trace" result is sufficient to start therapy in individuals with known or suspected HIV infection and in children, and for the diagnosis of EPTB. To mitigate the risk of overtreatment in HIV-negative adults, Xpert Ultra should be repeated on a fresh specimen, with a second "trace" positive result being sufficient to make a diagnosis of PTB, unless there is a recent history of TB [4].

Loop-mediated isothermal amplification

A TB-LAMP assay for the detection of MTBC has been developed by Eiken Chemical Company (Tokyo, Japan). It is based on a rapid nucleic acid amplification method that occurs at a constant temperature of ~65°C. The assay leads to results in <1 h, does not require special reagents or sophisticated equipment and has the potential to be applied in peripheral facilities. Following a review of the latest evidence, in 2016 the WHO issued a policy guideline recommending the use of TB-LAMP as a replacement for smear microscopy in adults and children with signs or symptoms consistent with TB, but not among people with HIV due to the lack of data [7]. TB-LAMP has limited application in settings with high rates of HIV and drug resistance.

Lateral flow urine lipoarabinomannan assay

The commercially available LF-LAM assay Determine TB LAM (Alere, Waltham, MA, USA) allows the presence of LAM antigen released from metabolically active or degenerating mycobacterial cells to be detected in the urine of people with active TB

https://doi.org/10.1183/2312508X.10021318

disease. This is a technically simple, instrument-free, low-cost, rapid and point-of-care assay easily implemented in remote health facilities in low-resource settings. Results from a meta-analysis showed a pooled sensitivity and specificity of LF-LAM for TB diagnosis of 56% and 90%, respectively, in participants with CD4 $\leqslant$100 cells·μL^{-1} *versus* 26% and 92%, respectively, in those with CD4 >100 cells·μL^{-1} [30]. The WHO released policy guidance in 2015 stating that the test may be used to assist the diagnosis of HIV-positive TB presumptive patients with very low CD4 counts (<100 cells·mm^{-3}) or who are seriously ill [8]. In 2016, a multicentre RCT conducted in Africa showed that LF-LAM-guided, prompt anti-TB treatment initiation could reduce all-cause 8-week mortality in HIV-positive hospital inpatients [31]. Despite the positive results of the trial and the WHO recommendations, no country has yet committed to using LAM testing on a large scale.

Abbott RealTime MTB assay

Abbott Molecular (Des Plaines, IL, USA) has recently launched an automated RealTime MTB assay for the detection of MTBC in respiratory specimens through the amplification of both the IS6110 sequence and the gene for protein antigen B. The company offers a fully automated system from DNA extraction, to amplification and detection, with a flexible throughput to up to 94 samples per run and ~7 h to complete the entire process. Published studies have reported good analytical performances with sensitivity ranging from 71.7% to 96.7% in smear-negative, culture-positive samples and specificity ranging from 97% to 100% [32–36].

Current methodologies for drug resistance detection

Phenotypic-based drug-susceptibility testing

Drug resistance is defined as a significant reduction in sensitivity to a specific drug leading to affected strains being unlikely to demonstrate clinical responsiveness to the drug. Resistance to anti-TB drugs, especially MDR- and XDR-TB, is an emerging problem worldwide, and effective management of DR-TB largely relies on rapid and accurate identification of resistant *M. tuberculosis* strains.

The principal objectives for DST include: 1) determination of the resistance/sensitivity pattern of individual *M. tuberculosis* strains to ensure adequate treatment and management of a TB case, 2) assessment of the need for institutional isolation of patients, and 3) assisting in drug resistance surveillance at various levels and/or determination of the scope of institutional and community outbreak investigations/interventions required [37, 38]. The implementation of the WHO End TB Strategy requires provision of access to DST for all patients with signs and symptoms of TB [39].

Culture-based phenotypic DST methods remain the gold standard for the detection of drug resistance despite being time consuming, labour intensive and requiring sophisticated laboratory infrastructure [38]. The currently employed indirect phenotypic methods are based on inoculation of mycobacteria grown in bacterial culture onto drug-containing solid media or liquid media followed by a direct observation of growth, or an indirect monitoring of growth through oxygen consumption. Prior identification of species to ensure purity of MTBC culture is very important as many NTM are intrinsically resistant to many anti-TB drugs, thus increasing the risk of false-resistance results.

The principal phenotypic DST methods endorsed by the WHO include liquid media and egg- or agar-based solid media assays [37, 40–43]. Three solid culture methods (*i.e.* the proportion method, the resistance ratio method and the absolute concentration method) are relatively inexpensive and remain in use worldwide, but have been standardised predominantly for testing of first-line drugs only (rifampicin, isoniazid, ethambutol and pyrazinamide) and require up to 8 weeks to produce DST results. Turnaround times for liquid culture methods are significantly shorter and DST results are usually obtainable within 2 weeks.

Automated liquid culture-based systems monitor mycobacteria growth through oxygen consumption, thus enabling accurate reading and interpretation of DST results. This method has been extensively validated and is proposed as the reference method for performing DST for the majority of anti-TB drugs, including second-line and novel drugs (bedaquiline and delamanid) [38]. Recently developed microtitre plate-based liquid culture methods (*e.g.* Sensititre MYCOTB; Thermo Fisher, Waltham, MA, USA) allow MICs for multiple drugs to be determined in one plate, thus achieving an unprecedented level of precision for phenotypic DST [44–46]. Details of both liquid and solid media-based methodologies are described elsewhere [11].

Modern phenotypic DST methods traditionally use critical concentrations of anti-TB agents to determine if an isolate is resistant or sensitive to a given drug, where the critical concentration is defined as the lowest concentration of a drug *in vitro* that inhibits the growth of a pre-defined (usually 99%) proportion of a wild-type MTBC strain [38, 47, 48]. Definitions and utility of critical concentrations as well as other cut-off values (clinical breakpoints, MICs and epidemiological cut-off values) in phenotypic DST have considerably evolved over the last decade and are considered in detail elsewhere [49–51]. The updated list of critical concentrations and clinical breakpoints for drugs recommended for treatment of DR-TB was published in 2018 [38].

Several noncommercial phenotypic assays, including the nitrate reductase (NRA), microscopic observation drug susceptibility (MODS) and colorimetric redox indictor (CRI) assays, could be considered as inexpensive and rapid alternatives to complex and technically demanding commercial assays, especially in resource-constrained settings. The WHO has endorsed the use of the NRA and MODS assays for direct DST, and the NRA, MODS and CRI assays for indirect DST, in reference laboratories under clearly defined operational conditions following strict laboratory protocols [52]. Performance characteristics and the current status of phenotypic DST assays are summarised in table 2.

Rapid molecular tools for detection of drug resistance

Line probe assays
LPAs are a family of DNA strip-based tests that allow the drug resistance profile to be determined through the binding of amplicons to probes targeting the most common mutations to first- and second-line drugs and to wild-type probes. They can be used for the direct testing of smear-positive sputum specimens as well as indirect testing on culture isolates. Given the moderate complexity of the assay, the necessity of multiple pieces of equipment and the laboratory infrastructure requirements, LPAs are usually implemented at upper- and middle-tier health facilities. Compared with phenotypic DST, the use of LPAs allows the drug susceptibility profile to be obtained within 24–48 h, and presents a

 https://doi.org/10.1183/2312508X.10021318

Table 2. Principal characteristics of phenotypic-based DST for *Mycobacterium tuberculosis*

Assay	Direct or indirect	Turnaround time	WHO status or recommendations	Cost	Labour intensity	Quantitative or qualitative
Solid media	Indirect	⩽8 weeks	First-line drugs only	++	+++	Qualitative
Liquid media: automated	Indirect	1–2 weeks	First, second, reserve drugs	+++	+++	Qualitative
Liquid media: plate based	Indirect	1–2 weeks	Not endorsed/ research in progress	+++	++	Quantitative
NRA	Direct/ indirect	Days	Conditional endorsement	++	++	Qualitative
MODS	Direct/ indirect	Days	Conditional endorsement	++	++	Qualitative
CRI	Indirect	Days	Conditional endorsement	++	++	Quantitative

NRA: nitrate reductase; MODS: microscopic observation drug susceptibility; CRI: colorimetric redox indictor.

lower biosafety risk and a higher throughput. In 2016, the WHO approved the use of several commercially available LPAs for the detection of MTBC and resistance to rifampicin and isoniazid, *i.e.* GenoType MTBDR*plus* versions 1 and 2 (Hain Lifescience, Nehren, Germany), and Nipro NTM+MDRTB detection kit 2 (Nipro, Osaka, Japan) [5], and a third LPA for the detection of resistance to SLIDs and fluoroquinolones, *i.e.* GenoType MTBDR*sl* versions 1 and 2 (Hain Lifescience) [6].

Line-probe assays for detection of resistance to first-line anti-tuberculosis drugs
The GenoType MTBDR*plus* and Nipro NTM+MDRTB detection kit 2 assays target mutations in the *inhA* promoter (from −15 to −8 nucleotides upstream) and *katG* regions (codon 315) to identify isoniazid resistance, and in the rifampicin resistance-determining region (RRDR) of the *rpoB* gene (from codon 505 to 533) for rifampicin resistance. The Nipro assay also differentiates *Mycobacterium avium*, *Mycobacterium intracellulare* and *Mycobacterium kansasii* from other NTM. A noninferiority study conducted by FIND showed equivalence among the three commercially available LPAs for detection of rifampicin and isoniazid resistance in smear-positive samples [53]. The overall pooled estimates of the sensitivity and specificity of the three LPAs for rifampicin resistance were 96.8% and 98.1%, respectively. For isoniazid, the pooled estimates of the sensitivity and specificity were 90.2% and 99.2%, respectively [5]. The WHO recommends the use of LPAs for persons with a sputum smear-positive specimen or a cultured isolate of MTBC, as the initial test, instead of phenotypic DST, to detect resistance to rifampicin and isoniazid [5]. However, given the different accuracy of detecting resistance to these two drugs, phenotypic DST for isoniazid may still be used when the LPA does not detect isoniazid resistance [5].

Line-probe assays for detection of resistance to second-line anti-tuberculosis drugs
The second version of GenoType MTBDR*sl* includes the *gyrA* and *gyrB* genes for detection of resistance to fluoroquinolones, and *rrs* and the *eis* promoter region for detection of resistance to SLIDs. In addition to culture isolates, the assay may be used on both smear-positive and smear-negative specimens. For fluoroquinolones, the sensitivity and specificity were 97% and 98% on smear-positive specimens and 80% and 100% on

smear-negative specimens, respectively [54]. For SLIDs, the sensitivity and specificity were 89% and 90% on smear-positive specimens and 80% and 100% on smear-negative specimens, respectively [55]. The WHO recommends the use of second-line LPAs for patients with confirmed RR-TB or MDR-TB, as the initial test, instead of phenotypic DST, to detect resistance to fluoroquinolones and to SLIDs. However, given the suboptimal sensitivity of the assay, culture and phenotypic DST is still required to completely exclude resistance to these classes of drugs as well as to other second-line drugs [6].

Line-probe assays for detection of resistance to pyrazinamide

The Genoscholar PZA-TB II assay (Nipro) is the first commercial molecular test available for the rapid detection of resistance to pyrazinamide starting from direct sample or culture isolates. The assay targets a 700-bp fragment covering the entire *pncA* coding region and 18 nucleotides upstream. The Genoscholar PZA-TB II assay comprises a total of 48 probes which recognise the wild-type sequence of the gene, while no specific mutant probes are included. Resistance is identified by the absence of probe binding. Two studies assessed the performance of the test, and reported a sensitivity ranging from 93.2% to 94.3% and a specificity ranging from 91.2% to 94.9% [55, 56]. The accuracy of the assay may be affected by the detection of mutations not causing resistance and this may vary depending on the regional context. In addition, the test has poor capacity in detecting heteroresistance and insertions. Despite these limitations, the Genoscholar PZA-TB II assay offers a valid alternative for rapid susceptibility testing for pyrazinamide.

Xpert MTB/RIF and Xpert Ultra

The Xpert MTB/RIF assay uses a molecular beacon technology to detect rifampicin resistance. A failure in, or delayed binding of one or more of the five probes to, the RRDR of the *rpoB* gene indicates potential rifampicin resistance. The pooled estimates for rifampicin resistance detection on pulmonary samples were 95% and 98% for sensitivity and specificity, respectively [22]. Despite the good analytical performance, the assay has some limitations including a poor sensitivity of specific probes in detecting certain mutations [57] or in the case of heteroresistance [58, 59] and may lead to false-positive results in the presence of some synonymous mutations [60] or in the case of paucibacillary samples or extrapulmonary samples [61].

The new version of the test, *i.e.* Xpert Ultra, provides more reliable detection of rifampicin resistance. Four sloppy molecular beacon probes targeting the RRDR of the *rpoB* gene have been designed to detect mutations by measurable shifts in melting temperature peaks. The assay allows a vast range of mutations to be identified, has improved capacity to detect resistant mutations at codon 533, correctly identifies mutations in mixed and paucibacillary samples, and differentiates synonymous mutations from other RRDR mutations [26]. Results from the multicentre diagnostic accuracy study showed comparable diagnostic performance of Xpert Ultra and Xpert MTB/RIF for detection of rifampicin resistance [27].

FluoroType MTBDR

The FluoroType MTBDR test (Hain Lifescience) is a fluorescence-based single-tube multiplex PCR for the rapid detection of MTBC and resistance to rifampicin and isoniazid directly from clinical samples. The assay combines LATE (linear-after-the-exponential)-PCR [62] together with specific probes using a lights-on/lights-off detection technology, where the presence of specific mutations is detected by shifts in the melting curves of the probes [63]. The test is semiautomated, with amplification and detection occurring in a closed system, and allows the simultaneous processing of up to 96 samples including an internal control. Results are generated within 3 h and are interpreted by software. Recent studies evaluated the

https://doi.org/10.1183/2312508X.10021318

performance of the test for rifampicin and isoniazid resistance detection on culture isolates and sputum specimens, showing very good results in terms of sensitivity and specificity for both drugs, and high accuracy for the identification of mutations in *rpoB*, *katG* and the *inhA* promoter [64, 65]. In theory, new mutations and the corresponding melting curve properties could be entered in the analytical software, potentially allowing the performance of the test to be improved.

BD MAX MDR-TB assay

BD has recently developed a multiplex real-time PCR assay (BD MAX MDR-TB assay) for the simultaneous detection of MTBC and mutations conferring resistance to rifampicin and isoniazid from sputum specimens [66]. The assay runs on a fully integrated platform, the BD MAX System, including automated DNA extraction and five-colour detection real-time PCR. Each run allows the simultaneous testing of up to 24 sputum specimens within 4 h, making the platform suitable for use in central laboratories. The assay has recently undergone evaluation for rapid detection of *M. tuberculosis* DNA and rifampicin and isoniazid resistance in a multicountry study, showing promising performance [67].

Next-generation sequencing

Whole-genome sequencing

WGS utilising high-throughput NGS technologies interrogates the entire bacterial genome, and can be used for a reliable prediction of drug-resistant or -sensitive phenotype through identification of single nucleotide polymorphisms and small insertions/deletions (indels) within regions associated with resistance to anti-TB drugs, thus offering completely new opportunities in TB diagnostics and clinical management [68–73].

Regardless of the platform and/or chemistry employed, WGS workflow can be broadly subdivided into four major steps: 1) DNA extraction, 2) library preparation (comprising fragmentation and adapter linkage), 3) automated NGS generating millions of reads and 4) data analysis. Existing chemistries (*e.g.* Illumina (San Diego, CA, USA), Ion Torrent (Thermo Fisher), Pacific Biosciences (Menlo Park, CA, USA) and MinION (Oxford Nanopore, Oxford, UK)) vary, sometimes considerably, in terms of read length, error rate, cost and other parameters [74]. The minimum concentration of genomic *M. tuberculosis* DNA required for good quality WGS is generally 5–10 ng·µL^{-1} but lower (>0.5 ng·µL^{-1}) concentrations could be acceptable, enabling successful WGS of mycobacteria from 1–2 mL of early MGIT cultures for the purposes of speciation, drug resistance prediction and relatedness [72]. DNA could be isolated using a variety of commercial and in-house methods. Details of wet laboratory procedures, including DNA extraction, quantification, library preparation and WGS, are described elsewhere [72, 75, 76].

WGS data analysis for drug resistance prediction predominantly involves identification of polymorphisms in genes associated with drug resistance using analytical pipelines [69, 70, 77]. This could be done using a variety of free online tools (*e.g.* TB Profiler, PhyReSE, Mykrobe, *etc.*) as well as commercial/proprietary software [78–81]. Online tools have the advantage of being free, but may need to be extensively validated in the laboratory to enable their use in routine diagnostic management.

Over 100 genes have been shown to be associated with resistance to anti-TB drugs, and the availability of high-quality curated up-to-date databases is of utmost importance for the correct interpretation and reporting of WGS DST results [68, 82]. While much is known about polymorphisms associated with resistance to principal first-line drugs, including rifampicin and isoniazid, molecular mechanisms of resistance to selected reserve and new drugs are yet to be fully understood, which may have an impact on the performance of WGS for some of these drugs [68, 78]. Importantly, the quality of phenotypic DST data plays a major role in establishing the associations between polymorphisms and phenotypic resistance [82]. Ideally, specific mutations should be linked to specific MICs, and WGS should be able to predict both resistant and sensitive phenotypes, thus enabling clinicians to adjust treatment regimens, including dosage, depending on whether specific mutations are associated with low or high levels of resistance [69, 70].

Implementation of WGS-based systems for routine diagnosis of TB in selected high-income settings in Europe and North America has already provided evidence about WGS methodology to inform clinical management of DR-TB [83, 84].

Targeted sequencing
One of the main goals for the near future is to move towards culture-free NGS for rapid DST. This requires the capacity to extract high-molecular-weight genomic DNA from an extremely low number of *M. tuberculosis* bacilli ($100-10^5$ cells·mL^{-1}) present in a complex matrix which contains large amounts (<99%) of both human and other bacterial DNA. A process of enrichment is thus required to increase the proportion of mycobacterial DNA to enhance the sequencing efficiency. Although in principle direct NGS from smear-positive clinical sputum samples has proven to be feasible [85, 86], the protocols are rather cumbersome or very expensive. A recent study presented a new method for extracting *M. tuberculosis* DNA directly from smear-positive respiratory samples, allowing sufficient data for antibiotic susceptibility prediction to be retrieved from >60% of the samples tested [87]. However, the bioinformatic analysis was computationally intensive as human DNA reads had to be removed *a priori*.

An alternative approach for the rapid sequencing of primary specimens is to perform targeted NGS (amplicon NGS), which allows the ultra-deep sequencing of specific genomic regions of interest, such as those associated to drug resistance and species identification. Although this method requires pre-existing knowledge of the targets, in principle it is easily customisable and scalable with the addition of new targets of interest. Only a few studies have evaluated the performance of amplicon sequencing of *M. tuberculosis* DNA from sputum specimens to provide rapid DST, showing a high level of concordance (97%) with phenotypic testing [88, 89]. Importantly, amplicon NGS allows the identification of resistant subpopulations with high accuracy thanks to the high coverage depth of the targets [89]. GenoScreen (Lille, France) has recently released the Deeplex-MycTB assay for research purposes, which is a 24-plexed amplicon mix allowing the simultaneous prediction of resistance to 13 anti-TB drugs, genotyping and mycobacterial identification, directly on primary specimens. The kit includes access to a secure, cloud-based application for the rapid analysis and interpretation of the sequencing data. Recently, the assay has been used for rapid DST of sputum specimens collected during the anti-TB drug resistance survey of Djibouti [90].

Future perspectives

Despite a promising pipeline in new diagnostics, major gaps remain in the diagnosis of TB and DR-TB, including 1) a highly sensitive low-cost triaging test perhaps with an acceptable lower specificity that could be used as a point-of-care test to exclude TB and 2) a biomarker for cure. A next generation of LAM assays working on sputum is under field trials and preliminary unpublished data seem really promising. Other biomarker assays are under development. At present none of them have been fully validated as able to be used as a marker of cure [66].

A "closer to point of need", fully portable and wireless device (Omni; Cepheid) compatible with Xpert Ultra cartridges is also close to commercialisation. If expectations are confirmed by performance data, the detection of TB and MDR-TB cases will be further decentralised. Other devices and portable platforms are in different stages of development. The ability to rapidly detect resistance to isoniazid has important implications, especially in light of the new WHO recommendations on the treatment of patients with confirmed rifampicin-susceptible, isoniazid-resistant TB [91]. Roll-out of molecular assays able to predict isoniazid monoresistance is needed to allow implementation of the WHO guidelines in high-burden countries: several platforms are in the pipeline or close to commercialisation in the European Union or global market, although the majority are designed for centralised work.

The Xpert XDR cartridge has been developed to complement the Xpert MTB/RIF assay, providing additional information on isoniazid, fluoroquinolone and SLID resistance of TB-positive samples [92, 93].

In the next few years we expect an increasing role of WGS/NGS-based technologies. These technologies have the incomparable advantage of providing "complete" sets of data, allowing us not only to predict drug resistance with higher sensitivity (interrogating larger numbers, full genes and relevant noncoding sequences), but also providing an indication of the transmission of the disease. Data on transmission of TB and MDR-TB should inform TB programme strategies in low- and medium-burden countries engaged in eliminating TB.

Molecular data coupled with the knowledge obtained by MIC data (now more easily obtainable using microtitre plates) will allow a truly personalised treatment to be designed. Phenotypic DST will not disappear soon; it may be restricted to a few molecules for which genomic data are insufficient for clear-cut interpretation.

Conclusion

The TB diagnostic pipeline has flourished in the past 5 years as never before with many companies becoming interested and new tests/platforms entering in the process. How many of the proposed tests will pass the "reality check" (*i.e.* high-level performance in high-burden settings at a competitive cost) and become reality is unknown. Phenotypic DST will be gradually replaced by molecular interpretation of mutations for some drugs, but not for all. With more information on drug MIC distribution becoming available, the use of a single critical concentration to categorise drugs as susceptible or resistant is insufficient to properly guide treatment. MIC values or "clinical concentration" tests should be provided for key drugs when alternative or less toxic regimens are not possible.

References

1.   World Health Organization. Global Tuberculosis Report 2016. Geneva, WHO, 2016.

2. Foundation for Innovative New Diagnostics. TB diagnostic pipeline. 2018. www.finddx.org/dx-pipeline-status Date last accessed: June 20, 2018.

3. World Health Organization. Automated Real-time Nucleic Acid Amplification Technology for Rapid and Simultaneous Detection of Tuberculosis and Rifampicin Resistance: Xpert MTB/RIF Assay for the Diagnosis of Pulmonary and Extrapulmonary TB in Adults and Children: Policy Update. Geneva, WHO, 2013.

4. World Health Organization. WHO Meeting Report of a Technical Expert Consultation: Non-inferiority Analysis of Xpert MTB/RIF Ultra Compared to Xpert MTB/RIF. Geneva, WHO, 2017.

5. World Health Organization. The Use of Molecular Line Probe Assays for the Detection of Resistance to Isoniazid and Rifampicin: Policy Update. Geneva, WHO, 2016.

6. World Health Organization. The Use of Molecular Line Probe Assays for the Detection of Resistance to Second-line Anti-tuberculosis Drugs: Policy Guidance. Geneva, WHO, 2016.

7. World Health Organization. The Use of Loop-mediated Isothermal Amplification (TB-LAMP) for the Diagnosis of Pulmonary Tuberculosis: Policy Guidance. Geneva, WHO, 2016.

8. World Health Organization. The Use of Lateral Flow Urine Lipoarabinomannan Assay (LF-LAM) for Diagnosis and Screening of Active Tuberculosis in People Living with HIV: Policy Guidance. Geneva, WHO, 2015.

9. World Health Organization. Implementing Tuberculosis Diagnostics: Policy Framework. Geneva, WHO, 2015.

10. Clinical and Laboratory Standards Institute. Laboratory Detection and Identification of Mycobacteria. Approved Guideline M48-A. Wayne, CLSI, 2008.

11. European Centre for Disease Prevention and Control. Handbook on TB Laboratory Diagnostic Methods for the European Union. Stockholm, ECDC, 2016.

12. Garcia LS, Isenberg HD, eds. Clinical Microbiology Procedures Handbook. 3rd Edn. Washington, ASM Press, 2010.

13. World Health Organization. Fluorescent Light Emitting Diode (LED) Microscopy for Diagnosis of Tuberculosis: WHO Policy Statement. Geneva, WHO, 2010.

14. World Health Organization. Approaches to Improve Sputum Smear Microscopy for Tuberculosis Diagnosis: Expert Group Meeting Report. Geneva, WHO, 2009.

15. Kvach JT, Veras JR. A fluorescent staining procedure for determining the viability of mycobacterial cells. *Int J Lepr Other Mycobact Dis* 1982; 50: 183–192.

16. Datta S, Sherman JM, Bravard MA, *et al.* Clinical evaluation of tuberculosis viability microscopy for assessing treatment response. *Clin Infect Dis* 2015; 60: 1186–1195.

17. Hanna BA, Ebrahimzadeh A, Elliott LB, *et al.* Multicenter evaluation of the BACTEC MGIT 960 system for recovery of mycobacteria. *J Clin Microbiol* 1999; 37: 748–752.

18. Tenover FC, Crawford JT, Huebner RE, *et al.* The resurgence of tuberculosis: is your laboratory ready? *J Clin Microbiol* 1993; 31: 767–770.

19. Tortoli E, Cichero P, Piersimoni C, *et al.* Use of BACTEC MGIT 960 for recovery of mycobacteria from clinical specimens: multicenter study. *J Clin Microbiol* 1999; 37: 3578–3582.

20. Helb D, Jones M, Story E, *et al.* Rapid detection of *Mycobacterium tuberculosis* and rifampin resistance by use of on-demand, near-patient technology. *J Clin Microbiol* 2010; 48: 229–237.

21. World Health Organization. Automated Real-time Nucleic Acid Amplification Technology for Rapid and Simultaneous Detection of Tuberculosis and Rifampicin Resistance: Xpert MTB/RIF System: Policy Statement. Geneva, WHO, 2011.

22. Steingart KR, Schiller I, Horne DJ, *et al.* Xpert MTB/RIF assay for pulmonary tuberculosis and rifampicin resistance in adults. *Cochrane Database Syst Rev* 2014; 1: CD009593.

23. Detjen AK, DiNardo AR, Leyden J, *et al.* Xpert MTB/RIF assay for the diagnosis of pulmonary tuberculosis in children: a systematic review and meta-analysis. *Lancet Respir Med* 2015; 3: 451–461.

24. Denkinger CM, Schumacher SG, Boehme CC, *et al.* Xpert MTB/RIF assay for the diagnosis of extrapulmonary tuberculosis: a systematic review and meta-analysis. *Eur Respir J* 2014; 44: 435–446.

25. Maynard-Smith L, Larke N, Peters JA, *et al.* Diagnostic accuracy of the Xpert MTB/RIF assay for extrapulmonary and pulmonary tuberculosis when testing non-respiratory samples: a systematic review. *BMC Infect Dis* 2014; 14: 709.

26. Chakravorty S, Simmons AM, Rowneki M, *et al.* The New Xpert MTB/RIF Ultra: improving detection of *Mycobacterium tuberculosis* and resistance to rifampin in an assay suitable for point-of-care testing. *MBio* 2017; 8: e00812-17.

27. Dorman SE, Schumacher SG, Alland D, *et al.* Xpert MTB/RIF Ultra for detection of *Mycobacterium tuberculosis* and rifampicin resistance: a prospective multicentre diagnostic accuracy study. *Lancet Infect Dis* 2018; 18: 76–84.

28. Bahr NC, Nuwagira E, Evans EE, *et al.* Diagnostic accuracy of Xpert MTB/RIF Ultra for tuberculous meningitis in HIV-infected adults: a prospective cohort study. *Lancet Infect Dis* 2018; 18: 68–75.

29. Nicol MP, Workman L, Prins M, *et al.* Accuracy of Xpert MTB/RIF Ultra for the diagnosis of pulmonary tuberculosis in children. *Pediatr Infect Dis J* 2018; 37: e261–e263.

30. Shah M, Hanrahan C, Wang ZY, *et al.* Lateral flow urine lipoarabinomannan assay for detecting active tuberculosis in HIV-positive adults. *Cochrane Database Syst Rev* 2016; 5: CD011420.

https://doi.org/10.1183/2312508X.10021318

31. Peter JG, Zijenah LS, Chanda D, *et al.* Effect on mortality of point-of-care, urine-based lipoarabinomannan testing to guide tuberculosis treatment initiation in HIV-positive hospital inpatients: a pragmatic, parallel-group, multicountry, open-label, randomised controlled trial. *Lancet* 2016; 387: 1187–1197.

32. Tang N, Frank A, Pahalawatta V, *et al.* Analytical and clinical performance of Abbott RealTime MTB, an assay for detection of *Mycobacterium tuberculosis* in pulmonary specimens. *Tuberculosis* 2015; 95: 613–619.

33. Hofmann-Thiel S, Molodtsov N, Antonenka U, *et al.* Evaluation of the Abbott RealTime MTB and RealTime MTB INH/RIF assays for direct detection of *Mycobacterium tuberculosis* complex and resistance markers in respiratory and extrapulmonary specimens. *J Clin Microbiol* 2016; 54: 3022–3027.

34. Hinić V, Feuz K, Turan S, *et al.* Clinical evaluation of the Abbott RealTime MTB Assay for direct detection of *Mycobacterium tuberculosis*-complex from respiratory and non-respiratory samples. *Tuberculosis* 2017; 104: 65–69.

35. Scott L, David A, Noble L, *et al.* Performance of the Abbott RealTime MTB and MTB RIF/INH assays in a setting of high tuberculosis and HIV coinfection in South Africa. *J Clin Microbiol* 2017; 55: 2491–2501.

36. Chen JH, She KK, Kwong TC, *et al.* Performance of the new automated Abbott RealTime MTB assay for rapid detection of *Mycobacterium tuberculosis* complex in respiratory specimens. *Eur J Clin Microbiol Infect Dis* 2015; 34: 1827–1832.

37. Drobniewski F, Rüsch-Gerdes S, Hoffner S, *et al.* Antimicrobial susceptibility testing of *Mycobacterium tuberculosis* (EUCAST document E.DEF 8.1) – report of the Subcommittee on Antimicrobial Susceptibility Testing of *Mycobacterium tuberculosis* of the European Committee for Antimicrobial Susceptibility Testing (EUCAST) of the European Society of Clinical Microbiology and Infectious Diseases (ESCMID). *Clin Microbiol Infect* 2007; 13: 1144–1156.

38. World Health Organization. Technical Report on Critical Concentrations for Drug Susceptibility Testing of Medicines Used in the Treatment of Drug-resistant Tuberculosis. Geneva, WHO, 2018.

39. World Health Organization. Global consultation on research for TB elimination opens today. 2014. www.who.int/tb/features_archive/researchforTBelimination_meeting/en Date last accessed: September 1, 2018.

40. World Health Organization. Guidelines for Surveillance of Drug Resistance in Tuberculosis. 5th Edn. Geneva, WHO, 2015.

41. Canetti G, Froman S, Grosset J, *et al.* Mycobacteria: laboratory methods for testing drug sensitivity and resistance. *Bull World Health Organ* 1963; 29: 565–578.

42. Krüüner A, Yates MD, Drobniewski FA. Evaluation of MGIT 960-based antimicrobial testing and determination of critical concentrations of first- and second-line antimicrobial drugs with drug-resistant clinical strains of *Mycobacterium tuberculosis*. *J Clin Microbiol* 2006; 44: 811–818.

43. Springer B, Lucke K, Calligaris-Maibach R, *et al.* Quantitative drug susceptibility testing of *Mycobacterium tuberculosis* by use of MGIT 960 and EpiCenter instrumentation. *J Clin Microbiol* 2009; 47: 1773–1780.

44. Lee J, Armstrong DT, Ssengooba W, *et al.* Sensititre MYCOTB MIC plate for testing *Mycobacterium tuberculosis* susceptibility to first- and second-line drugs. *Antimicrob Agents Chemother* 2014; 58: 11–18.

45. Xia H, Zheng Y, Zhao B, *et al.* Assessment of a 96-well plate assay of quantitative drug susceptibility testing for *Mycobacterium tuberculosis* complex in China. *PLoS One* 2017; 12: e0169413.

46. Rancoita PMV, Cugnata F, Gibertoni Cruz AL, *et al.* Validating a 14-drug microtiter plate containing bedaquiline and delamanid for large-scale research susceptibility testing of *Mycobacterium tuberculosis*. *Antimicrob Agents Chemother* 2018; 62: e00344-18.

47. Ängeby K, Juréen P, Kahlmeter G, *et al.* Challenging a dogma: antimicrobial susceptibility testing breakpoints for *Mycobacterium tuberculosis*. *Bull World Health Organ* 2012; 90: 693–698.

48. Werngren J, Sturegård E, Juréen P, *et al.* Reevaluation of the critical concentration for drug susceptibility testing of *Mycobacterium tuberculosis* against pyrazinamide using wild-type MIC distributions and *pncA* gene sequencing. *Antimicrob Agents Chemother* 2012; 56: 1253–1257.

49. Schön T, Miotto P, Köser CU, *et al.* *Mycobacterium tuberculosis* drug-resistance testing: challenges, recent developments and perspectives. *Clin Microbiol Infect* 2017; 23: 154–160.

50. Heyckendorf J, Andres S, Köser CU, *et al.* What is resistance? Impact of phenotypic versus molecular drug resistance testing on therapy for multi- and extensively drug-resistant tuberculosis. *Antimicrob Agents Chemother* 2018; 62: e01550-17.

51. Köser CU, Javid B, Liddell K, *et al.* Drug-resistance mechanisms and tuberculosis drugs. *Lancet* 2015; 385: 305–307.

52. World Health Organization. Noncommercial Culture and Drug-susceptibility Testing Methods for Screening Patients at Risk for Multidrug-resistant Tuberculosis: Policy Statement. Geneva, WHO, 2011.

53. Foundation for Innovative New Diagnostics. Non-inferiority evaluation of Nipro NTM+MDRTB and Hain GenoType MTBDRplus V2 line probe assays. Version 4.1. 2015. www.finddx.org/wp-content/uploads/2016/04/LPA-report_noninferiority-study_oct2015.pdf Date last accessed: September 1, 2018.

54. Theron G PJ, Richardson M, Warren R, *et al.* GenoType MTBDR assay for resistance to second-line anti-tuberculosis drugs. *Cochrane Database Syst Rev* 2016; 9: CD010705.

55. Driesen M, Kondo Y, de Jong BC, *et al.* Evaluation of a novel line probe assay to detect resistance to pyrazinamide, a key drug used for tuberculosis treatment. *Clin Microbiol Infect* 2018; 24: 60–64.

56. Willby MJ, Wijkander M, Havumaki J, *et al.* Detection of *Mycobacterium tuberculosis pncA* mutations by the Nipro Genoscholar PZATB II assay compared to conventional sequencing. *Antimicrob Agents Chemother* 2018; 62: e01871-17.

57. Rufai SB, Kumar P, Singh A, *et al.* Comparison of Xpert MTB/RIF with line probe assay for detection of rifampin-monoresistant *Mycobacterium tuberculosis. J Clin Microbiol* 2014; 52: 1846–1852.

58. Zetola NM, Shin SS, Tumedi KA, *et al.* Mixed *Mycobacterium tuberculosis* complex infections and false-negative results for rifampin resistance by GeneXpert MTB/RIF are associated with poor clinical outcomes. *J Clin Microbiol* 2014; 52: 2422–2429.

59. Blakemore R, Story E, Helb D, *et al.* Evaluation of the analytical performance of the Xpert MTB/RIF assay. *J Clin Microbiol* 2010; 48: 2495–2501.

60. Köser CU, Comas I, Feuerriegel S, *et al.* Genetic diversity within *Mycobacterium tuberculosis* complex impacts on the accuracy of genotypic pyrazinamide drug-susceptibility assay. *Tuberculosis* 2014; 94: 451–453.

61. Williamson DA, Basu I, Bower J, *et al.* An evaluation of the Xpert MTB/RIF assay and detection of false-positive rifampicin resistance in *Mycobacterium tuberculosis. Diagn Microbiol Infect Dis* 2012; 74: 207–209.

62. Sanchez JA, Pierce KE, Rice JE, *et al.* Linear-after-the-exponential (LATE)-PCR: an advanced method of asymmetric PCR and its uses in quantitative real-time analysis. *Proc Natl Acad Sci USA* 2004; 101: 1933–1938.

63. Rice LM, Reis AH, Wangh LJ. Virtual Barcoding using LATE-PCR and Lights-On/Lights-Off probes: identification of nematode species in a closed-tube reaction. *Mitochondrial DNA A DNA Mapp Seq Anal* 2016; 27: 1358–1363.

64. Hillemann D, Haasis C, Andres S, *et al.* Validation of the FluoroType MTBDR assay for detection of rifampin and isoniazid resistance in *Mycobacterium tuberculosis* complex isolates. *J Clin Microbiol* 2018; 56: e00072-18.

65. de Vos M, Derendinger B, Dolby T, *et al.* Diagnostic accuracy and utility of FluoroType MTBDR, a new molecular assay for multidrug-resistant tuberculosis. *J Clin Microbiol* 2018; 56: e00531-18.

66. UNITAID, World Health Organization. Tuberculosis diagnostic technology landscape. 5th Edn. 2017. https://unitaid.eu/assets/2017-Unitaid-TB-Diagnostics-Technology-Landscape.pdf Date last accessed: September 1, 2018.

67. Stefan Z, Alexander D, Patrick M, *et al.* Pre-validation of the BD MAX MDR-TB assay for the rapid detection of MTBc DNA and mutations associated with rifampin and isoniazid resistance. 2018. www.escmid.org/escmid_publications/escmid_elibrary/material/?mid=61376 Date last accessed: September 1, 2018.

68. Papaventsis D, Casali N, Kontsevaya I, *et al.* Whole genome sequencing of *Mycobacterium tuberculosis* for detection of drug resistance: a systematic review. *Clin Microbiol Infect* 2017; 23: 61–68.

69. Walker TM, Merker M, Kohl TA, *et al.* Whole genome sequencing for M/XDR tuberculosis surveillance and for resistance testing. *Clin Microbiol Infect* 2017; 23: 161–166.

70. Satta G, Lipman M, Smith GP, *et al. Mycobacterium tuberculosis* and whole-genome sequencing: how close are we to unleashing its full potential? *Clin Microbiol Infect* 2018; 24: 604–609.

71. Walker TM, Kohl TA, Omar SV, *et al.* Whole-genome sequencing for prediction of *Mycobacterium tuberculosis* drug susceptibility and resistance: a retrospective cohort study. *Lancet Infect Dis* 2015; 15: 1193–1202.

72. Pankhurst LJ, Del Ojo Elias C, Votintseva AA, *et al.* Rapid, comprehensive, and affordable mycobacterial diagnosis with whole-genome sequencing: a prospective study. *Lancet Respir Med* 2016; 4: 49–58.

73. Witney AA, Gould KA, Arnold A, *et al.* Clinical application of whole-genome sequencing to inform treatment for multidrug-resistant tuberculosis cases. *J Clin Microbiol* 2015; 53: 1473–1483.

74. Kwong JC, McCallum N, Sintchenko V, *et al.* Whole genome sequencing in clinical and public health microbiology. *Pathology* 2015; 47: 199–210.

75. Satta G, Atzeni A, McHugh TD. *Mycobacterium tuberculosis* and whole genome sequencing: a practical guide and online tools available for the clinical microbiologist. *Clin Microbiol Infect* 2017; 23: 69–72.

76. Votintseva AA, Pankhurst LJ, Anson LW, *et al.* Mycobacterial DNA extraction for whole-genome sequencing from early positive liquid (MGIT) cultures. *J Clin Microbiol* 2015; 53: 1137–1143.

77. Dookie N, Rambaran S, Padayatchi N, *et al.* Evolution of drug resistance in *Mycobacterium tuberculosis*: a review on the molecular determinants of resistance and implications for personalized care. *J Antimicrob Chemother* 2018; 73: 1138–1151.

78. Coll F, McNerney R, Preston MD, *et al.* Rapid determination of anti-tuberculosis drug resistance from whole-genome sequences. *Genome Med* 2015; 7: 51.

79. Feuerriegel S, Schleusener V, Beckert P, *et al.* PhyResSE: a web tool delineating *Mycobacterium tuberculosis* antibiotic resistance and lineage from whole-genome sequencing data. *J Clin Microbiol* 2015; 53: 1908–1914.

80. Schleusener V, Köser CU, Beckert P, *et al. Mycobacterium tuberculosis* resistance prediction and lineage classification from genome sequencing: comparison of automated analysis tools. *Sci Rep* 2017; 7: 46327.

81. Bradley P, Gordon NC, Walker TM, *et al.* Rapid antibiotic-resistance predictions from genome sequence data for *Staphylococcus aureus* and *Mycobacterium tuberculosis. Nat Commun* 2015; 6: 10063.

82. Miotto P, Tessema B, Tagliani E, *et al.* A standardised method for interpreting the association between mutations and phenotypic drug resistance in *Mycobacterium tuberculosis. Eur Respir J* 2017; 50: 1701354.

83. Cabibbe AM, Trovato A, De Filippo MR, *et al.* Countrywide implementation of whole genome sequencing: an opportunity to improve tuberculosis management, surveillance and contact tracing in low incidence countries. *Eur Respir J* 2018; 51: 1800387.

https://doi.org/10.1183/2312508X.10021318

84. Shea J, Halse TA, Lapierre P, *et al.* Comprehensive whole-genome sequencing and reporting of drug resistance profiles on clinical cases of *Mycobacterium tuberculosis* in New York State. *J Clin Microbiol* 2017; 55: 1871–1882.

85. Doughty EL, Sergeant MJ, Adetifa I, *et al.* Culture-independent detection and characterisation of *Mycobacterium tuberculosis* and *M. africanum* in sputum samples using shotgun metagenomics on a benchtop sequencer. *PeerJ* 2014; 2: e585.

86. Brown AC, Bryant JM, Einer-Jensen K, *et al.* Rapid whole-genome sequencing of *Mycobacterium tuberculosis* isolates directly from clinical samples. *J Clin Microbiol* 2015; 53: 2230–2237.

87. Votintseva AA, Bradley P, Pankhurst L, *et al.* Same-day diagnostic and surveillance data for tuberculosis via whole-genome sequencing of direct respiratory samples. *J Clin Microbiol* 2017; 55: 1285–1298.

88. Daum LT, Rodriguez JD, Worthy SA, *et al.* Next-generation ion torrent sequencing of drug resistance mutations in *Mycobacterium tuberculosis* strains. *J Clin Microbiol* 2012; 50: 3831–3837.

89. Colman RE, Anderson J, Lemmer D, *et al.* Rapid drug susceptibility testing of drug-resistant *Mycobacterium tuberculosis* isolates directly from clinical samples by use of amplicon sequencing: a proof-of-concept study. *J Clin Microbiol* 2016; 54: 2058–2067.

90. Tagliani E, Hassan MO, Waberi Y, *et al.* Culture and next-generation sequencing-based drug susceptibility testing unveil high levels of drug-resistant-TB in Djibouti: results from the first national survey. *Sci Rep* 2017; 7: 17672.

91. World Health Organization. WHO Treatment Guidelines for Isoniazid-resistant Tuberculosis: Supplement to the WHO Treatment Guidelines for Drug-resistant Tuberculosis. Geneva, WHO, 2018.

92. Chakravorty S, Roh SS, Glass J, *et al.* Detection of isoniazid-, fluoroquinolone-, amikacin-, and kanamycin-resistant tuberculosis in an automated, multiplexed 10-color assay suitable for point-of-care use. *J Clin Microbiol* 2017; 55: 183–198.

93. Dorman S. An Xpert assay for detection of resistance to INH, FQ, SLIDs. 2017. www.uitb.cat/wp-content/uploads/2017/12/Taller-TB-2017_sdorman2.pdf Date last accessed: September 1, 2018.

Disclosures: None declared.

Chapter 8

Imaging for diagnosis and management

Dumitru Chesov[1,2] and Victor Botnaru[1]

The importance of imaging in the diagnosis and management of TB has varied over time. Chest radiography, in particular, has moved from its role as a key diagnostic test in all cases to one where it is now recognised as an efficient method of early TB detection. This has arisen in part due to the introduction of new digital radiographic approaches (both in performance and reading) as well as changes in global TB policies to detect all TB cases irrespective of their infectiousness. Combined with clinical and microbiological data, radiography remains helpful in both TB diagnosis and follow-up in a large number of patients. However, in some cases imaging tools with a higher specificity are required, *e.g.* computed tomography or magnetic resonance imaging. These may be particularly useful in EPTB, paucibacillary and immunocompromised patients. The relatively high cost of modern imaging diagnostics remains a barrier to their wider adoption in high-burden TB settings.

Cite as: Chesov D, Botnaru V. Imaging for diagnosis and management. *In:* Migliori GB, Bothamley G, Duarte R, *et al.*, eds. Tuberculosis (ERS Monograph). Sheffield, European Respiratory Society, 2018; pp. 116–136 [https://doi.org/10.1183/2312508X.10021217].

@ERSpublications
Combined with clinical and microbiological data, radiography complemented by other imaging tools is indispensable for proper diagnosis and follow-up of both PTB and EPTB. http://ow.ly/cfVQ30lqCfE

Imaging tests, particularly chest radiography, have a long history of being used for the clinical management of TB. Between the 1930s and 1960s, chest radiography was at the forefront of TB detection in industrialised and developing countries. It was widely used for mass TB screening campaigns [1, 2]. However, in the mid-1970 s the WHO endorsed symptom screening and bacteriological testing as the cornerstone of TB detection and follow-up [3]. These recommendations led to an (unintended) decline in interest in the use of imaging in TB patients [4].

A recent shift in global TB priorities from detection of the most contagious TB patients to early diagnosis of all active disease cases, even asymptomatic, has driven a resurgence of

[1]Division of Pneumology and Allergology, "Nicolae Testemitanu" State University of Medicine and Pharmacy, Chisinau, Republic of Moldova. [2]Division of Clinical Infectious Diseases, Research Center Borstel, Borstel, Germany.

Correspondence: Dumitru Chesov, Division of Pneumology and Allergology, "Nicolae Testemitanu" State University of Medicine and Pharmacy, 165 Stefan cel Mare, 2004 Chisinau, Republic of Moldova. E-mail: dumitru.chesov@usmf.md

interest in imaging strategies. Modern imaging modalities offer prompt detection of TB-associated lesions as well as assessment of disease activity and patient follow-up [5].

Role of imaging diagnostics

Radiography is the most accessible and commonly used imaging test for the clinical management of TB, but it is not the only available tool. Existing evidence suggests that a wide variety of modern imaging diagnostics may be useful at various stages of TB clinical care or research.

Radiography

Radiography for tuberculosis screening and triage

Due to its high sensitivity (87–98%) chest radiography is recognised as a powerful screening tool that has a higher accuracy than symptoms-based approaches, particularly in the detection of early TB [6]. Recent data suggest that over half of patients with bacteriologically confirmed TB and abnormal chest radiographs would be missed by symptoms-based screening [6]. Chest radiography allows rapid screening for a range of medical conditions beyond TB. However, its low specificity (46–89%) and high interreader variability are also well known [7]. These deficiencies could be overcome by inclusion of a high-specificity bacteriological test into the TB screening algorithm [8]. Use of chest radiography as part of screening practice can also reduce the number of persons tested by relatively expensive microbiological diagnostics [9]. Its value is also dependent on the situation, being more expensive and logistically challenging when used as a screening intervention for active TB outside of medical centres in comparison with its role in symptomatic patients attending medical services [1, 6].

The accuracy of radiographic screening depends on many factors, such as TB prevalence in the screened population, quality of clinical assessment, and quality of the radiographs and their interpretation. The latter may be improved through standardisation using imaging scores. Currently proposed radiographic TB scores are sufficiently sensitive (~96%), but have a low specificity (~45%) [10]. There is also concern regarding their applicability in outpatient settings and in patients with HIV. An alternative and more attractive approach for the improvement of radiograph interpretation in TB patients is computer-aided detection, which uses machine learning methods and could aid or replace radiologists or other healthcare personnel in reading radiographs, and thus help to scale-up radiology for systematic TB screening or triaging [11]. Several successful computer-aided detection implementations in resource-limited settings have been reported [12, 13].

Radiography for tuberculosis diagnosis

As a TB diagnostic tool, radiography is extremely useful in persons in whom active disease is clinically suspected. Particular radiographic signs associated with TB disease can be described for each site of the human body affected by TB. Due to the low specificity, a bacteriological confirmation of disease should always be attempted, even in patients with radiographic lesions highly suggestive for TB. Nevertheless, after repeated negative bacteriological tests a positive TB diagnosis could be concluded using a combination of history, clinical signs and radiological data [6]. Worldwide, the overall proportion of PTB cases diagnosed using clinical and radiological criteria ranges between 22% and 62% [14]. Imaging-based diagnosis is particularly relevant in patients with a low sensitivity for bacteriological tests (immunocompromised persons or EPTB) or in those with difficult sample collection (young children), as well as in critically ill patients in whom treatment delay may be fatal [15, 16]. At the same time, if the patient is not critically ill, it may be reasonable to postpone the diagnostic decision and to consider a follow-up with microbiological and radiological re-evaluation.

In clinical practice, high-quality images and specialist interpretation are essential for accurate radiological diagnosis. Multidisciplinary clinical rounds and/or implementation of peer review procedures are recommended to help achieve this [6].

Radiography for assessment of treatment response and follow-up

Radiography should be part of treatment monitoring in all PTB cases as it provides valuable information on the therapeutic response [6, 17]. However, the predictive value of initial radiographic findings on TB treatment outcome is controversial [18–20]. The chest radiograph may appear unchanged in the first few months of treatment or show only slight improvement, especially in paediatric patients or in those with chronic pulmonary lesions [21]. The evidence is also equivocal regarding the value of end-of-treatment imaging to predict TB disease relapse [22, 23].

The optimal frequency of radiographic monitoring during treatment for PTB is unclear. Pragmatically, where there is drug-sensitive (DS)-TB, it seems reasonable to perform radiography at the end of the intensive phase and at treatment completion. In MDR-TB, radiographic assessment every 6 months of treatment is recommended [24]. Chest radiography should also be performed whenever the patient's clinical condition worsens; however, it is less useful when monitoring treatment response in EPTB.

Computed tomography

Computed tomography (CT) is a more accurate imaging modality than radiography for PTB, with a sensitivity up to 91% and a specificity of 76% [25]. It is commonly used in patients with suspected TB and a normal radiograph or ill-defined radiographic lesions (*e.g.* small cavities, fuzzy opacities or tiny nodules) [26]. Indications for CT assessment are less precise in children and adolescents, where there may be issues regarding radiation dosing. CT can be helpful in suspected TB with negative microbiological tests or pre-existing lesions [27, 28]. Several CT-based PTB screening scores have been proposed that can be used before microbiological test results become available; however, these have not yet been validated in large cohorts [29–31].

CT is largely accepted as a technique of choice for diagnosis of mediastinal lymphadenopathy, but it is also useful for the detection of other sites of extrapulmonary involvement [32, 33].

In patients with diagnosed TB, a CT scan is frequently requested in cases with persistence or worsening of radiographic lesions. CT is an essential method for assessing the extent of active TB disease prior to surgical intervention and for the detection of some complications of PTB, such as bronchiectasis or fungal balls [34, 35]. Relatively high costs could preclude CT use in some resource-limited settings.

Ultrasound

Ultrasound is a readily available imaging modality in many settings [35]. It is especially useful for rapid diagnosis and follow-up of EPTB lesions (pleural, lymph nodes and

https://doi.org/10.1183/2312508X.10021217

parenchymal abdominal organs), but could also be of use in some pulmonary cases [36, 37]. During the past decade the quality of ultrasound imaging has substantially improved, and the size and cost of equipment have significantly decreased. As a result, ultrasound is increasingly used as a point-of-care tool for imaging diagnosis and follow-up of EPTB. It is particularly efficient in HIV patients and paediatric populations in TB-endemic areas [38, 39]. A common impediment for large-scale implementation of ultrasound is the lack of medical personnel trained in ultrasound imaging. This could be overcome by implementation of focused protocols that have shown their efficiency in some high-burden TB settings [40, 41].

Magnetic resonance imaging

Magnetic resonance imaging (MRI) plays a crucial role in the diagnosis of central nervous system and musculoskeletal TB by providing better quality images than CT [42]. It also could be indicated for the assessment of other extrapulmonary sites, especially in paediatric or pregnant patients in whom ionising radiation should be avoided [43, 44]. For improved lesion visualisation, conventional T1- and T2-weighted images are combined with diffusion-weighted and subtracted contrast-enhanced imaging [45]. MRI of the lung is a promising technique that is starting to enter clinical practice. Some of the existing data suggest that MRI is superior to noncontrast CT in lymph node characterisation [46, 47] and assessment of PTB disease activity [48]. However, its high cost and lack of local availability are common issues.

Positron emission tomography/computed tomography

Due to its ability to assess anatomical and biological aspects of TB lesions, positron emission tomography (PET) combined with CT (PET/CT) is among the newest imaging tools proposed for assessment of TB. ^{18}F-fluorodeoxyglucose (FDG) is the most commonly used tracer for PET/CT scanning in TB patients [49]. Due to avid uptake of FDG by TB granulomas, FDG-PET/CT has been reported to be useful for the assessment of TB disease activity and the identification of individuals with subclinical TB at risk of progression to clinically manifest disease [50, 51]. Similar uptake of FDG by both PTB and EPTB foci provides the opportunity to assess the extrapulmonary extent of disease, especially when there is no possibility of sampling for microbiological or morphological analysis [52]. Unfortunately, FDG-PET/CT fails to distinguish between TB and other FDG-avid lesions, such those from sarcoidosis, NTM and HIV-associated lymphadenopathy [52, 53]. A particular challenge is differentiating PET/CT abnormalities seen in TB from malignancy [53]. In an attempt to overcome these limitations, dual-tracing imaging or dual-time-point imaging have been proposed, but their added value is not yet clear [52]. FDG-PET/CT has been suggested to be used to assess treatment efficacy in the first months of TB medication, treatment completion and relapse prediction during follow-up [54, 55]. This may be particularly relevant for MDR-TB patients in whom this may reduce the use of ineffective and toxic treatment regimens, plus also prevent the emergence of additional resistance, as well as in EPTB cases [55, 56].

Despite these promising results, considerable limitations for the use of PET/CT in clinical practice are its unaffordability in many high-burden TB settings and the associated high doses of radiation patients receive. The latter could be potentially overcome by PET/MRI [57].

Specific organ imaging and differential diagnosis

Respiratory tuberculosis

Respiratory TB refers to PTB and pleural TB. Traditionally, two distinctive imaging patterns are described in patients with respiratory TB. The first corresponds to primary TB disease that develops after initial exposure to infection [58]. The second pattern characterises post-primary TB that occurs due to reactivation of "dormant" infection in a previously healed focus [59]. It is assumed, even it is not always the case, that primary TB is a paediatric disease, while reactivated disease is more an adult type [60]. In this categorisation, radiological findings in primary TB mainly include lymphadenopathy (figure 1) and parenchymal consolidation, while upper lung zone patchy consolidation, cavitation and signs of airway spread of the infection are the main features of reactivation (figure 2) [61]. Lesions such as pleural effusion and miliary nodules can be seen in both primary and post-primary TB [59].

During the past couple of decades the classical concept of distinctive imaging patterns in primary and post-primary TB has been challenged. This is based on emerging evidence

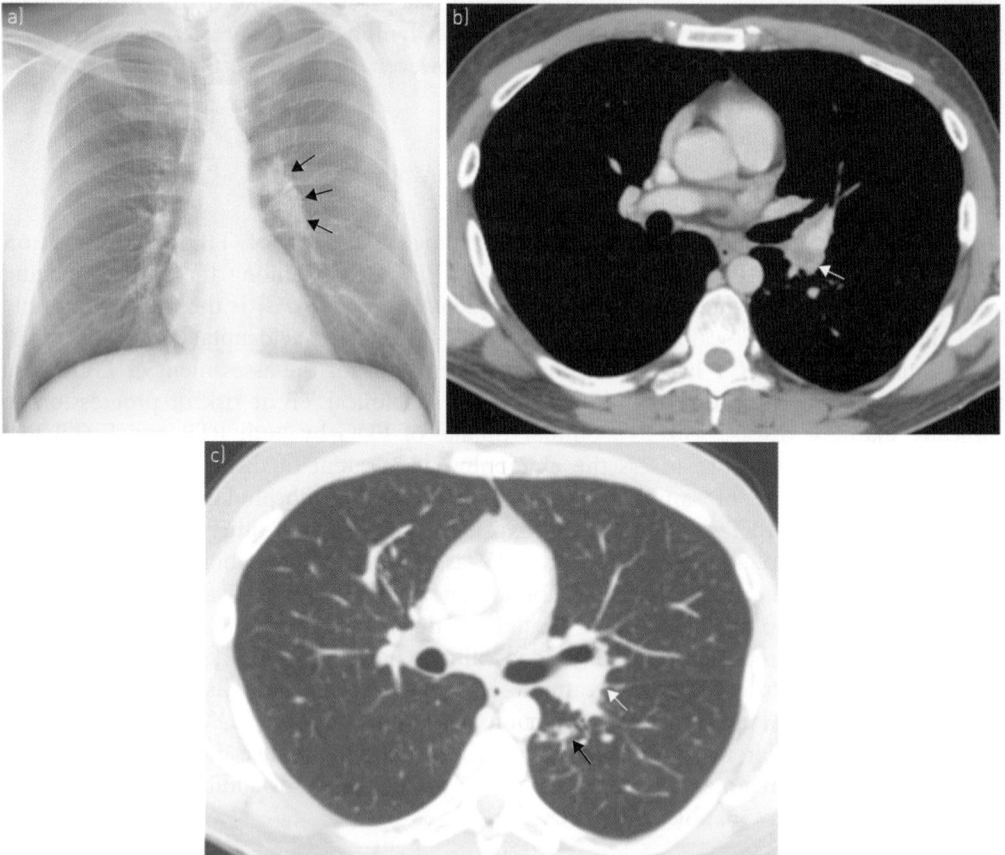

Figure 1. Primary TB imaging pattern. a) Posteroanterior chest radiograph of a 35-year-old male shows a left hilar mass (arrows). b, c) Transverse computed tomography scans of the same patient, at the level of the main bronchi, show an enlarged lymph node with central low attenuation (white arrows) and a small zone of parenchymal consolidation (black arrow).

https://doi.org/10.1183/2312508X.10021217

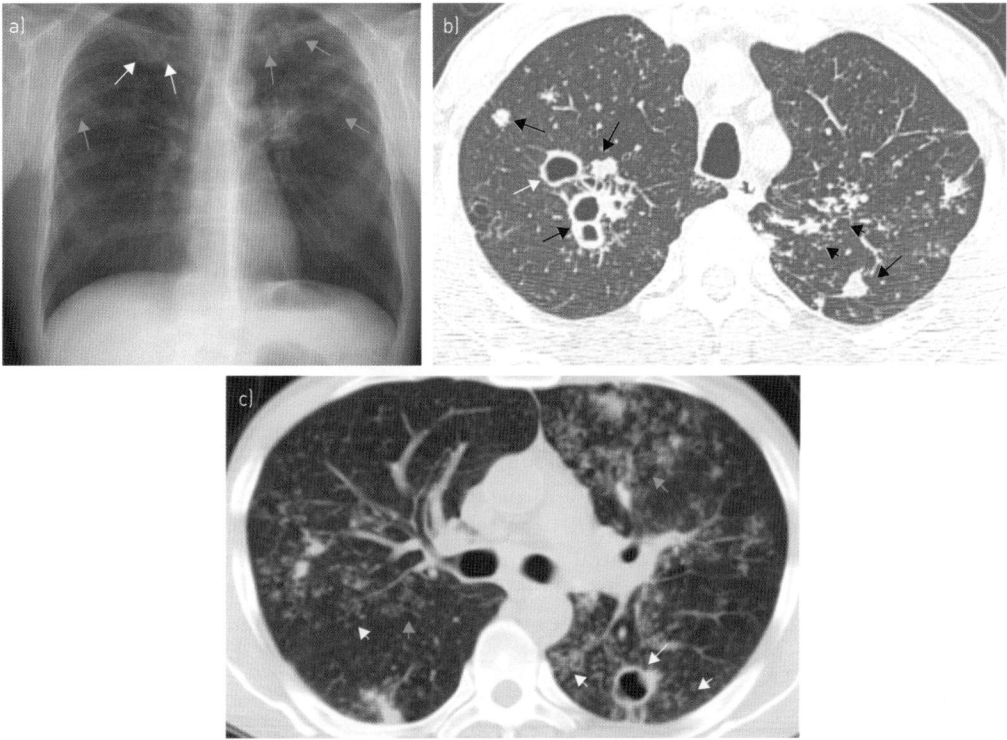

Figure 2. Post-primary TB imaging pattern. a) Posteroanterior chest radiograph of a 53-year-old male shows ill-defined, confluent nodular opacities (grey arrows) in the upper zone of both lungs and small foci of parenchymal destruction (white arrows). b, c) Chest computed tomography scans of the same patient, at the level of b) the proximal descending aorta and c) the main bronchi, show several bilateral thick-walled cavities (long white arrows), irregular patchy consolidations (long black arrows) and bilateral multiple acinar nodules (short black or grey arrows): signs of airway dissemination. Note branching linear and clustered nodular opacities: "tree-in-bud" sign (short white arrows).

from several studies that assessed the type of TB disease (primary or reactivated) not by seroconversion, as was typically done before, but by DNA genotyping of the *Mycobacterium tuberculosis* strains [62, 63]. The data suggest that the main determinant of radiological appearances in TB patients is not the time from infection acquisition to the development of TB disease, but the potency of the immune response of the human host. The classical primary TB pattern is associated with an immunocompromised status, whereas the reactivation type of radiographic lesion is seen in immunocompetent patients [64]. In line with this are data that demonstrate transition from the reactivation to primary TB imaging pattern in HIV patients as blood CD4 counts decline [65]. Similarly, a primary TB radiological pattern is more commonly seen in patients with impaired immunity due to DM [66, 67] or anti-tumour necrosis factor-α therapy [68].

Imaging features of respiratory MDR-TB do not differ significantly from those in DS-TB. Although large nodules as well as parenchymal and lymph node calcification have been reported as being more common in DS-TB, patients with MDR-TB receiving treatment for the first time had a greater frequency of cavitation and bronchiectasis [69, 70]. Some limited data suggest that MDR-TB cases with no history of previous treatment tend to have a more primary TB-like imaging appearance, while retreatment MDR cases resemble reactivation disease [71].

Primary tuberculosis imaging pattern

Parenchymal lesions

Parenchymal lesions are often represented by homogeneous segmental or lobar lung consolidation, with a predilection for the lower and middle lobes [58, 72]. Consolidation is similar to that in bacterial pneumonia. However, the presence of lymphadenopathy and lack of improvement on conventional antibiotics may suggest TB as the cause of consolidation [73]. Cavitary lesions are very rare in primary TB, usually coexisting with consolidation, and are known as progressive-type primary disease [74, 75]. It is thought that only a minority of patients (~15%) have a radiologically identifiable Ghon focus, comprising parenchymal fibrotic or calcified scars following resolution of consolidation [73].

Thoracic lymphadenopathy

Thoracic lymphadenopathy is the most common radiological sign of primary TB, seen in up to 95% of paediatric cases and 42% of adult cases [61]. It is often unilateral with a right side predilection, involving the hilum and paratracheal region. It may be accompanied by parenchymal or pleural lesions. CT can reveal central low attenuation and rim enhancement, both features of central caseous necrosis (itself highly suggestive of active disease) [76]. MRI is an alternative method to assess lymphadenopathy [77]. Residual calcification of normal sized lymph nodes can be present after resolution of active disease, although it occurs in many granulomatous conditions, including sarcoidosis and fungal diseases [78].

Post-primary tuberculosis (reactivation) imaging pattern

Parenchymal lesions

Parenchymal lesions associated with reactivated pulmonary disease at their onset are expressed radiologically by focal or patchy, ill-defined lung opacities mainly with an apical and posterior distribution [60]. Usually more than one lung segment is affected and bilateral involvement is common [73]. Cavitary lesions are the distinctive feature of post-primary disease and are present in more than half of patients [61]. Multiple cavities of different sizes can occur within areas of consolidation. Thick irregular walls that become smooth and thin on effective treatment are typical of TB cavities [79]. Air-fluid levels are rarely present and are more suggestive of an associated bacterial infection [80]. In ~5% of cases, parenchymal lesions are represented by a tuberculoma (a single round nodular opacity 0.5–4 cm in diameter), sometimes surrounded by satellite nodules [73].

Airway involvement

Airway involvement is manifest by signs of endobronchial spread of TB infection and bronchial stenosis. The former is detected on CT in ~25% of cases. It is seen as poorly defined clusters of nodules [81]. These may be accompanied by branching linear opacities known as the "tree-in-bud" sign [82]. However, it is nonspecific, and may also be seen in NTM, sarcoidosis, lymphoma, infectious bronchiolitis, lung malignancies and gastro-oesophageal aspiration [83]. Bronchial stenosis is detected by CT in 10–40% of active TB cases, and is characterised by long segment narrowing, irregular wall thickening and luminal obstruction [69]. Bronchial involvement is more common in females from high-burden TB countries in their second or third decades of life as well as the Western elderly population [84, 85]. Parenchymal abnormalities secondary to bronchial stenosis such as collapse, hyperinflation or hypoventilation pneumonia may also be present [69].

      https://doi.org/10.1183/2312508X.10021217

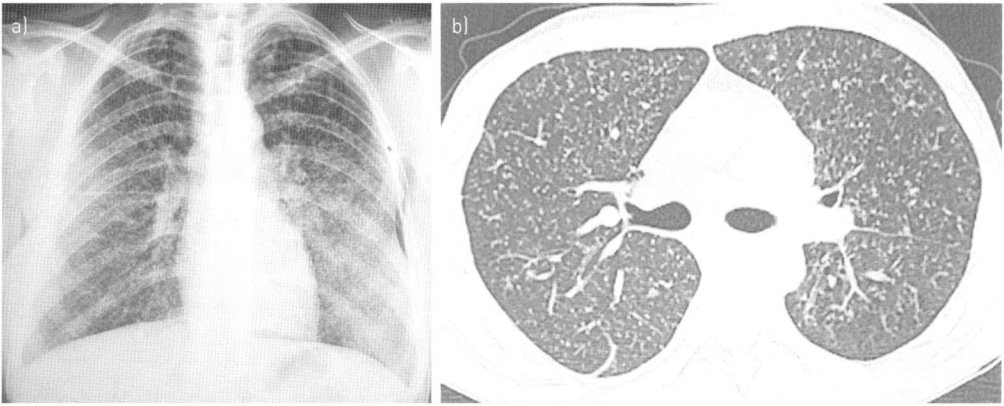

Figure 3. Miliary TB. a) Posteroanterior radiograph of a 27-year-old female shows multiple diffuse miliary nodules with basal predominance in both lungs. b) Transversal chest computed tomography scan, at the level of the main bronchi, in a different patient shows bilateral randomly distributed micronodules.

Miliary tuberculosis

Miliary TB can occur in both primary and reactivated disease (figure 3). It results from haematogenous dissemination of the infection [86]. Miliary TB is considerably more common in infants and immunocompromised persons [87]. Chest radiography and CT reveal randomly distributed small 1–3 mm micronodules (miliary nodules) with a slight lower lobe predominance [87]. In cases of extrapulmonary dissemination, miliary nodules could be detected in any organ. In 15% of cases chest radiography may be normal, particularly in the early stage of the disease [88]. Associated thickening of the interlobular septa, thin reticular opacities and ground-glass opacity can be present [89]. With appropriate treatment, miliary TB resolves without scaring [73]. The differential diagnoses include other pulmonary disseminated diseases, such as sarcoidosis, fungal disease, hypersensitivity pneumonia, pneumoconiosis and malignant metastases.

Pleural effusion

Pleural effusion due to TB is usually unilateral and is described in ~40% of primary TB cases [58]. Frequently it is the single expression of primary disease. Pleural effusion can also be diagnosed in patients with reactivated disease (~20%). Here it is usually associated with parenchymal lesions (figure 4) [59]. Ultrasound can be helpful in initial patient assessment as well as follow-up [90]. Detection of pleural enhancement on CT (the pleura split sign) is suggestive of empyema, although it is not specific for TB [91]. Severe complications such as empyema or fistulation are rare, but residual pleural thickening, calcification or even fibrothorax can be detected on follow-up chest radiography [92, 93]. Discriminating TB from other causes of a lymphocytic exudate such as malignancy, lymphoma and rheumatoid arthritis relies on pleural fluid and pleural biopsy microbiology, culture and molecular testing for TB, as well as tissue histology [94].

Extrarespiratory tuberculosis

Extrathoracic lymphadenopathy

Lymphadenopathy is the most common extrarespiratory manifestation of TB. Cervical and abdominal lymph nodes are usually involved [71]. An accurate imaging assessment of the enlarged TB lymph nodes can be easily performed by ultrasound [95]. TB adenitis is

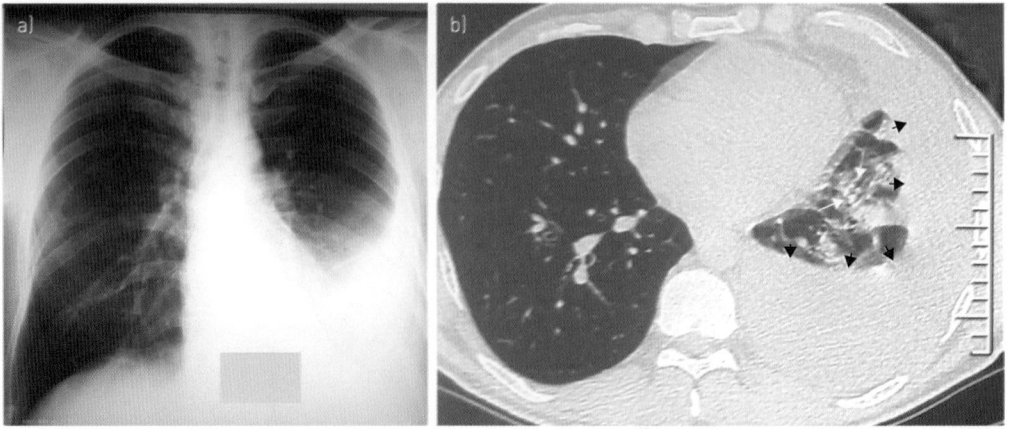

Figure 4. Tuberculous pleural effusion. a) Anonymised posteroanterior chest radiograph shows a left-side pleural effusion in a 43-year-old patient with close contact with a known TB patient. b) Computed tomography scan of the same patient that, in addition to pleural effusion (short black arrows), reveals nodular opacities in the lung parenchyma (long white arrows).

usually characterised by round, moderately increased hypoechogenic lymph nodes with a regularly thickened cortex [95]. Matting and surrounding oedema are useful clues for ultrasonic differentiation from malignant lymphoma or metastatic lymphadenopathy [95]. CT assessment shows low attenuation and rim enhancement [76]. Similar rim enhancement with central hypo- or hyperdensity in T1- and T2-weighted images is seen on MRI [96]. FDG-PET/CT shows an increased metabolic activity (figure 5a) [97]. Residual calcification could be found in cured cases [98].

Liver and spleen

Hepatosplenic involvement is frequent in patients with disseminated TB [99]. Micronodular (miliary) lesions are the most common finding in liver and spleen TB, which are often missed due to insufficient resolution on ultrasound or CT [100]. In such cases, hepatomegaly may be the single imaging abnormality. Ultrasound can identify tiny hypoechoic lesions, in some cases with a "bright liver" pattern [101]. Macronodular lesions of the liver and spleen are rare [102]. Macronodules appear as hypoechoic masses on ultrasound or as hypoattenuating zones with rim enhancement on CT. Both micro- and macronodular lesions are nonspecific, and differential diagnoses include metastatic disease, pyogenic abscesses, sarcoidosis and fungal infection [99]. In case of macronodules, a primary liver malignancy should be considered. Presence of parenchymal calcifications is often used as an argument in favour of TB [100]. An imaging-guided biopsy may be required for a definitive diagnosis [103].

Gastrointestinal tract

The gastrointestinal tract is affected by TB less frequently than parenchymal abdominal organs [104]. Barium studies and CT scanning are used for the imaging assessment of the TB-induced intestinal lesions. The ileocaecal junction is the most commonly involved bowel segment (~90%) [105]. In advanced disease, a pulled-up shrunken caecum can be observed on barium radiography or CT. Involvement of the small bowel is revealed by mural thickening and luminal narrowing with potential proximal dilatation. The changes

https://doi.org/10.1183/2312508X.10021217

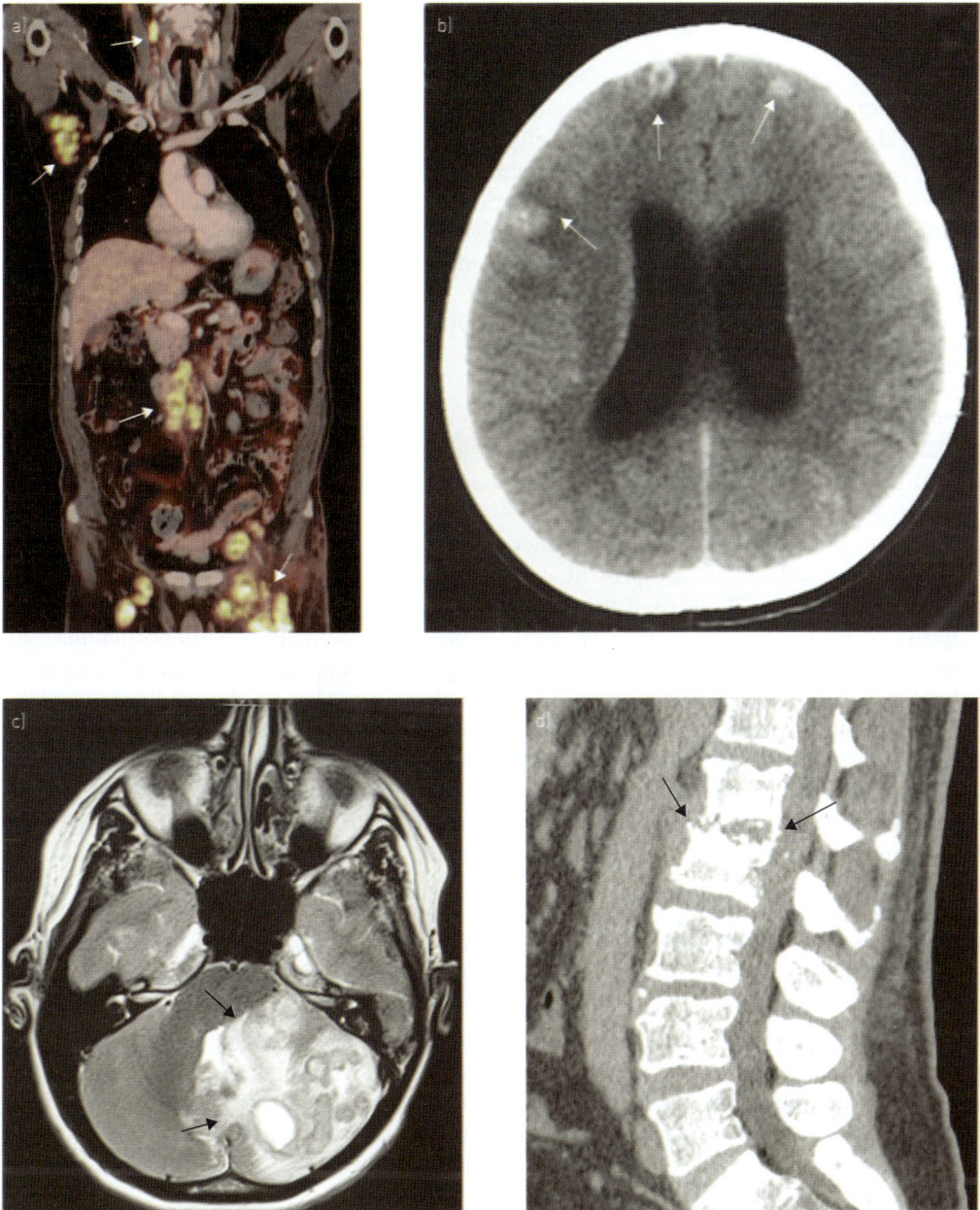

Figure 5. EPTB involvement. a) Coronal positron emission tomography/computed tomography (CT) showing avid tracer uptake by multiple axillary, abdominal and inguinal lymph nodes (arrows) in a male adult diagnosed with TB adenopathy. Hypometabolic zones detected in the nodes are suggestive of caseation. b) Contrast-enhanced CT scan shows several caseating and noncaseating tuberculomas (arrows) and significant ventricular enlargement in a 24-year-old female. c) Contrast-enhanced T1-weighted magnetic resonance imaging of the same patient shows a huge cerebellar tuberculous lesion with a mixture of hyper- and hyposignal intensities (arrows) with a mass effect on the adjacent brain structures. There is also mild meningeal enhancement. d) Sagittal CT scan image of a 52-year-old male diagnosed with tuberculous spondylitis shows extensive involvement of L1–L2 vertebrae (arrows).

are not specific and need to be differentiated from inflammatory bowel disease and malignancies [104].

Peritoneum

Peritoneal TB involvement is most frequently unmasked by free or loculated ascites [106]. Other associated imaging signs are peritoneal thickening, omental caking, matting and thickening of the intestinal loops and lymphadenopathy [107]. Both CT and ultrasound can be used successfully to assess peritoneal involvement [108]. Ultrasound is more sensitive than CT in detecting diffuse peritoneal thickening in the presence of significant ascites [109]. Similar imaging abnormalities may result from disseminated malignancy, mesothelioma and nontuberculous peritonitis [99].

Genitourinary system

TB of the genitourinary system constitutes up to 40% of extrarespiratory TB, with a higher prevalence in high-burden TB countries and is more common in older males [110]. Any of the genitourinary system organs could be affected by TB [111].

Specific imaging clues suggestive of kidney involvement can be seen in various imaging tests. Foci of calcifications are present in 20–50% of plain radiographs and CT scans in patients with renal TB [112]. Intravenous urography (IVU) appears abnormal in the majority of renal TB cases (90–95%) [113]. A broad spectrum of IVU abnormalities has been described, such as moth-eaten calyces, parenchymal scars, irregular caliectasis, "phantom" calyx and hydronephrosis. Similar lesions can also be detected by CT [114, 115]. Ultrasound-specific signs of renal TB include loss of corticomedullary differentiation, focal lesions, masses with cavitation, irregular cavities and hydronephrosis [116]. However, a TB-affected kidney may have a normal ultrasound appearance if there is diffuse involvement or if masses have a similar echogenicity to the renal parenchyma [101]. Ultrasound could be reliably used for fine needle biopsy guidance [117].

Both IVU and CT can demonstrate wall thickening and ureteric strictures. Bladder involvement is revealed by reduced bladder volume, thickened walls, filling defects, scarring and calcification [116].

Imaging assessment of genital TB in females is done by hysterosalpingography. This usually reveals multiple areas of obstruction and/or constriction of the uterine tubes, endometrial adhesion or deformities of the uterine cavity [118]. In males, genital TB is usually confined to the prostate and seminal glands. Contrast-enhanced CT shows hypoattenuating prostatic lesions, expression of caseous necrosis and inflammation [119].

Central nervous system

TB meningitis and parenchymal lesions (tuberculomas, abscesses and cerebritis) are the main types of central nervous system TB [99].

CT scans in TB meningitis reveal intensely, usually homogeneously, enhanced meninges with typical basal predominance. Extension to the surface of the cerebral hemispheres can also be seen [120]. On MRI, the meninges are hyperintense on the pre-contrast T1-weighted images and continue to enhance on post-contrast images [121]. The magnetisation transfer ratio (MTR) can be useful to distinguish TB from viral meningitis (MTR is lower than in TB), fungal or pyogenic meningitis (MTR is lower in TB) [122, 123]. Common TB meningitis complications potentially detectable by imaging are

https://doi.org/10.1183/2312508X.10021217

communicating or noncommunicating hydrocephalus, ischaemic infarcts (20–40%) and cranial nerve involvement (17–70%) [124, 125].

Cerebral tuberculomas may vary in number and size from large unique lesions to multiple miliary foci. Common distribution is in the frontal or parietal zones. At CT, tuberculomas appear as high- or low-attenuation round or lobulated masses [126]. Rim enhancement is common (figure 5b and c). A particular but not pathognomonic finding is the target sign appearance (central calcification or punctate enhancement with surrounding hypoattenuation and ring enhancement) [127]. MRI images of tuberculomas depend on their morphological status [128]. Noncaseating granulomas are hypodense relative to grey matter in T1-weighted images and hyperdense in T2-weighted images with homogeneous enhancement. Caseating granulomas with a solid centre are isointense to hypointense in T1- and T2-weighted images. Caseating tuberculomas with a liquid centre are hypointense on T1-weighted images and centrally hyperintense on T2-weighted images, with a peripheral hypointense rim that represents the capsule. FDG-PET/CT shows a "doughnut" appearance of tuberculomas with intense peripheral and low central tracer uptake [129]. Cerebral tuberculomas can completely resolve on treatment, although residual calcifications are present in up to a quarter of patients [73, 130]. TB cerebral abscess are uncommon and are characterised by similar imaging as liquid caseating tuberculomas, except that they tend to be larger and often are multiloculate. TB cerebritis is very rare and has nonspecific features [73].

Musculoskeletal system

The diagnosis of skeletal TB is particularly difficult and it is frequently associated with a significant diagnostic delay [127]. Histological and microbiological examination of the affected tissue is often impossible; therefore, despite low specificity, imaging assessment is of particular importance in this type of TB disease.

The spine is the most common site of skeletal TB (~50%), with the lower thoracic and upper lumbar levels being frequently affected [131]. MRI or CT are the preferred techniques for the assessment of tuberculous spondylitis. Features suggestive of TB aetiology include involvement of multiple vertebral levels, relative initial sparing of the intervertebral disc space, predominant involvement of the anterior structures of the column including the development of an anterior spinal collection and presence of calcified paravertebral masses (figure 5d) [127]. Untreated TB spondylitis leads to vertebral collapse and anterior wedging (gibbus deformity) [131]. TB spondylitis should be differentiated from metastatic disease, sarcoidosis, fungal infection and pyogenic infection.

TB arthritis is a large-joint monoarthritis. The hip or knee joints are mostly affected. Imaging findings include severe osteoporosis, marginal erosion and gradual articular space narrowing (Phemister triad) [11]. Differential diagnoses include other forms of erosive arthritis. MRI imaging and examination of synovial fluid may prove helpful in this regard [132]. The presence of calcification or abscesses of the periarticular soft tissues suggests a possible TB aetiology. Bone sequestration can occur with progression of the infection. The final result is usually fibrous ankylosis of the joint [132].

Tuberculous osteomyelitis most frequently affects the femur, tibia, and short bones of the feet and hands [133]. It is usually associated with TB arthritis. Suggestive imaging signs are unspecific: metaphysis osteopenia, lytic foci (which are rare) and minimal sclerosis. An increased FDG uptake may be seen on PET/CT [134].

https://doi.org/10.1183/2312508X.10021217

Cardiac

Cardiac TB usually involves the pericardium and much less frequently the myocardium. Endocardial lesions are very rare. An imaging finding typical of pericardial involvement is irregular thickening by >3 mm detectable by ultrasound or CT [135]. On cardiac MRI, T1- and T2-weighted images can show isointense nodular lesions with mild enhancement post-gadolinium [136]. About one-fifth of patients with pericardial effusion develop pericardial calcifications, which can also be seen on chest radiography, although MRI and CT are much more sensitive for this purpose [137, 138]. Confirmation of TB aetiology is challenging due to paucibacillary pericardial effusions plus the inaccessibility of biopsy in many high-burden settings.

Imaging features of cured tuberculosis

The initial TB imaging abnormalities typically regress with treatment, although complete resolution is not always observed. The imaging assessment of patients with a past history of TB frequently demonstrates variable residual lesions, often calcification and fibrosis. In clinical practice, particularly in high-burden TB countries, imaging changes suggestive of healed TB can be detected incidentally in persons with no prior history of active TB or treatment for this. It is assumed that these have had a "self-healed" oligosymptomatic episode of TB. However, other aetiologies with similar imaging should be considered (*e.g.* NTM and chronic pulmonary aspergillosis) [139, 140]. A microbiological work-up to exclude disease reactivation is recommended in patients with post-TB sequelae and clinical symptoms suggestive of TB. Clinical and imaging signs of disease activity should not be disregarded (table 1). At least 6 months of residual lesion stability on imaging is suggested as an indicator of disease inactivity if microbiological investigations are not performed [141].

Calcifications

Calcification is a typical mode of healing of infectious granulomas. Calcified foci of lung parenchyma are detected in 20–30% of cases of previous TB (figure 6a and b) [60]. Some classical appearances of the lung calcification associated with healed primary TB are well known. These include the Ranke complex and Simons foci. The first represents a calcified Ghon complex, while Simon foci describe apical calcified nodules that result from haematogenous spread of primary TB infection [142]. Calcification may not only be

Table 1. Imaging signs suggestive of active or inactive (cured) respiratory TB

Active TB	Inactive TB
Centrilobular, clustered nodules, tree-in-bud sign	Fibrotic bands, reticulonodular scarring
Miliary nodules	Calcified parenchymal nodules
Thick-walled cavities	Calcified lymph nodes
Consolidation	Thin-walled cavities with or without mycetoma
Pleural effusion, empyema (split pleura sign)	Bronchiectasis
Enlarged lymph nodes with signs of central necrosis (central low attenuation, rim enhancement)	Pleural thickening

  https://doi.org/10.1183/2312508X.10021217

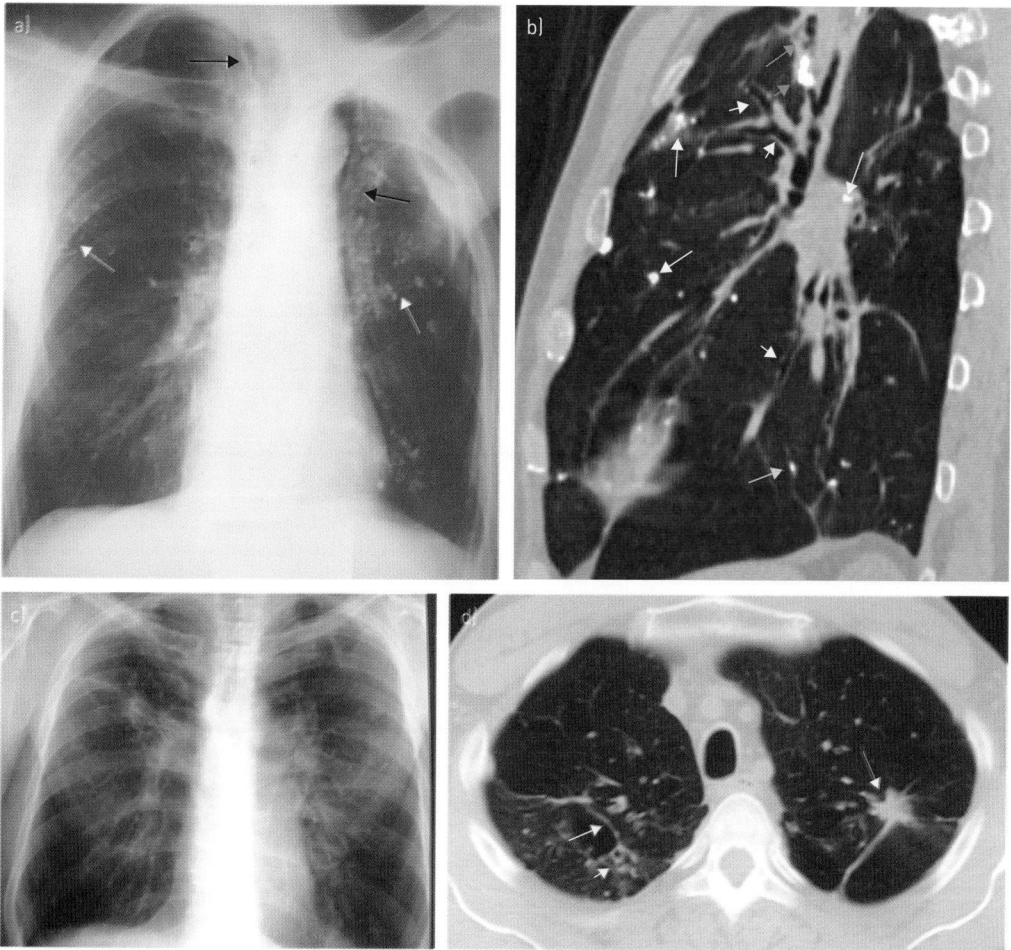

Figure 6. Residual imaging lesions in healed TB. a) Anonymised posteroanterior chest radiograph of a 68-year-old male with three known prior episodes of cured PTB and segmental resection of the upper left lobe shows reduced left lung volume and multiple bilateral calcifications (white arrows) and fibrotic sequelae (black arrows) in the apical zones of the both lungs. b) Computed tomography (CT) scan of the same patient (sagittal reconstruction) shows reduced volume of the left lung, fibrotic scars (long grey arrow), bronchiectasis (short white arrows), parenchymal and lymph node calcification (long white arrows) as well as calcified masses in bronchial lumen: broncholithiasis (short grey arrow). c) Posteroanterior chest radiograph and d) CT scan of a 50-year-old male with a history of cured PTB shows fibrotic scars in both upper lobes (long arrows) and cylindrical bronchiectasis (short arrow).

detected in the lung parenchyma, but also in any organ where granulomas develop [143]. They can be frequently seen in lymph nodes, pleura, pericardium, liver and spleen of the patient with healed TB. A varying degree of calcification may occur in any of these organs. Multiple-site involvement can be present in the same patient. Decalcification may be observed in the case of infection reactivation [144].

Fibrosis and associated parenchymal lesions

Fibrosis is another mode of granuloma healing. About 40% of patients with post-primary TB have important fibrotic changes on their follow-up radiographs (figure 6c and d) [145].

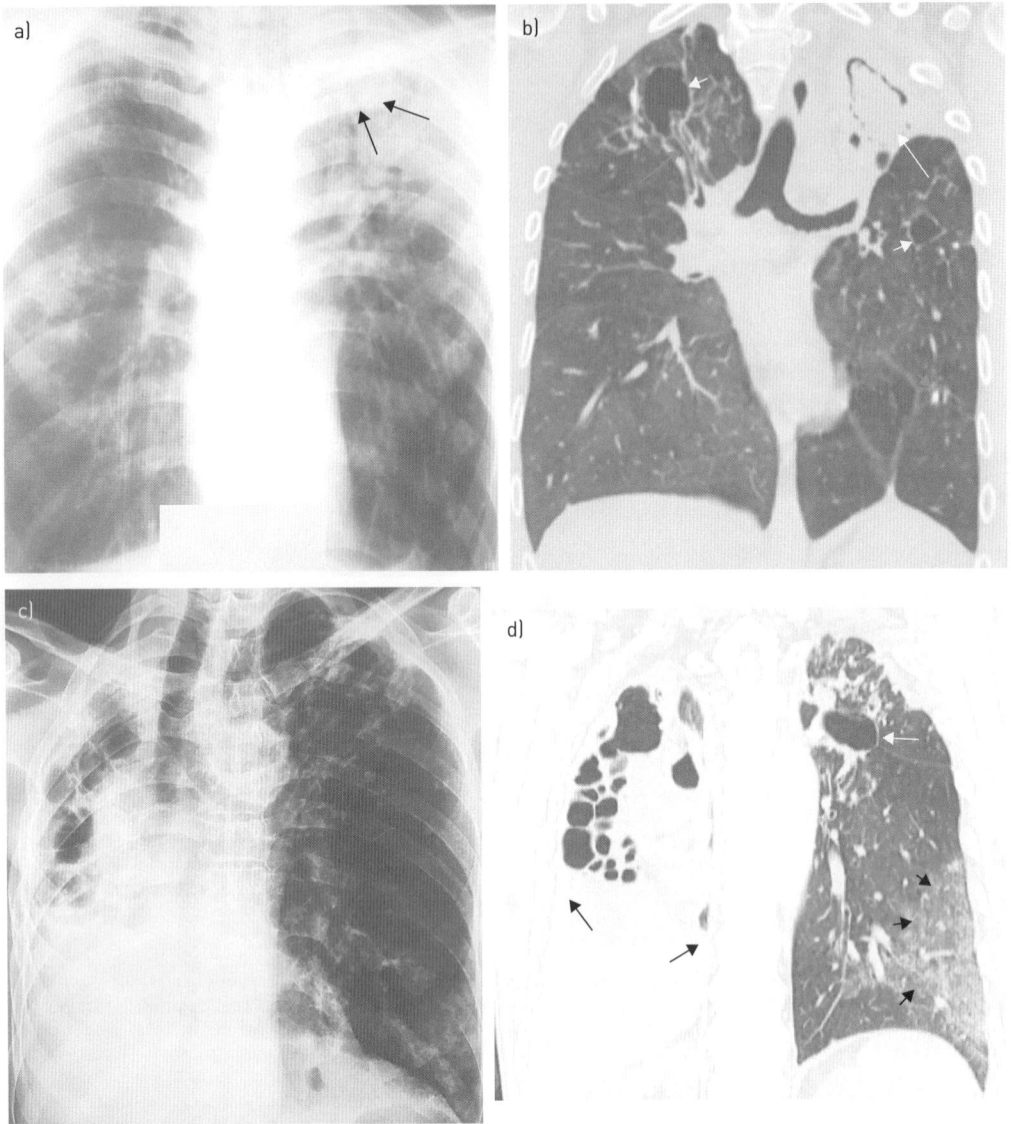

Figure 7. Advanced PTB sequelae. a) Anonymised posteroanterior radiograph of a 28-year-old male with a history of cured TB shows fibrotic changes in both upper lobes, parenchymal calcinates, thin-walled cavities and the meniscus sign in a cavitary lesion of the left upper lobe (arrows). b) Computed tomography (CT) scan of the same patient (coronary reconstruction) proving fibrotic sequelae, thin-walled cavities (short white arrow), calcification (short grey arrow), traction bronchiectasis (long grey arrow) and left upper lobe mycetoma (long white arrow). c) Posteroanterior chest radiograph and d) CT scan (coronary reconstruction) of a 66-year-old male with a past history of PTB shows a completely destroyed right lung with multiple cavities, pleural calcification (long black arrows) and right pulled mediastinum as well as multiple thin-walled cavities (white arrow), fibrotic nodules and a zone of ground-glass in the left lung (short black arrows).

TB-associated fibrotic change is nonspecific and includes any of the following: parenchymal fibrotic bands, lung lobe volume reduction, compensatory lower lobe hyperinflation, hilum retraction, mediastinal shift toward the affected lung, apical pleural thickening and secondary bronchiectasis [146]. Residual single or multiple cavities could be seen in some patients with microbiologically cured TB [147]. However, the healed status of these cases is

https://doi.org/10.1183/2312508X.10021217

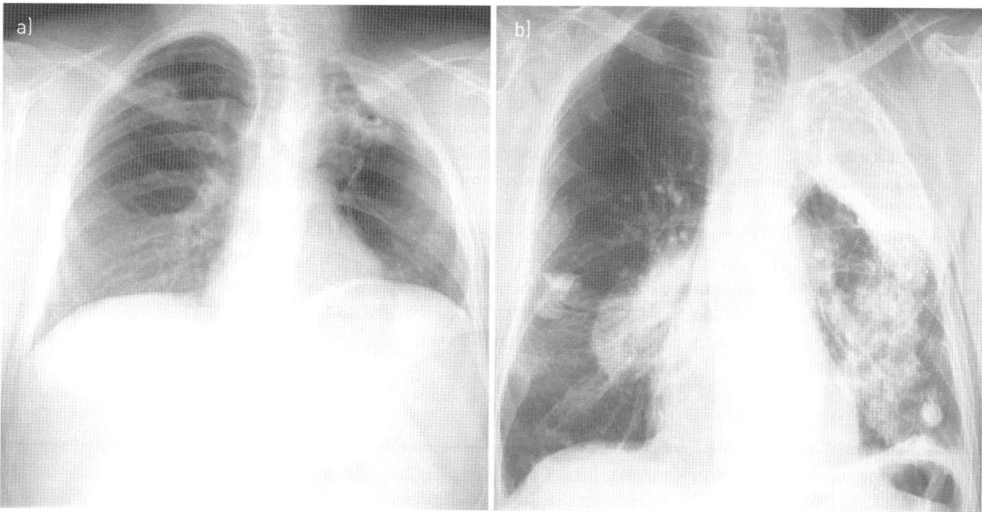

Figure 8. Surgical treatment-associated sequalae. a) Left upper lobectomy with thoracoplasty in a 36-year-old male with MDR-TB treatment failure. b) Left side oleothorax in a 94-year-old male with a past history of TB at age 34 years.

questionable. Residual cavities provide proper conditions for further fungal, NTM or pyogenic superinfection (figure 7a and b). Complete destruction of an entire lung or a major part of it can occur in patients with a prolonged process of cavitation and subsequent fibrosis (figure 7c and d) [148].

Particular TB treatment-associated sequalae can be seen in patients who undergo thoracic surgery (lobe/lungectomy or thoracoplasty) or lung collapse inducing methods (artificial pneumothorax, oleothorax or plombage) (figure 8). These were largely used in the pre-antibiotic era and their residual lesions occasionally could be identified in persons with an old history of TB [146]. However, post-surgical sequalae can be seen in recently treated patients as well, following the reintroduction of surgery for the treatment of some MDR/XDR-TB cases.

Conclusion

A broad spectrum of imaging diagnostics is currently available to assist in the diagnostic work-up and clinical management of TB. Despite its limitations, such as low specificity and interreader variability, radiography remains the most commonly used tool for imaging screening and follow-up of TB patients. Digital approaches and computer-assisted technology offer new solutions for overcoming classical limitations associated with radiography and to scale-up radiography-based screening with an increased detection of early-stage TB. Specific clinical scenarios, such as complicated PTB, EPTB, immunocompromised hosts or assessment of disease reactivation, require the application of tools with a higher diagnostic accuracy, e.g. ultrasound, CT or MRI. However, access to these modalities in many high-burden TB areas is still quite limited. Combined assessment of morphological and physiological features of TB lesions by PET/CT makes it an attractive tool for determining TB process activity, extension and even cure in clinical or research settings. However, its large-scale clinical implementation does not seem feasible at this point.

References

1.   Dobler CC. Screening strategies for active tuberculosis: focus on cost-effectiveness. *Clinicoecon Outcomes Res* 2016; 8: 335–347.

2.   Hermans SM, Andrews JR, Bekker L-G, *et al.* The mass miniature chest radiography programme in Cape Town, South Africa, 1948–1994: the impact of active tuberculosis case finding. *S Afr Med J* 2016; 106: 1263–1269.

3.   World Health Organization. WHO Expert Committee on Tuberculosis. Ninth Report. Geneva, WHO, 1974.

4.   Raviglione MC, Pio A. Evolution of WHO policies for tuberculosis control, 1948–2001. *Lancet* 2002; 359: 775–780.

5.   Uplekar M, Weil D, Lonnroth K, *et al.* WHO's new End TB Strategy. *Lancet* 2015; 385: 1799–1801.

6.   World Health Organization. Chest Radiography in Tuberculosis Detection. Summary of Current WHO Recommendations and Guidance on Programmatic Approaches. Geneva, WHO, 2016.

7.   De Villiers RV, Andronikou S, Van de Westhuizen S. Specificity and sensitivity of chest radiographs in the diagnosis of paediatric pulmonary tuberculosis and the value of additional high-kilovolt radiographs. *Australas Radiol* 2004; 48: 148–153.

8.   World Health Organization. Systematic Screening for Active Tuberculosis: Principles and Recommendations. Geneva, WHO, 2013.

9.   Somashekar N, Chadha VK, Praseeja P, *et al.* Role of pre-Xpert screening using chest X-ray in early diagnosis of smear-negative pulmonary tuberculosis. *Int J Tuberc Lung Dis* 2014; 18: 1243–1244.

10.   Pinto LM, Pai M, Dheda K, *et al.* Scoring systems using chest radiographic features for the diagnosis of pulmonary tuberculosis in adults: a systematic review. *Eur Respir J* 2013; 42: 480–494.

11.   Ahmad Khan F, Pande T, Tessema B, *et al.* Computer-aided reading of tuberculosis chest radiography: moving the research agenda forward to inform policy. *Eur Respir J* 2017; 50: 1700953.

12.   Pande T, Cohen C, Pai M, *et al.* Computer-aided detection of pulmonary tuberculosis on digital chest radiographs: a systematic review. *Int J Tuberc Lung Dis* 2016; 20: 1226–1230.

13.   Rahman MT, Codlin AJ, Rahman MM, *et al.* An evaluation of automated chest radiography reading software for tuberculosis screening among public- and private-sector patients. *Eur Respir J* 2017; 49: 1602159.

14.   World Health Organization. WHO Global Tuberculosis Report 2017. Geneva, WHO, 2017.

15.   Tewolde E, Atnafu A, Kebede T, *et al.* Evaluating the validity and reliability of chest radiography in the diagnosis of tuberculosis among smear negative pulmonary tuberculosis patients. *Ethiop Med J* 2015; 53: 83–89.

16.   Ebrahimzadeh A, Mohammadifard M, Naseh G. Comparison of chest X-ray findings of smear positive and smear negative patients with pulmonary tuberculosis. *Iran J Radiol* 2014; 11: e13575.

17.   Ryu YJ. Diagnosis of pulmonary tuberculosis: recent advances and diagnostic algorithms. *Tuberc Respir Dis* 2015; 78: 64–71.

18.   Thiel BA, Bark CM, Nakibali JG, *et al.* Reader variability and validation of the Timika X-ray score during treatment of pulmonary tuberculosis. *Int J Tuberc Lung Dis* 2016; 20: 1358–1363.

19.   Pefura-Yone EW, Kuaban C, Assamba-Mpom SA, *et al.* Derivation, validation and comparative performance of a simplified chest X-ray score for assessing the severity and outcome of pulmonary tuberculosis. *Clin Respir J* 2015; 9: 157–164.

20.   Kriel M, Lotz JW, Kidd M, *et al.* Evaluation of a radiological severity score to predict treatment outcome in adults with pulmonary tuberculosis. *Int J Tuberc Lung Dis* 2015; 19: 1354–1360.

21.   World Health Organization. Companion Handbook to the WHO Guidelines for the Programmatic Management of Drug-resistant Tuberculosis. Geneva, WHO, 2014.

22.   Hamilton CD, Stout JE, Goodman PC, *et al.* The value of end-of-treatment chest radiograph in predicting pulmonary tuberculosis relapse. *Int J Tuberc Lung Dis* 2008; 12: 1059–1064.

23.   Seon HJ, Kim YI, Lim SC, *et al.* Clinical significance of residual lesions in chest computed tomography after anti-tuberculosis treatment. *Int J Tuberc Lung Dis* 2014; 18: 341–346.

24.   World Health Organization. WHO Treatment Guidelines for Drug-resistant Tuberculosis 2016 Update. Geneva, WHO, 2016.

25.   Lee KS, Hwang JW, Chung MP, *et al.* Utility of CT in the evaluation of pulmonary tuberculosis in patients without AIDS. *Chest* 1996; 110: 977–984.

26.   Hashemian SM, Tabarsi P, Karam MB, *et al.* Radiologic manifestations of pulmonary tuberculosis in patients of intensive care units. *Int J Mycobacteriol* 2015; 4: 233–238.

27.   Jeon KN, Ha JY, Park MJ, *et al.* Pulmonary tuberculosis in patients with emphysema. *J Comput Assist Tomogr* 2016; 40: 912–916.

28.   Nakanishi M, Demura Y, Ameshima S, *et al.* Utility of high-resolution computed tomography for predicting risk of sputum smear-negative pulmonary tuberculosis. *Eur J Radiol* 2010; 73: 545–550.

29.   Feng F, Shi Y-X, Xia G-L, *et al.* Computed tomography in predicting smear-negative pulmonary tuberculosis in AIDS patients. *Chin Med J* 2013; 126: 3228–3233.

30.   Yeh J-J, Neoh C-A, Chen C-R, *et al.* A high resolution computer tomography scoring system to predict culture-positive pulmonary tuberculosis in the emergency department. *PLoS One* 2014; 9: e93847.

https://doi.org/10.1183/2312508X.10021217

31. Yeh J-J, Chen SC-C, Chen C-R, *et al.* A high-resolution computed tomography-based scoring system to differentiate the most infectious active pulmonary tuberculosis from community-acquired pneumonia in elderly and non-elderly patients. *Eur Radiol* 2014; 24: 2372–2384.

32. Theron S, Andronikou S. Comparing axillary and mediastinal lymphadenopathy on CT in children with suspected pulmonary tuberculosis. *Pediatr Radiol* 2005; 35: 854–858.

33. Sah SK, Zeng C, Li X, *et al.* CT characterization of hepatic tuberculosis. *Radiol Infect Dis* 2017; 4: 143–149.

34. Jin J, Li S, Yu W, *et al.* Emphysema and bronchiectasis in COPD patients with previous pulmonary tuberculosis: computed tomography features and clinical implications. *Int J Chron Obstruct Pulmon Dis* 2018; 13: 375–384.

35. Sapienza LG, Gomes MJL, Maliska C, *et al.* Hemoptysis due to fungus ball after tuberculosis: a series of 21 cases treated with hemostatic radiotherapy. *BMC Infect Dis* 2015; 15: 546.

36. von Hahn T, Bange F-C, Westhaus S, *et al.* Ultrasound presentation of abdominal tuberculosis in a German tertiary care center. *Scand J Gastroenterol* 2014; 49: 184–190.

37. Agostinis P, Copetti R, Lapini L, *et al.* Chest ultrasound findings in pulmonary tuberculosis. *Trop Doct* 2017; 47: 320–328.

38. Weber SF, Bélard S, Gehring S, *et al.* Point-of-care ultrasound for extrapulmonary tuberculosis in India: a prospective cohort study in HIV-positive and HIV-negative presumptive tuberculosis patients. *Am J Trop Med Hyg* 2018; 98: 266–273.

39. Bélard S, Heuvelings CC, Banderker E, *et al.* Utility of point-of-care ultrasound in children with pulmonary tuberculosis. *Pediatr Infect Dis J* 2018; 37: 637–642.

40. Janssen S, Basso F, Giordani MT, *et al.* Sonographic findings in the diagnosis of HIV-associated tuberculosis: image quality and inter-observer agreement in FASH vs. remote-FASH ultrasound. *J Telemed Telecare* 2013; 19: 491–493.

41. Heller T, Wallrauch C, Brunetti E, *et al.* Changes of FASH ultrasound findings in TB-HIV patients during anti-tuberculosis treatment. *Int J Tuberc Lung Dis* 2014; 18: 837–839.

42. Sawlani V, Chandra T, Mishra RN, *et al.* MRI features of tuberculosis of peripheral joints. *Clin Radiol* 2003; 58: 755–762.

43. Schloß M, Heckrodt J, Schneider C, *et al.* Magnetic resonance imaging of the lung as an alternative for a pregnant woman with pulmonary tuberculosis. *J Radiol Case Rep* 2015; 9: 7–13.

44. Uysal G, Köse G, Güven A, *et al.* Magnetic resonance imaging in diagnosis of childhood central nervous system tuberculosis. *Infection* 2001; 29: 148–153.

45. Kioumehr F, Dadsetan MR, Rooholamini SA, *et al.* Central nervous system tuberculosis: MRI. *Neuroradiology* 1994; 36: 93–96.

46. Shao H, Yang Z-G, Xu G-H, *et al.* Tuberculosis in the abdominal lymph nodes: evaluation with contrast-enhanced magnetic resonance imaging. *Int J Tuberc Lung Dis* 2013; 17: 90–95.

47. De Backer AI, Mortelé KJ, Deeren D, *et al.* Abdominal tuberculous lymphadenopathy: MRI features. *Eur Radiol* 2005; 15: 2104–2109.

48. Rizzi EB, Schinina' V, Cristofaro M, *et al.* Detection of pulmonary tuberculosis: comparing MR imaging with HRCT. *BMC Infect Dis* 2011; 11: 243.

49. Ankrah AO, van der Werf TS, de Vries EFJ, *et al.* PET/CT imaging of *Mycobacterium tuberculosis* infection. *Clin Transl Imaging* 2016; 4: 131–144.

50. Boshomane G, Lawal I, Lengana T, *et al.* ^{18}F-FDG PET/CT for the assessment of disease extension and activity in patients with tuberculosis: preliminary results of a prospective study. *J Nucl Med* 2017; 58: Suppl., 591–591.

51. Esmail H, Lai RP, Lesosky M, *et al.* Characterization of progressive HIV-associated tuberculosis using 2-deoxy-2-[^{18}F]fluoro-D-glucose positron emission and computed tomography. *Nat Med* 2016; 22: 1090–1093.

52. Park YH, Yu CM, Kim ES, *et al.* Monitoring therapeutic response in a case of extrapulmonary tuberculosis by serial F-18 FDG PET/CT. *Nucl Med Mol Imaging* 2012; 46: 69–72.

53. Lee SH, Min J-W, Lee CH, *et al.* Impact of parenchymal tuberculosis sequelae on mediastinal lymph node staging in patients with lung cancer. *J Korean Med Sci* 2011; 26: 67–70.

54. Lin PL, Maiello P, Gideon HP, *et al.* PET CT identifies reactivation risk in cynomolgus macaques with latent *M. tuberculosis*. *PLoS Pathog* 2016; 12: e1005739.

55. Chen RY, Dodd LE, Lee M, *et al.* PET/CT imaging correlates with treatment outcome in patients with multidrug-resistant tuberculosis. *Sci Transl Med* 2014; 6: 265ra166.

56. Tian G, Xiao Y, Chen B, *et al.* FDG PET/CT for therapeutic response monitoring in multi-site non-respiratory tuberculosis. *Acta Radiol* 2010; 51: 1002–1006.

57. Thomas BA, Molton JS, Leek F, *et al.* A comparison of ^{18}F-FDG PET/MR with PET/CT in pulmonary tuberculosis. *Nucl Med Commun* 2017; 38: 971–978.

58. Leung AN, Müller NL, Pineda PR, *et al.* Primary tuberculosis in childhood: radiographic manifestations. *Radiology* 1992; 182: 87–91.

59. Choyke PL, Sostman HD, Curtis AM, *et al.* Adult-onset pulmonary tuberculosis. *Radiology* 1983; 148: 357–362.

60.   Lee KS, Song KS, Lim TH, *et al.* Adult-onset pulmonary tuberculosis: findings on chest radiographs and CT scans. *AJR Am J Roentgenol* 1993; 160: 753–758.

61.   Jeong YJ, Lee KS. Pulmonary tuberculosis: up-to-date imaging and management. *AJR Am J Roentgenol* 2008; 191: 834–844.

62.   Geng E, Kreiswirth B, Burzynski J, *et al.* Clinical and radiographic correlates of primary and reactivation tuberculosis: a molecular epidemiology study. *JAMA* 2005; 293: 2740–2745.

63.   Jones BE, Ryu R, Yang Z, *et al.* Chest radiographic findings in patients with tuberculosis with recent or remote infection. *Am J Respir Crit Care Med* 1997; 156: 1270–1273.

64.   Rozenshtein A, Hao F, Starc MT, *et al.* Radiographic appearance of pulmonary tuberculosis: dogma disproved. *AJR Am J Roentgenol* 2015; 204: 974–978.

65.   Jones BE, Young SMM, Antoniskis D, *et al.* Relationship of the manifestations of tuberculosis to CD4 cell counts in patients with human immunodeficiency virus infection. *Am Rev Respir Dis* 1993; 148: 1292–1297.

66.   Pérez-Guzman C, Torres-Cruz A, Villarreal-Velarde H, *et al.* Atypical radiological images of pulmonary tuberculosis in 192 diabetic patients: a comparative study. *Int J Tuberc Lung Dis* 2001; 5: 455–461.

67.   Huang L-K, Wang H-H, Lai Y-C, *et al.* The impact of glycemic status on radiological manifestations of pulmonary tuberculosis in diabetic patients. *PLoS One* 2017; 12: e0179750.

68.   Huang L-K, Wu M-H, Chang S-C. Radiological manifestations of pulmonary tuberculosis in patients subjected to anti-TNF-α treatment. *Int J Tuberc Lung Dis* 2014; 18: 95–101.

69.   Im JG, Itoh H, Shim YS, *et al.* Pulmonary tuberculosis: CT findings – early active disease and sequential change with antituberculous therapy. *Radiology* 1993; 186: 653–660.

70.   Li D, He W, Chen B, *et al.* Primary multidrug-resistant tuberculosis *versus* drug-sensitive tuberculosis in non-HIV-infected patients: comparisons of CT findings. *PLoS One* 2017; 12: e0176354.

71.   Gao XW, Qian Y. Prediction of multidrug-resistant TB from CT pulmonary images based on deep learning techniques. *Mol Pharm* 2018; 15: 4236–4335.

72.   Kim WS, Moon WK, Kim IO, *et al.* Pulmonary tuberculosis in children: evaluation with CT. *AJR Am J Roentgenol* 1997; 168: 1005–1009.

73.   Burrill J, Williams CJ, Bain G, *et al.* Tuberculosis: a radiologic review. *Radiographics* 2007; 27: 1255–1273.

74.   Smith DT. Progressive primary tuberculosis in the adult and its differentiation from lymphomas and mycotic infections. *N Engl J Med* 1949; 241: 198–202.

75.   Dempers J, Sens MA, Wadee SA, *et al.* Progressive primary pulmonary tuberculosis presenting as the sudden unexpected death in infancy: a case report. *Forensic Sci Int* 2011; 206: e27–e30.

76.   Pombo F, Rodríguez E, Mato J, *et al.* Patterns of contrast enhancement of tuberculous lymph nodes demonstrated by computed tomography. *Clin Radiol* 1992; 46: 13–17.

77.   Moon WK, Im JG, Yu IK, *et al.* Mediastinal tuberculous lymphadenitis: MR imaging appearance with clinicopathologic correlation. *AJR Am J Roentgenol* 1996; 166: 21–25.

78.   Gawne-Cain ML, Hansell DM. The pattern and distribution of calcified mediastinal lymph nodes in sarcoidosis and tuberculosis: a CT study. *Clin Radiol* 1996; 51: 263–267.

79.   Gadkowski LB, Stout JE. Cavitary pulmonary disease. *Clin Microbiol Rev* 2008; 21: 305–333.

80.   Hadlock FP, Park SK, Awe RJ, *et al.* Unusual radiographic findings in adult pulmonary tuberculosis. *AJR Am J Roentgenol* 1980; 134: 1015–1018.

81.   Lee JY, Lee KS, Jung KJ, *et al.* Pulmonary tuberculosis: CT and pathologic correlation. *J Comput Assist Tomogr* 2000; 24: 691–698.

82.   Rossi SE, Franquet T, Volpacchio M, *et al.* Tree-in-bud pattern at thin-section CT of the lungs: radiologic-pathologic overview. *Radiographics* 2005; 25: 789–801.

83.   Terhalle E, Günther G. "Tree-in-bud": thinking beyond infectious causes. *Respiration* 2015; 89: 162–165.

84.   Van den Brande PM, Van de Mierop F, Verbeken EK, *et al.* Clinical spectrum of endobronchial tuberculosis in elderly patients. *Arch Intern Med* 1990; 150: 2105–2108.

85.   Jung S-S, Park H-S, Kim J-O, *et al.* Incidence and clinical predictors of endobronchial tuberculosis in patients with pulmonary tuberculosis. *Respirology* 2015; 20: 488–495.

86.   Sharma SK, Mohan A. Miliary tuberculosis. *Microbiol Spectr* 2017; 5: TNMI7-0013-2016.

87.   McGuinness G, Naidich DP, Jagirdar J, *et al.* High resolution CT findings in miliary lung disease. *J Comput Assist Tomogr* 1992; 16: 384–390.

88.   Kwong JS, Carignan S, Kang EY, *et al.* Miliary tuberculosis. Diagnostic accuracy of chest radiography. *Chest* 1996; 110: 339–342.

89.   Kim JY, Jeong YJ, Kim K-I, *et al.* Miliary tuberculosis: a comparison of CT findings in HIV-seropositive and HIV-seronegative patients. *Br J Radiol* 2010; 83: 206–211.

90.   Akhan O, Demirkazik FB, Ozmen MN, *et al.* Tuberculous pleural effusions: ultrasonic diagnosis. *J Clin Ultrasound* 1992; 20: 461–465.

91.   Kim JS, Shim SS, Kim Y, *et al.* Chest CT findings of pleural tuberculosis: differential diagnosis of pleural tuberculosis and malignant pleural dissemination. *Acta Radiol* 2014; 55: 1063–1068.

https://doi.org/10.1183/2312508X.10021217

92. Al-Kattan KM. Management of tuberculous empyema. *Eur J Cardiothorac Surg* 2000; 17: 251–254.

93. Barbas CS, Cukier A, de Varvalho CR, *et al.* The relationship between pleural fluid findings and the development of pleural thickening in patients with pleural tuberculosis. *Chest* 1991; 100: 1264–1267.

94. Du J, Huang Z, Luo Q, *et al.* Rapid diagnosis of pleural tuberculosis by Xpert MTB/RIF assay using pleural biopsy and pleural fluid specimens. *J Res Med Sci* 2015; 20: 26–31.

95. Moon IS, Kim DW, Baek HJ. Ultrasound-based diagnosis for the cervical lymph nodes in a tuberculosis-endemic area. *Laryngoscope* 2015; 125: 1113–1117.

96. King AD, Ahuja AT, Metreweli C. MRI of tuberculous cervical lymphadenopathy. *J Comput Assist Tomogr* 1999; 23: 244–247.

97. Ding R-L, Cao H-Y, Hu Y, *et al.* Lymph node tuberculosis mimicking malignancy on ^{18}F-FDG PET/CT in two patients: a case report. *Exp Ther Med* 2017; 13: 3369–3373.

98. Kara I, Yeler D, Yeler H, *et al.* Panoramic radiographic appearance of massive calcification of tuberculous lymph nodes. *J Contemp Dent Pract* 2008; 9: 108–114.

99. MacLean KA, Becker AK, Chang SD, *et al.* Extrapulmonary tuberculosis: imaging features beyond the chest. *Can Assoc Radiol J* 2013; 64: 319–324.

100. Kakkar C, Polnaya AM, Koteshwara P, *et al.* Hepatic tuberculosis: a multimodality imaging review. *Insights Imaging* 2015; 6: 647–658.

101. Goblirsch S, Bahlas S, Ahmed M, *et al.* Ultrasound findings in cases of extrapulmonary TB in patients with HIV infection in Jeddah, Saudi Arabia. *Asian Pacific J Trop Dis* 2014; 4: 14–17.

102. Huang W-T, Wang C-C, Chen W-J, *et al.* The nodular form of hepatic tuberculosis: a review with five additional new cases. *J Clin Pathol* 2003; 56: 835–839.

103. Ghoneim I, Zuhdi Z, Arrifin AC, *et al.* Mistaking primary hepatic tuberculosis for malignancy: could surgery have been avoided? *Formos J Surg* 2015; 48: 94–97.

104. Joyati Tarafder A, Mahtab M-A, Ranjan Das S, *et al.* Abdominal tuberculosis: a diagnostic dilemma. *Euroasian J Hepatogastroenterol* 2015; 5: 57–59.

105. Balthazar EJ, Gordon R, Hulnick D. Ileocecal tuberculosis: CT and radiologic evaluation. *AJR Am J Roentgenol* 1990; 154: 499–503.

106. Poyrazoglu OK, Timurkaan M, Yalniz M, *et al.* Clinical review of 23 patients with tuberculous peritonitis: presenting features and diagnosis. *J Dig Dis* 2008; 9: 170–174.

107. Na-ChiangMai W, Pojchamarnwiputh S, Lertprasertsuke N, *et al.* CT findings of tuberculous peritonitis. *Singapore Med J* 2008; 49: 488–491.

108. Demirkazik FB, Akhan O, Özmen MN, *et al.* US and CT findings in the diagnosis of tuberculous peritonitis. *Acta Radiol* 1996; 37: 517–520.

109. Corneja-Egwolf AL, Suresh C, Espinar MA. Role of ultrasound in the diagnosis of extrapulmonary TB: an overview. *TB Corner* 2016; 2 (4): 1–10.

110. Figueiredo AA, Lucon AM, Srougi M. Urogenital tuberculosis. *Microbiol Spectr* 2017; 5: TNMI7-0015-2016.

111. Engin G, Acunaş B, Acunaş G, *et al.* Imaging of extrapulmonary tuberculosis. *Radiographics* 2000; 20: 471–488.

112. Kollins SA, Hartman GW, Carr DT, *et al.* Roentgenographic findings in urinary tract tuberculosis. *Am J Roentgenol Radium Ther Nucl Med* 1974; 121: 487–499.

113. Ericsson NO, Lindbom A. Intravenous urography in renal tuberculosis. *Br J Urol* 1950; 22: 201–207.

114. Wang L-J, Wu C-F, Wong Y-C, *et al.* Imaging findings of urinary tuberculosis on excretory urography and computerized tomography. *J Urol* 2003; 169: 524–528.

115. Sankhe A, Joshi AR. Multidetector CT in renal tuberculosis. *Curr Radiol Rep* 2014; 2: 69.

116. Vijayaraghavan SB, Kandasamy S V, Arul M, *et al.* Spectrum of high-resolution sonographic features of urinary tuberculosis. *J Ultrasound Med* 2004; 23: 585–594.

117. Das KM, Vaidyanathan S, Rajwanshi A, *et al.* Renal tuberculosis: diagnosis with sonographically guided aspiration cytology. *AJR Am J Roentgenol* 1992; 158: 571–573.

118. Grace GA, Devaleenal DB, Natrajan M. Genital tuberculosis in females. *Indian J Med Res* 2017; 145: 425–436.

119. Kulchavenya E. Urogenital tuberculosis: definition and classification. *Ther Adv Infect Dis* 2014; 2: 117–122.

120. Ozateş M, Kemaloglu S, Gürkan F, *et al.* CT of the brain in tuberculous meningitis. A review of 289 patients. *Acta Radiol* 2000; 41: 13–17.

121. Abdelmalek R, Kanoun F, Kilani B, *et al.* Tuberculous meningitis in adults: MRI contribution to the diagnosis in 29 patients. *Int J Infect Dis* 2006; 10: 372–377.

122. Azad R, Tayal M, Azad S, *et al.* Qualitative and quantitative comparison of contrast-enhanced fluid-attenuated inversion recovery, magnetization transfer spin echo, and fat-saturation T1-weighted sequences in infectious meningitis. *Korean J Radiol* 2017; 18: 973.

123. Gupta RK, Kathuria MK, Pradhan S. Magnetization transfer MR imaging in CNS tuberculosis. *AJNR Am J Neuroradiol* 1999; 20: 867–875.

124. Malhotra HS, Garg RK. Vascular complications of tuberculous meningitis. *In:* Turgut M, Akhaddar A, Turgut AT, *et al.*, eds. Tuberculosis of the Central Nervous System. Cham, Springer, 2017; pp. 139–155.

125. Sharma P, Garg RK, Verma R, *et al.* Incidence, predictors and prognostic value of cranial nerve involvement in patients with tuberculous meningitis: a retrospective evaluation. *Eur J Intern Med* 2011; 22: 289–295.

126. Konsuoglu SS, Ozcan C, Ozmenoglu M, *et al.* Intracranial tuberculoma: clinical and computerized tomographic findings. *Isr J Med Sci* 1994; 30: 153–157.

127. Bargalló J, Berenguer J, García-Barrionuevo J, *et al.* The "target sign": is it a specific sign of CNS tuberculoma? *Neuroradiology* 1996; 38: 547–550.

128. Gupta R, Trivedi R, Saksena S. Magnetic resonance imaging in central nervous system tuberculosis. *Indian J Radiol Imaging* 2009; 19: 256–265.

129. Harkirat S, Anand S, Indrajit I, *et al.* Pictorial essay: PET/CT in tuberculosis. *Indian J Radiol Imaging* 2008; 18: 141–147.

130. Garg RK. Tuberculosis of the central nervous system. *Postgrad Med J* 1999; 75: 133–140.

131. Rasouli MR, Mirkoohi M, Vaccaro AR, *et al.* Spinal tuberculosis: diagnosis and management. *Asian Spine J* 2012; 6: 294–308.

132. Pigrau-Serrallach C, Rodríguez-Pardo D. Bone and joint tuberculosis. *Eur Spine J* 2013; 22: Suppl. 4, 556–566.

133. Hakimi M, Hashemi F, Zare Mirzaie A, *et al.* Tuberculous osteomyelitis of the long bones and joints. *Indian J Pediatr* 2008; 75: 505–508.

134. Lebowitz D, Wolter L, Zenklusen C, *et al.* TB determined: tuberculous osteomyelitis. *Am J Med* 2014; 127: 198–201.

135. Faria D, Freitas A. Tuberculous pericarditis. *N Engl J Med* 2018; 378: e27.

136. Jagia P, Gulati GS, Sharma S, *et al.* MRI features of tuberculoma of the right atrial myocardium. *Pediatr Radiol* 2004; 34: 904–907.

137. Yetkin U, Ilhan G, Calli AO, *et al.* Severe calcific chronic constrictive tuberculous pericarditis. *Texas Heart Inst J* 2008; 35: 224–225.

138. Groves R, Chan D, Zagurovskaya M, *et al.* MR imaging evaluation of pericardial constriction. *Magn Reson Imaging Clin N Am* 2015; 23: 81–87.

139. Dabó H, Santos V, Marinho A, *et al.* Nontuberculous mycobacteria in respiratory specimens: clinical significance at a tertiary care hospital in the north of Portugal. *J Bras Pneumol* 2015; 41: 292–294.

140. Okoi C, Anderson STB, Antonio M, *et al.* Non-tuberculous mycobacteria isolated from pulmonary samples in sub-Saharan Africa – a systematic review and meta analyses. *Sci Rep* 2017; 7: 12002.

141. American Thoracic Society, Centers for Disease Control and Prevention. Diagnostic standards and classification of tuberculosis in adults and children. *Am J Respir Crit Care Med* 2000; 161: 1376–1395.

142. Saldanha P, Saldanha J. Eponyms in tuberculosis. *Arch Med Heal Sci* 2016; 4: 287–289.

143. Kim HY, Song K-S, Goo JM, *et al.* Thoracic sequelae and complications of tuberculosis. *Radiographics* 2001; 21: 839–858.

144. Palmer PES. The Imaging of Tuberculosis: With Epidemiological, Pathological, and Clinical Correlation. Berlin, Springer, 2002.

145. Ravimohan S, Kornfeld H, Weissman D, *et al.* Tuberculosis and lung damage: from epidemiology to pathophysiology. *Eur Respir Rev* 2018; 27: 170077.

146. Hicks A, Muthukumarasamy S, Maxwell D, *et al.* Chronic inactive pulmonary tuberculosis and treatment sequelae: chest radiographic features. *Int J Tuberc Lung Dis* 2014; 18: 128–133.

147. Varona Porres D, Persiva O, Pallisa E, *et al.* Radiological findings of unilateral tuberculous lung destruction. *Insights Imaging* 2017; 8: 271–277.

148. Menon B, Nima G, Dogra V, *et al.* Evaluation of the radiological sequelae after treatment completion in new cases of pulmonary, pleural, and mediastinal tuberculosis. *Lung India* 2015; 32: 241–245.

Disclosures: None declared.

https://doi.org/10.1183/2312508X.10021217

Chapter 9

Bronchoscopy and other invasive procedures for diagnosis

Angshu Bhowmik[1] and Felix J.F. Herth[2]

Examination of the sputum, either spontaneous or induced, for acid- and alcohol-fast bacilli smear and culture for *Mycobacterium* remains the first choice for diagnosing TB. If sputum cannot be obtained, bronchoscopic procedures such as bronchoalveolar lavage may be required, targeting areas of radiographic abnormality. If endobronchial lesions are seen, biopsies are helpful. Endobronchial ultrasound (EBUS)-guided needle aspiration is recommended for the diagnosis of paratracheal, subcarinal and hilar lymphadenopathy. Endoscopic ultrasound helps to diagnose lower mediastinal lymphadenopathy, left adrenal disease, and accessible parts of the mesentery and omentum. Transbronchial lung biopsy, bronchial brushings and blind transbronchial needle aspiration are less useful nowadays, unless EBUS is not available. Image-guided biopsy, thoracoscopy and surgical biopsy have a role in undiagnosed lesions, particularly when peripheral. Pleural aspiration is required for pleural effusion but thoracoscopy with pleural biopsy may increase yield. Closed pleural biopsy may improve yield in resource-poor areas. Gastric lavage may be useful for diagnosis in children.

Cite as: Bhowmik A, Herth FJF. Bronchoscopy and other invasive procedures for diagnosis. *In*: Migliori GB, Bothamley G, Duarte R, *et al.*, eds. Tuberculosis (ERS Monograph). Sheffield, European Respiratory Society, 2018; pp. 137–151 [https://doi.org/10.1183/2312508X.10020518].

@ERSpublications
The first choice for diagnosing TB is sputum, induced if necessary, for AFB culture. Bronchial washings or lavage help when sputum is not available. EBUS-TBNA±EUS-B is increasingly becoming the investigation of choice in mediastinal lymphadenopathy. http://ow.ly/cfVQ30lqCfE

Examination of the sputum has been the primary method of confirming the diagnosis of TB since Robert Koch first described *Mycobacterium tuberculosis* in 1882. While the presence of acid- and alcohol-fast bacilli in the sputum was considered adequate for the purpose of deciding to start anti-TB chemotherapy, the emergence of resistance to first-line anti-TB drugs has meant that obtaining material for TB culture and DST, rather than merely aiding in the decision whether or not to commence therapy, has become the overriding concern [1]. Sputum is often not expectorated by patients with TB and sometimes sputum samples that are obtained are not diagnostic. Sputum induction by the inhalation of

[1]Dept of Respiratory Medicine, Homerton University Hospital, London, UK. [2]Dept of Pneumology and Critical Care Medicine, Thoraxklinik and Translational Lung Research Center, University of Heidelberg, Heidelberg, Germany.

Correspondence: Angshu Bhowmik, Dept of Respiratory Medicine, Homerton University Hospital NHS Foundation Trust, Homerton Row, London, E9 6SR, UK. E-mail: a.bhowmik@nhs.net

hypertonic saline has been used for half a century as a method to aid diagnosis in those patients who do not produce sputum spontaneously [2]. As more advanced techniques such as bronchoscopy were developed, studies in various population groups revealed that bronchoscopy could provide the diagnosis in many cases of suspected TB that were negative on sputum microscopy and culture [3]. Bronchial washing, bronchoalveolar lavage (BAL), bronchial brushing, endobronchial biopsy, transbronchial biopsy (TBB), transbronchial needle aspiration (TBNA) and endobronchial ultrasound (EBUS)-guided TBNA (EBUS-TBNA) have gradually grown in popularity as methods for obtaining samples for microbiological, histological, cytopathological, immunological, biological, genetic and molecular analysis. When sputum, either spontaneous or induced, is not available for performing the vital tests for drug sensitivity, bronchoscopic procedures are the next port of call [4].

Bronchoscopy

General considerations

The European Respiratory Society/American Thoracic Society statement on interventional pulmonology provides guidance on all bronchoscopic procedures and gives information about training requirements and safety considerations [5].

Preparation of the patient

Thorough explanation and the opportunity for a detailed and open discussion about what to expect are vital prior to obtaining informed written consent. Topical lignocaine was found to reduce the cough frequency and the total dose of sedative required during bronchoscopy [6], and is therefore recommended for all bronchoscopic procedures by the American College of Chest Physicians [7]. Lignocaine gel is preferred over lignocaine nasal spray for bronchoscopic procedures *via* the nasal route [8]. Historically, bronchoscopic procedures were performed without sedation, but it is now generally agreed that sedative, analgesic and antitussive medicines improve the tolerability of bronchoscopic procedures for patients, and make it easier for the operator to perform more complex and lengthy procedures such as EBUS. Various drug combinations have been tried and tested for delivering optimal sedation during bronchoscopy. Usually, a combination of a benzodiazepine (*e.g.* midazolam) and an opiate (*e.g.* fentanyl) is used. Propofol has been found to have advantages in some studies, but some countries do not allow the use of propofol by non-anaesthetists, leading to increased cost of the procedure if it is used [9].

Guidelines recommend that antiplatelet and anticoagulant medicines should be withheld prior to undertaking bronchial biopsies and TBNA. However, one study of 12 patients on clopidogrel concluded that in cases where the risk of thrombosis outweighed the risk of bleeding, EBUS-TBNA could safely be undertaken in patients taking clopidogrel [10] and thus it is possible that antiplatelet agents may not be as dangerous as commonly feared.

Preparation of the procedure environment

The risk of invasive procedures, such as bronchoscopy, in the transmission of TB should not be forgotten. Using a questionnaire survey of TST status of pulmonary physicians in training, MALASKY *et al.* [11] found that seven out of 62 (11%) pulmonary fellows at risk converted their TST as opposed to one out of 42 (2.4%) infectious disease fellows. Although the evidence base for the recommendation is limited, bronchoscopy should be performed in a negative-pressure room in order to avoid contamination of other adjoining

https://doi.org/10.1183/2312508X.10020518

clinical areas where staff and patients may be present [12], and FFP3 (filtering facepiece class 3) masks should be worn by all staff in the room with splash guards or eye protection for anyone involved in the procedure. A pilot study looking at the use of an ultrathin bronchoscope for diagnosing solitary pulmonary lesions found no advantages with this technique over standard bronchoscopy [13].

Bronchoscopic sampling techniques

Bronchoalveolar lavage

Pulmonary lavage was described as a method for obtaining microbiological samples for the diagnosis of TB as early as 1946 [14]. DE GRACIA et al. [15] used fibreoptic bronchoscopes to obtain BAL, bronchial washings, and post-bronchoscopy sputum smears and cultures in 20 patients, finding that BAL was the best way to diagnose TB (in 17 out of the 20 patients), although they recommended that post-bronchoscopy sputum smears might also have an additional role.

While gastric lavage (discussed later in this chapter) may be useful in children, NORRMAN et al. [16] found in 63 patients with suspected TB that 13 out of 62 BALs were culture-positive while only seven out of 60 gastric lavages provided a positive result, confirming the superiority of BAL. Other studies have confirmed the diagnostic utility of bronchoscopy, and in particular BAL, in diagnosing smear-negative TB or disease in those unproductive of sputum [17–19].

Although the details of PCR nucleic acid amplification tests (NAATs) are not discussed in this chapter, it is worth noting that several studies have shown that BAL culture with PCR NAATs improved the diagnostic yield of bronchoscopy [17, 20–26]. THERON et al. [23] showed BAL smear positivity of 58% with NAATs 93%. In the study by TUELLER et al. [20], these figures were 47% and 78%, for BARNARD et al. [22], 41% and 92%, and for LEE et al. [21], 13% and 82%, respectively. However, it is also worth pointing out that these studies were performed before the widespread use of EBUS, which has changed the paradigm of the diagnostic pathway. Bronchial aspiration and BAL have become the standard approaches to investigating suspected TB in the absence of a diagnostic spontaneous or induced sputum culture and even for assuring adequate sampling for subsequent DST prior to commencing therapy in smear-negative patients [27, 28], in the absence of mediastinal lymphadenopathy accessible by the other techniques discussed later in this chapter.

Various studies have looked at the sensitivity of BAL compared with sputum. BAUGHMANN et al. [29] found that sputum was smear-positive in six out of 47 (34%) and culture-positive in 24 out of 47 (51%) diagnosed patients, while bronchoscopy was smear-positive in 34 out of 50 (68%) and culture-positive in 46 out of 50 (92%). However, CONDE et al. [30] studied 251 patients with suspected PTB, diagnosing the disease in 143 (57%), of whom 17% were HIV-positive. They found no difference between the sensitivities of induced sputum and BAL for acid-fast bacilli smear or culture positivity. ANDERSON et al. [31] found that induced sputum provided samples as good as, if not better than, bronchoscopic samples, suggesting that sputum induction is an appropriate first diagnostic test for suspected PTB in the absence of spontaneous sputum positivity [30] and if induced sputum cannot be obtained, BAL should be the next step.

Bronchial brushings

In 1975, KOVNAT et al. [32] described two cases of TB, out of 44 patients with undiagnosed peripheral lung lesions, diagnosed by bronchial brushings alone. FANG et al. [33] made a diagnosis of TB by cytological features in 23 out of 746 bronchoscopic brush specimens. HOU *et al.* [34] found bronchial brushing smears positive for acid-fast bacilli in 29 out of 74 cases and CHAWLA *et al.* [35] found positive brush smears in 28 out of 45 patients. It is worth noting that HOU *et al.* [34] found that PCR NAATs significantly increased the yield to 66 out of 74 cases. However, there are not many larger studies to support bronchial brushings alone and we would not usually perform blind bronchial brushings with the aim of diagnosing TB in the absence of visible lesions.

Bronchial biopsy

Bronchial biopsies were reported in the diagnosis of TB as far back as 1958 [36]. As with other sampling techniques, the main use of the biopsy samples is for culture and determining anti-TB drug sensitivity. Several case series have demonstrated the use of bronchial biopsies in diagnosing TB [35, 37–40]. Bronchial biopsies are particularly useful in diagnosing endobronchial TB, where lesions are visible endobronchially (figure 1) although they may not necessarily be seen on radiographs [37, 41]. LEE and CHUNG [42] described 81 cases of endobronchial TB and noted that there were seven subtypes: caseating, fibrostenotic, oedematous-hyperaemic, tumourous, ulcerative, granular and nonspecific bronchitic according to the bronchoscopic features. Bronchial biopsies were used to establish the diagnosis and also to follow-up and monitor the course and cure [42]. Histological features have often been studied in order to differentiate TB from other causes of granulomatous inflammation, but although the presence of necrosis is a strong indicator of TB, necrosis has often been found to be absent. Moreover, necrosis was seen in some cases where the final diagnosis of sarcoidosis was made [43]. The addition of PCR methods has added to the diagnostic yield of bronchial biopsy, making it more sensitive than

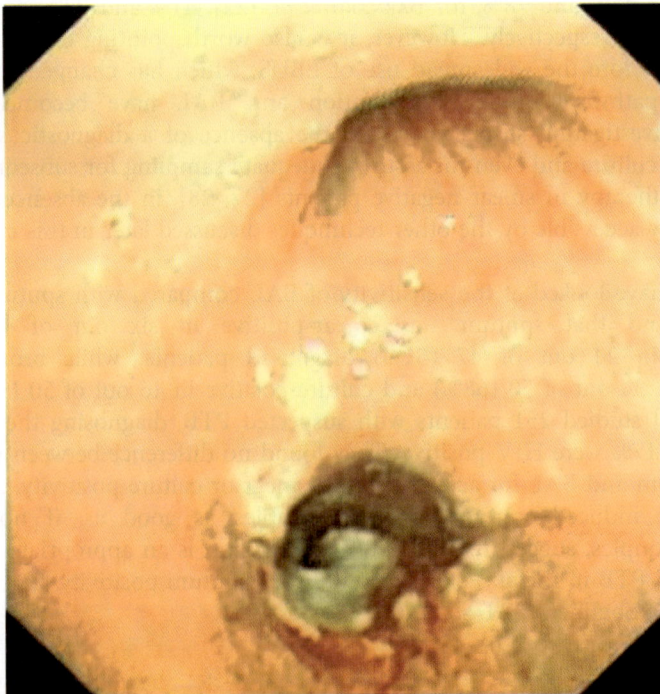

Figure 1. Appearance of endobronchial TB in the bronchus intermedius.

https://doi.org/10.1183/2312508X.10020518

sputum smears and bronchial brush smears [34]. Apart from standard biopsies, reports have described cases where cryobiopsies have also led to the diagnosis of TB [44, 45].

Transbronchial lung biopsy

Although bronchial washings have been used routinely in sputum-negative cases of suspected TB, there are cases which cannot be diagnosed even using this technique. An early study of TBB was not promising: only two out of 12 patients with culture-positive TB were found to have positive TBB culture [46]. However, other studies reported that TBB has a higher sensitivity than BAL. Levy et al. [47] reported 35 cases of TB diagnosed by TBB where bronchial washing was only positive on culture in 18 out of 34 of those cases in which it was performed. Other studies also support the additional diagnostic yield of TBB over BAL alone [17, 18, 48–50]. However, Mok et al. [51] compared the yield of BAL with Xpert MTB/RIF and concluded that the PCR technique might obviate the need for TBB. In our practice, we rarely perform TBB purely for the purpose of confirming a diagnosis of TB, but only do it if the clinical likelihood of an alternative diagnosis is high.

Transbronchial needle aspiration

TBNA was first described in 1949 by Schieppati [52] and he noted that the technique could be used to diagnose granulomatous disease [53]. In 1990, in a Japanese article, Watanabe et al. [54] wrote that TBNA and bronchial lavage were useful in the diagnosis of PTB and NTM disease. TBNA has been used particularly in the diagnosis of peripheral pulmonary lesions; in one study of 87 patients it increased the diagnostic yield of bronchoscopy from 35% to 51% [55]. The role of rapid on-site cytological evaluation (ROSE) has been examined by some groups [56, 57], but there is insufficient evidence to suggest that ROSE is necessary for better outcomes in suspected TB.

Endobronchial ultrasound-guided needle aspiration

Lymph nodes are the structures most likely to be involved in EPTB [58, 59]. The diagnosis of lymph node enlargement has previously presented a significant clinical dilemma. "Blind" TBNA helped in the diagnosis of numerous patients, but many groups found it difficult to raise yields much above the 50% mark [55, 60, 61], although some did record somewhat higher diagnostic yields [62, 63]. A definite diagnosis or even reliable sampling of mediastinal lymph nodes required an invasive mediastinoscopy in a thoracic surgical unit. In many cases, such an invasive procedure may have been felt to be unjustified, leading to the risk of diagnostic delays.

The introduction of EBUS-TBNA to routine practice around the turn of the last century had an enormous impact on the diagnosis of mediastinal lymphadenopathy [64].

There have been many studies looking at whether or not malignancy or benign disease can be diagnosed on the basis of ultrasonographic features of lymph nodes. One study showed that well-defined margins, presence of central hilar structure and presence of nodal conglomeration are predictors of benign disease [65]. Presence of hypoechoic areas representing necrotic nodes (figure 2a) or calcification (figure 2b) may be found in tuberculous lymphadenopathy.

Cytological features have also been found to be useful in the diagnosis of TB more quickly than TB culture would allow, especially in the presence of granulomas with visible necrosis [66].

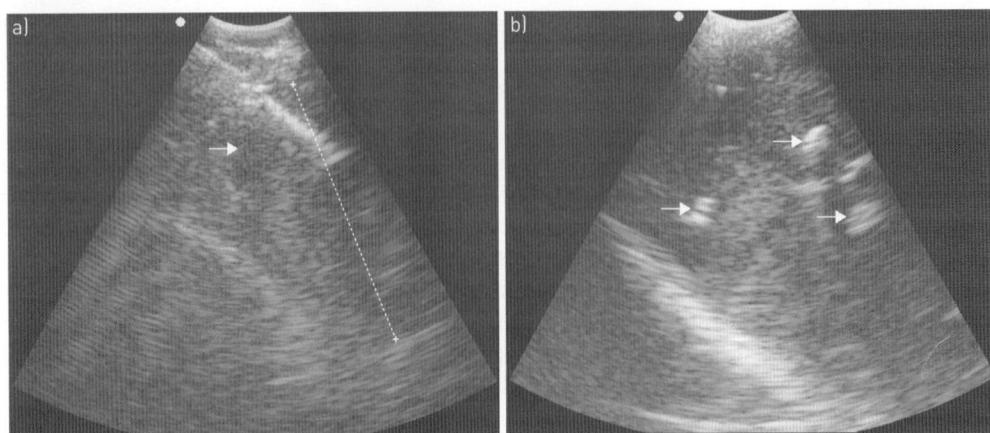

Figure 2. Endobronchial ultrasound appearance of a) heterogeneous echotexture (the arrow shows the hypoechoic region; the dashed line shows the maximal accessible diameter of the lymph node) in keeping with lymph node necrosis and b) heterogeneous echotexture in keeping with lymph node calcification (the arrows show the hyperechoic regions).

However, the greatest value of EBUS-TBNA is in obtaining microbiological samples for TB culture and DST with sensitivity rates >95% in some series [67]. The role of EBUS-TBNA as the initial diagnostic tool for mediastinal lymphadenopathy has been studied. One study of 56 patients found an overall diagnostic accuracy of 83.9%, with that for TB being 50% [68]. Another study showed a sensitivity of 85% with a diagnostic accuracy of 90% [66]. In a larger study by NAVANI et al. [69], EBUS-TBNA provided samples for the diagnosis of TB with mediastinal lymphadenopathy in 94% of cases. A meta-analysis showed an 80% sensitivity with 100% specificity for EBUS-TBNA in the diagnosis of intrathoracic TB [70]. GEAKE et al. [71] concluded from 159 patients who had EBUS-TBNA that the procedure was safe and well tolerated, and demonstrated a sensitivity of 62% for a microbiological diagnosis of isolated mediastinal lymphadenitis. They suggested that EBUS-TBNA should be considered the procedure of choice for patients in whom lymph node TB was suspected [71].

The question of whether ROSE for EBUS-TBNA specimens is required has been addressed by several researchers. OKI et al. [72] found that ROSE reduced the number additional bronchoscopic procedures and the number of node punctures required. One study showed that the addition of ROSE did not add any benefits for diagnosing cancer [73]. A systemic review by SEHGAL et al. [74] of five studies involving 618 subjects came to similar conclusions and added that ROSE did not improve diagnostic yield nor did it reduce the procedure time. Overall, the personnel and administrative costs of having a cytologist on standby seem to outweigh the benefits. For TB, there is no evidence that ROSE presents any advantages over the sampling and transport of samples which appear adequate on inspection to a remote laboratory, and this is our practice.

The role of PCR in the early diagnosis of TB has been discussed elsewhere. Performing PCR NAATs improves the diagnostic yield of bronchoscopic samples and this is increased further by the use of EBUS [75, 76]. The WHO has advised that Xpert MTB/RIF be used for bronchoscopic samples in order to optimise speed of diagnosis and early detection of rifampicin resistance [1]. LEE et al. [77] showed that the addition of Xpert MTB/RIF increased the yield of TB diagnoses. DHASMANA et al. [78] showed a sensitivity of 72.6% for

https://doi.org/10.1183/2312508X.10020518

a single Xpert MTB/RIF assay for culture-positive TB. SENTURK *et al.* [79] showed that PCR had a sensitivity of 56.7%, while GEAKE *et al.* [71] demonstrated a sensitivity of 38%. We recommend requesting Xpert MTB/RIF for all EBUS-TBNA samples.

Radial endobronchial ultrasound

A study in Singapore, with a high TB incidence, showed that radial EBUS-guided TBB had a 77% sensitivity for TB [80]. We did not find any published trials of radial EBUS in the diagnosis of TB, but the role of radial EBUS in the diagnosis of pulmonary nodules has been well established and biopsies obtained using this method may reveal the presence of TB in some patients [81].

Endobronchial ultrasound with endoscopic ultrasound-guided fine needle aspiration

Following the description by HERTH *et al.* [82] of the use of the EBUS scope for the combined procedure of EBUS and endoscopic ultrasound-guided fine needle aspiration (EUS-FNA) of mediastinal lymph nodes in the diagnosis and staging of lung cancer, this combined procedure using a single EBUS bronchoscope (EUS-B-FNA) has also been found to be useful in the diagnosis of TB. MEDFORD and AGRAWAL [83] wrote in a letter that in their first five cases of the use of EBUS-TBNA/EUS-B-FNA using a single scope for TB, three cases were diagnosed using the EUS-B-FNA samples alone. BAL was negative in all cases.

Role of bronchoscopy in HIV

There are many studies evaluating the role of bronchoscopic sampling in patients with HIV infection. Clearly, TB is one of the most common serious co-infections seen in HIV infection. However, in general, the diagnostic process remains the same as for non-HIV-infected individuals. Bronchial washings, BAL, endobronchial biopsy and TBB have all been shown to be valuable in the diagnosis of TB with HIV [84, 85]. However, some have argued that the addition of bronchoscopy and BAL may not be of the highest priority in resource-poor areas with a high prevalence of TB [86].

Other procedures

Gastric lavage

In adults unable to expectorate spontaneous sputum, BROWN *et al.* [87] studied 140 subjects of whom 107 produced three induced sputum samples and three gastric lavage samples. Induced sputum gave a result of TB in 39%, while gastric lavage provided the answer in 30%. BAL in selected patients did not increase the detection rate. While BAL and TBB seem to have definite advantages over gastric lavage in adults, the latter procedure is useful in the diagnosis of childhood TB, with one study of three consecutive daily gastric lavages providing a sensitivity of 50% *versus* 10% for a single BAL [88]. Other studies have drawn similar conclusions [89, 90]. Another retrospective analysis found that while BAL was superior to gastric lavage, the addition of gastric lavage increased the diagnosis rate from 34% to 38% [91].

Endoscopic ultrasound

In the same way that the diagnosis of mediastinal and hilar lymphadenopathy has been problematic, the diagnosis of lower mediastinal and abdominal lymphadenopathy has also previously been difficult, with a reluctance to undertake potentially hazardous surgical procedures on patients with relatively small-volume lymphadenopathy. However, there has been a growing body of evidence confirming the role of EUS-FNA in this scenario [92] and with more evidence for the diagnosis of TB in areas of high prevalence [93]. There have been several case reports of peripancreatic abdominal lymphadenopathy diagnosed as TB. There have even been some case reports of splenic lesions diagnosed using EUS-FNA [94]. The EUS features that are suggestive of a diagnosis of TB have been described and, as in EBUS, include hypoechoic echotexture, patchy anechoic/hypoechoic areas, calcification, sharply demarcated borders, pus-like material on aspirate and conglomeration of lymph nodes [95]. The addition of PCR techniques to cytology and culture improved the yield of EUS-FNA in diagnosing TB [96]. One study described 20 patients who first had TBNA and ROSE. If samples were inadequate, EUS-FNA was performed. This approach led to a diagnostic yield of 90% [97]. In one study in a high-prevalence area, 76% of 130 patients who had EUS-FNA for abdominal lymphadenopathy were found to have cytopathological features of TB [98]. Another series showed that 21 out of 53 cases of benign abdominal lymphadenopathy were due to TB [99]. FRITSCHER-RAVENS et al. [100] showed that EUS-FNA provided a useful and reliable method of obtaining samples to differentiate TB from sarcoidosis using microbiological methods in addition to cytopathological examination.

Pleural aspiration and closed pleural biopsy

One study of 51 patients with undiagnosed pleural effusions compared pleural aspiration, bronchial washing, closed pleural biopsy and thoracoscopic sampling. The final diagnosis was TB in 42 patients. The sensitivity of combined histology and culture was 79% for closed needle biopsy and 100% for thoracoscopy [101]. A study in Nigeria of 37 patients with pleural effusions who underwent Abrams needle pleural biopsy revealed TB in 22% [102]. It has been suggested that at least six biopsy specimens are required to optimise yield [103]. Abrams needle pleural biopsy is now performed increasingly rarely, and training and competence in this procedure are also becoming less prevalent. In the vast majority of cases, thoracoscopic pleural biopsy is superior. However, Abrams biopsies are performed in low-resource settings where access to medical thoracoscopy or video-assisted thoracoscopic surgery (VATS) may be limited and in rare situations where thoracoscopy may not be feasible for other reasons.

Percutaneous fine needle aspiration or biopsy

There have been several reports and case series describing the use of ultrasound or computed tomography (CT)-guided biopsy of bone, liver, spleen, pancreas, adrenal gland, omentum, mediastinum and lungs in the diagnosis of unidentified lesions, resulting in a diagnosis of TB [104–118]. More recently, the addition of NAATs has been found to provide a more early and accurate diagnosis of TB from percutaneous lung biopsy specimens [119].

Thoracoscopic biopsy

The procedure of medical thoracoscopy in the diagnosis of pleural disease, particularly pleural effusions, has been well documented [120, 121]. BEHESHTIROUY et al. [122] described their experience in Iran of performing VATS in 26 patients for undiagnosed exudative pleural effusions where they found TB in 30.8% of cases. They did not observe any mortality or complications of these procedures. GEORGHIOU et al. [123] described 18 cases of pericardial effusion in Israel. VATS was used to perform pericardial drainage and biopsy, and TB was diagnosed histologically in two cases despite all other tests being negative [123].

https://doi.org/10.1183/2312508X.10020518

VATS has also been used effectively in the diagnosis of mediastinal disease, including lymph nodes, thymic tumours, cysts and other tumours [124]. Two out of 15 patients who had VATS for hilar and mediastinal lymphadenopathy were found to have TB in a high-incidence area in Taiwan [125]. VATS was used for the diagnosis and treatment of TB in 62 patients over 5 years in Hong Kong [126]. As with other procedures described here, thoracoscopy and VATS are not primarily tests for TB, but for pleural, lung and mediastinal diseases not accessible by less invasive means. They play a role in the diagnosis of such disease processes and inevitably lead to a diagnosis of TB in a percentage of cases, depending on the background prevalence.

Mediastinoscopy and surgical biopsy

Mediastinoscopy was described in 1978 as the method of diagnosis of TB in 14 patients [127]. In 1985, FARROW et al. [128] studied 41 Asian immigrants in whom a final diagnosis of TB was made on the basis of pathology, microbiology or response to treatment. Mediastinoscopy led to a confirmed diagnosis in 24, but complications included a severe haemorrhage and two cases of chronic sinus formation. They concluded that the use of mediastinoscopy is unlikely to change management in most patients and should be reserved only for cases in which there is additional clinical doubt. However, with the rise in drug resistance, the need for obtaining material for DST has to be considered. There have been several retrospective studies describing the role of mediastinoscopy and thoracic surgery in the diagnosis of TB. SALOMAA et al. [129] analysed 33 patients in Finland and found that in only three of them could TB have been diagnosed without mediastinoscopy. One study in the UK of 1252 cases of TB showed that 160 had mediastinal TB and of these, 37 were diagnosed using mediastinoscopy [130]. A review of 88 patients in Pakistan who underwent mediastinoscopy for the diagnosis of mediastinal disease found 26 with TB [131] and a Saudi Arabian group found that 20 out of 72 patients who had a surgical biopsy (mediastinoscopy, anterior mediastinotomy or thoracoscopy) had TB [132]. Another Saudi group found that in 22 patients with mediastinal TB, CT-guided FNA revealed the diagnosis in 66%, bronchoscopy in 20%, mediastinoscopy in 75% and thoracotomy in 100% [118]. A Turkish study showed that 16 out of 315 patients with confirmed cancer also had TB diagnosed by mediastinoscopy or thoracotomy [133]. A French review of 240 mediastinoscopies revealed only four cases of TB, emphasising that pre-test probability is likely the major factor when considering the utility of any diagnostic test [134].

A small prospective study of 35 patients in Kuwait showed that bronchoscopy and biopsy revealed TB in three patients, while all were diagnosed by mediastinoscopy. However, BAL did not seem to have been performed [135]. The largest prospective study available, by PORTE et al. [136] in France, found that in 398 patients who had mediastinoscopy, TB was found in 16 with a sensitivity of 94%.

Conclusion

Several procedures have been used to diagnose TB (figure 3). While tests of spontaneous and induced sputum as well as bronchial washings/BAL are often performed with the prime intention of confirming the type and drug sensitivity in people with clinically suspected TB, other more invasive bronchoscopic techniques such as bronchial biopsies, TBB and EBUS-TBNA are often performed to establish the pathological cause of anatomical abnormalities or to obtain material for TB culture and sensitivity, and may reveal

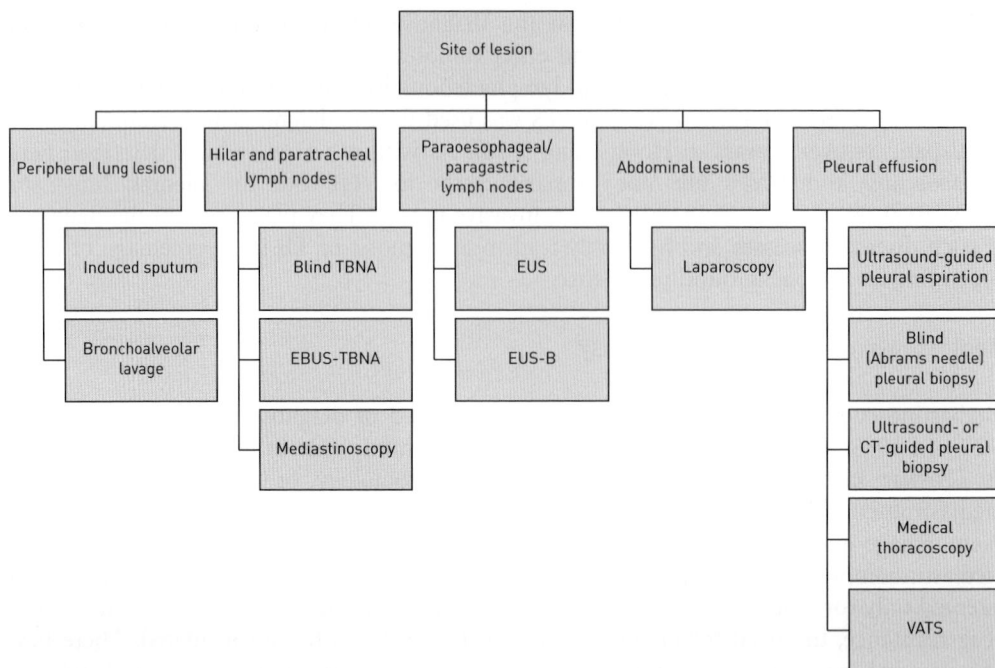

Figure 3. Algorithm for choosing the appropriate diagnostic test in suspected TB. TBNA: transbronchial needle aspiration; EBUS: endobronchial ultrasound; EUS: endoscopic ultrasound; EUS-B: EUS with an EBUS scope; CT: computed tomography; VATS: video-assisted thoracoscopic surgery.

malignancy, sarcoidosis or TB. Other procedures including EUS-FNA, mediastinoscopy, thoracoscopy/VATS and percutaneous biopsies also have a role in the diagnosis of TB, but are not primary investigations to look for this disease, rather they often incidentally reveal the diagnosis of TB when performed to search for malignancy or other conditions. In recent years, EBUS-TBNA has rapidly become a useful and highly successful tool for the diagnosis of mediastinal and hilar lymphadenopathy, particularly in obtaining samples for establishing drug resistance patterns. It has replaced mediastinoscopy in a large proportion of cases.

References

1.   World Health Organization. Global Tuberculosis Report 2017. Geneva, WHO, 2017.
2.   Carr DT, Karlson AG, Stilwell GG. A comparison of cultures of induced sputum and gastric washings in the diagnosis of tuberculosis. *Mayo Clin Proc* 1967; 42: 23–25.
3.   Schoch OD, Rieder P, Tueller C, *et al.* Diagnostic yield of sputum, induced sputum, and bronchoscopy after radiologic tuberculosis screening. *Am J Respir Crit Care Med* 2007; 175: 80–86.
4.   Lewinsohn DM, Leonard MK, LoBue PA, *et al.* Official American Thoracic Society/Infectious Diseases Society of America/Centers for Disease Control and Prevention Clinical Practice Guidelines: Diagnosis of Tuberculosis in Adults and Children. *Clin Infect Dis* 2017; 64: 111–115.
5.   Bolliger CT, Mathur PN. ERS/ATS statement on interventional pulmonology. *Eur Respir J* 2002; 19: 356–373.
6.   Antoniades N, Worsnop C. Topical lidocaine through the bronchoscope reduces cough rate during bronchoscopy. *Respirology* 2009; 14: 873–876.
7.   Wahidi MM, Jain P, Jantz M, *et al.* American College of Chest Physicians consensus statement on the use of topical anesthesia, analgesia, and sedation during flexible bronchoscopy in adult patients. *Chest* 2011; 140: 1342–1350.
8.   Webb AR, Woodhead MA, Dalton HR, *et al.* Topical nasal anaesthesia for fibreoptic bronchoscopy: patients' preference for lignocaine gel. *Thorax* 1989; 44: 674–675.

https://doi.org/10.1183/2312508X.10020518

9. José RJ, Shaefi S, Navani N. Sedation for flexible bronchoscopy: current and emerging evidence. *Eur Respir Rev* 2013; 22: 106–116.

10. Stather DR, Maceachern P, Chee A, *et al*. Safety of endobronchial ultrasound-guided transbronchial needle aspiration for patients taking clopidogrel: a report of 12 consecutive cases. *Respiration* 2012; 83: 330–334.

11. Malasky C, Jordan T, Potulski F, *et al*. Occupational tuberculous infections among pulmonary physicians in training. *Am Rev Respir Dis* 1990; 142: 505–507.

12. Culver DA, Gordon SM, Mehta AC. Infection control in the bronchoscopy suite. *Am J Respir Crit Care Med* 2003; 167: 1050–1056.

13. Franzen D, Diacon AH, Freitag L, *et al*. Ultrathin bronchoscopy for solitary pulmonary lesions in a region endemic for tuberculosis: a randomised pilot trial. *BMC Pulm Med* 2016; 16: 62.

14. De Abreu M. Pulmonary lavage; a method for demonstrating tubercle bacilli. *Am Rev Tuberc* 1946; 53: 570–574.

15. de Gracia J, Curull V, Vidal R, *et al*. Diagnostic value of bronchoalveolar lavage in suspected pulmonary tuberculosis. *Chest* 1988; 93: 329–332.

16. Norrman E, Keistinen T, Uddenfeldt M, *et al*. Bronchoalveolar lavage is better than gastric lavage in the diagnosis of pulmonary tuberculosis. *Scand J Infect Dis* 1988; 20: 77–80.

17. Tamura A, Shimada M, Matsui Y, *et al*. The value of fiberoptic bronchoscopy in culture-positive pulmonary tuberculosis patients whose pre-bronchoscopic sputum specimens were negative both for smear and PCR analyses. *Intern Med* 2010; 49: 95–102.

18. Jacomelli M, Silva PRAA, Rodrigues AJ, *et al*. Bronchoscopy for the diagnosis of pulmonary tuberculosis in patients with negative sputum smear microscopy results. *J Bras Pneumol* 2012; 38: 167–173.

19. Willcox PA, Benatar SR, Potgieter PD. Use of the flexible fibreoptic bronchoscope in diagnosis of sputum-negative pulmonary tuberculosis. *Thorax* 1982; 37: 598–601.

20. Tueller C, Chhajed PN, Buitrago-Tellez C, *et al*. Value of smear and PCR in bronchoalveolar lavage fluid in culture positive pulmonary tuberculosis. *Eur Respir J* 2005; 26: 767–772.

21. Lee HY, Seong MW, Park SS, *et al*. Diagnostic accuracy of Xpert MTB/RIF on bronchoscopy specimens in patients with suspected pulmonary tuberculosis. *Int J Tuberc Lung Dis* 2013; 17: 917–921.

22. Barnard DA, Irusen EM, Bruwer JW, *et al*. The utility of Xpert MTB/RIF performed on bronchial washings obtained in patients with suspected pulmonary tuberculosis in a high prevalence setting. *BMC Pulm Med* 2015; 15: 103.

23. Theron G, Peter J, Meldau R, *et al*. Accuracy and impact of Xpert MTB/RIF for the diagnosis of smear-negative or sputum-scarce tuberculosis using bronchoalveolar lavage fluid. *Thorax* 2013; 68: 1043–1051.

24. Ullah I, Javaid A, Masud H, *et al*. Rapid detection of *Mycobacterium tuberculosis* and rifampicin resistance in extrapulmonary tuberculosis and sputum smear-negative pulmonary suspects using Xpert MTB/RIF. *J Med Microbiol* 2017; 66: 412–418.

25. Chavalertsakul K, Boonsarngsuk V, Saengsri S, *et al*. TB-PCR and drug resistance pattern in BALF in smear-negative active pulmonary TB. *Int J Tuberc Lung Dis* 2017; 21: 1294–1299.

26. Jafari C, Olaru ID, Daduna F, *et al*. Rapid diagnosis of pulmonary tuberculosis by combined molecular and immunological methods. *Eur Respir J* 2018; 51: 1702189.

27. Khoo KK, Meadway J. Fibreoptic bronchoscopy in rapid diagnosis of sputum smear negative pulmonary tuberculosis. *Respir Med* 1989; 83: 335–338.

28. Chan HS, Sun AJ, Hoheisel GB. Bronchoscopic aspiration and bronchoalveolar lavage in the diagnosis of sputum smear-negative pulmonary tuberculosis. *Lung* 1990; 168: 215–220.

29. Baughman RP, Dohn MN, Loudon RG, *et al*. Bronchoscopy with bronchoalveolar lavage in tuberculosis and fungal infections. *Chest* 1991; 99: 92–97.

30. Conde MB, Soares SL, Mello FC, *et al*. Comparison of sputum induction with fiberoptic bronchoscopy in the diagnosis of tuberculosis: experience at an acquired immune deficiency syndrome reference center in Rio de Janeiro, Brazil. *Am J Respir Crit Care Med* 2000; 162: 2238–2240.

31. Anderson C, Inhaber N, Menzies D. Comparison of sputum induction with fiber-optic bronchoscopy in the diagnosis of tuberculosis. *Am J Respir Crit Care Med* 1995; 152: 1570–1574.

32. Kovnat DM, Rath GS, Anderson WM, *et al*. Bronchial brushing through the flexible fiberoptic bronchoscope in the diagnosis of peripheral pulmonary lesions. *Chest* 1975; 67: 179–184.

33. Fang X, Ma B, Yang X. Bronchial tuberculosis. Cytologic diagnosis of fiberoptic bronchoscopic brushings. *Acta Cytol* 1997; 41: 1463–1467.

34. Hou G, Zhang T, Kang D, *et al*. Efficacy of real-time polymerase chain reaction for rapid diagnosis of endobronchial tuberculosis. *Int J Infect Dis* 2014; 27: 13–17.

35. Chawla R, Pant K, Jaggi OP, *et al*. Fibreoptic bronchoscopy in smear-negative pulmonary tuberculosis. *Eur Respir J* 1988; 1: 804–806.

36. Andrews NC, Britt CI, Pratt PC. An analysis of preoperative bronchial biopsy in one hundred patients with pulmonary tuberculosis. *Am Rev Tuberc* 1958; 78: 839–847.

https://doi.org/10.1183/2312508X.10020518

37. Altin S, Cikrikçioğlu S, Morgül M, *et al.* 50 endobronchial tuberculosis cases based on bronchoscopic diagnosis. *Respiration* 1997; 64: 162–164.

38. Zainudin BM, Wahab Sufarlan A, Rassip CN, *et al.* The role of diagnostic fiberoptic bronchoscopy for rapid diagnosis of pulmonary tuberculosis. *Med J Malaysia* 1991; 46: 309–313.

39. Ip MS, So SY, Lam WK, *et al.* Endobronchial tuberculosis revisited. *Chest* 1986; 89: 727–730.

40. So SY, Lam WK, Yu DY. Rapid diagnosis of suspected pulmonary tuberculosis by fiberoptic bronchoscopy. *Tubercle* 1982; 63: 195–200.

41. Aggarwal AN, Gupta D, Joshi K, *et al.* Endobronchial involvement in tuberculosis: a report of 24 cases diagnosed by flexible bronchoscopy. *J Bronchol* 1999; 6: 247–250.

42. Lee JH, Chung HS. Bronchoscopic, radiologic and pulmonary function evaluation of endobronchial tuberculosis. *Respirology* 2000; 5: 411–417.

43. Danila E, Zurauskas E. Diagnostic value of epithelioid cell granulomas in bronchoscopic biopsies. *Intern Med* 2008; 47: 2121–2126.

44. Chou C-L, Wang C-W, Lin S-M, *et al.* Role of flexible bronchoscopic cryotechnology in diagnosing endobronchial masses. *Ann Thorac Surg* 2013; 95: 982–986.

45. Dhooria S, Bal A, Sehgal IS, *et al.* Transbronchial lung biopsy with a flexible cryoprobe: first case report from India. *Lung India* 2016; 33: 64–68.

46. Stenson W, Aranda C, Bevelaqua FA. Transbronchial biopsy culture in pulmonary tuberculosis. *Chest* 1983; 83: 883–884.

47. Levy H, Feldman C, Kallenbach JM. The diagnostic yield of prebronchoscopy sputa and bronchial washings in patients with biopsy-proven pulmonary tuberculosis. *S Afr Med J* 1989; 75: 527–528.

48. Kennedy DJ, Lewis WP, Barnes PF. Yield of bronchoscopy for the diagnosis of tuberculosis in patients with human immunodeficiency virus infection. *Chest* 1992; 102: 1040–1044.

49. Charoenratanakul S, Dejsomritrutai W, Chaiprasert A. Diagnostic role of fiberoptic bronchoscopy in suspected smear negative pulmonary tuberculosis. *Respir Med* 1995; 89: 621–623.

50. Wallace JM, Deutsch AL, Harrell JH, *et al.* Bronchoscopy and transbronchial biopsy in evaluation of patients with suspected active tuberculosis. *Am J Med* 1981; 70: 1189–1194.

51. Mok Y, Tan TY, Tay TR, *et al.* Do we need transbronchial lung biopsy if we have bronchoalveolar lavage Xpert MTB/RIF? *Int J Tuberc Lung Dis* 2016; 20: 619–624.

52. Schieppati E. La puncion mediastinal a traves de la carina traqueal. [Mediastinal puncture thru the tracheal carina.] *Rev Asoc Med Argent* 1949; 63: 497–499.

53. Schieppati E. Mediastinal lymph node puncture through the tracheal carina. *Surg Gynecol Obstet* 1958; 107: 243–246.

54. Watanabe K, Inoue Y, Shimoda T, *et al.* [Diagnostic usefulness of transbronchial aspiration and bronchial lavage for pulmonary tuberculosis.] *Kekkaku* 1990; 65: 227–230.

55. Reichenberger F, Weber J, Tamm M, *et al.* The value of transbronchial needle aspiration in the diagnosis of peripheral pulmonary lesions. *Chest* 1999; 116: 704–708.

56. Mondoni M, Carlucci P, Di Marco F, *et al.* Rapid on-site evaluation improves needle aspiration sensitivity in the diagnosis of central lung cancers: a randomized trial. *Respiration* 2013; 86: 52–58.

57. Gasparini S, Ferretti M, Secchi EB, *et al.* Integration of transbronchial and percutaneous approach in the diagnosis of peripheral pulmonary nodules or masses. Experience with 1027 consecutive cases. *Chest* 1995; 108: 131–137.

58. Yang SO, Lee YI, Chung DH, *et al.* Detection of extrapulmonary tuberculosis with gallium-67 scan and computed tomography. *J Nucl Med* 1992; 33: 2118–2123.

59. Hayati IN, Ismail Y, Zurkurnain Y. Extrapulmonary tuberculosis: a two-year review of cases at the General Hospital Kota Bharu. *Med J Malaysia* 1993; 48: 416–420.

60. Baran R, Tor M, Tahaoğlu K, *et al.* Intrathoracic tuberculous lymphadenopathy: clinical and bronchoscopic features in 17 adults without parenchymal lesions. *Thorax* 1996; 51: 87–89.

61. Barthwal MS, Rajan KE, Deoskar RB, *et al.* Extrapulmonary tuberculosis in human immunodificiency virus infection. *Med J Armed Forces India* 2005; 61: 340–341.

62. Cetinkaya E, Yildiz P, Kadakal F, *et al.* Transbronchial needle aspiration in the diagnosis of intrathoracic lymphadenopathy. *Respiration* 2002; 69: 335–338.

63. Bilaçeroğlu S, Günel O, Eriş N, *et al.* Transbronchial needle aspiration in diagnosing intrathoracic tuberculous lymphadenitis. *Chest* 2004; 126: 259–267.

64. Herth F, Becker HD, LoCicero J, *et al.* Endobronchial ultrasound in therapeutic bronchoscopy. *Eur Respir J* 2002; 20: 118–121.

65. Ayub II, Mohan A, Madan K, *et al.* Identification of specific EBUS sonographic characteristics for predicting benign mediastinal lymph nodes. *Clin Respir J* 2018; 12: 681–690.

66. Sun J, Teng J, Yang H, *et al.* Endobronchial ultrasound-guided transbronchial needle aspiration in diagnosing intrathoracic tuberculosis. *Ann Thorac Surg* 2013; 96: 2021–2027.

https://doi.org/10.1183/2312508X.10020518

67. Kiral N, Caglayan B, Salepci B, et al. Endobronchial ultrasound-guided transbronchial needle aspiration in diagnosing intrathoracic tuberculous lymphadenitis. Med Ultrason 2015; 17: 333–338.

68. Choi YR, An JY, Kim MK, et al. The diagnostic efficacy and safety of endobronchial ultrasound-guided transbronchial needle aspiration as an initial diagnostic tool. Korean J Intern Med 2013; 28: 660–667.

69. Navani N, Molyneaux PL, Breen RA, et al. Utility of endobronchial ultrasound-guided transbronchial needle aspiration in patients with tuberculous intrathoracic lymphadenopathy: a multicentre study. Thorax 2011; 66: 889–893.

70. Ye W, Zhang R, Xu X, et al. Diagnostic efficacy and safety of endobronchial ultrasound-guided transbronchial needle aspiration in intrathoracic tuberculosis: a meta-analysis. J Ultrasound Med 2015; 34: 1645–1650.

71. Geake J, Hammerschlag G, Nguyen P, et al. Utility of EBUS-TBNA for diagnosis of mediastinal tuberculous lymphadenitis: a multicentre Australian experience. J Thorac Dis 2015; 7: 439–448.

72. Oki M, Saka H, Kitagawa C, et al. Rapid on-site cytologic evaluation during endobronchial ultrasound-guided transbronchial needle aspiration for diagnosing lung cancer: a randomized study. Respiration 2013; 85: 486–492.

73. Griffin AC, Schwartz LE, Baloch ZW. Utility of on-site evaluation of endobronchial ultrasound-guided transbronchial needle aspiration specimens. Cytojournal 2011; 8: 20.

74. Sehgal IS, Dhooria S, Aggarwal AN, et al. Impact of rapid on-site cytological evaluation (ROSE) on the diagnostic yield of transbronchial needle aspiration during mediastinal lymph node sampling: systematic review and meta-analysis. Chest 2018; 153: 929–938.

75. Lin S-M, Ni Y-L, Kuo C-H, et al. Endobronchial ultrasound increases the diagnostic yields of polymerase chain reaction and smear for pulmonary tuberculosis. J Thorac Cardiovasc Surg 2010; 139: 1554–1560.

76. Eom JS, Mok JH, Lee MK, et al. Efficacy of TB-PCR using EBUS-TBNA samples in patients with intrathoracic granulomatous lymphadenopathy. BMC Pulm Med 2015; 15: 166.

77. Lee J, Choi SM, Lee C-H, et al. The additional role of Xpert MTB/RIF in the diagnosis of intrathoracic tuberculous lymphadenitis. J Infect Chemother 2017; 23: 381–384.

78. Dhasmana DJ, Ross C, Bradley CJ, et al. Performance of Xpert MTB/RIF in the diagnosis of tuberculous mediastinal lymphadenopathy by endobronchial ultrasound. Ann Am Thorac Soc 2014; 11: 392–396.

79. Senturk A, Arguder E, Hezer H, et al. Rapid diagnosis of mediastinal tuberculosis with polymerase chain reaction evaluation of aspirated material taken by endobronchial ultrasound-guided transbronchial needle aspiration. J Investig Med 2014; 62: 885–889.

80. Chan A, Devanand A, Low SY, et al. Radial endobronchial ultrasound in diagnosing peripheral lung lesions in a high tuberculosis setting. BMC Pulm Med 2015; 15: 90.

81. Xu C-H, Yu L-K, Cao L, et al. Value of radial probe endobronchial ultrasound-guided localization of solitary pulmonary nodules with the combination of ultrathin bronchoscopy and methylene blue prior to video-assisted thoracoscopic surgery. Mol Clin Oncol 2016; 5: 279–282.

82. Herth FJF, Krasnik M, Kahn N, et al. Combined endoscopic-endobronchial ultrasound-guided fine-needle aspiration of mediastinal lymph nodes through a single bronchoscope in 150 patients with suspected lung cancer. Chest 2010; 138: 790–794.

83. Medford ARL, Agrawal S. Single bronchoscope combined endoscopic-endobronchial ultrasound-guided fine-needle aspiration for tuberculous mediastinal nodes. Chest 2010; 138: 1274.

84. Calpe JL, Chiner E, Larramendi CH. Endobronchial tuberculosis in HIV-infected patients. AIDS 1995; 9: 1159–1164.

85. Albino JA, Shapiro JM. Early bronchoscopic diagnosis of concomitant tuberculosis and Pneumocystis carinii pneumonia in patients with human immunodeficiency virus infection. J Assoc Acad Minor Phys 1996; 7: 99–103.

86. Daley CL, Mugusi F, Chen LL, et al. Pulmonary complications of HIV infection in Dar es Salaam, Tanzania. Role of bronchoscopy and bronchoalveolar lavage. Am J Respir Crit Care Med 1996; 154: 105–110.

87. Brown M, Varia H, Bassett P, et al. Prospective study of sputum induction, gastric washing, and bronchoalveolar lavage for the diagnosis of pulmonary tuberculosis in patients who are unable to expectorate. Clin Infect Dis 2007; 44: 1415–1420.

88. Abadco DL, Steiner P. Gastric lavage is better than bronchoalveolar lavage for isolation of Mycobacterium tuberculosis in childhood pulmonary tuberculosis. Pediatr Infect Dis J 1992; 11: 735–738.

89. Somu N, Swaminathan S, Paramasivan CN, et al. Value of bronchoalveolar lavage and gastric lavage in the diagnosis of pulmonary tuberculosis in children. Tuber Lung Dis 1995; 76: 295–299.

90. Singh M, Moosa NV, Kumar L, et al. Role of gastric lavage and broncho-alveolar lavage in the bacteriological diagnosis of childhood pulmonary tuberculosis. Indian Pediatr 2000; 37: 947–951.

91. Dickson SJ, Brent A, Davidson RN, et al. Comparison of bronchoscopy and gastric washings in the investigation of smear-negative pulmonary tuberculosis. Clin Infect Dis 2003; 37: 1649–1653.

92. Berzosa M, Tsukayama DT, Davies SF, et al. Endoscopic ultrasound-guided fine-needle aspiration for the diagnosis of extra-pulmonary tuberculosis. Int J Tuberc Lung Dis 2010; 14: 578–584.

93. Dhir V, Mathew P, Bhandari S, et al. Endosonography-guided fine needle aspiration cytology of intra-abdominal lymph nodes with unknown primary in a tuberculosis endemic region. J Gastroenterol Hepatol 2011; 26: 1721– 1724.

94. Fritscher-Ravens A, Mylonaki M, Pantes A, *et al.* Endoscopic ultrasound-guided biopsy for the diagnosis of focal lesions of the spleen. *Am J Gastroenterol* 2003; 98: 1022–1027.

95. Bodh V, Choudhary NS, Puri R, *et al.* Endoscopic ultrasound characteristics of tubercular lymphadenopathy in comparison to reactive lymph nodes. *Indian J Gastroenterol* 2016; 35: 55–59.

96. Nieuwoudt M, Lameris R, Corcoran C, *et al.* Polymerase chain reaction amplifying mycobacterial DNA from aspirates obtained by endoscopic ultrasound allows accurate diagnosis of mycobacterial disease in HIV-positive patients with abdominal lymphadenopathy. *Ultrasound Med Biol* 2014; 40: 2031–2038.

97. Khoo K-L, Ho K-Y, Nilsson B, *et al.* EUS-guided FNA immediately after unrevealing transbronchial needle aspiration in the evaluation of mediastinal lymphadenopathy: a prospective study. *Gastrointest Endosc* 2006; 63: 215–220.

98. Puri R, Mangla R, Eloubeidi M, *et al.* Diagnostic yield of EUS-guided FNA and cytology in suspected tubercular intra-abdominal lymphadenopathy. *Gastrointest Endosc* 2012; 75: 1005–1010.

99. Wang J, Chen Q, Wu X, *et al.* Role of endoscopic ultrasound-guided fine-needle aspiration in evaluating mediastinal and intra-abdominal lymphadenopathies of unknown origin. *Oncol Lett* 2018; 15: 6991–6999.

100. Fritscher-Ravens A, Ghanbari A, Topalidis T, *et al.* Granulomatous mediastinal adenopathy: can endoscopic ultrasound-guided fine-needle aspiration differentiate between tuberculosis and sarcoidosis? *Endoscopy* 2011; 43: 955–961.

101. Diacon AH, Van de Wal BW, Wyser C, *et al.* Diagnostic tools in tuberculous pleurisy: a direct comparative study. *Eur Respir J* 2003; 22: 589–591.

102. Ezemba N, Eze JC, Anyanwu CH. Percutaneous needle pleural biopsies in pleural effusion of uncertain aetiology in a Nigerian teaching hospital. *Trop Doct* 2006; 36: 112–114.

103. Kirsch CM, Kroe DM, Azzi RL, *et al.* The optimal number of pleural biopsy specimens for a diagnosis of tuberculous pleurisy. *Chest* 1997; 112: 702–706.

104. Joo E-J, Yeom J-S, Ha YE, *et al.* Diagnostic yield of computed tomography-guided bone biopsy and clinical outcomes of tuberculous and pyogenic spondylitis. *Korean J Intern Med* 2016; 31: 762–771.

105. Türkel Küçükmetin N, Ince U, Ciçek B, *et al.* Isolated hepatic tuberculosis: a rare cause of hepatic mass lesions. *Turk J Gastroenterol* 2014; 25: 110–112.

106. Watt JP, Davis JH. Percutaneous core needle biopsies: the yield in spinal tuberculosis. *S Afr Med J* 2013; 104: 29–32.

107. Wang J, Gao L, Tang S, *et al.* A retrospective analysis on the diagnostic value of ultrasound-guided percutaneous biopsy for peritoneal lesions. *World J Surg Oncol* 2013; 11: 251.

108. Lee JK, Baek SY, Lim SM, *et al.* Reticular infiltrations alone without mass in the mesentery and omentum identified at contrast-enhanced CT: efficacy of US-guided percutaneous core biopsy. *Radiology* 2011; 261: 311–317.

109. Tan K-K, Chen K, Liau K-H, *et al.* Pancreatic tuberculosis mimicking pancreatic carcinoma: series of three cases. *Eur J Gastroenterol Hepatol* 2009; 21: 1317–1319.

110. Bhatia P, Srinivasan R, Rajwanshi A, *et al.* 5-year review and reappraisal of ultrasound-guided percutaneous transabdominal fine needle aspiration of pancreatic lesions. *Acta Cytol* 2008; 52: 523–529.

111. Yuan A, Yang PC, Chang DB, *et al.* Ultrasound guided aspiration biopsy for pulmonary tuberculosis with unusual radiographic appearances. *Thorax* 1993; 48: 167–170.

112. Yang PC, Chang DB, Yu CJ, *et al.* Ultrasound guided percutaneous cutting biopsy for the diagnosis of pulmonary consolidations of unknown aetiology. *Thorax* 1992; 47: 457–460.

113. Kiranantawat N, Srisala N, Sungsiri J, *et al.* Transthoracic imaging-guided biopsy of lung lesions: evaluation of benign non-specific pathologic diagnoses. *J Med Assoc Thai* 2015; 98: 501–507.

114. Tangthangtham A, Subhannachart P, Tungsagunwattana S. Transthoracic aspiration cytology for the diagnosis of thoracic infection. *J Med Assoc Thai* 2001; 84: 688–692.

115. Liatsikos EN, Kalogeropoulou CP, Papathanassiou Z, *et al.* Primary adrenal tuberculosis: role of computed tomography and CT-guided biopsy in diagnosis. *Urol Int* 2006; 76: 285–287.

116. Pombo F, Rodriguez E, Martin R, *et al.* CT-guided core-needle biopsy in omental pathology. *Acta Radiol* 1997; 38: 978–981.

117. Das DK, Pant CS, Pant JN, *et al.* Transthoracic (percutaneous) fine needle aspiration cytology diagnosis of pulmonary tuberculosis. *Tuber Lung Dis* 1995; 76: 84–89.

118. Khan J, Akhtar M, von Sinner WN, *et al.* CT-guided fine needle aspiration biopsy in the diagnosis of mediastinal tuberculosis. *Chest* 1994; 106: 1329–1332.

119. Jiang F, Huang W, Wang Y, *et al.* Nucleic acid amplification testing and sequencing combined with acid-fast staining in needle biopsy lung tissues for the diagnosis of smear-negative pulmonary tuberculosis. *PLoS One* 2016; 11: e0167342.

120. Rodríguez-Panadero F. Medical thoracoscopy. *Respiration* 2008; 76: 363–372.

121. Mathur PN, Loddenkemper R. Medical thoracoscopy. Role in pleural and lung diseases. *Clin Chest Med* 1995; 16: 487–496.

https://doi.org/10.1183/2312508X.10020518

122. Beheshtirouy S, Kakaei F, Mirzaaghazadeh M. Video assisted rigid thoracoscopy in the diagnosis of unexplained exudative pleural effusion. *J Cardiovasc Thorac Res* 2013; 5: 87–90.

123. Georghiou GP, Stamler A, Sharoni E, *et al.* Video-assisted thoracoscopic pericardial window for diagnosis and management of pericardial effusions. *Ann Thorac Surg* 2005; 80: 607–610.

124. Kitami A, Suzuki T, Usuda R, *et al.* Diagnostic and therapeutic thoracoscopy for mediastinal disease. *Ann Thorac Cardiovasc Surg* 2004; 10: 14–18.

125. Chen JS, Chang YL, Cheng HL, *et al.* Video-assisted thoracoscopic surgery for the diagnosis of patients with hilar and mediastinal lymphadenopathy. *J Formos Med Assoc* 2001; 100: 213–216.

126. Yim AP, Izzat MB, Lee TW. Thoracoscopic surgery for pulmonary tuberculosis. *World J Surg* 1999; 23: 1114–1117.

127. Cameron EW. Tuberculosis and mediastinoscopy. *Thorax* 1978; 33: 117–120.

128. Farrow PR, Jones DA, Stanley PJ, *et al.* Thoracic lymphadenopathy in Asians resident in the United Kingdom: role of mediastinoscopy in initial diagnosis. *Thorax* 1985; 40: 121–124.

129. Salomaa ER, Liippo K, Puhakka HJ, *et al.* Indispensability of mediastinoscopy in intrathoracic tuberculosis. *ORL J Otorhinolaryngol Relat Spec* 1992; 54: 275–277.

130. Jacob B, Parsa R, Frizzell R, *et al.* Mediastinal tuberculosis in Bradford, United Kingdom: the role of mediastinoscopy. *Int J Tuberc Lung Dis* 2011; 15: 240–245.

131. Hasan SB, Khan FW, Hashmi S, *et al.* Cervical mediastinoscopy in the diagnosis of lymphadenopathy in South Asia. *J Pak Med Assoc* 2016; 66: Suppl. 3, S16–S18.

132. Hajjar W, Elmedany Y, Bamousa A, *et al.* Diagnostic yield of mediastinal exploration. *Med Princ Pract* 2002; 11: 210–213.

133. Solak O, Sayar A, Metin M, *et al.* The coincidence of mediastinal tuberculosis lymphadenitis in lung cancer patients. *Acta Chir Belg* 2005; 105: 180–182.

134. Venissac N, Alifano M, Mouroux J. Video-assisted mediastinoscopy: experience from 240 consecutive cases. *Ann Thorac Surg* 2003; 76: 208–212.

135. Ayed AK, Behbehani NA. Diagnosis and treatment of isolated tuberculous mediastinal lymphadenopathy in adults. *Eur J Surg* 2001; 167: 334–338.

136. Porte H, Roumilhac D, Eraldi L, *et al.* The role of mediastinoscopy in the diagnosis of mediastinal lymphadenopathy. *Eur J Cardiothorac Surg* 1998; 13: 196–199.

Disclosures: F.J.F. Herth reports receiving personal fees from the following, outside the submitted work: AstraZeneca, GSK, Chiesi, Novartis, Boehringer Ingelheim, Olympus, Uptake, Erbe, BTG and Pulmonx.

| Chapter 10

Treatment of drug-susceptible and drug-resistant tuberculosis

José A. Caminero[1,2], Anna Scardigli[3], Tijp van der Werf[4] and
Marina Tadolini[5]

The treatment of TB, both drug-susceptible and drug-resistant forms, should be based on two principles: 1) the combination of drugs (at least four) to avoid selection pressure resulting in the emergence of DR-TB strains and 2) the need for prolonged treatment in order to sterilise all infectious sites and thus cure the patient and prevent relapses. The selection of drugs should be based on their bactericidal and sterilising properties, their ability to prevent drug resistance and their safety profile. Based on these principles, and on the mode of action of the different drugs, this chapter describes in detail anti-TB treatment, the most appropriate choice of drugs based on *in vitro* susceptibility testing, starting with drug-susceptible TB (DS-TB), and a proposal to standardise as much as possible the difficult-to-manage patients with DR-TB. The chapter delineates the recommended treatment for DS-TB, mono- and polyresistant TB, MDR-TB, XDR-TB and forms of TB beyond XDR-TB. Special attention is given to the 2018 WHO guidelines regarding the revised grouping of second-line TB drugs recommended for use in longer MDR-TB regimens, the shorter MDR-TB regimens, the possibility of designing a standardised pre-XDR and XDR-TB regimen adapted to the country, and some relevant management issues.

Cite as: Caminero JA, Scardigli A, van der Werf T, *et al.* Treatment of drug-susceptible and drug-resistant tuberculosis. *In:* Migliori GB, Bothamley G, Duarte R, *et al.*, eds. Tuberculosis (ERS Monograph). Sheffield, European Respiratory Society, 2018; pp. 152–178 [https://doi.org/10.1183/2312508X.10021417].

🐦 @ERSpublications
A review of the bacteriological fundaments of TB treatment, and a discussion of the principles involved in designing a regimen to treat all TB cases, including those with extensive patterns of resistance. http://ow.ly/cfVQ30lqCfE

T he basic principles guiding effective TB treatment were tested and confirmed between 1948 and 1976 [1]. Several decades later, after TB had become an almost universally curable disease (successful outcome of 83% in 2015), the emergence of strains of

[1]Dept of Pneumology, University Hospital of Gran Canaria "Dr Negrín", Las Palmas de Gran Canaria, Spain. [2]International Union against Tuberculosis and Lung Disease (The Union), Paris, France. [3]The Global Fund to Fight AIDS, Tuberculosis and Malaria, Geneva, Switzerland. [4]Depts of Pulmonary Diseases and Tuberculosis, and Internal Medicine, Division of Infectious Diseases, University of Groningen, University Medical Center Groningen, Groningen, The Netherlands. [5]Unit of Infectious Diseases, Dept of Medical and Surgical Sciences, Alma Mater Studiorum, University of Bologna, Bologna, Italy.

Correspondence: José A. Caminero, Dept of Pneumology, University Hospital of Gran Canaria "Dr Negrín", Barranco de la Ballena s/n, 35010 Las Palmas de Gran Canaria, Spain. E-mail: jcamlun@gobiernodecanarias.org

https://doi.org/10.1183/2312508X.10021417

Mycobacterium tuberculosis resistant to the most active drugs available made TB once again a major threat and a challenge to global public health [2]. The WHO has highlighted that the estimated number of patients with RR-TB and/or MDR-TB, a form of TB resistant to at least isoniazid (H) and rifampicin (R), is increasing over time. The poor prognosis has hardly improved, with a successful outcome for only ~54% of patients started on treatment [2]. This prognosis is even worse for patients with XDR-TB (forms of MDR-TB with additional resistance to any fluoroquinolone and any of the three SLIDs: kanamycin, amikacin and capreomycin), where globally just a 26% successful outcome is being achieved [2].

Fortunately, the successful outcome of new and relapsed TB cases at the global level is much better, achieving 83% in 2015 [2]. There are also recent promising publications not only showing a successful treatment outcome (80–85%) with a shorter (9–11 months) MDR-TB regimen [3–9], but also estimating the association of treatment success and death with the use of individual drugs, as well the optimal number and duration of those drugs in DR-TB [10, 11]. However, the situation does not seem to improve for XDR-TB patients, who still have a very poor prognosis. For this reason, it is necessary to improve the management of XDR-TB patients, trying to design adequate regimens and, of course, including the new and repurposed anti-TB drugs [10–12].

Here, we review the bacteriological fundaments of TB treatment, and discuss the principles involved in designing a regimen to treat even cases of TB with extensive patterns of resistance, with the possibility of curing most patients [13–17].

Bacteriological basis of tuberculosis treatment

All TB treatments should be based on two important bacteriological considerations: 1) the need to use combinations of drugs to avoid the development of resistance and 2) the need for prolonged chemotherapy to cure the disease and prevent disease relapse [15–20]. This applies to all forms of TB, both drug-susceptible TB (DS-TB) and DR-TB, regardless of the pattern of *M. tuberculosis* drug resistance and TB localisation. The number of drugs in a combination regimen and the total duration of treatment depend on the efficacy of the drugs utilised in the regimen [14–17].

The need for drug combinations to prevent selection of drug-resistant tuberculosis strains

How many drugs are needed to treat TB [15, 16]? Spontaneous natural mutants of *M. tuberculosis* arise during successive bacillary divisions as a random event, including mutations in genes that determine antibiotic drug susceptibility and resistance. The probability of these mutations occurring is a chance event, depending on the number of cell divisions, and is therefore driven by the number of replicating bacilli present at the site of replication. The selection of resistant mutants is due to drug selection pressure. Depending on the specific genetic target, 10^5–10^8 cell divisions with an equally large bacterial load are necessary for the appearance of a natural mutant resistant to any of the anti-TB drugs. These mutations are independent for each drug, as different genetic targets are involved for the different drugs. For this reason, the probability of resistance to two drugs developing simultaneously is equal to the product of their single respective mutation rates. It takes 10^{12}–10^{14} bacilli for mutations to isoniazid plus rifampicin to appear, a bacillary load that would be incompatible with life for the human host.

Therefore, if *M. tuberculosis* is fully susceptible to all anti-TB drugs, the use of two very active drugs (*e.g.* isoniazid plus rifampicin) could cure practically all susceptible cases of TB [15–22]. Unfortunately, there are already a considerable number of *M. tuberculosis* strains with resistance to isoniazid or another drug circulating in the community. Moreover, some anti-TB drugs are weaker. This is the reason why the programme recommendation is to use at least four or five new, or likely to be effective, anti-TB drugs, in order to try to cure all patients in the field [10, 11, 15–17, 19, 23, 24]. This recommendation is valid for all forms of TB, including cases of cavitary TB (with the highest bacillary load) and isoniazid or other monoresistances. When rapid DST to isoniazid and rifampicin is available, as a proxy for *in vitro* phenotypic DST results, molecular tests with a rapid laboratory turnaround time will clearly help in this respect. With the results available before the start of treatment, only three drugs (isoniazid, rifampicin and pyrazinamide (Z)) might be sufficient and effective [15, 17, 21, 22]. This principle can also apply to a regimen with second-line drugs if these drugs have good bactericidal and/or sterilising activity [15, 17].

In summary, the first premise of any anti-TB treatment is that a combination of at least four to five drugs not used previously or with a high likelihood of being effective is recommended.

The need for prolonged treatments: bactericidal *versus* sterilising activity of anti-tuberculosis drugs

The second premise for the treatment of TB is the need for prolonged treatment in order to enable the drugs to kill *M. tuberculosis* in all its different growth phases, not only the metabolically active bacilli that produce symptoms and are responsible for transmission but also the dormant or semi-dormant (persisting) bacilli responsible for relapses [15–20].

The capacity of an anti-TB drug to eliminate metabolically active mycobacteria (located within cavitary lesions, where the conditions of oxygen pressure and pH are ideal for growth) is referred to as bactericidal activity [14–18]. Therefore, drugs with a good bactericidal activity will be essential to obtain clinical improvement and to reduce transmission.

In contrast, the capacity of drugs to eliminate persisting organisms is referred as sterilising activity [14–18]. These persisting bacilli, also referred to as dormant or semi-dormant bacilli, have switched on a genetically controlled programme operated by the DosR regulon that enables the organisms to survive in the solid caseum with low metabolic activity and only sporadic replications. As persisting or dormant bacilli are few (10^3–10^5 bacilli) and largely escape the immune system, they do not drive inflammation with symptoms, and they do not have a role in transmission. Therefore, in the first phase of TB treatment, the priority is not to kill these persistent bacilli; however, if not eradicated, they can produce relapses after completion of therapy [1, 14–20]. As they divide very slowly, most bactericidal drugs (acting on replicating bacilli) cannot kill them, and for this reason, if the TB regimen does not contain sterilising drugs, it is necessary to administer bactericidal drugs for a long time to ensure that the organisms are killed during replication. Therefore, only sterilising drugs will be able to shorten the duration of TB treatment and avoid relapses [1, 14–20].

https://doi.org/10.1183/2312508X.10021417

Objectives of tuberculosis treatment

There are three main objectives of all forms of TB treatment: 1) to reduce the risk of death (the highest priority when a patient is diagnosed with TB), to alleviate the symptoms and to reduce the risk of transmission, using drugs with bactericidal activity, 2) to prevent the selection of drug-resistant organisms, which requires a combination of at least four to five drugs, and 3) to eventually obtain relapse-free cure, which requires drugs with sterilising activity (table 1) [12, 16, 17].

Minimal requirements for tuberculosis treatment

Based on the three objectives of TB treatment, the minimal requirements for all TB treatments should be as follows [12, 16, 17]:

1) At least four to five "new" drugs (*i.e.* drugs not previously used in this patient, or drugs with probable efficacy) are needed to obtain a cure and to avoid the possible selection or amplification of drug-resistant organisms. Molecular rapid DST must support the selection of these drugs.

2) Of these four to five drugs, two or three should be core drugs, at least one or two with good bactericidal activity, and one or two with good sterilising activity to obtain a relapse-free cure. The sterilising drugs should be administered throughout the treatment duration.

Table 1. The three main objectives of TB treatment

To reduce mortality and morbidity for affected patients and avoid the risk of further transmission	To achieve these objectives, drugs with bactericidal activity are needed for their ability to kill the rapidly dividing, metabolically active bacilli found in the cavities and sputum of patients with microscopy smear-positive PTB Bactericidal drugs include: isoniazid, rifampicin, fluoroquinolones (levofloxacin, moxifloxacin), SLIDs (kanamycin, amikacin, capreomycin), linezolid, bedaquiline, delamanid and meropenem (imipenem)+amoxicillin–clavulanic acid
To avoid the selection of drug-resistant mutant bacilli	To achieve this objective, it is necessary to administer drug combinations of at least four new (or likely to be effective) drugs
To avoid relapses	To achieve this objective, drugs with sterilising activity are needed for their ability to kill persisting, dormant or intermittently active bacilli, responsible for relapses; rapid sterilisation will lead to the shortening of treatment duration Sterilising drugs include: rifampicin, pyrazinamide, levofloxacin/moxifloxacin, linezolid, clofazimine, bedaquiline and delamanid

3) The other one to two drugs should be companion drugs to protect the action of the core drugs. Usually, companion drugs are only necessary until smear and culture conversion has been achieved.

4) The drugs should be administered for a prolonged period of time, to achieve a relapse-free cure, as only drugs with better sterilising activity (rifampicin, pyrazinamide, moxifloxacin) can reduce the duration of treatment.

Selection of anti-tuberculosis drugs: core *versus* companion drugs

The selection of anti-TB drugs for any TB treatment should be based on the drug characteristics. The desirable properties of anti-TB drugs are: 1) bactericidal activity, 2) sterilising activity, 3) prevention of resistance when provided in combination with other anti-TB drugs and 4) minimal toxicity. These characteristics are shown in figure 1 [15, 17]. Core drugs are those with bactericidal and/or sterilising activity. They are the drugs that kill the bacilli, cure the patient and avoid relapses. However, there are other anti-TB drugs with very little or no bactericidal and sterilising activity, but with a good capacity to prevent resistance to the core drugs. These are called companion drugs. They should be included in the anti-TB regimen simply to protect the action of the core drugs [12, 14–17]. Although these definitions of core and companion drugs are generally accepted, they are not completely true because sometimes the evidence can re-allocate a possible companion drug to a core drug.

Isoniazid and rifampicin have the best overall bactericidal activity [1, 14–18, 20]. Among the second-line drugs, the fluoroquinolones (especially the new-generation ones) and the SLIDs have good bactericidal activity. According to the currently available data, linezolid, bedaquiline, delamanid and the carbapenems plus amoxicillin–clavulanic acid also have good bactericidal activity [14–17]. If a bactericidal drug cannot be used due to toxicity and/or proven resistance, this drug should be replaced with another with similar bactericidal activity [14–16].

Activity	Prevention of resistance	Bactericidal activity	Sterilising activity	Toxicity	
High ↓	Rifampicin Isoniazid Ethambutol	Isoniazid Rifampicin Lfx/Mfx	Rifampicin Pyrazinamide Mfx/Lfx	Ethambutol Rifampicin Isoniazid FQs	Low ↓
Moderate ↓	Injectables FQs Ethionamide Cycloserine PAS Linezolid?	Injectables Linezolid Bedaquiline Delamanid Carbapenems	Linezolid Bedaquiline Delamanid	Bedaquiline Delamanid Pyrazinamide Linezolid	Moderate ↓
Low	Pyrazinamide	Ethionamide Pyrazinamide	Clofazimine	Injectables Rest	High

Figure 1. The four desirable characteristics of anti-TB drugs. Lfx: levofloxacin; Mfx: moxifloxacin; FQ: fluoroquinolone. Reproduced and modified from [17] and [25] with permission.

https://doi.org/10.1183/2312508X.10021417

The drugs with the strongest sterilising action are rifampicin and pyrazinamide, while isoniazid has a lower sterilising capacity [1, 14–18, 20]. The fluoroquinolones, especially high-dose moxifloxacin and gatifloxacin, also have a good sterilising capacity. Other drugs with sterilising activity are clofazimine, linezolid, bedaquiline and delamanid [1, 14–17]. However, this action is rather limited for streptomycin and other SLIDs [1, 14–19]. In the same way, if a sterilising drug cannot be used because of toxicity and/or proven resistance, this drug should be replaced with another with similar sterilising activity [14–16].

Although the doses of all anti-TB drugs have been standardised [2, 4, 24], the ideal is to adjust these doses according to TDM, aiming for the best efficacy and to reduce the likelihood of any adverse events [26]. Basically, the driver of successful treatment is the equation of exposure of each drug divided by the MIC of the *M. tuberculosis* isolate *in vitro* [27]. The field of TDM is changing rapidly. With TDM, drug concentration is measured by pharmacokinetic blood specimens over time. However, simplified schedules with limited sampling (sometimes accompanied by using finger-prick blood samples) can be used. The samples are stored and sent to reference laboratories under ambient temperature and humidity conditions [28]. This approach makes TDM feasible and potentially accessible for vulnerable populations and low-resource settings [26]. Ultimately, with a gradual increase in MICs of *M. tuberculosis* over time, and with the increasing epidemic of obesity, the need to apply TDM principles is likely to become more important [27, 29].

Intensive and continuation phases in tuberculosis treatment

The ideal treatment regimen for TB should have two phases: the intensive phase when the bacillary load is very high, with four to five new drugs (two to three core and one to two accompanying) until the bacillary load has been reduced to a minimum [10, 11, 14–17, 19], and the continuation phase, when the bacillary load is largely reduced and when the accompanying drugs can therefore be stopped. The best indicator that the bacillary load has been reduced to a minimum, and that the intensive phase can safely be replaced by the continuation phase, is the sputum smear reversion to negative [15, 16]. Although some authors prefer to use culture conversion as a proxy of bactericidal activity, most experts agree that sputum smear conversion is an appropriate proxy for bactericidal activity [6, 7, 15, 16]. Following sputum smear conversion, two potent drugs (three to four if they are weaker) in the continuation phase should be enough to cure the patient [10, 11, 14–17, 19].

Treatment of drug-susceptible tuberculosis

The best treatment for TB caused by drug-susceptible strains of *M. tuberculosis* should include isoniazid, rifampicin and pyrazinamide in the first 2 months (2HRZ), followed by isoniazid and rifampicin for another 4 months (4HR). It is advisable also to include ethambutol (E) in the intensive phase to cover the possibility that the patient is infected by isoniazid-monoresistant TB (HMR-TB) bacilli [15–17, 21]. Nevertheless, when isoniazid primary resistance was very uncommon worldwide, the recommendations to treat TB were only with the HRZ or HR regimens in the intensive phase [21, 22]. Similarly, ethambutol can be avoided in cases where susceptibility to isoniazid and rifampicin is known before starting the treatment or <1–2 weeks after starting treatment [15].

As ethambutol is given to protect against the possibility that the patient has been infected by bacilli resistant to isoniazid, it should not be stopped until DST shows that the

M. tuberculosis isolate is susceptible to isoniazid and rifampicin, or at least until the sputum smears have converted to negative [15–17, 30]. However, if the sputum smear is still positive at the end of the second month, it is better to continue the treatment with an HRZE regimen until the sputum smear has converted to negative or until the laboratory reports susceptibility to isoniazid and rifampicin. Persistent sputum smear positivity >2 months after the start of treatment conceivably reflects a high initial bacillary load, and it is therefore possible that the continuation of pyrazinamide may have added value in this context [15–17, 30]. It can also mean too low a drug exposure, resulting in a slow response and, for this reason, TDM should be recommended [29].

Although the continuation phase with 4HR is usually enough to cure most patients with DS-TB, patients with extensively advanced or cavitary TB and/or those with a delayed smear and/or culture conversion may benefit from prolongation of the continuation phase to reduce the chance of a relapse. In these patients, we recommend maintaining the continuation phase for ⩾4 months following sputum smear conversion [15–17, 30].

This treatment regimen (2HRZE/4HR) offers potent bactericidal and sterilising action (with the support of ethambutol as a companion drug), curing >95–98% of patients, with few relapses (<1–2%) and few adverse events (<5%).

The entire treatment should be administered daily, using fixed-dose combinations [24, 31]. The same treatment regimen should be utilised for all forms of EPTB and for patients with HIV and other comorbidities [24, 31]. However, the American Thoracic Society (ATS) and Infectious Diseases Society of America (IDSA) recommend extending the duration of therapy for patients with central nervous system TB (12 months) or bone-joint disease (9 months), but with the same 2 months of intensive phase with HRZE [31].

Steroids are indicated only in the treatment of severe forms of TB such as meningeal, miliary or pericardial TB, where their anti-inflammatory properties can be helpful in the acute phase and, perhaps, to reduce the chance of sequelae [16, 19, 31]. However, one large multicentre trial in Africa failed to show any benefit of steroids in TB pericarditis [32]; similarly, a large trial conducted in Vietnam failed to confirm any benefit from steroids in TB pericarditis [33]. The use of steroids in TB meningitis is generally accepted as the standard of care [24, 33].

Treatment of mono- and polyresistance to isoniazid but with susceptibility to rifampicin

TB mono- and polyresistance to isoniazid but with susceptibility to rifampicin is relatively commonly observed in all national TB programmes [2]. The WHO [34] recommends treatment with rifampicin, pyrazinamide, ethambutol and levofloxacin (Lfx) for 6 months, for patients with HMR-TB. Fixed-dose combinations with HRZE may be used (as there is no approved RZE fixed-dose combination available), to limit the need for using single drugs. Drug susceptibility to fluoroquinolones should preferably be confirmed prior to the start of treatment. However, the WHO also accepts a regimen with only 6 months of RZE (or HRZE if fixed-dose combinations are used) in some special cases, such as when RR-TB cannot be excluded, in case of suspected fluoroquinolone resistance or intolerance, for known or suspected risk for a prolonged QT interval, and during pregnancy or breastfeeding (although this is not considered an absolute contraindication) [34].

 https://doi.org/10.1183/2312508X.10021417

The WHO 2018 HMR-TB recommendations are based on the recent meta-analysis by FREGONESE *et al.* [35] where the addition of a fluoroquinolone to ≥6 months of (H)RZE treatment was associated with significantly greater treatment success (adjusted (a)OR 2.8, 95% CI 1.1–7.3), but with no significant effect on mortality (aOR 0.7, 95% CI 0.4–1.1) or acquired rifampicin resistance (aOR 0.1, 95% CI 0.0–1.2). However, the authors highlighted that the quality of the evidence was very low for all outcomes and treatment regimens assessed, owing to the observational nature of most of the data, the diverse settings and the imprecision of estimates.

The recommendation to add levofloxacin to the RZE (or HRZE) regimen to treat HMR-TB refers to cases for whom HMR-TB is known before starting the treatment or soon after because, in this case, levofloxacin is working from the beginning (or immediately after), together with the other drugs [34]. However, in the case where HMR-TB is diagnosed later during treatment, after >1–2 months of therapy with HRZE, the introduction of levofloxacin translates into the addition of just one drug to a regimen possibly not working very well because of the isoniazid monoresistance, especially if the patient then becomes smear/culture positive after these 1–2 months. In this situation, levofloxacin can easily be compromised over time, even with a new confirmation of rifampicin susceptibility, leading to the development of further resistance.

For this reason, it would be best to test susceptibility to isoniazid before the start of treatment and initiate a regimen of 6(H)RZE plus a fluoroquinolone for all those with confirmed isoniazid monoresistance. DST for isoniazid, better if implemented with a rapid molecular test, should be carried out for all cases. However, for patients in whom isoniazid monoresistance is discovered later during treatment, as well as for all patients with intolerance or contraindications to the use of fluoroquinolone, a regimen of 6–9H*RZE (*=high dose, 15–20 mg·kg^{-1}) should be considered. Ideally, this would be 6 months for patients with limited disease and early smear conversion to negative (within 2 months of the start of treatment), and 9 months in all other HMR-TB patients [17].

With the 6–9H*RZE regimen, not only is the risk of fluoroquinolone resistance amplification avoided, but these patients also receive a highly effective regimen, which is also recommended by the WHO in special circumstances [34]. This 6–9H*RZE regimen is also supported by two other meta-analyses published recently [36, 37]. This regimen follows the three conclusions of the meta-analysis by STAGG *et al.* [36]. In addition, the meta-analysis by GEGIA *et al.* [37] showed that the outcomes with 6–9RZE were practically the same for patients with HMR-TB as for those with DS-TB, with practically no failures (1% in both group of patients: HMR-TB and isoniazid-susceptible TB), few relapses (7% *versus* 6%, respectively) and negligible acquired drug resistance (0.3% *versus* 0.1%, respectively).

These two meta-analyses support a core regimen of RZE to cure practically all HMR-TB patients [36, 37]. Adding high-dose isoniazid for all patients should be considered for two reasons. First, it can facilitate administration in the field using fixed-dose combinations (and adding only extra isoniazid), and second, many of the isoniazid-resistant strains could respond to high-dose isoniazid [38, 39].

In conclusion, a regimen of 6RZE (or HRZE)+Lfx is the preferred option in patients for whom isoniazid resistance is known before starting the treatment [17, 34]. However, if the HMR-TB result is known after 1–2 months of HRZE therapy and/or if fluoroquinolones are not available or not tolerated, the recommended HMR-TB regimen should be 6–9H*RZE [17].

Treatment of mono- and polyresistance to rifampicin but with susceptibility to isoniazid

This situation is very uncommon in the field, as >80–90% of cases with RR-TB are actually true MDR-TB [2]. Moreover, as the prognosis of TB is linked to the possible resistance to rifampicin, all mono- and polyresistant RR-TB cases should be managed like MDR-TB patients [3, 11, 17], following the premises discussed in the next section. Isoniazid should be included in the regimen but should not be counted as one of the four new or probably effective drugs [17].

Treatment of multidrug-resistant tuberculosis

The conventional MDR-TB regimen mostly used worldwide to date is represented by a 20–24-month therapy with at least five drugs considered to be effective, comprising a fluoroquinolone (levofloxacin or moxifloxacin), a thioamide (usually ethionamide or prothionamide), cycloserine (or terizidone) or two other drugs of group C of the WHO 2016 classification (table 2), and pyrazinamide, adding also an SLID (usually kanamycin, but also sometimes amikacin or capreomycin) in the first 8 months (intensive phase) [3, 40–42]. Although this regimen had all the previously mentioned principles [14–17], it did not achieve success rates >55–70%, particularly due to high dropout rates [2, 3, 9, 43], mainly associated with the extensive duration of treatment and the poor tolerability resulting from high toxicity. Success rates are higher when a more personalised MDR-TB treatment is chosen, including TDM [44]. Therefore, this individualised MDR-TB treatment should be the first choice if there are enough resources and well-trained physicians [11, 44]. The WHO is now also recommending that this individualised approach is preferably used, proposing a revised grouping of TB medicines for use in longer MDR-TB regimens (table 3) [11]. The revised grouping of TB drugs has been elaborated after doing an individual patient data meta-analysis correlating the association of treatment success and death with use of individual drugs in longer MDR-TB regimens [10].

According to the new WHO guidelines, drugs to be prioritised (group A) are: levofloxacin/moxifloxacin, bedaquiline and linezolid [10, 11, 14]. The medicines to be added next (group B) are clofazimine and cycloserine/terizidone [11]. Finally, the medicines to be included to complete the regimens and when agents from groups A and B cannot be used (group C) are: ethambutol, delamanid, pyrazinamide, imipenem–cilastatin, meropenem, amikacin (streptomycin), ethionamide/prothionamide and PAS [11]. Medicines no longer recommended are kanamycin and capreomycin, given the increased risk of treatment failure and relapse associated with their use in longer MDR-TB regimens [11].

While WHO understanding is that it will not be immediately possible to achieve the new standards of care in every individual MDR-TB patient, strategic planning should start immediately to enable rapid implementation of these upcoming new WHO guidelines [10]. It is clear, in fact, that this individualised approach currently is not feasible in many burdened countries, and therefore, while waiting to build the new standards, and also in view of promising results obtained with 9–11-month MDR-TB regimens [4–9] recommended in the 2016 WHO guidelines for MDR/RR-TB patients [3], a shorter regimen remains a valid option. This shorter MDR/RR-TB regimen is in fact still considered in the new 2018 guidelines [10], but replaces kanamycin with amikacin for patients who do not have any of the following conditions: 1) resistance or suspected ineffectiveness to a medicine

https://doi.org/10.1183/2312508X.10021417

Table 2. Antimycobacterial drugs recommended for the treatment of MDR/RR-TB

Group A: fluoroquinolones	Group B: SLIDs	Group C: other core second-line drugs	Group D: add-on agents
Levofloxacin Moxifloxacin Gatifloxacin	Amikacin Capreomycin Kanamycin (Streptomycin)	Ethionamide/ prothionamide Cycloserine/terizidone Clofazimine[#] Linezolid[#]	D1: pyrazinamide, ethambutol, high-dose isoniazid D2: bedaquiline, delamanid D3: PAS[¶], imipenem/meropenem[+], amoxicillin/clavulanic acid, (thioacetazone)

[#]: clofazimine and linezolid were moved from a previous group 5 designation to group C. [¶]: PAS was moved from a previous group 4 designation to group D3. [+]: carbapenems should be combined with clavulanic acid, which is available as amoxicillin–clavulanic acid. Reproduced and modified from [3] with permission.

Table 3. The WHO 2018 grouping of medicines recommended for use in longer MDR-TB regimens

Group A: include all three medicines (unless they cannot be used)	Group B: add both medicines (unless they cannot be used)	Group C: add to complete the regimen and when medicines from groups A and B cannot be used
Levofloxacin or moxifloxacin Bedaquiline[#,¶] Linezolid[+]	Clofazimine Cycloserine or terizidone	Ethambutol Delamanid[§,¶] Pyrazinamide[f] Imipenem–cilastatin or meropenem[##] Amikacin (or streptomycin)[¶¶] Ethionamide or prothionamide PAS

[#]: evidence on the safety and effectiveness of bedaquiline for >6 months was insufficient for review; extended bedaquiline use in individual patients will need to follow "off-label" use best practices. [¶]: evidence on concurrent use of bedaquiline and delamanid was insufficient for review. [+]: the optimal duration of use of linezolid is not established; use for $\geqslant$6 months was shown to be highly effective, although toxicity may limit its use. [§]: the position of delamanid will be re-assessed once individual patient data from the Otsuka trial 213 has been reviewed; these data were not available for the evidence assessment; evidence on the safety and effectiveness of delamanid for >6 months was insufficient for review; extended use of delamanid in individual patients will need to follow "off-label" use best practices. [f]: pyrazinamide is only counted as an effective agent when DST results confirm susceptibility. [##]: amoxicillin–clavulanic acid is administered with every dose of imipenem–cilastatin or meropenem but is not counted as a separate agent and should not be used as a separate agent. [¶¶]: amikacin and streptomycin are only to be considered if DST results confirm susceptibility and high-quality audiology monitoring for hearing loss can be ensured; streptomycin is to be considered only if amikacin cannot be used and if DST results confirm susceptibility (streptomycin resistance is not detectable with second-line molecular line probe assays, and phenotypic DST is required). Reproduced and modified from [11] with permission.

included in the shorter MDR-TB regimen (except isoniazid resistance), 2) exposure to one or more second-line drugs in the regimen for >1 month (unless susceptibility to these second-line drugs is confirmed), 3) intolerance to any medicine in the shorter MDR-TB regimen or risk of toxicity (*e.g.* drug–drug interactions), 4) pregnancy or 5) disseminated, meningeal or central nervous system TB, or any extrapulmonary disease in HIV patients.

The shorter MDR/RR-TB regimen consists of an intensive phase of 4 months (or until sputum smears become negative, but not >6 months) with amikacin, high-dose moxifloxacin, clofazimine, ethionamide/prothionamide, pyrazinamide, ethambutol and high-dose isoniazid. The continuation phase consists of 5 months of high-dose moxifloxacin, clofazimine, ethambutol and pyrazinamide. Patients must be closely monitored for possible adverse effects, especially possible prolongation of the corrected QT (QTc) interval on ECG, related to high moxifloxacin doses and clofazimine [3, 17, 45, 46].

The shorter MDR/RR-TB regimens can be used also in children and people living with HIV (excluding patients with any extrapulmonary disease). Concerning the shorter regimen exclusion criteria mentioned previously [3, 10], the first (resistance or suspected ineffectiveness to a medicine included in the shorter MDR-TB regimen (except isoniazid resistance)) should be analysed critically, especially because of the poor reliability of DST to drugs such as ethambutol, pyrazinamide and ethionamide/prothionamide. Moreover, recent publications have showed that resistance to any of these drugs has no influence on the final successful outcome [8]. Therefore, only confirmed resistance to the fluoroquinolones and/or SLIDs represent absolute exclusion criteria for the shorter MDR/RR-TB regimen [8, 46].

A recent systematic review and meta-analysis of the shorter MDR/RR-TB regimens found that the successful outcome of these regimens was 83%, much better than the 54% achieved with the conventional longer MDR/RR-TB regimens [2, 9]. Risk factors for poor treatment outcomes included fluoroquinolone resistance (OR 46, 95% CI 8–273), followed by use of moxifloxacin rather than gatifloxacin (OR 9, 95% CI 4–22), pyrazinamide resistance (OR 8, 95% CI 2–38) and no culture conversion after 2 months (OR 7, 95% CI 3–202). When death was compared with survival, people living with HIV were five times more likely to die than HIV-negative patients.

In conclusion, although an individualised longer MDR/RR-TB regimen following the new WHO 2018 guidelines should be prioritised for these patients, the shorter MDR/RR-TB regimens (9–11 months) can be also considered for patients with MDR/RR-TB who have not previously received fluoroquinolones or SLIDs for >1 month and with adequate capacity for monitoring drug safety (especially ototoxicity) [3, 10, 45, 46]. The previous use of or confirmed resistance to fluoroquinolones and/or SLIDs may limit the applicability of the shorter regimen, especially in settings where patients have more resistant forms of TB (including to fluoroquinolones and/or SLIDs) and are more treatment experienced (*e.g.* in reference centres in Europe) [47, 48]. Nevertheless, confirmation of susceptibility to fluoroquinolones and SLIDs, by molecular testing, should be done as soon as possible, regardless of the chosen regimen.

Treatment of pre-XDR-TB, XDR-TB and beyond XDR-TB

While the treatment success rates achieved globally with MDR/RR-TB patients are suboptimal, barely exceeding 50% [2, 43], this proportion decreases much further to ⩽26% in

https://doi.org/10.1183/2312508X.10021417

patients with XDR-TB and beyond XDR-TB [2, 12, 43]. Moreover, currently many XDR-TB cases are patients failing the MDR-TB standardised regimen, or new TB patients who are contacts of these cases. Therefore, *M. tuberculosis* strains in these patients often carry a very similar pattern of extended resistance, including the drugs prescribed previously (ethionamide/prothionamide and cycloserine/terizidone, among others) [12]. Thus, taking into account the possible pattern of resistance of most current XDR-TB patients, an empirical treatment can be designed trying to cover most of the patients with pre-XDR-TB, XDR-TB and beyond XDR-TB. This regimen should therefore include the following anti-TB drugs [12]:

1) Linezolid. This is a core drug with bactericidal and sterilising capacity [12, 14, 17, 49].

2) Bedaquiline. This is also a potential core drug with bactericidal and sterilising characteristics [12, 14, 17]. Some countries may value the use of delamanid instead of bedaquiline, as it also has the features of a core drug [12, 14, 17]. In selected cases, the combination of bedaquiline and delamanid can be considered (*e.g.* in those settings where the use of carbapenems is not possible), but strict monitoring of patients must be ensured, as experience is still limited at the global level, and the concomitant use of these two drugs is not yet recommended [50].

3) Clofazimine. This is considered a core drug because of its sterilising capacity [12, 14, 17]. If the patient has previously received clofazimine in a failing regimen (*e.g.* a shorter MDR/RR-TB regimen or another conventional regimen), this drug should be replaced by cycloserine (playing the role of a companion drug).

4) A carbapenem-class antibiotic, plus amoxicillin–clavulanic acid [51–54]. These are also core drugs because of their likely bactericidal activity [12, 14, 17]. However, given the need for parenteral administration with carbapenems, delamanid is also a potential choice (although ECG monitoring will be required).

5) Additionally, there is the need to re-inforce and protect the four drugs in the previous steps with more "supporting" drugs (important for some XDR-TB cases and even more so for pre-XDR-TB):

- A fluoroquinolone, different from that used in the MDR-TB regimen [12]. In the case of pre-XDR-TB due to SLID resistance, the fluoroquinolone would play a key role in the regimen [12]. However, even in the case of XDR-TB, the fluoroquinolone may still play a role, especially considering there is no complete cross resistance among the new fluoroquinolones [55, 56]. If the result of conventional DST demonstrates resistance to all fluoroquinolones, including high concentrations of moxifloxacin, this fluoroquinolone should be discontinued. If moxifloxacin or levofloxacin is used, strict QTc ECG control must be ensured.

- Amikacin if this drug has not been used before and DST shows susceptibility to this drug [12]. Many pre-XDR or XDR-TB patients have received kanamycin or capreomycin previously, but there is no total cross resistance among SLIDs [56, 57]. If DST shows resistance to amikacin or if there are adverse reactions to this drug, it should be stopped [12].

- High-dose isoniazid (15–20 mg·kg^{-1}) may have a role in cases with low-level resistance [12, 38, 39].

A summary of the possible designs for a standardised regimen for patients with pre-XDR-TB or XDR-TB is presented in table 4 [12]. However, when the recent 2018 WHO recommendations have been applied widely throughout the world, this proposal of empirical pre-XDR and XDR-TB will be not a valid option because some of the core drugs of this regimen (linezolid, bedaquiline) will have been used previously in the MDR-TB regimen. In this situation, individualised management will again be the best option.

Because of the composition of the proposed regimen (which includes two to three sterilising core drugs), the total duration of the regimen might be 15–18 months, with at least up to 12 months treatment following culture conversion. All drugs are necessary throughout the treatment (particularly those that are new and the core drugs, such as linezolid, bedaquiline and/or delamanid), with the exception of SLIDs and high-dose isoniazid, which could be discontinued after 4 months of treatment [12, 58]. If sputum smear microscopy and culture remain positive at the end of the sixth month of treatment, treatment failure should be accepted and the case should be re-evaluated to undergo an individualised regimen [12]. If a carbapenem is included in the regimen, it could be discontinued after 6 months following bacteriological conversion [12]. As bedaquiline and delamanid are considered core drugs in this regimen, these agents should conceivably be administered for the whole treatment duration (and not only for 6 months as current guidelines suggest) [12, 58]. This extended use has already been used successfully in some settings, although it is not yet globally recommended [12, 50, 58–60]. Nevertheless, as fluoroquinolones, bedaquiline, delamanid and clofazimine can prolong the QTc interval during an ECG, close monitoring must be undertaken when some of these drugs are used.

Management of tuberculosis and drug-resistant tuberculosis in special situations

Some situations may be considered "special" because the clinical management requires more careful consideration. Paediatric cases of TB or MDR-TB, patients who are contacts of a case of TB or MDR-TB, and patients with TB or MDR-TB who have special conditions such pregnancy or comorbidities such as HIV infection and DM may require different management strategies. These are summarised in table 5.

Surgery in the treatment of tuberculosis and multidrug-resistant/extensively drug-resistant tuberculosis

Surgical resection of infected lung tissue may be indicated in selected patients with PTB, including in some patients with MDR/RR/XDR-TB [3, 16, 19, 62–64]. This topic will be addressed in depth in another chapter in this *Monograph* [65].

Treatment of tuberculosis when one anti-tuberculosis drug cannot be used because of adverse reactions

Toxicity preventing the use of certain TB drugs is largely similar to the situation where drug resistance prohibits their use: 1) if isoniazid cannot be used due to toxicity, a 6–9RZE regimen, with or without a fluoroquinolone, can be enough to cure patients with DS-TB,

https://doi.org/10.1183/2312508X.10021417

Table 4. Summary of the options to design an empirical standardised regimen for patients with pre-XDR-TB or XDR-TB receiving the shorter MDR-TB regimen or the longer 2016 WHO MDR-TB regimen

Regimen composition	Drug	Activity	Proposed recommendations
1) Two core drugs (always in the regimen)	Linezolid	Bactericidal and sterilising	Delamanid could replace linezolid or bedaquiline if: • one of these drugs has been used previously • there is confirmed resistance to one of these drugs • there is severe toxicity
	Bedaquiline	Bactericidal and sterilising	Bedaquiline: potentially QT-prolonging drug ECG monitoring is needed
2a) One companion drug (one of the following)	Clofazimine (core drug, first choice)	Sterilising	To be given if never administered before; especially useful in MDR-TB patients failing a conventional 20–24-month MDR-TB regimen Potentially QT-prolonging drug
	Cycloserine	Nonbactericidal and nonsterilising	To be given if never administered before, and when clofazimine was administered in a previous failing regimen (shorter 9–12-month MDR/RR-TB regimen or other regimen)
2b) One companion drug (one of the following)	One carbapenem +amoxicillin–clavulanic acid	Bactericidal	Three options: • meropenem (first choice) • imipenem–cilastatin • ertapenem
	Delamanid	Bactericidal and sterilising	ECG monitoring needed
3) Three supporting drugs: one FQ, one SLID and high-dose isoniazid	One FQ (moxifloxacin)[#]	Bactericidal and sterilising	Dependent on patient's previous treatment history Indicated in pre-XDR or XDR-TB patients not previously treated for TB with an FQ Close monitoring of QTc interval required if used with bedaquiline and clofazimine
	One FQ (high-dose moxifloxacin)[#]	Bactericidal and sterilising	Use if levofloxacin has been used previously to treat TB; if possible, it is important to assure high exposure is achieved (TDM)

Continued

https://doi.org/10.1183/2312508X.10021417

Table 4. Continued

Regimen composition	Drug	Activity	Proposed recommendations
3) Three supporting drugs: one FQ, one SLID and high-dose isoniazid (cont.)	One FQ (high-dose levofloxacin)#	Bactericidal and sterilising	Use if moxifloxacin has been used previously to treat TB; if possible, it is important to assure high exposure is achieved (TDM)
	One SLID (amikacin)¶	Bactericidal	Use in a pre-XDR or XDR-TB patient not previously treated for TB with an SLID Use if kanamycin or capreomycin have been used previously to treat TB
	High-dose isoniazid	Bactericidal	Dose: 15–20 mg·kg⁻¹ Isoniazid is discontinued when: • high level of resistance is confirmed in vitro • when a line probe assay demonstrates mutation in katG and inhA

This proposal does not apply when the pre-XDR or XDR-TB patient has received a longer MDR/RR-TB regimen following the 2018 WHO recommendations. FQ: fluoroquinolone; QTc: corrected QT interval. #: if DST shows resistance to levofloxacin and moxifloxacin, the FQ will be discontinued from the regimen. ¶: if DST shows resistance to all the SLDs, this drug will be discontinued from the regimen. Reproduced and modified from [12] with permission.

https://doi.org/10.1183/2312508X.10021417

Table 5. TB and MDR-TB management in special situations

TB in contacts of TB/ DR-TB patients	• Contacts of patients with TB, and who develop TB, are very likely to have susceptible TB as well. Contacts of MDR-TB patients, and who develop active TB, are very likely to have MDR-TB as well (65–85% of cases) • However, in some cases, contacts may show a different pattern of resistance from the index case. They can have a completely susceptible TB, MDR-TB or even XDR-TB, depending on when and where the infection occurred and the prevalence of TB and DR-TB in the community, as there is the possibility that this happened in the community with a different source • In MDR-TB contacts who develop TB, GeneXpert (Cepheid, Sunnyvale, CA, USA) should be used, followed by culture and DST. While awaiting the final results, patients should receive the same MDR-TB regimen as the index case. The regimen should then be adjusted later according to the DST results
TB/MDR-TB and HIV coinfection	• HIV is the strongest risk factor for active TB disease, especially in the absence of ART and TB preventative therapy. All HIV patients should be screened regularly for TB and tested with GeneXpert if TB is suspected, and TB treatment should be started as soon as the disease is diagnosed. However, ART should be initiated in TB/HIV patients irrespective of CD4$^+$ cell count as early as possible (within the first 8 weeks, or even earlier in the case of TB meningitis or very low CD4$^+$ cell counts) following the initiation of anti-TB treatment • Unsuccessful TB treatment outcomes are more common in patients coinfected with HIV than in HIV-negative patients • Rifampicin is a potent cytochrome P450 and other enzymes inducer, and rifabutin and rifapentine are cytochrome P450 3A4 substrates and inducers. Therefore, they can accelerate the metabolism of several drugs, resulting in a significant reduction in antiretroviral drug exposure. The anti-retroviral drugs most affected are the protease inhibitors and the NNRTIs, but also other drugs such the integrase strand transfer inhibitors elvitegravir, the CCR5 antagonist maraviroc, and also dolutegravir, raltegravir and tenofovir alafenamide. In contrast to other NNRTIs (etravirine and rilpivirine), efavirenz concentration is not much affected by rifampicin, and this anti-retroviral drug is generally part of the ART used for TB/HIV coinfected patients. Recently, the WHO has included dolutegravir (an integrase inhibitor)-based HIV treatment as an alternative first-line regimen, but the limited experience with specific groups, such as TB/HIV coinfected patients, has prevented the WHO from being able to recommend these antiretroviral drugs across all populations • These interactions with rifamycins are not relevant in the case of MDR-TB, since by definition it is resistant to rifampicin and does not need to include rifampicin in the regimen. However, overlapping toxicity, increased side-effects and drug–drug interactions can occur during MDR- and XDR-TB/HIV cotreatment, *e.g.* potential hepatotoxicity (protease inhibitors, NNRTIs and thionamides), nephrotoxicity (tenofovir and SLIDs), psychiatric disturbances (efavirenz and cycloserine), myelosuppression and mitochondrial toxicity (nucleoside reverse transcriptase inhibitors such as didanosine, stavudine, azidothymidine and linezolid) and others

Continued

Table 5. Continued

	• No significant drug–drug interactions between delaminid and antiretroviral drugs have been observed so far. However, the concentration of bedaquiline could be affected by some antiretroviral drugs (efavirenz, nevirapine, ritonavir) and should be used with caution in HIV patients receiving antiretroviral drugs, due to limited available information • The composition of the treatment regimen for MDR-TB does not differ for patients with HIV coinfection, including shorter MDR-TB regimens. Thioacetazone should not be used in HIV patients • Immuno-reconstitution inflammatory syndrome might appear more frequently, as soon as the ART is initiated in patients receiving anti-TB drugs
TB/DR-TB and DM	• Similarly to HIV, but at much lower scale, DM increases the risk of TB (3-fold on average) by weakening the immune system and impairing host defences. DM is also a risk factor for atypical presentation of TB disease and for worse outcomes (death, failures and relapses) • However, TB may complicate the management of DM because of drug–drug interactions and because of its effect on glucose regulation. Many drugs for DM are metabolised by the cytochrome P450 enzymatic system in the liver, and thus rifampicin can reduce their concentration. Enzyme induction effects can last for 2–4 weeks after discontinuation of rifampicin. The levels of glucose should be monitored, and oral hypoglycaemic drugs should be re-adjusted at the end of TB treatment • TB patients should be screened for DM, and screening for TB should be performed in DM patients to allow early TB detection and prompt access to treatment • Patients with TB and DM require close follow-up, given the increased risk of side-effects, especially renal failure and neuropathy
TB/MDR-TB and pregnancy	• Initial pregnancy testing should be carried out for all women of child-bearing age with TB/MDR-TB. If untreated, TB in pregnancy increases maternal and fetal mortality (especially if there is HIV coinfection), and is a cause of low birthweight, premature birth and transmission to the baby • Anti-TB drugs may have some risk to the fetus, but knowledge about potential teratogenesis and toxicity of second-line drugs is limited. Only ethambutol and amoxicillin–clavulanic acid are in FDA drug safety class B; isoniazid, rifampicin, pyrazinamide, capreomycin, fluoroquinolones, ethionamide, cycloserine and clofazimine are in class C, and streptomycin, kanamycin and amikacin are all in class D. As there are no data on the safety of bedaquiline and delamanid in pregnancy, these drugs are not currently indicated in pregnant women. Capreomycin and kanamycin are no longer recommended for the treatment of DR-TB • In the case of MDR-TB, treatment should ideally be avoided during the first trimester, but the risks and benefits need to be evaluated. If there are life-threatening conditions such advanced disease, respiratory failure or HIV coinfection, MDR-TB treatment should be considered, regardless of the trimester. The MDR-TB

Continued

https://doi.org/10.1183/2312508X.10021417

Table 5. Continued

	regimen should be individualised and started in sufficient time to achieve smear conversion before delivery. Shorter MDR-TB regimens are not currently recommended for pregnant women, given the lack of sufficient data in this group • Nausea and vomiting can be increased by ethionamide, which should therefore be avoided if possible
TB/MDR-TB and children	• A bacteriologically confirmed diagnosis of TB is difficult in children, especially in young children, due to the low bacillary load and the difficulty in obtaining specimens. GeneXpert should be used to diagnose TB in children, given its higher sensitivity than microscopy, and since it also allows early detection of RR-TB. The DST pattern of the index case should be used if no isolates are available from the child and the possible index case is known • New paediatric formulations (fixed-dose combinations) have recently been developed in line with the revised dosing to achieve the appropriate therapeutic levels, and are preferred. These child-friendly fixed-dose combinations are dispersible in water, taste nice for children and allow more precise dosages • In the case of MDR-TB treatment, the criteria for designing a regimen are mostly the same as in adults, including shorter regimens. However, in children with mild forms of the disease, the side-effects associated with the group B medications (SLIDs) outweigh the benefits, and thus group B drugs should be excluded from their regimen • In 2016, the delamanid interim policy was extended to children aged 6–17 years • Most children tolerate second-line drugs well and treatment outcomes are good; this is also the case in HIV high-prevalence settings
EPTB/MDR-TB	• EPTB should be treated as for PTB; however, some experts recommend longer treatment when there is involvement of the central nervous system or bone-joint disease • Extrapulmonary MDR-TB is not very frequent

NNRTIs: nonnucleoside reverse transcriptase inhibitors; FDA: US Food and Drug Administration. Reproduced and modified from [61] with permission.

2) when pyrazinamide cannot be used, the initial regimen simply needs to be prolonged to 9 months (2HRE/7HR) [1, 17, 19], 3) if ethambutol cannot be used, there is no problem if there is confirmed susceptibility to isoniazid and rifampicin, and a regimen of 2HRZ/4HR can cure practically all patients [19] or 4) regarding SLIDs, the management is very similar when the drugs cannot be used due to resistance or toxicity, simply by changing this drug for another with bactericidal activity.

The situation is different for rifampicin, because when there is confirmed resistance to this drug, >80–90% of strains also have resistance to isoniazid [2] and ~50% have resistance to pyrazinamide [2, 66–68]. In addition, as DST is not reliable for these two drugs (it is very reliable for isoniazid but has poor reliability for pyrazinamide), when a patient has RR-TB, they should be treated as for MDR-TB, as explained previously. In this situation, isoniazid and pyrazinamide should be added to the regimen, but they should not be counted among the four new drugs needed in the treatment.

When rifampicin cannot be used because of toxicity, rifampicin can be replaced by rifabutin, if well tolerated. In these cases, isoniazid and pyrazinamide should be used and counted as new and core drugs and, for this reason, a regimen of HZE plus rifabutin (if tolerated) or a fluoroquinolone can be a reasonably good alternative regimen. The duration should be 6 months if rifabutin can be used, or 9 months when high-dose moxifloxacin is in the regimen.

Adverse events and their management

A more detailed discussion of the management of the adverse events is provided in another chapter in this *Monograph* [69]. However, table 6 provides a summary of the most frequent adverse events to the different anti-TB drugs and their respective management options. Adequate identification and management of adverse drug reactions is essential in the management of patients with TB, especially in those with MDR/RR/XDR-TB.

Active drug safety monitoring and management (aDSM) should be organised to provide active and systematic clinical and laboratory assessment of patients, and also to ensure adequate and timely detection, management, and reporting of suspected or confirmed drug toxicity.

Management issues

There are some important clinical and operational management issues that need to be addressed to maximise the possibility of treatment success. In order to select the most appropriate treatment for patients with TB, training is essential. Indeed, in-depth knowledge is essential about the role of the different diagnostic procedures, adequate interpretation of DST results including the interpretation of possible discordant results, and the role of the different anti-TB drugs and how to identify and manage the possible adverse events as early as possible. However, there are also important operational management issues, such as accessibility to different diagnostic procedures, an uninterrupted drug supply, aDSM and pharmacology including pharmacokinetics, as well as drug–drug interactions. All of these factors taken together are essential for a successful TB treatment outcome and are addressed in other chapters in this *Monograph*. Finally, it is important to identify the most appropriate model of care in each given setting. Considering the long duration of treatment, especially for MDR/XDR-TB, the risk of adverse reactions and the essentiality of good compliance, the model of care should as far as possible be "person centred", as this provides important detailed information for the patient [11]. Moreover, programmes and their stakeholders should start transitioning towards implementation of the upcoming new WHO guidelines at the earliest opportunity [11].

Tuberculosis consilium

The management of patients with MDR/RR-TB, and especially those with pre-XDR-TB, XDR-TB and beyond XDR-TB, is very challenging. For this reason, it is advisable to discuss the management of each case in a consilium composed of a team of expert physicians.

https://doi.org/10.1183/2312508X.10021417

Table 6. Common adverse effects and management options

System	Adverse effect	Suggested drugs	Management options
Gastrointestinal	Nausea and vomiting	**Eto/Pto**, **PAS**, H, E, Z, Dlm, Bdq, Lzd	1) Assess for dehydration; initiate re-hydration if indicated 2) Initiate antiemetic therapy 3) Lower the dose of suspected agent if this can be done without compromising the regimen (rarely necessary)
	Gastritis	**PAS, Eto/Pto**	1) H$_2$-blockers, proton-pump inhibitors or antacids (cannot be given with FQs) 2) Stop suspected agent(s) for short periods of time (e.g. 1–7 days) 3) Lower the dose of suspected agent, if this can be done without compromising the regimen 4) Discontinue and/or replace suspected agent if this can be done without compromising the regimen
	Diarrhoea	**PAS, Eto/Pto**, FQs, Bdq, Lzd	1) Provide hydration, in hospital if severe 2) Provide antidiarrhoeal agent as needed 3) Search for other causes of diarrhoea, such as infections 4) Lower the dose of suspected agent, if this can be done without compromising the regimen 5) Discontinue and/or replace suspected agent if this can be done without compromising the regimen
	Hepatitis	**Z**, **H**, **R**, Eto/Pto, PAS, E, FQs, Bdq, Lzd	1) Stop all drugs pending resolution of hepatitis 2) Explore and address other potential causes of hepatitis 3) Consider suspending drugs, one at a time, with the most hepatotoxic agents first, while monitoring liver function
Cardiac	Prolonged QTc	**FQs, Bdq, Dlm, Cfm**	1) Stop medications if QTc >500 m 2) Monitor electrolytes and serum albumin, and correct if required 3) Possible synergistic effect on QTc if more than one of these drugs are used
Musculoskeletal	Joint pain	**Z**, FQs	1) Initiate therapy with NSAIDs 2) Lower the dose of suspected agent if this can be done without compromising the regimen 3) Discontinue and/or replace suspected agent if this can be done without compromising the regimen

Continued

Table 6. Continued

System	Adverse effect	Suggested drugs	Management options
Otological	Hearing loss and vestibular disturbances	S, **Km, Am**, Cm	1) Document hearing loss and compare with baseline audiometry if available 2) Change parenteral treatment to Cm if patient has documented susceptibility to Cm 3) Decrease frequency and/or lower the dose of suspected agent if this can be done without compromising the regimen (consider administration three times per week) 4) Discontinue and/or replace suspected agent if this can be done without compromising the regimen
Endocrine	Hypothyroidism	**PAS, Eto/Pto**	1) Initiate levothyroxine therapy
Ophthalmic	Optic neuritis	**E**, Eto/Pto, Lzd	1) Stop the drug involved 2) Refer patient to an ophthalmologist
Haematological disorders	Pancytopenia	**Lzd**	1) Reduce dose and ensure close control 2) Evaluate transfusion
Neurological	Seizures	**Cs**, H, FQs	1) Suspend the suspected agent pending resolution of seizures 2) Initiate anticonvulsant therapy (e.g. phenytoin, valproic acid) 3) Increase pyridoxine to maximum daily dose (200 mg·day^{-1}) 4) Restart suspected agent, or re-initiate suspected agent at a lower dose if essential to the regimen 5) Discontinue and/or replace suspected agent if this can be done without compromising regimen
	Peripheral neuropathy	**Lzd, Cs, H**, S, Km, Am, Cm, Eto/Pto, FQs	1) Increase pyridoxine to maximum daily dose (200 mg·day^{-1}) 2) Initiate therapy with tricyclic antidepressants such as amitriptyline. NSAIDs or acetaminophen may help alleviate symptoms 3) Lower dose of suspected agent if this can be done without compromising the regimen 4) Discontinue and/or replace suspected agent if this can be done without compromising the regimen

Continued

https://doi.org/10.1183/2312508X.10021417

Table 6. Continued

System	Adverse effect	Suggested drugs	Management options
Neurological (cont.)	Psychotic symptoms	**Cs, H,** FQs, Eto/Pto	1) Stop suspected agent for a short period of time (1–4 weeks) while psychotic symptoms are brought under control 2) Initiate antipsychotic therapy 3) Lower dose of suspected agent if this can be done without compromising the regimen 4) Discontinue and/or replace suspected agent if this can be done without compromising the regimen
	Depression	**Cs,** FQs H, Eto/Pto	1) Address socioeconomic issues; consider financial support 2) Offer group or individual counselling 3) Initiate antidepressant therapy 4) Lower dose of suspected agent if this can be done without compromising the regimen 5) Discontinue and/or replace suspected agent if this can be done without compromising the regimen
Renal	Nephrotoxicity	**S, Km, Am, Cm**	1) Discontinue suspected agent 2) Consider using Cm if an aminoglycoside has not been the prior injectable in the regimen 3) Consider dosing two to three times per week if the drug is essential to the regimen and the patient can tolerate this (close monitoring of creatinine) 4) Adjust all anti-TB medications according to the creatinine clearance
	Electrolyte disturbances (hypokalaemia and hypomagnesaemia)	**Cm,** Km, Am, S	1) Check potassium levels 2) If potassium is low, also check magnesium (and calcium if hypocalcaemia is suspected) 3) Replace electrolytes as needed

Note that drugs in bold are more strongly associated with the adverse effect than drugs not in bold. Eto/Pto: ethionamide/prothionamide; H: isoniazid; E: ethambutol; Z: pyrazinamide; Dlm: delamanid; Bdq: Bedaquiline; Lzd: linezolid; FQ: fluoroquinolone; R: rifampicin; QTc: corrected QT interval; Cfm: clofazimine; NSAID: nonsteroidal anti-inflammatory drug; S: streptomycin; Km: kanamycin; Cm: capreomycin; Cs: cycloserine; Am: amikacin. Reproduced and modified from [70] with permission.

https://doi.org/10.1183/2312508X.10021417

Table 7. Principles in designing MDR, RR and XDR-TB regimens

Step	Considerations
1) Diagnosis	Perform Xpert MTB/RIF, as the initial diagnosis, in all patients suspected of having TB If MDR/RR-TB (GeneXpert or LPA), perform LPA (GenoType) for FQs and SLIDs, to inform the selection of the ideal MDR/RR/XDR-TB regimen Analyse the following information: • History of drugs taken by the patient: at least 1 month of monotherapy or adding one drug to a failing regimen is a strong predictor of resistance • Phenotypic and molecular DST: reliable for R, H, FQs and SLID. Not reliable for E, Z, Eto, Cs/Tz and PAS. Not available for and/or validated for new and repurposed drugs. The result of the reliable DST should be followed Perform HIV test: if positive, initiate CPT immediately and combination ART for all TB patients within the first 8 weeks after initiation of anti-TB treatment
2) Number of drugs	At least four to five effective drugs that have not been used in the past and/or are susceptible by DST, taking into account the DST reliability and cross resistance At least one to two bactericidal and one to two sterilising drugs
3) Drug selection	Preferable follow individualised regimens following the 2018 WHO regrouping of TB medicines (see table 3) The short-course regimen can also be recommended if all conditions are met: 4 months of Am, high-dose Mfx (Gfx), Cfz, Pto (Eto), Z, E and high-dose H, plus 5 months of high-dose Mfx (Gfx), Cfz, Z and E For longer (21–24 months) MDR/RR-TB treatment, a regimen with at least five effective TB medicines during the intensive phase is recommended, following the new WHO regrouping of TB medicines (see table 3) It is very important to select the ideal dose for each drug
4) Duration of TB treatment	Short MDR/RR-TB regimen: 9–12 months Minimum length of treatment is 21 months in the longer regimen: • Intensive phase: 4 months or until smear negative in the shorter regimens (9–12 months) and 8 months and ⩾6 months after culture conversion in the conventional regimen; longer if three effective drugs are not available during the continuation phase • Continuation phase: minimum of 5 months in the shorter regimens and 12 months in the conventional regimens
5) Surgery	Consider only if few effective drugs are available, localised pulmonary lesions are present and the patient has sufficient respiratory reserve Consider especially in MDR-TB cases with additional resistance to the FQs and beyond

LPA: line probe assay; FQ: fluoroquinolone; R: rifampicin; H: isoniazid; E: ethambutol; Z: pyrazinamide; Eto: ethionamide; Cs/Tz: cycloserine/terizidone; CPT: cotrimoxazole preventative therapy; Am: amikacin; Mfx: moxifloxacin; Gfx: gatifloxacin; Cfz: clofazimine; Pto: prothionamide; Eto: ethionamide. Reproduced and modified from [72] with permission.

This would ensure the choice of the most appropriate anti-TB regimen according to the clinical picture, the history of TB treatment and the pattern of resistance. For this reason, all countries should have a national consilium to discuss the most difficult TB cases. In 2012,

https://doi.org/10.1183/2312508X.10021417

the European Respiratory Society (ERS) launched a web-based platform called the ERS/ WHO TB Consilium to provide technical assistance to clinicians dealing with difficult-to-treat cases [71]. The ERS/WHO TB Consilium consists of a free-to-access, internet-based consultation system available in four languages (English, Spanish, Russian and Portuguese) able to provide suggestions on the clinical management of complicated TB cases with a turnaround time of ~48 h. The launch of the initiative was followed by a call for experts including TB clinicians but also other professionals relevant for patient management. The expert applications have been reviewed and validated by an ERS/WHO/European Centre for Disease Prevention and Control (ECDC) review team based on strict criteria. A panel of 57 global experts was selected and is available for consultation.

Between 2013 and June 2018, 393 cases were discussed in the ERS/WHO TB Consilium. Requests for expert advice originated from 42 countries (with India, South Africa, Italy, the UK, the Russian Federation and the Philippines among the main requesting countries). Drug-resistant cases comprised 275 requests (74.7%); of these 160 were XDR-TB, 88 MDR-TB and 27 pre-XDR. The core clinical questions posed to the experts concerned the most appropriate treatment regimen and/or duration, advice on the introduction of one new drug (delamanid or bedaquiline), advice on the introduction of delamanid for compassionate use, and advice on the combination of delamanid and bedaquiline. The mean time to upload a new case was approximately 20 min and the average response time was 49.4 h.

The ERS/WHO TB Consilium, which works in parallel with national TB consilia wherever available, shepherded clinicians dealing with particularly challenging cases, greatly contributing to their positive treatment outcomes and adverse event management.

Conclusion

With appropriate clinical and operational management, most TB patients can be cured, even those with extensive drug resistance, because, although resistance to TB drugs complicates treatment and reduces the chances of success, careful selection of a regimen based on the basic rules described in this chapter can lead to good treatment outcomes. The basic principles and a summary of most of these fundamental principles can be found in table 7 [61]. This chapter reflects the current evidence behind recommendations for the treatment of patients with TB and different levels of *M. tuberculosis* drug resistance.

References

1. Fox W, Ellard GA, Mitchison DA. Studies on the treatment of tuberculosis undertaken by the British Medical Research Council Tuberculosis Units, 1946–1986, with relevant subsequent publications. *Int J Tuberc Lung Dis* 1999; 3: Suppl. 2, S231–S279.
2. WHO. Global Tuberculosis Report 2017. Document WHO/HTM/TB/2017.23. Geneva, WHO, 2017. http://www. who.int/tb/publications/global_report/gtbr2017_main_text.pdf
3. WHO. WHO Treatment Guidelines for Drug-resistant Tuberculosis. 2016 Update. Document WHO/HTM/TB/ 2016.04. Geneva, WHO, 2016. www.who.int/tb/areas-of-work/drug-resistant-tb/treatment/resources/en/
4. Van Deun A, Kya Jai Maug A, Halim MA, *et al.* Short, highly effective, and inexpensive standardized treatment of multidrug-resistant tuberculosis. *Am J Respir Crit Care Med* 2010; 182: 684–692.
5. Aung KJM, Van Deun A, Declercq E, *et al.* Successful '9-month Bangladesh regimen' for multidrug-resistant tuberculosis among over 500 consecutive patients. *Int J Tuberc Lung Dis* 2014; 18: 1180–1187.
6. Kuaban C, Noeske J, Rieder HL, *et al.* High effectiveness of a 12-month regimen for MDR-TB patients in Cameroon. *Int J Tuberc Lung Dis* 2015; 19: 517–524.

7.   Piubello A, Hassane Harouna S, Souleymane MB, *et al.* High cure rate with standardised short-course multidrug-resistant tuberculosis treatment in Niger: no relapses. *Int J Tuberc Lung Dis* 2014; 18: 1188–1194.

8.   Trébucq A, Schwoebel V, Kashongwe Z, *et al.* Treatment outcome with a short multidrug-resistant tuberculosis regimen in nine African countries. *Int J Tuberc Lung Dis* 2018; 22: 17–25.

9.   Ahmad Khan F, Salim MAH, du Cros P, *et al.* Effectiveness and safety of standardised shorter regimens for multidrug-resistant tuberculosis: individual patient data and aggregate data meta-analysis. *Eur Respir J* 2017; 50: 1700061.

10. Ahmad N, Ahuja SD, Akkerman OW, *et al.* Treatment correlates of successful outcomes in pulmonary multidrug-resistant tuberculosis: an individual patient data meta-analysis of 12,030 patients from 25 countries. *Lancet* 2018; 392: 821–834.

11. WHO. Rapid Communication: Key Changes to Treatment of Multidrug- and Rifampicin-resistant Tuberculosis (MDR/RR-TB). Document WHO/CDS/TB/2018.18. Geneva, WHO, 2018. www.who.int/tb/publications/2018/rapid_communications_MDR/en/

12. Caminero JA, Piubello A, Scardigli A, *et al.* Proposal for a standardised treatment regimen to manage pre- and extensively drug-resistant tuberculosis cases. *Eur Respir J* 2017; 50: 1700648.

13. Caminero JA, Matteelli A, Loddenkemper R. Tuberculosis: are we making it incurable? *Eur Respir J* 2013; 42: 5–8.

14. Caminero JA, Scardigli A. Classification of anti-TB drugs: a new potential proposal based on the most recent evidence. *Eur Respir J* 2015; 46: 887–893.

15. Caminero JA, Matteelli A, Lange C. Treatment of TB. *In:* Lange C, Migliori GB, eds. Tuberculosis (ERS Monograph). Sheffield, European Respiratory Society, 2012; pp. 154–166.

16. Caminero JA, Van Deun A, Fujiwara PI, *et al.* Guidelines for Clinical and Operational Management of Drug-resistant Tuberculosis. Paris, IUATLD, 2013.

17. Caminero JA, Cayla JA, García-García JM, *et al.* Diagnosis and treatment of drug-resistant tuberculosis. *Arch Bronconeumol* 2017; 53: 501–509.

18. Mitchison DA. Basic mechanisms of chemotherapy. *Chest* 1979; 76: 771–781.

19. Caminero JA. A Tuberculosis Guide for Specialist Physicians. Paris, Imprimerie Chirat, 2004.

20. Canetti G, le Lirzin M, Porven G, *et al.* Some comparative effects of rifampicin and isoniazid. *Tubercle* 1968; 49: 367–376.

21. American Thoracic Society/CDC. Treatment of tuberculosis and tuberculosis infection in adults and children. *Am Rev Respir Dis* 1986; 134: 355–363.

22. WHO. Guidelines for Tuberculosis Treatment in Adults and Children in National Tuberculosis Programmes. Document WHO/TUB/91.161. Geneva, WHO, 1991.

23. Caminero JA. Treatment of multidrug-resistant tuberculosis: evidence and controversies. *Int J Tuberc Lung Dis* 2006; 10: 829–37.

24. WHO. Guidelines for Treatment of Drug-susceptible Tuberculosis and Patient Care. 2017 Update. Document WHO/HTM/TB/2017.05. Geneva, WHO, 2017. www.who.int/tb/publications/2017/dstb_guidance_2017/en/

25. Caminero Luna JA. Actualización en el diagnóstico y tratamiento de la tuberculosis pulmonar. *Rev Clin Esp* 2016; 216: 76–84.

26. Mota L, Al-Efraij K, Campbell JR, *et al.* Therapeutic drug monitoring in anti-tuberculosis treatment: a systematic review and meta-analysis. *Int J Tuberc Lung Dis* 2016; 20: 819–826.

27. Zignol M, Cabibbe AM, Dean AS, *et al.* Genetic sequencing for surveillance of drug resistance in tuberculosis in highly endemic countries: a multi-country population-based surveillance study. *Lancet Infect Dis* 2018; 18: 675–683.

28. Bolhuis MS, Tiberi S, Sotgiu G, *et al.* Is there still room for therapeutic drug monitoring of linezolid in patients with tuberculosis? *Eur Respir J* 2016; 47: 1288–1290.

29. van der Burgt EPM, Sturkenboom MGG, Bolhius MS, *et al.* End TB with precision treatment. *Eur Respir J* 2016; 47: 680–682.

30. Caminero JA. Likelihood of generating MDR-TB and XDR-TB under adequate National Tuberculosis Programme implementation. *Int J Tuberc Lung Dis* 2008; 12: 869–877.

31. Nahid P, Dorman SE, Alipanah N, *et al.* Official American Thoracic Society/Centers for Disease Control and Prevention/Infectious Diseases Society of America clinical practice guidelines: treatment of drug-susceptible tuberculosis. *Clin Infect Dis* 2016; 63: 853–867.

32. Mayosi BM, Ntsekhe M, Smieja M. Immunotherapy for tuberculous pericarditis. *N Engl J Med* 2014; 371: 1121–1130.

33. Prasad K, Singh MB, Ryan H. Corticosteroids for managing tuberculous meningitis. *Cochrane Database Syst Rev* 2016; 4: CD002244.

34. WHO. WHO Treatment Guidelines for Isoniazid-resistant Tuberculosis. Supplement to the WHO Treatment Guidelines for Drug-resistant Tuberculosis. Document WHO/CDS/TB/2018.7. Geneva, WHO, 2018. www.who.int/tb/publications/2018/WHO_guidelines_isoniazid_resistant_TB/en/

35. Fregonese F, Ahuja SD, Akkerman OW, *et al.* Comparison of different treatments for isoniazid-resistant tuberculosis: an individual patient data meta-analysis. *Lancet Respir Med* 2018; 6: 265–275.

https://doi.org/10.1183/2312508X.10021417

36. Stagg HR, Harris RJ, Hatherell HA, *et al.* What are the most efficacious treatment regimens for isoniazid-resistant tuberculosis? A systematic review and network meta-analysis. *Thorax* 2016; 71: 940–949.

37. Gegia M, Winters N, Benedetti A, *et al.* Treatment of isoniazid-resistant tuberculosis with first-line drugs: a systematic review and meta-analysis. *Lancet Infect Dis* 2017; 17: 223–234.

38. Cambau E, Viveiros M, Machado D, *et al.* Revisiting susceptibility testing in MDR-TB by a standardized quantitative phenotypic assessment in a European multicentre study. *J Antimicrob Chemother* 2015; 70: 686–696.

39. Rieder HL, Van Deun A. Rationale for high-dose isoniazid in the treatment of multidrug-resistant tuberculosis. *Int J Tuberc Lung Dis* 2017; 21: 123–124.

40. WHO. Guidelines for the Programmatic Management of Drug-resistant Tuberculosis. Document WHO/HTM/TB/ 2006.361. Geneva, WHO, 2006. www.who.int/tb/areas-of-work/drug-resistant-tb/programmatic_guidelines_for_ mdrtb/en/

41. WHO. Guidelines for the Programmatic Management of Drug-resistant Tuberculosis. Emergency Update 2008. Document WHO/HTM/TB/2008.402. Geneva, WHO, 2008. www.who.int/tb/challenges/mdr/programmatic_ guidelines_for_mdrtb/en/

42. WHO. Guidelines for the Programmatic Management of Drug-resistant Tuberculosis. 2011 Update. Document WHO/ HTM/TB/2011.6. Geneva, WHO, 2011. www.who.int/tb/challenges/mdr/programmatic_guidelines_for_mdrtb/en/

43. Bastos ML, Lanz Z, Menzies D. An updated systematic review and meta-analysis for treatment of multidrug-resistant tuberculosis. *Eur Respir J* 2017; 49: 1600803.

44. van Altena R, de Vries G, Haar CH, *et al.* Highly successful treatment outcome of multidrug-resistant tuberculosis in the Netherlands, 2000–2009. *Int J Tuberc Lung Dis* 2015; 19: 406–412.

45. WHO. Position Statement on the Continued Use of the Shorter MDR-TB Regimen Following an Expedited Review of the STREAM Stage 1 Preliminary Results. Document WHO/CDS/TB/2018.2. Geneva, WHO, 2018. www.who. int/tb/publications/2018/Position_statement_shorter_MDR_TB_regimen/en/

46. WHO. Frequently Asked Questions About the Implementation of the New WHO Recommendation on the Use of the Shorter MDR-TB Regimen Under Programmatic Conditions. Geneva, WHO, 2016. www.who.int/tb/ areas-of-work/drug-resistant-tb/treatment/FAQshorter_MDR_regimen.pdf

47. Heldal E, van Deun A, Chiang CY, *et al.* Shorter regimens for multidrug-resistant tuberculosis should also be applicable in Europe. *Eur Respir J* 2017; 49: 1700228.

48. Sotgiu G, Tiberi S, D'Ambrosio L, *et al.* Faster for less: the new "shorter" regimen for multidrug-resistant tuberculosis. *Eur Respir J* 2016; 48: 1503–1507.

49. Sotgiu G, Pontali E, Migliori GB. Linezolid to treat MDR-/XDR-tuberculosis: available evidence and future scenarios. *Eur Respir J* 2015; 45: 25–29.

50. Pontali E, Sotgiu G, Tiberi S, *et al.* Combined treatment of drug-resistant tuberculosis with bedaquiline and delamanid: a systematic review. *Eur Respir J* 2018; 52: 1800934.

51. Tiberi S, Sotgiu G, D'Ambrosio L, *et al.* Comparison of effectiveness and safety of imipenem/clavulanate- *versus* meropenem/clavulanate-containing regimens in the treatment of MDR- and XDR-TB. *Eur Respir J* 2016; 47: 1758– 1766.

52. Sotgiu G, D'Ambrosio L, Centis R, *et al.* Carbapenems to treat multidrug and extensively drug-resistant tuberculosis: a systematic review. *Int J Mol Sci* 2016; 17: 373.

53. Tiberi S, Payen MC, Sotgiu G, *et al.* Effectiveness and safety of meropenem/clavulanate-containing regimens in the treatment of MDR- and XDR-TB. *Eur Respir J* 2016; 47: 1235–1243.

54. Tiberi S, Sotgiu G, D'Ambrosio L, *et al.* Effectiveness and safety of imipenem-clavulanate added to an optimized background regimen (OBR) *versus* OBR control regimens in the treatment of multidrug-resistant and extensively drug-resistant tuberculosis. *Clin Infect Dis* 2016; 62: 1188–1190.

55. Zignol M, Dean AS, Alikhanova N, *et al.* Population-based resistance of *Mycobacterium tuberculosis* isolates to pyrazinamide and fluoroquinolones: results from a multicountry surveillance project. *Lancet Infect Dis* 2016; 16: 1185–1192.

56. WHO. The Use of Molecular Line Probe Assays for the Detection of Resistance to Second-line Anti-tuberculosis Drugs. Policy Guidance. Geneva, WHO, 2016. www.who.int/tb/publications/policy-guidance-molecular-line/en/

57. Georghiou SB, Magana M, Garfein RS, *et al.* Evaluation of genetic mutations associated with *Mycobacterium tuberculosis* resistance to amikacin, kanamycin and capreomycin: a systematic review. *PLoS One* 2012; 7: e33275.

58. Caminero JA, Piubello A, Scardigli A, *et al.* Bedaquiline: how to better use it. *Eur Respir J* 2017; 50: 1701670.

59. Guglielmetti L, Le Dû D, Jachym M, *et al.* Compassionate use of bedaquiline for the treatment of multidrug-resistant and extensively drug-resistant tuberculosis: interim analysis of a French cohort. *Clin Infect Dis* 2015; 60: 188–194.

60. Lewis JM, Hine P, Walker J, *et al.* First experience of effectiveness and safety of bedaquiline for 18 months within an optimised regimen for XDR-TB. *Eur Respir J* 2016; 47: 1581–1584.

61. Scardigli A, Caminero JA. Management of drug-resistant tuberculosis. *Curr Respir Care Rep* 2013; 2: 208–217.

62. Freixinet J, Rivas JJ, Rodriguez de Castro F, *et al.* Role of surgery in pulmonary tuberculosis. *Med Sci Monit* 2002; 8: CR782–CR786.

63. Marrone MT, Venkataramana V, Goodman M, *et al.* Surgical interventions for drug-resistant tuberculosis: a systematic review and meta-analysis. *Int J Tuberc Lung Dis* 2013; 17: 6–16.

64. Chan ED, Iseman MD. Surgery for MDR-TB? *Int J Tuberc Lung Dis* 2013; 17: 710.

65. Olland A, Falcoz P-E, Guinard S, *et al.* Surgery as a treatment. *In:* Migliori GB, Bothamley G, Duarte R, *et al.*, eds. Tuberculosis (ERS Monograph). Sheffield, European Respiratory Society, 2018; pp. 228–233.

66. Xia Q, Zhao LL, Li F, *et al.* Phenotypic and genotypic characterization of pyrazinamide resistance among multidrug-resistant *Mycobacterium tuberculosis* isolates in Zhejiang, China. *Antimicrob Agents Chemother* 2015; 59: 1690–1695.

67. Mphahlele M, Syre H, Valvatne H, *et al.* Pyrazinamide resistance among South African multidrug-resistant *Mycobacterium tuberculosis* isolates. *J Clin Microbiol* 2008; 46: 3459–3464.

68. Kurbatova EV, Cavanaugh JS, Dalton T, *et al.* Epidemiology of pyrazinamide-resistant tuberculosis in the United States, 1999–2009. *Clin Infect Dis* 2013; 57: 1081–1093.

69. Caminero JA, Lasserra P, Piubello A, *et al.* Adverse anti-tuberculosis drug events and their management. *In:* Migliori GB, Bothamley G, Duarte R, *et al.*, eds. Tuberculosis (ERS Monograph). Sheffield, European Respiratory Society, 2018; pp. 205–227.

70. Daley CL, Caminero JA. Management of multidrug-resistant tuberculosis. *Sem Respir Crit Care Med* 2018; 39: 310–324.

71. Blasi F, Dara M, van der Werf MJ, *et al.* Supporting TB clinicians managing difficult cases: the ERS/WHO Consilium. *Eur Respir J* 2013; 41: 491–494.

72. Monedero I, Caminero JA. Management of multidrug-resistant tuberculosis: an update. *Ther Adv Respir Dis* 2010; 4: 117–127.

Disclosures: None declared.

Acknowledgements: The authors alone are responsible for the views expressed in this chapter, and they do not necessarily represent the decisions or policies of their institutions.

https://doi.org/10.1183/2312508X.10021417

Chapter 11

New and repurposed drugs

Maria Krutikov[1], Judith Bruchfeld[2,3], Giovanni Battista Migliori [4],
Sergey Borisov[5] and Simon Tiberi[1,6]

Rates of resistance to antimicrobial agents that are used to treat *Mycobacterium tuberculosis* infection have risen in recent years and account for a growing number of TB deaths worldwide. DR-TB often necessitates long treatment times with toxic drug combinations that are poorly tolerated. Research is focusing on repurposing existing agents for use in TB treatment and on the discovery of new compounds. There are many new agents in the TB drug development pipeline that have shown great promise. Bedaquiline is the first new drug to be licensed for treatment of TB in 40 years. Trials are researching different drug combinations in order to shorten treatment duration and reduce toxicity. This chapter will summarise the evidence around these new and repurposed agents, and their action and adverse effects, and will discuss new potential drug combinations that may soon be recommended.

Cite as: Krutikov M, Bruchfeld J, Migliori GB, *et al*. New and repurposed drugs. *In:* Migliori GB, Bothamley G, Duarte R, *et al*., eds. Tuberculosis (ERS Monograph). Sheffield, European Respiratory Society, 2018; pp. 179–204 [https://doi.org/10.1183/2312508X.10021517].

@ERSpublications

Although the incidence of DR-TB is rising, many new and re-purposed drugs are in the pipeline. These may enable shorter, less toxic and more tolerable treatment regimens. http://ow.ly/cfVQ30lqCfE

*M*ycobacterium tuberculosis is a slow-growing, aerobic micro-organism with a Gram-positive structure characterised by a rich lipid and fatty mycolic acid wall that resists Gram staining and requires other "acid-fast" stains for visualisation. The very abundant fatty acids in the cell wall of mycobacteria and the propensity of these micro-organisms to develop resistance to antimicrobials, as well as their slow replication, challenge drug development and necessitate clinical trials of long duration to determine the efficacy of treatment.

Treatment of mycobacteria requires a combination of antimicrobials to ensure efficacy and reduce the likelihood of acquiring resistance and of treatment failure. Drug-susceptible tuberculosis (DS-TB) is treated with a classic oral standard quadruple regimen of isoniazid,

[1]Division of Infection, Royal London Hospital, Barts Health NHS Trust, London, UK. [2]Infectious Diseases Unit, Dept of Medicine, Solna (MedS), K2, Group A Färnert, B3:03, Karolinska Universitetssjukhuset, Solna, Stockholm, Sweden. [3]Dept of Infectious Diseases, Karolinska University Hospital, Solna, Sweden. [4]Istituti Clinici Scientifici Maugeri IRCCS, Tradate, Italy. [5]Moscow Research and Clinical Center for TB Control, Moscow Government's Health Dept, Moscow, Russian Federation. [6]Blizard Institute, Barts and The London School of Medicine and Dentistry, Queen Mary University of London, London, UK.

Correspondence: Simon Tiberi, Division of Infection, Royal London Hospital, Barts Health NHS Trust, 80 Newark Street, London E1 2ES, UK. E-mail: simon.tiberi@bartshealth.nhs.uk

Copyright ©ERS 2018. Print ISBN: 978-1-84984-099-6. Online ISBN: 978-1-84984-100-9. Print ISSN: 2312-508X. Online ISSN: 2312-5098.

rifampicin, pyrazinamide and ethambutol, which, if taken appropriately, guarantees a high success rate of >90%. It is also cheap; a 6-month course costs <US$20.

The emergence of drug resistance through the HIV epidemic and systemic failures in the programmatic delivery of the standard quadruple regimen has led to a significant rise in DR-TB. MDR-TB, defined as TB that is resistant to isoniazid and rifampicin, requires a minimum of four active drugs for 18–20 months or a combination of several drugs for a shorter course of 9–12 months.

A significant majority of resistant cases of TB can be managed and treated successfully with individualised therapy, which may or may not include surgery and rehabilitation. The high cost and complexity required for the delivery of individualised therapy limit the dissemination of this form of treatment where it is most needed, mainly in resource-limited and high-incidence settings. Without treatment, two-thirds of affected patients will die, and the remaining one-third are likely to suffer from chronic sequelae.

New oral TB drugs that are more active and less toxic are desperately needed to build new regimens that can be disseminated rapidly and successfully to the many people affected by MDR-TB in low-resource settings [1–5].

In this chapter, we will list and describe the novel antimycobacterial drugs that have joined the armamentarium and those currently in the development pipeline. Figure 1 depicts the new drug classes under development and their relevant sites and mechanisms of action.

Nitroimidazoles

Nitroimidazoles are novel anti-TB agents that have become more widely available for use in the treatment of MDR-TB or XDR-TB (resistance to at least four of the core anti-TB drugs, including isoniazid and rifampicin) over the last few years. Their primary action is through inhibition of cell wall synthesis and respiration.

Pretomanid (PA-824)

Action
Pretomanid is a pro-drug that is activated by deazaflavin-dependent nitroreductase (Ddn) and forms des-nitroimidazole, which in turn inhibits cell wall lipid biosynthesis. Des-nitroimidazole contributes to mycobacterial killing through its role in the production of reactive nitrogen species such as nitric oxide in the host macrophage. It is also considered to affect cell respiration by an undefined mechanism. It is active against both replicating and nonreplicating mycobacteria [7].

Resistance
Mutations in the *ddn* gene and in the *fgd1* gene encoding F420-dependent glucose-6-phosphate dehydrogenase have been found in pretomanid-resistant species. These enzymes are both involved in biosynthesis of the F420 coenzyme.

Mycobacterium canettii has also been found to be intrinsically resistant to pretomanid.

https://doi.org/10.1183/2312508X.10021517

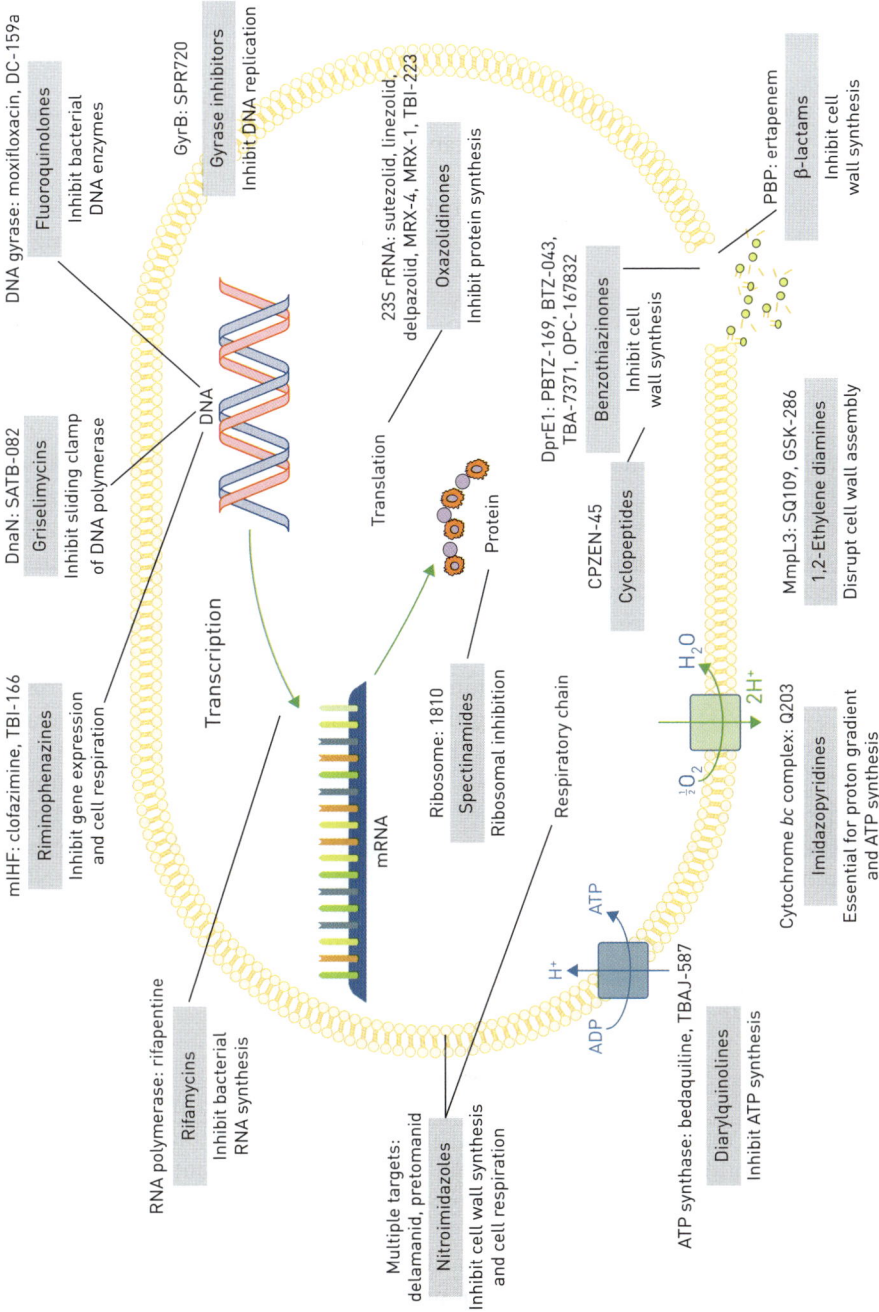

Figure 1. Sites and mechanisms of action of new and repurposed antimicrobials for *Mycobacterium tuberculosis*. For each drug group, the target and individual drugs are indicated. mIHF: mycobacterial integration host factor; GyrB: DNA gyrase subunit B; rRNA: ribosomal RNA; DprE1: decaprenylphosphoryl-β-D-ribose oxidase; MmpL3: mycolic acid transporter; PBP: penicillin-binding protein. Reproduced and modified from [6] with permission.

Evidence

The NC-002 (New Combination 2) trial, completed in 2013, was a phase IIb study investigating the efficacy of 8 weeks of pretomanid, pyrazinamide and moxifloxacin for drug-susceptible and drug-resistant PTB. The study demonstrated superior bactericidal activity within the first 56 days of treatment in DS-TB when compared with standard therapy, and did not show an increased rate of adverse events [8].

Adverse effects

At present, no significant adverse effects have been reported with the use of pretomanid.

Clinical use

This drug is currently not licensed for use anywhere in the world but is available on a compassionate basis. Based on clinical trials, the recommended dosage is 200 mg once daily.

Future trials

There are a number of ongoing trials to assess the use of pretomanid in the treatment of DR- and DS-TB (NC-005, STAND NC-006, NiX-TB, TB PRACTECAL, ZeNiX NC-007, SimpliciTB NC-008). The NC-005 trial (ClinicalTrials.gov identifier NCT02193776) conducted by the TB Alliance has just completed. Patients with DS-TB were randomised to either the standard treatment arm or a regimen of bedaquiline, pretomanid and pyrazinamide (BPaZ) for 8 weeks. Those with DR-TB were given the BPaZ regime with the addition of moxifloxacin (BPaMZ). Preliminary results showed the BPaMZ regimen to be the most effective, with sputum culture conversion in 78–96% of patients and culture conversion times that were three times faster than the other regimens; standard therapy was the least effective [8]. This suggests that it may be possible to reduce total treatment durations in DS-TB. A further trial is planned (SimpliciTB NC-008; ClinicalTrials.gov identifier NCT03338621) to investigate using this combination to shorten total therapy to 4 months in DS-TB and 6 months in MDR-TB. The promising NiX-TB phase III study (ClinicalTrials.gov identifier NCT02333799) is investigating the use of pretomanid, linezolid and bedaquiline in the treatment of XDR- or MDR-TB and has demonstrated auspicious results with high treatment success rates in MDR- and XDR-TB patients with this 6–9-month regimen. The NiX-TB study has now continued into the ZeNiX NC-007 trial (ClinicalTrials.gov identifier NCT03086486), where different doses of linezolid will be evaluated to determine the most tolerated and efficacious dosing schedule for this drug [9].

Delamanid (OPC-67683)

Action

Delamanid inhibits the synthesis of methoxy-mycolic acid and keto-mycolic acids, both components of the mycobacterial cell wall. Similarly to pretomanid, its pro-drug is activated by Ddn forming a metabolite from delamanid and desnitro-imidazooxazole, which is involved in inhibition of the production of mycolic acid.

Given both the bactericidal and sterilising properties of delamanid, it is considered a core drug in the treatment of *M. tuberculosis* infections [10, 11].

Resistance

Mutations in any of the five coenzyme F420 genes (*fgd1*, *ddn*, *fbiA*, *fbiB* and *fbiC*) have been associated with resistance to delamanid. The highest likelihood of resistance to

https://doi.org/10.1183/2312508X.10021517

delamanid has been found with the mutation *fbiA* D49Y. Mutations in *ddn* or *fgd1* have been found to encode resistance to both delamanid and pretomanid [6].

Evidence

In a phase IIb RCT in 2012, delamanid or placebo was added to standard therapy in patients with pulmonary MDR-TB for 2 months [11]. At 2 months, 45.4% of the treatment arm had culture converted, compared with 29.6% in the placebo group (p=0.008); however, QT interval prolongation was significantly associated with delamanid treatment. This cohort was subsequently followed up for 24 months in an observational study that showed lower mortality and higher rates of treatment success in those patients who were treated with delamanid for at least 6 months [12, 13].

Adverse effects

The main concern with clinical usage has been the QT interval prolongation associated with delamanid. This has not been reported in the compassionate-use setting. In addition, delamanid has been found to cause nausea, vomiting or dizziness in up to 33% of patients.

Clinical use

The European Medicines Agency has officially approved the usage of delamanid for the treatment of MDR-TB as part of an appropriate combination of anti-TB drugs. This is only in cases where the currently approved regimen cannot be used as a result of drug resistance or intolerability. Following a paediatric safety and efficacy trial, this has also been extended to use in children.

The currently recommended dose is 100 mg twice daily taken with food, for 6 months.

Future trials

As a result of the promising preliminary results, the phase III Otsuka 213 trial was performed (ClinicalTrials.gov identifier NCT01424670). The preliminary findings of this were presented at the 48th Union World Conference on Lung Health in Mexico in October 2017 [14]. This was a multicentre noninferiority open-label study that compared a shorter delamanid-containing 9–11-month regimen with standard prolonged treatment for MDR-TB. The study failed to demonstrate noninferiority, as the control arm showed much higher success rates than anticipated. There were no significant differences in cure rates (77.6% for control *versus* 77.1% for treatment), mortality (4.7% for control *versus* 5.3% for treatment) or culture conversion at 6 months (86.1% for control *versus* 87.6% for treatment). This may be due to closer monitoring for adverse drug effects in all subjects as a result of the study, therefore improving outcomes for the control arm. Further subgroup analyses are ongoing at present. In response to this, the WHO issued a statement in January 2018 reiterating the consideration of delamanid only in circumstances where there are no other treatment options.

Diarylquinolines

Bedaquiline (TMC207 and R207910)

Action

Bedaquiline inhibits mycobacterial ATP synthase, an enzyme required for ATP synthesis in *M. tuberculosis* but not in mammalian cells. This leads to disruption of the intracellular metabolism and bacterial death but does not affect host cells. Bedaquiline has been found to be effective against mycobacteria both during active replication and in the dormant phase [15].

Resistance

Mutations in the *atpE* gene have been associated with bedaquiline resistance in *M. tuberculosis*. This gene encodes the membrane-bound subunit c of F_0ATP synthase. However, resistance has been seen in mycobacteria that do not express mutation in this gene or any of the other genes known to encode ATP synthase components, suggesting that other mechanisms of resistance also exist. Of note, mutations in the transcriptional regulator Rv0678 have been associated with cross resistance between clofazimine and bedaquiline [6, 16].

Evidence

A large double-blinded RCT in 2009 was designed in two phases and showed that, in the first phase, of the 47 patients with pulmonary MDR-TB enrolled, 48% in the bedaquiline arm had culture converted after 8 weeks compared with 9% in the placebo arm [17]. In the second phase, the median time to culture conversion in those receiving bedaquiline in addition to standard treatment was 83 days, compared with 125 days in the placebo arm, which was statistically significant ($p<0.001$) [18].

Adverse effects

The largest RCT of bedaquiline use in treating TB infections found an unexplained higher number of deaths in the bedaquiline arm of the study (11.4% bedaquiline *versus* 2.5% placebo), although these all occurred after 6 months of treatment and may have been unrelated [19]. This trial also found an increased risk of QT prolongation, a finding that has not been replicated in subsequent trials [19]. The increased risk of QT prolongation has been the main trigger for the US Food and Drug Administration's (FDA) black box warning regarding the use of bedaquiline. The FDA and WHO have advised that bedaquiline should only be used in patients who have no other treatment options [19].

Clinical use

Despite the aforementioned therapeutic concerns, bedaquiline remains a valuable treatment in patients with TB infections with high levels of drug resistance. It is the first drug to be approved by the FDA for the treatment of TB in >40 years. It has been found to be highly active against MDR- and XDR-TB strains. Provisional recommendations issued by the WHO and CDC in 2013 outlined the use of this drug in MDR- and XDR-TB treatment regimens, including for children and pregnant women [20, 21]. Bedaquiline should only be used in an effective regimen consisting of pyrazinamide and four second-line medications. However, such a regimen cannot be used if there is documented resistance to fluoroquinolones in the presence of multidrug resistance. These guidelines also suggest that bedaquiline should not be prescribed for >6 months unless there are extenuating circumstances.

The recommended dose is 400 mg once daily for the first 2 weeks and is then reduced to 200 mg three times weekly for the remaining 22 weeks [22].

Future trials

A phase III trial, STREAM 2 (Short-course treatment for multidrug-resistant tuberculosis), is currently in progress (ClinicalTrials.gov identifier NCT02409290). This will compare a

https://doi.org/10.1183/2312508X.10021517

6- and 9-month bedaquiline-containing regimen against the WHO and the shorter Bangladesh regimen, and is expected complete in 2021.

TBAJ-587

Similarly to bedaquiline, this drug also inhibits *M. tuberculosis* ATP synthase. However, animal models have shown that TBAJ-587 has better efficacy and more potent activity than bedaquiline.

The drug is currently undergoing pre-clinical trials led by the University of Auckland and the TB Alliance [23].

Rifamycins

These are bactericidal macrocyclic antibiotics that bind to DNA-dependent RNA polymerase, inhibiting bacterial RNA synthesis. Examples include rifampicin, rifapentine and rifabutin.

Rifapentine

Action
Rifapentine is a semi-synthetic cyclopentyl rifampicin derivative that was first synthesised in 1965. The cyclopentyl ring side chain allows increased protein binding and subsequently a longer drug half-life of approximately 13–14 h, which means that it can be administered weekly in the treatment of TB infection. Due to its potent intracellular activity, rifapentine accumulates in human granulomas at concentrations that are four to five times higher than rifampicin; however, it exhibits poor cavity penetration. Unlike rifampicin, rifapentine binds to DNA-dependent RNA polymerase but does not bind to polymerase in mammalian cells.

Resistance
Due to the infrequency of administration, concerns have been raised about the high potential for development of resistance if given at an insufficient dose.

Cross resistance between rifampicin and rifapentine has been found in all resistant isolates. A single nucleotide mutation in the β-subunit of the RNA polymerase gene *rpoB* is the primary gene that has been found to confer resistance to rifapentine.

Evidence
An RCT with three treatment arms, conducted in HIV-positive patients in four southern African countries, was published in 2014 [24]. This study looked at replacing rifampicin with rifapentine for a shorter duration, either weekly at a higher dose or twice weekly at a lower dose in addition to moxifloxacin. Giving higher doses of rifapentine less frequently was shown to be noninferior to the control group (standard treatment), suggesting that the drug, if administered at a high enough dose, has a long enough half-life to protect against resistance. A phase III study looking at LTBI treatment in more than 7000 patients was completed in 2011 and showed noninferiority between weekly rifapentine and isoniazid for 3 months compared with daily isoniazid for 9 months [25].

Adverse effects

Rifapentine is a potent enzyme inducer; however, the lower frequency of administration results in lower rates of inhibition of concomitant drugs, such as fluoroquinolones and protease inhibitors, than with the more conventionally used rifampicin.

Clinical use

Rifapentine was approved by the FDA in 1998 for the treatment of PTB. It is recommended by the WHO for treatment of PTB in those with noncavitatory, culture-positive, drug-susceptible disease who are HIV negative. Unlike rifampicin, high-fat meals increase the bioavailability of rifapentine; therefore, the advice is to take with a meal. The oral dosage recommendation in adults is 600 mg twice weekly for the intensive phase (2 months), followed by 600 mg once weekly in the continuation phase (4 months) [26].

Future trials

Given the long half-life of rifapentine, it may be an excellent alternative therapy for treatment of LTBI as it can be administered just once weekly. This is the focus of most current trials of rifapentine, particularly in the HIV-infected population, for whom drug interactions are especially pertinent. The Tuberculosis Trials Consortium (TBTC) Study 31 (ClinicalTrials.gov identifier NCT02410772) is a phase III open-label RCT that will recruit 2500 patients with active drug-susceptible PTB and replace rifampicin for daily rifapentine and ethambutol for moxifloxacin over a total duration of 4 months; it is expected to complete in 2019 [9]. The poor cavity penetration of rifapentine may prove to be a limitation in the treatment of active disease [27].

Oxazolidinones

Oxazolidinones are a class of antibiotics that inhibit protein synthesis. First-generation drugs such as linezolid were originally approved for the treatment of drug-resistant Gram-positive infections, but long-term use has been associated with severe neurological and haematological toxicity; therefore, use in TB treatment is with caution. However, newer generations of these drugs have lower toxicity profiles and have been the focus of research into DR-TB treatment [28, 29].

Linezolid

Action

Linezolid is a first-generation oxazolidinone that binds to 23S ribosomal RNA (rRNA) adjacent to the ribosomal 50S subunit, inhibiting protein synthesis. Linezolid has excellent oral bioavailability.

Former uses

Linezolid was initially licensed in 2000 for the treatment of resistant Gram-positive infections such as methicillin-resistant *Staphylococcus aureus* and vancomycin-resistant enterococci.

Resistance

The mutations G2061T and G2576T in the 23S rRNA of *M. tuberculosis* have been shown to correlate with high-level resistance to linezolid. However, no mutations are seen in the 23S rRNA of mutants that exhibit low-level linezolid resistance. These low-level resistance

https://doi.org/10.1183/2312508X.10021517

mutants have been found to have mutations in the *rplC*-encoded ribosomal protein L3 (T460C mutation).

A study in China found that 11% of circulating MDR-TB strains were linezolid resistant but that only 30% of these mutants had 23S rRNA or *rplC* gene mutations [29]. This suggests that there is an alternative mechanism of resistance that is yet to be established [6].

Evidence

A prospective RCT published in 2012 enrolled patients with XDR-TB who had already failed conventional treatment. The addition of linezolid to their treatment regimen resulted in culture conversion in 87% of patients within 6 months [30].

A meta-analysis by Sotgiu *et al.* [31] in 2012 showed that the rate of adverse effects with linezolid was substantially higher when >600 mg of linezolid was administered once daily (adverse events in 63 out of 107 patients). Additionally, treatment with 600 mg four times daily did not lead to statistically significant differences in bacteriological conversion rates when compared with twice daily dosing, suggesting that lower doses of linezolid may be adequate. A study by Alffenaar *et al.* [32] suggested that splitting the 600 mg daily dose to 300 mg twice daily may prevent the peaks in serum concentration of linezolid that may account for the haematological and neurological toxicity. They also showed that, in these patients, the serum concentration was sufficiently high to be effective in 87.5% of patients.

Adverse effects

Long-term use is associated with severe adverse effects that can be classified into haematological and neurological. Haematological effects include severe reversible anaemia and bone marrow suppression. Neurological effects are peripheral neuropathy, taste disturbance and optic neuritis. Mild gastrointestinal symptoms, deranged LFTs and discoloration of the tongue can also occur. Rare adverse effects include severe bullous drug reactions such as Stevens–Johnson syndrome.

Clinical use

Linezolid is a group C drug from the recent WHO MDR-TB guidelines, but its use in these circumstances is still off-label. Coadministration with monoamine oxidase inhibitors is contraindicated, and caution should be exercised with selective serotonin reuptake inhibitors, tricyclic antidepressants and opioid analgesics due to increased risk of serotonin syndrome. Although clarithromycin boosts serum linezolid concentration, there is recent evidence suggesting that this may allow the use of lower linezolid doses and limit the known associated adverse effects. Dosage in the treatment of DR-TB is 600 mg once daily orally or intravenously, and a full blood count should be carried out and LFTs monitored.

Future trials

The ZeNiX NC-007 phase III trial (ClinicalTrials.gov identifier NCT03086486) is currently enrolling patients with XDR- and MDR-TB to assess the efficacy of different doses and durations of linezolid in combination with bedaquiline and pretomanid. In a double-blinded design, four groups of patients will be randomised to different linezolid doses and durations of treatment. It is postulated that linezolid could be cycled to reduce toxicity. Further trials are investigating the addition of linezolid to other agents in MDR- and XDR-TB in an attempt to reduce treatment duration and avoid injectable agents (ClinicalTrials.gov identifiers NCT02454205, NCT02754765 and NCT02454205).

Sutezolid (PNU-100480)

Action

Sutezolid is an analogue drug of linezolid that has been in development since 1996 and has a better *in vitro* antimycobacterial action and safety profile.

Resistance

Mutations in the *rrl* gene and RplC ribosomal protein L3 of 23S rRNA are associated with resistance to sutezolid. Cross resistance with other oxazolidinones has been reported [33].

Evidence

Trials in mouse models have shown a more rapid reduction in pulmonary bacterial burden, resulting in shorter treatment duration. A phase IIa trial in 2013 showed that at a dose of 600 mg twice daily patients experienced no neurological or haematological complications after 28 days of treatment [34]. Studies have also suggested that bactericidal activity may be improved when sutezolid is combined with bedaquiline in the treatment of *M. tuberculosis* infection [35–38].

Adverse effects

Sutezolid is considered to have a reduced propensity for toxicity [34]; however, more studies are required to verify this.

Clinical use

Sutezolid has received orphan drug designation in the USA and EU. The recommended dose is 600 mg twice daily.

Future trials

Sequella has recently acquired the drug development licence for sutezolid [38], and a phase IIb study is awaited. Due to changes in licensing, some earlier studies may need to be repeated.

TBI-223

TBI-223 is an oxazolidinone that is currently under development and has promising potential. The reasons for this include its stability in hepatocytes and microsomes, the low incidence of neurological and haematological toxicity associated with its use in mice and because it does not inhibit cytochrome P450 enzymes in humans. This means that it does not interact with other drugs that share this enzymatic pathway and is therefore a safer treatment option.

TBI-223 is currently in pre-clinical development but has the potential to be a safer alternative to linezolid in treatment-shortening regimens for *M. tuberculosis* infection [39, 40].

Delpazolid (LCB01-0371)

This is a novel oxazolidinone that has been shown to be more active than linezolid in *in vitro* studies, particularly in the treatment of *Mycobacterium abscessus* infections [30]. A recent publication from ZONG *et al.* [41] concluded that *in vitro* activity against

https://doi.org/10.1183/2312508X.10021517

M. tuberculosis is similar between linezolid and delpazolid. A single-dose study is currently in progress (ClinicalTrials.gov identifier NCT01554995) [42].

MRX-4

MRX-4 is available in injectable and oral forms and is the pro-drug of MRX-1, an oral drug currently in phase III trials in China. The discovery of MRX-1 was initially reported in 2014 as a novel oxazolidinone with an improved safety profile and a lower rate of drug interactions. MRX-4 has the potential to expand the use of this drug through *i.v.* administration and is in phase I dose escalation clinical trials in the USA (ClinicalTrials.gov identifier NCT03033329) [43–45].

Imidazopyridines

Q203

The imidazopyridine Q203 targets the cytochrome *b* subunit that works within the mycobacterial respiratory electron transport chain, which is required for the synthesis of ATP. This means that intracellular ATP is destroyed within active mycobacteria cells and synthesis is interrupted in dormant cells [46].

This drug is currently undergoing phase I clinical trials (ClinicalTrials.gov identifier NCT03563599).

Fluoroquinolones

Fluoroquinolones are antibiotics that inhibit the bacterial enzymes DNA gyrase and topoisomerase IV, which are required for cell replication, transcription, recombination and chromosomal supercoiling.

Moxifloxacin

Former uses
Moxifloxacin has been licensed as a broad-spectrum antibiotic for the treatment of Gram-negative and Gram-positive infections and has good penetration of the blood–brain barrier.

Resistance
Mutations associated with resistance have been found in the *gyrA* and *gyrB* genes, both of which disrupt the drug-binding site in the DNA gyrase enzyme. A combination of both *gyrA* and *gyrB* mutations has been shown to have higher rates of drug resistance than either mutation alone.

Evidence
Studies dating back to 2004 have shown that moxifloxacin is a suitable replacement for isoniazid in the treatment of *M. tuberculosis* infections in mouse models as it has good bactericidal activity [47].

https://doi.org/10.1183/2312508X.10021517

A meta-analysis in 2017 included nine studies that used moxifloxacin in addition to standard TB therapy [48]. Concerning sputum culture conversion rates, the study found a significant improvement with the addition of moxifloxacin in the first 2 months of treatment (OR 1.895; p=0.000). They also found that moxifloxacin can reduce the rate of relapse in the first year after treatment (OR 0.516; p=0.022). The rate of adverse events was not increased with the addition of moxifloxacin (OR 1.001, p=0.989) [49, 50].

Adverse effects

The use of moxifloxacin has been associated with increased risk of a prolonged QT interval and sudden death. Prolonged use has been associated with tendonitis and increased risk of tendon rupture. It has also been found to cause profound nausea and vomiting. As with all fluoroquinolones, the risk of *Clostridium difficile* infection is increased, especially with prolonged use.

Clinical use

Treatment is recommended with doses of 400–800 mg once daily. TDM with serum concentrations and ECGs is advised.

Future trials

Moxifloxacin is currently being used as part of a regimen in several trials that are investigating shortening the duration and toxicity profile of MDR- and XDR-TB treatment (ClinicalTrials.gov identifiers NCT03338621, NCT02409290 and NCT02589782). A multicentre observational study is being conducted to assess the feasibility of centralised TDM to improve access to safe administration of these drugs in low-resource settings (ClinicalTrials.gov identifier NCT03409315).

DC-159a

Due to historical use of fluoroquinolones in the treatment of TB, resistance is often class-wide. DC-159a is a novel fluoroquinolone that has been shown to have activity against quinolone-resistant strains of *M. tuberculosis in vitro*. Mouse models have shown it to be superior to moxifloxacin with regard to treatment duration. This may be because the drug has a very rapid uptake and can reach high concentrations within the lungs [51–53].

Benzothiazinones

Benzothiazinones are inhibitors of the DprE1 (decaprenylphosphoryl-β-D-ribose oxidase) enzyme, which is involved in the synthesis of the mycobacterial cell wall, and has been identified as one of the most attractive targets for TB drug development.

The benzothiazinones BTZ-043 and PBTZ-169 inhibit cell wall arabinan synthesis, provoking cell lysis and death. These drugs are in the most advanced stages of development out of the DprE1 inhibitors [54, 55].

BTZ-043

BTZ-043 has been found to be active against MDR- and XDR-TB species, and even has potential synergistic effects when used with bedaquiline and rifampicin. It has a low

https://doi.org/10.1183/2312508X.10021517

side-effect profile and few interactions with cytochrome P450 enzymes, allowing ease of coadministration with other drugs. It is currently planned for phase I trials [55, 56].

Macozinone (PBTZ-169)

This is a piperazino-benzothiazinone derivative that acts in a similar way to BTZ-043 but is easier to synthesise chemically. Similarly, it has been shown to have synergistic effects when used with bedaquiline and clofazimine. A phase IIa early bactericidal activity study has recently been completed in Russia and Belarus in DS-TB showing good drug safety and efficacy (ClinicalTrials.gov identifier NCT03334734). The Bill and Melinda Gates Foundation has funded a phase I clinical trial to start in Switzerland in healthy volunteers [57].

Other DprE1 inhibitors

The DprE1 inhibitor TBA-7371 is currently undergoing phase I clinical trials (ClinicalTrials.gov identifier NCT03199339) [58].

OPC-167832 is a novel DprE1 inhibitor has been developed to be used in combination with delamanid to shorten treatment duration. This is currently undergoing human trials after being granted FastTrack status [59].

β-lactams

For many years, carbapenems have been used to treat MDR- and XDR-TB, despite a distinct lack of published evidence for their efficacy. More recently, *in vitro* work on *M. tuberculosis*, including MDR- and XDR-TB strains, has suggested that the addition of clavulanate and amoxicillin to meropenem can reduce the MIC of meropenem required to kill each of these mycobacterial strains. This is likely to be because *M. tuberculosis* has an inherent β-lactamase encoded by the *blaC* gene. This can be overcome by clavulanate when studied *in vitro*. This has led to the use of amoxicillin/clavulanate in clinical studies in addition to carbapenems in the treatment of resistant *M. tuberculosis* infections [60–64].

Meropenem/clavulanate

Action
This regimen requires two separate drugs, meropenem and clavulanate (only available in combination with amoxicillin). Meropenem is a broad-spectrum β-lactam that acts against Gram-negative, Gram-positive and anaerobic bacteria. β-lactams are a class of drugs that act on cell wall synthesis. They contain a β-lactam ring that is sterically similar to a protein used in cell wall synthesis, and are therefore mistakenly bound by penicillin-binding proteins, rendering these proteins unable to catalyse further reactions and stopping cell wall synthesis. This eventually leads to cell lysis and death. Bacterial production of β-lactamases leads to resistance of the bacteria to the action of penicillins and other β-lactams.

Clavulanate, the first β-lactamase inhibitor discovered, was initially isolated from a *Streptomyces* sp. in the 1970s. When used in conjunction with a β-lactam, it significantly lowered the concentration of drug required to inhibit bacterial growth.

Evidence

Large observational trials have examined the use of meropenem with the addition of amoxicillin/clavulanate for the treatment of TB infections. A study conducted by the International Carbapenems Study Group (ICSG) included 17 centres in six countries in Europe and Latin America [59]. It was found to be noninferior regarding sputum smear and culture conversion rates and treatment success. A further similar retrospective observational study in five centres found no significant difference in sputum smear and culture conversion times between those exposed to meropenem with amoxicillin/clavulanate and those not exposed [60]. However, the study did find that those given meropenem and amoxicillin/clavulanate were more likely to have a more severe resistance profile (including XDR), as the drugs were more likely to be added in when other treatment options were unavailable. A significant drawback of these studies is that neither was powered to give statistically significant outcomes and both were retrospective; therefore, no randomisation was possible. One significant drawback of the use of meropenem is that it is only available in *i.v.* form and requires a three-times-daily dosing, which would have a severe impact on quality of life. In addition, in many countries, meropenem is costly and there is some difficulty with its acquisition; therefore, further work is needed to evaluate the use of this drug economically.

Adverse effects

Penicillin drug allergy has a prevalence of 10% in the USA and UK, although, due to over-reporting, only 10% of these patients are likely to have a true allergy. Severe anaphylactic reactions are seen in 1 in 10 000 penicillin administrations. Other less severe effects include gastrointestinal upset, transaminitis and, rarely, leukopenia and neutropenia. In a study of patients using meropenem/clavulanate as part of their TB treatment regimen, only six out of 94 patients reported adverse events related to the drug, and four of these patients were able to restart treatment after an interruption.

Clinical use

Meropenem is not currently licensed in the treatment of TB. When used, it should only be counted as half of a drug in a regime. Dosage is 1 g *i.v.* given three times daily with oral amoxicillin/clavulanate 500 mg/125 mg three times daily.

Further trials

Two phase II trials are underway, and one has been completed, investigating the bactericidal activity, safety and tolerability of meropenem and amoxicillin/clavulanate when administered early on in treatment (ClinicalTrials.gov identifiers NCT02381470, NCT02349841 and NCT03174184). These trials will also be looking into the use of faropenem (oral penem) with amoxicillin/clavulanate in the same conditions.

Ertapenem/clavulanate

Ertapenem/clavulanate has a similar mechanism of action and treatment profile to other β-lactams and β-lactamase inhibitor combination drugs. In contrast to meropenem/clavulanate, ertapenem is administered *i.v.* just once daily [65].

In 2017, a hollow-fibre model that used Monte Carlo simulations to emulate the lung found that the optimum ertapenem dose for the treatment of *M. tuberculosis* infection was 2 g once daily, which was able to sterilise 96% of infections [66]. This once-daily dosing has a significant advantage over meropenem regarding ease of administration.

https://doi.org/10.1183/2312508X.10021517

Imipenem/clavulanate

Trials comparing imipenem/clavulanate with meropenem/clavulanate found that time to smear and culture conversion was shorter in the meropenem group, and the success rate was also higher in this group (77.5% *versus* 59.7%) and was statistically significant (p=0.03) [59].

Ceftazidime/avibactam

Action
This is a third-generation cephalosporin (ceftazidime) combined with a non-β-lactam β-lactamase inhibitor (avibactam). Ceftazidime is bactericidal against Gram-positive and Gram-negative bacteria through binding to penicillin-binding proteins. Avibactam protects ceftazidime from degradation, therefore prolonging its half-life [67].

Former uses
This drug was licensed for use in complicated urinary tract infections and intra-abdominal infections by the FDA in 2015.

Evidence
Since its discovery, ceftazidime/avibactam has also been found to have high bactericidal activity against most strains causing XDR-, MDR- and DS-TB in human macrophage cells. Hollow-fibre models that can replicate the human lung have shown that it has greater activity against *M. tuberculosis* than the first-line drugs isoniazid and pyrazinamide [68].

Resistance
Mutations in the *ponA1* gene encoding the penicillin-binding protein 1A, which is involved in cell wall remodelling, have been associated with resistance to ceftazidime/avibactam *in vitro*.

Further trials
There are currently no trials investigating the use of ceftazidime/avibactam in *M. tuberculosis*.

Riminophenazines

Clofazimine

Clofazimine is a fat-soluble riminophenazine dye that has been used in the treatment of leprosy. It was initially synthesised as a drug to treat TB in 1954. However, studies that showed poor activity in monkeys prevented this drug from being widely implemented.

Action
The exact mechanism of antimycobacterial action is not fully understood; however, it has been shown to compete for electrons with menaquinone, the substrate for type 2 NADH:quinone oxidoreductase involved in the mycobacterial respiratory chain, thereby interrupting cell respiration, and has potent activity against drug-resistant strains of *M. tuberculosis* both intra- and extracellularly. This has led to the recent addition of clofazimine to group C of the WHO recommendations on treatment of DR-TB [69].

Former uses

Clofazimine has been used since the 1970s in the treatment of leprosy; however, serious skin pigmentation and prolongation of the QT interval have been the main drawbacks in its use.

Resistance

In a recent *in vitro* study, isolates with no prior exposure to clofazimine were tested [70]. Out of 90 isolates from China, five were found to have clofazimine resistance; four had the *Rv0678* mutation, which also demonstrated cross resistance with bedaquiline, and one had the *Rv1979c* mutation associated with isoniazid resistance.

Evidence

Clofazimine was reintroduced into the drug regimen for the treatment of MDR-TB in an observational study in Bangladesh in 2004 [71]. Clofazimine-containing drug regimens showed a cure rate of 69%. In an RCT in China in 2015, 105 patients with pulmonary MDR-TB were prospectively enrolled and allocated to either the clofazimine or the control arm [72]. Sputum culture conversion was earlier in the clofazimine arm, and 73.6% of patients had treatment success in this arm (53.8% in the control arm; p=0.035). A retrospective observational study conducted in Brazil compared patients treated for MDR-TB with a clofazimine-containing regimen against those treated with a pyrazinamide-containing regimen [73]. They found similar success rates (880 out of 1446, 60.9%, *versus* 708 out of 1096, 64.6%; p=0.054) but more TB-related deaths in the clofazimine group (314 out of 1446, 21.7%, *versus* 120 out of 1096, 10.9%).

Adverse effects

The most commonly experienced adverse reaction is skin hyperpigmentation due to the extremely long half-life of this drug, resulting in accumulation in tissues and skin. In a study where 861 patients with XDR- or MDR-TB received clofazimine, only 0.1% had to discontinue treatment due to adverse reactions, while 5.1% experienced adverse reactions [74]. This was most frequently skin discoloration and rash. Both of these are reversible after treatment is discontinued. Other adverse effects are gastrointestinal upset and photosensitivity, and these should be monitored. A prolonged QT interval and ventricular tachyarrhythmia have been described in a few case reports; thus, patients should be monitored with regular ECGs. The Brazil study described previously reviewed 1446 patients treated with clofazimine-containing TB regimens and found no difference in rates of adverse events reported when compared with pyrazinamide-containing regimens (1096 patients) [73]. These adverse events consisted mainly of hyperpigmentation, gastrointestinal upset and neurological disturbance.

Clinical use

Clofazimine remains unlicensed for the treatment of TB by any regulatory body; however, it is frequently used off-label. The recommended daily dosage is 100 mg daily, and it is only available in oral formulations [75, 76].

Future trials

Several large multicentre trials are currently recruiting patients for evaluation of the use of clofazimine as part of a drug regimen in the treatment of DR-TB, focusing particularly on shortening treatment duration and improving treatment success rates (ClinicalTrials.gov identifiers NCT02589782, NCT02409290, NCT02754765, NCT03057756, NCT03604848, NCT03474198, NCT03237182 and NCT03625739).

https://doi.org/10.1183/2312508X.10021517

TBI-166

TBI-166 is a riminophenazine compound that has been developed with the aim of reducing the side-effect profile seen in clofazimine use, while maintaining its excellent sterilising and bactericidal action. This has undergone clinical development and is in phase I clinical trials in China [77].

Gyrase inhibitors

SPR720

GyrB is a subunit of DNA gyrase and is needed for bacterial replication. SPR720 inhibits GyrB and has been shown to be effective in a murine *M. tuberculosis* infection model with low drug–drug interactions [78–80].

Spectinamides

1810

This is a semi-synthetic spectinomycin analogue that has been synthesised to have selective ribosomal inhibition and therefore a narrow spectrum of anti-TB activity. Spectinamides are particularly designed to evade the efflux pump that is upregulated in MDR strains of *M. tuberculosis* that are involved with macrophage-induced drug tolerance. Lee 1810 has shown the most potential in the murine model due to its excellent safety profile and synergy with pyrazinamide and rifampicin; it has therefore been selected for pre-clinical trials [81].

1,2 Ethylene diamines

SQ109

SQ109 is a 1,2-ethylene diamine small-molecule drug related to ethambutol that is metabolised by cytochrome P450 enzymes. So far, the main mechanisms of action have been shown to be disruption of cell wall assembly through inhibition of a monomycolate transporter (MmpL3), and inhibition of efflux systems and energy production. It has been shown to be synergistic when administered with rifampicin, bedaquiline, isoniazid and sutezolid, and to shorten treatment duration *in vitro*. This drug has undergone three phase I trials in the USA, two phase II trials in Africa and one phase IIb-3 trial in Russia [82–85]. The last trial found the culture conversion rate at 24 weeks (end of intensive phase) in the SQ109 group to be higher than in the placebo plus optimised background regimen group (80.0% *versus* 61.0%), which was statistically significant ($p=0.04$) [80].

GSK-286

GSK-286 is a novel compound that can kill intracellular mycobacteria through cholesterol catabolism. It has been shown to penetrate necrotic lesions and can also reduce inflammation through its action on macrophages. It is currently undergoing human clinical trials.

Griselimycins

SATB-082

SATB-082 is a synthetic analogue of griselimycin, a natural cyclic peptide produced by *Streptomyces* spp. that inhibits the DNA polymerase sliding clamp DnaN. This drug has been shown to have excellent bactericidal activity against *M. tuberculosis* in mice [86].

Cyclopeptides

Caprazene nucleoside (CPZEN-45)

CPZEN-45 is a caprazamycin that is usually produced by *Streptomyces* spp. It is a nucleoside antibiotic that uses a novel target to inhibit cell wall synthesis and is active against replicating and nonreplicating *M. tuberculosis*. It has been shown to be effective against XDR strains of *M. tuberculosis* in a murine model, particularly when used in combination with other drugs [87–89].

Other drugs

Mefloquine

This is a synthetic quinine analogue that has traditionally been used in the treatment and prophylaxis of malaria. It also has bactericidal activity against Gram-positive bacteria. Recent data has also shown that mefloquine has good *in vitro* activity against *M. tuberculosis* and especially against MDR-TB strains. There is some evidence that it may be synergistic when used with other anti-TB drugs. There are, however, concerns about side-effects, as the incidence of these has previously been reported as 47–90%, consisting mainly of nausea, vertigo and dizziness. In order to reduce this risk, it may be possible to administer the drug weekly once high initial intracellular concentrations are achieved [90, 91].

Co-trimoxazole

This is a combination of two antimicrobials: trimethoprim and sulfamethoxazole. They work synergistically and interfere with folic acid synthesis in bacteria. Co-trimoxazole has been widely used in prophylaxis against *Pneumocystis jirovecii* pneumonia in patients with HIV and also in the treatment of urinary tract infections. *In vitro* studies have shown that 98% of laboratory isolates of *M. tuberculosis* are sensitive to co-trimoxazole [92]. Several clinical studies looking at the use of co-trimoxazole in patients with HIV as prophylaxis against TB have shown good results and tolerance [92]. As this drug has excellent oral bioavailability and distribution within body fluids including cerebrospinal fluid, it has been considered as a potential candidate for the treatment of TB meningitis [92].

New drug combinations

Given the rapidly rising numbers of patients infected with DR-TB worldwide, there is much focus on developing novel drug combinations that are noninjectable, will allow a shorter treatment duration and have a lower toxicity profile.

https://doi.org/10.1183/2312508X.10021517

Table 1. Research and development pipeline for new anti-TB drugs

Discovery: lead optimisation	Pre-clinical development		Clinical development		
	Early stage development	Good laboratory practice toxicology studies	Phase I	Phase II	Phase III
Diarylquinolines DprE1 inhibitors InhA inhibitors Macrolides Mycobacterial gyrase inhibitors Pyrazinamide analogues Ruthenium (II) complexes	Caprazene nucleoside CPZEN-45 SATB-082 Spectinamide 1810 (targets protein synthesis) Fluoroquinolone DC-159a Gyrase inhibitor SPR-720 Pyrazolopyridine carboxamide TB-47	BTZ-043[#] (targets cell wall DprE1) TBAJ-587 (targets ATP synthase) TBI-223 (targets protein synthesis) GSK-286	Q203[¶] (targets QcrB) PBTZ-169[#] (targets cell wall DprE1) OPC-167832 TBI-166 (targets cell respiration) TBA-7371 (targets cell wall DprE1) GSK-656 (070) (targets protein synthesis) Contezolid (MRX-4/MRX-1) (targets protein synthesis)	Sutezolid[+] (PNU-100480) (targets protein synthesis) Linezolid[+] EBA and dose-ranging (targets protein synthesis) SQ109 (targets MmpL3) High-dose rifampicin[§] for DS-TB Bedaquiline[¶]/pretomanid[##]/pyrazinamide (moxifloxacin [BPaZ and BPaMZ NC005 trial; ClinicalTrials.gov NCT02193776] Levofloxacin[f] with OBR for MDR-TB [OPTI-Q trial; ClinicalTrials.gov NCT01918397]	Rifapentine[§]/moxifloxacin[f] for DS-TB [CDC TBTC-31 trial] Delamanid[##] (OPC-67683) with OBR for MDR-TB Pretomanid[##]/moxifloxacin[f] pyrazinamide regimen [STAND trial; ClinicalTrials.gov NCT02342886] Bedaquiline[¶]/pretomanid[##]/linezolid[+] [NiX-TB regimen] Bedaquiline[¶] STREAM MDR-TB trial stage 2 [with OBR 9 months or OBR with injectable 6 months] [targets ATP synthase] Bedaquiline[¶]/linezolid[+] with OBR for MDR-TB High-dose rifampicin[§] [RIFASHORT trial; ClinicalTrials.gov NCT02581527]

Continued

Table 1. Continued

Discovery: lead optimisation	Pre-clinical development		Clinical development		
	Early stage development	Good laboratory practice toxicology studies	Phase I	Phase II	Phase III
Inhibitors of MmpL3, translocase-1, Clp and PKS13 Pyrimidines DprE1 Aryl sulfonamides Squaramides Diarylthiazoles				PBTZ-169# (targets cell wall DprE1) Bedaquiline¶¶/delamanid## (ACTG 5343) Nitazoxanide β-lactams (meropenem/ clavulanate and rifampicin§) High-dose rifampicin§ (PanACEA trial; ClinicalTrials. gov NCT01785186) TB PRACTECAL trial (ClinicalTrials.gov NCT02589782): regimens including bedaquiline¶¶/ pretomanid## and linezolid⁺)	

QcrB: cytochrome *bc1* complex cytochrome *b* subunit; DS-TB: drug-sensitive TB; DprE1: decaprenylphosphoryl-β-D-ribose oxidase; EBA: early bactericidal activity; OBR: optimised background regimen; MmpL3; mycolic acid transporter; BPaZ: bedaquiline, pretomanid and pyrazinamide; BPaMZ: bedaquiline, pretomanid, pyrazinamide and moxifloxacin; PKS13: polyketide synthase 13. Drug groups as follows. #: benzothiazinones; ¶: imidazopyridines; ⁺: oxazolidinones; §: rifamycins; ᶠ: fluoroquinolones; ##: nitroimidazoles; ¶¶: diarylquinolines. Reproduced and modified from [5] with permission.

https://doi.org/10.1183/2312508X.10021517

The 9-month Bangladesh regimen that uses high-dose gatifloxacin, clofazimine, ethambutol and pyrazinamide with the addition of prothionamide, kanamycin and high-dose isoniazid during the 4-month intensive phase showed an 87.9% treatment success rate [71]. In view of this and subsequent studies that have confirmed this finding, the WHO published new guidelines using a shortened 9-month drug treatment in 2016 that is similar to the Bangladesh regimen but replaces gatifloxacin with moxifloxacin [93]. More details on this regimen are available in another chapter in this *Monograph* [94].

Notable ongoing and recent trials investigating the optimisation of these regimens include the STREAM 1 trial (ClinicalTrials.gov identifier NCT02409290), which compared the 2011 WHO recommended regimen of 20–24 months with the more recently issued 9-month regimen. Although this did not show inferiority of the older regime, the trial demonstrated very high success rates of >78% in both groups, suggesting that careful monitoring of patients can lead to better outcomes, regardless of the regime used [95, 96]. STREAM 2 will build on these results and compare a bedaquiline-containing 6- and 9-month entirely oral regime with the WHO's 18-month regimen. If successful, this will be a major breakthrough for MDR- and XDR-TB treatment, allowing better accessibility and safety. The NeXT trial (ClinicalTrials.gov identifier NCT02454205) has a similar aim and will compare the standard WHO regime with an oral 6–9-month combination of bedaquiline, levofloxacin, pyrazinamide and linezolid with high-dose isoniazid, ethionamide or terizidone. The NiX-TB trial is looking at reducing pill burden by giving a 6-month course of pretomanid, bedaquiline and linezolid, and has so far reported cure in 87% of patients [97].

Coadministration of bedaquiline and delamanid

Based on the lack of clear safety evidence, the WHO does not currently recommend coadministration of these two drugs, because of the possible drug–drug interactions and potential adverse events [69]. The main concern is represented by the prolongation of the QT interval, as both drugs and several others that often comprise the regimen of difficult-to-treat cases (*e.g.* fluoroquinolones, clofazimine) have QT prolongation effects. However, more evidence is becoming available on the limited problems caused by the combined administration of bedaquiline and delamanid [98, 99]. A recent systematic review of all published cases treated with bedaquiline showed that <5% of the total number of cases reported QT prolongation and <1% had to interrupt the drug use because of this [100].

While waiting for more evidence, salvage treatment with both drugs needs to be undertaken in highly specialised centres, where, under best practice of care, adequate QT monitoring is available, accurate and detailed pharmacovigilance is in place, and informed consent is provided [101].

Conclusion

Since the first antimycobacterial agents were discovered in the 1950s and 1960s, there has been a relative paucity of new discoveries. Dramatically rising rates of TB drug resistance, treatment toxicity and TB-related deaths have been a great concern for the global TB community. Some of the proposed new treatments are new chemicals altogether, and some are old drugs that have been repurposed for use in TB treatment. A summary of the research and development pipeline for new anti-TB drugs is shown in table 1. As a result of much research and lobbying, there are finally several drugs in the TB pipeline.

Bedaquiline is the first new drug to be licensed for the treatment of TB in >40 years and heralds an exciting prospect for shortening lengthy and toxic conventional treatments. Many of the repurposed and new agents have already been included in the WHO recommendations, but use is still off-label on a compassionate basis. This means that use is expensive and only available in better-resourced areas, often with the lowest burden of drug resistance. Drug development and identification of new compounds is ongoing. Several phase III trials are currently in progress to establish safer, better-tolerated treatment regimens. These are crucial to ensure that treatment is available and tolerable for the millions of people affected by DR-TB worldwide.

References

1.   DR-TB STAT. Country updates. http://drtb-stat.org/country-updates/ Date last accessed: May 28, 2018. Date last updated: May 24, 2018.
2.   WHO. Antibacterial Agents in Clinical Development: an Analysis of the Antibacterial Clinical Development Pipeline, Including Tuberculosis. Geneva, WHO, 2017.
3.   Lessem E, Low M. The tuberculosis treatment pipeline. *In*: Claydon P, Collins S, Frick M, *et al.*, eds. 2016 Pipeline report: HIV and TB, drugs, diagnostics, vaccines, preventive technologies, cure research, and immune-based and gene therapies in development. New York, Treatment Action Group, 2016; pp. 129–142.
4.   Tiberi S, D'Ambrosio L, De Lorenzo S, *et al.* Tuberculosis elimination, patients' lives and rational use of new drugs: revisited. *Eur Respir J* 2016; 47: 664–667.
5.   Working Group on New TB Drugs. Clinical pipeline. www.newtbdrugs.org/pipeline/clinical. Date last accessed: May 28, 2018. Date last updated: 2016.
6.   Lohrasbi V, Talebi M, Bialvaei AZ, *et al.* Trends in the discovery of new drugs for *Mycobacterium tuberculosis* therapy with a glance at resistance. *Tuberculosis* 2018; 109: 17–27.
7.   Li SY, Tasneen R, Soni H, *et al.* Bactericidal and sterilizing activity of a novel regimen with bedaquiline, pretomanid, moxifloxacin, and pyrazinamide in a murine model of tuberculosis. *Antimicrob Agents Chemother* 2017; 61: e00913-17.
8.   Dawson R, Harris K, Conradie A, *et al.* Efficacy of bedaquiline, pretomanid, moxifloxacin and PZA (BPAMZ) against DS- and MDR-TB. *In*: Conference on Retroviruses and Opportunistic Infections, Seattle, February 13–16, 2017. Abstract 724LB.
9.   Tiberi S, du Plessis N, Walzl G, *et al.* Tuberculosis: progress and advances in development of new drugs, treatment regimens, and host-directed therapies. *Lancet Infect Dis* 2018; 18: e183–e198.
10.   Wells CD, Gupta R, Hittel N, *et al.* Long-term mortality assessment of multidrug-resistant tuberculosis patients treated with delamanid. *Eur Respir J* 2015; 45: 1498–1501.
11.   Gler MT, Skripconoka V, Sanchez-Garavito E, *et al.* Delamanid for multidrug-resistant pulmonary tuberculosis. *N Engl J Med* 2012; 366: 2151–2160.
12.   Skripconoka V, Danilovits M, Pehme L, *et al.* Delamanid improves outcomes and reduces mortality in multidrug-resistant tuberculosis. *Eur Respir J* 2013; 41: 1393–1400.
13.   Xavier AS, Lakshmanan M. Delamanid: a new armor in combating drug-resistant tuberculosis. *J Pharmacol Pharmacother* 2014; 5: 222–224.
14.   DR-TB STAT. Phase III Clinical Trial Results at the 48th Union World Conference on Lung Health: Implications for the Field. Geneva, WHO, 2017. http://drtb-stat.org/wp-content/uploads/2017/11/Updated_November_12_2017_STAT_phaseIII_Union_summary-002.pdf
15.   Haagsma AC, Abdillahi-Ibrahim R, Wagner MJ, *et al.* Selectivity of TMC207 towards mycobacterial ATP synthase compared with that towards the eukaryotic homologue. *Antimicrob Agents Chemother* 2009; 53: 1290–1292.
16.   Koul A, Vranckx L, Dhar N, *et al.* Delayed bactericidal response of *Mycobacterium tuberculosis* to bedaquiline involves remodelling of bacterial metabolism. *Nat Commun* 2014; 5: 3369.
17.   Diacon AH, Pym A, Grobusch M, *et al.* The diarylquinoline TMC207 for multidrug-resistant tuberculosis. *N Engl J Med* 2009; 360: 2397–2405.
18.   Diacon AH, Pym A, Grobusch MP, *et al.* Multidrug-resistant tuberculosis and culture conversion with bedaquiline. *N Engl J Med* 2014; 371: 723–732.
19.   Pontali E, Sotgiu G, D'Ambrosio L, *et al.* Bedaquiline and multidrug-resistant tuberculosis: a systematic and critical analysis of the evidence. *Eur Respir J* 2016; 47: 394–402.
20.   CDC. Provisional CDC guidelines for the use and safety monitoring of bedaquiline fumarate (Sirturo) for the treatment of multidrug-resistant tuberculosis. *MMWR Recomm Rep* 2013; 62: 1–12.

https://doi.org/10.1183/2312508X.10021517

21. WHO. The Use of Bedaquiline in the Treatment of Multidrug-resistant Tuberculosis. Interim Policy Guidance. Geneva, WHO, 2013. http://apps.who.int/iris/bitstream/handle/10665/84879/9789241505482_eng.pdf;jsessionid= 2F2758FAB6F3C2CFB494072505C7C111?sequence=1

22. Ndjeka N, Conradie F, Schnippel K, et al. Treatment of drug-resistant tuberculosis with bedaquiline in a high HIV prevalence setting: an interim cohort analysis. Int J Tuberc Lung Dis 2015; 19: 979–985.

23. Working Group on New TB Drugs. TBAJ-587, diarylquinoline. www.newtbdrugs.org/pipeline/compound/ tbaj-587-diarylquinoline Date last accessed: May 28, 2018. Date last updated: 2016.

24. Jindani A, Harrison TS, Nunn AJ, et al. High-dose rifapentine with moxifloxacin for pulmonary tuberculosis. N Eng J Med 2014; 371: 1599–1608.

25. Sterling TR, Villarino ME, Borisov AS, et al. Three months of rifapentine and isoniazid for latent tuberculosis infection. N Engl J Med 2011; 365: 2155–2566.

26. Dorman SE, Savic RM, Goldberg S, et al. Daily rifapentine for treatment of pulmonary tuberculosis. a randomized, dose-ranging trial. Am J Respir Crit Care Med 2015; 191: 333–343.

27. Rifat D, Prideaux B, Savic RM, et al. Pharmacokinetics of rifapentine and rifampin in a rabbit model of tuberculosis and correlation with clinical trial data. Sci Transl Med 2018; 10: eaai7786.

28. Bialvaei AZ, Rahbar M, Yousefi M, et al. Linezolid: a promising option in the treatment of Gram-positives. J Antimicrob Chemother 2017; 72: 354–364.

29. Zhang Z, Pang Y, Wang Y, et al. Beijing genotype of Mycobacterium tuberculosis is significantly associated with linezolid resistance in multidrug-resistant and extensively drug-resistant tuberculosis in China. Int J Antimicrob Agents 2014; 43: 231–235.

30. Lee M, Lee J, Carroll MW, et al. Linezolid for treatment of chronic extensively drug-resistant tuberculosis. N Engl J Med 2012; 367: 1508–1518.

31. Sotgiu G, Centis R, D'Ambrosio L, et al. Efficacy, safety and tolerability of linezolid containing regimens in treating MDR-TB and XDR-TB: systematic review and meta-analysis. Eur Respir J 2012; 40: 1430–1442.

32. Alffenaar JW, van Altena R, Harmelink IM, et al. Comparison of the pharmacokinetics of two dosage regimens of linezolid in multidrug-resistant and extensively drug-resistant tuberculosis patients. Clin Pharmacokinet 2010; 49: 559–565.

33. McNeil MB, Dennison DD, Shelton CD, et al. In vitro isolation and characterization of oxazolidinone-resistant Mycobacterium tuberculosis. Antimicrob Agents Chemother 2017; 61: e01296-17.

34. Wallis RS, Jakubiec W, Kumar V, et al. Biomarker-assisted dose selection for safety and efficacy in early development of PNU-100480 for tuberculosis. Antimicrob Agents Chemother 2011; 55: 567–574.

35. Wallis RS, Dawson R, Friedrich SO, et al. Mycobactericidal activity of sutezolid (PNU-100480) in sputum (EBA) and blood (WBA) of patients with pulmonary tuberculosis. PLoS One 2014; 9: e94462.

36. Wallis RS, Jakubiec W, Mitton-Fry M, et al. Rapid evaluation in whole blood culture of regimens for XDR-TB containing PNU-100480 (sutezolid), TMC207, PA-824, SQ109, and pyrazinamide. PLoS One 2012; 7: e30479.

37. Andrews J. To be or not to be exclusive: the sutezolid story. Lancet Glob Health 2016; 4: e89–e90.

38. Sequella, Inc. Sutezolid for the Treatment of Tuberculosis. Rockville, Sequella, Inc., 2010. www.sequella.com/docs/ Sequella_1sheet_Sutezolid_v1.pdf

39. Working Group on New TB Drugs. TBI-223. www.newtbdrugs.org/pipeline/compound/tbi-223 Date last accessed: May 28, 2018. Date last updated: 2016.

40. Mdluli K, Cooper C, Yang T, et al. TBI-223: a safer oxazolidinone in pre-clinical development for tuberculosis. In: ASM Microbe 2017 Meeting, New Orleans, June 1–5, 2017. Abstract 6174.

41. Zong Z, Jing W, Shi J, et al. Comparison of in vitro activity and MIC distributions between the novel oxazolidinone delpazolid and linezolid against multidrug-resistant and extensively drug-resistant Mycobacterium tuberculosis in China. Antimicrob Agents Chemother 2018; 62: e00165-18.

42. Kim TS, Choe JH, Kim YJ, et al. Activities of LCB01-0371, a novel oxazolidinone, against Mycobacterium abscessus. Antimicrob Agents Chemother 2017; 61: e02752-16.

43. Li CR, Zhai QQ, Wang XK, et al. In vivo antibacterial activity of MRX-I, a new oxazolidinone. Antimicrob Agents Chemother 2014; 58: 2418–2421.

44. Gordeev MF, Yuan ZY. New potent antibacterial oxazolidinone (MRX-I) with an improved class safety profile. J Med Chem 2014; 57: 4487–4497.

45. MicurRx Pharmaceuticals. MicuRx initiates phase 1 clinical trial in U.S. for novel antibiotic agent MRX-4. http:// micurx.com/2016/11/30/micurx-initiates-phase-1-clinical-trial-in-u-s-for-novel-antibiotic-agent-mrx-4/ Date last accessed: May 28, 2018. Date last updated: November 30, 2016.

46. Pethe K, Bifani P, Jang J, et al. Discovery of Q203, a potent clinical candidate for the treatment of tuberculosis. Nat Med 2013; 19: 1157–1160.

47. Nuermberger EL, Yoshimatsu T, Tyagi S, et al. Moxifloxacin-containing regimen greatly reduces time to culture conversion in murine tuberculosis. Am J Respir Crit Care Med 2004; 169: 421–426.

48. Xu P, Chen H, Xu J, et al. Moxifloxacin is an effective and safe candidate agent for tuberculosis treatment: a meta-analysis. Int J Infect Dis 2017; 60: 35–41.

49. Thee S, Garcia-Prats AJ, Draper HR, *et al.* Pharmacokinetics and safety of moxifloxacin in children with multidrug-resistant tuberculosis. *Clin Infect Dis* 2015; 60: 549–556.

50. Burman WJ, Goldberg S, Johnson JL, *et al.* Moxifloxacin *versus* ethambutol in the first 2 months of treatment for pulmonary tuberculosis. *Am J Respir Crit Care Med* 2006; 174: 331–338.

51. Working group on New TB Drugs. DC-159a. www.newtbdrugs.org/pipeline/compound/dc-159a Date last accessed: May 28, 2018. Date last updated: 2016.

52. Disratthakit A, Doi N. *In vitro* activities of DC-159a, a novel fluoroquinolone, against *Mycobacterium* species. *Antimicrob Agents Chemother* 2009; 54: 2684–2686.

53. Nakamura H, Horita Y, Doi N. Comparative evaluation of new respiratory quinolone DC-159a or moxifloxacin containing regimens in a murine TB model. *In:* ASM Microbe 2017 Meeting, New Orleans, June 1–5, 2017. Poster 38.

54. Gao C, Peng C, Shi Y, *et al.* Benzothiazinethione is a potent preclinical candidate for the treatment of drug-resistant tuberculosis. *Sci Rep* 2016; 6: 29717.

55. Makarov V, Manina G, Mikusova K, *et al.* Benzothiazinones kill *Mycobacterium tuberculosis* by blocking arabinan synthesis. *Science* 2009; 324: 801–804.

56. BusinessWire. Otsuka awarded grant to advance development of novel anti-tuberculosis compound OPC-167832 with delamanid. www.businesswire.com/news/home/20180129005073/en/Otsuka-Awarded-Grant-Advance-Development-Anti-Tuberculosis-Compound Date last accessed: May 28, 2018. Date last updated: January 29, 2018.

57. Makarov V, Lechartier B, Zhang M, *et al.* Towards a new combination therapy for tuberculosis with next generation benzothiazinones. *EMBO Mol Med* 2014; 6: 372–383.

58. TB Alliance. TBA-7371/DprE1 inhibitor. www.tballiance.org/portfolio/compound/tba-7371-dpre1-inhibitor Date last accessed: May 28, 2018.

59. Otsuka Pharmaceutical Co. Updates in the Development of Delamanid, OPC 167832. Tokyo, Otsuka Pharmaceutical Co., 2018. www.cptrinitiative.org/wp-content/uploads/2017/05/Jeffrey_Hafkin_CPTR2017_JH.pdf

60. Tiberi S, Sotgiu G, D'Ambrosio L, *et al.* Comparison of effectiveness and safety of imipenem/clavulanate- *versus* meropenem/clavulanate-containing regimens in the treatment of multidrug and extensively drug-resistant tuberculosis. *Eur Respir J* 2016; 47: 1758–1766.

61. Tiberi S, Payen MC, Sotgiu G, *et al.* Effectiveness and safety of meropenem/clavulanate-containing regimens in the treatment of MDR- and XDR-TB. *Eur Respir J* 2016; 47: 1235–1243.

62. Sotgiu G, D'Ambrosio L, Centis R, *et al.* Carbapenems to treat multidrug and extensively drug-resistant tuberculosis: a systematic review. *Int J Mol Sci* 2016; 17: 373.

63. Gonzalo X, Drobniewski F. Is there a place for β-lactams in the treatment of multidrug-resistant/extensively drug-resistant tuberculosis? Synergy between meropenem and amoxicillin/clavulanate. *J Antimicrob Chemother* 2013; 68: 366–369.

64. Drawz SM, Bonomo RA. Three Decades of β-lactamase inhibitors. *Clin Microbiol Rev* 2010; 23: 160–201.

65. Tremblay LW, Fan F, Blanchard JS. Biochemical and structural characterization of *Mycobacterium tuberculosis* β-lactamase with the carbapenems ertapenem and doripenem. *Biochemistry* 2010; 49: 3766–3773.

66. Van Rijn SP, Srivastava S, Wessels MA, *et al.* Sterilizing effect of ertapenem-clavulanate in a hollow-fiber model of tuberculosis and implications on clinical dosing. *Antimicrob Agents Chemother* 2017; 61: e02039-16.

67. Mosley JF, Smith LL, Parke CK, *et al.* Ceftazidime-avibactam (Avycaz): for the treatment of complicated intra-abdominal and urinary tract infections. *P T* 2016; 41: 479–483.

68. Deshpande D, Srivastava S, Chapagain M, *et al.* Ceftazidime-avibactam has potent sterilizing activity against highly drug-resistant tuberculosis. *Sci Adv* 2017; 3: e1701102.

69. Falzon D, Schünemann HJ, Harausz E, *et al.* World Health Organization treatment guidelines for drug-resistant tuberculosis, 2016 update. *Eur Resp J* 2017; 49: 1602308.

70. Xu J, Wang B, Hu M, *et al.* Primary clofazimine and bedaquiline resistance among isolates from patients with multidrug-resistant tuberculosis. *Antimicrob Agents Chemother* 2017; 61: e00239-17.

71. Van Deun A, Salim MA, Das AP, *et al.* Results of a standardised regimen for multidrug-resistant tuberculosis in Bangladesh. *Int J Tuberc Lung Dis* 2004; 8: 560–567.

72. Tang S, Yao L, Hao X, *et al.* Clofazimine for the treatment of multidrug-resistant tuberculosis: prospective, multicenter, randomized controlled study in China. *Clin Infect Dis* 2015; 60: 1361–1367.

73. Dalcolmo M, Gayoso R, Sotgiu G, *et al.* Effectiveness and safety of clofazimine in multidrug-resistant tuberculosis: a nationwide report from Brazil. *Eur Respir J* 2017; 49: 1602445.

74. Hwang TJ, Dotsenko S, Jafarov A, *et al.* Safety and availability of clofazimine in the treatment of multidrug and extensively drug-resistant tuberculosis: analysis of published guidance and meta-analysis of cohort studies. *BMJ Open* 2014; 4: e004143.

75. WHO. WHO Treatment Guidelines for Drug-resistant Tuberculosis; 2016 Update. Geneva, WHO, 2016. http://apps.who.int/iris/bitstream/handle/10665/250125/9789241549639-eng.pdf;jsessionid=02167FEFD3846B38563CA942 E55EB5DE?sequence=1

https://doi.org/10.1183/2312508X.10021517

76. Brouqui P, Quenard F, Drancourt M. Old antibiotics for emerging multidrug-resistant/extensively drug-resistant tuberculosis (MDR/XDR-TB). *Int J Antimicrob Agents* 2017; 49: 554–557.

77. Zhang D, Lu Y, Liu K, *et al.* Identification of less lipophilic riminophenazine derivatives for the treatment of drug-resistant tuberculosis. *J Med Chem* 2012; 55: 8409–8417.

78. Working Group on New TB Drugs. SPR720. www.newtbdrugs.org/pipeline/compound/spr720 Date last accessed: May 28, 2018. Date last updated: 2016.

79. Shoen C, Pucci M, De Stefano M, *et al.* Efficacy of SPR720 and SPR750 gyrase inhibitors in a mouse *Mycobacterium tuberculosis* infection model. *In*: ASM Microbe 2017 Meeting, New Orleans, June 1–5, 2017. Poster 43.

80. Pucci MJ. A novel gyrase inhibitor for the treatment of drug-susceptible and multidrug-resistant *Mycobacterium tuberculosis* infections. https://sbirsource.com/sbir/awards/167445-a-novel-gyrase-inhibitor-for-the-treatment-of-drug-susceptible-and-multidrug-resistant-mycobacterium-tuberculosis-infections Date last accessed: May 28, 2018. Date last updated: 2018.

81. Robertson GT, Scherman MS, Bruhn DF, *et al.* Spectinamides are effective partner agents for the treatment of tuberculosis in multiple mouse infection models. *J Antimicrob Chemother* 2017; 72: 770–777.

82. Tahlan K, Wilson R, Kastrinsky DB, *et al.* SQ109 targets MmpL3, a membrane transporter of trehalose monomycolate involved in mycolic acid donation to the cell wall core of *Mycobacterium tuberculosis. Antimicrob Agents Chemother* 2012; 56: 1797–1809.

83. Heinrich N, Dawson R, du Bois J, *et al.* Early phase evaluation of SQ109 alone and in combination with rifampicin in pulmonary TB patients. *J Antimicrob Chemother* 2015; 70: 1558–1566.

84. Sacksteder KA, Protopopova M, Barry CE, *et al.* Discovery and development of SQ109: a new antitubercular drug with a novel mechanism of action. *Future Microbiol* 2012; 7: 823–837.

85. Borisov SE, Bogorodskaya EM, Volchenkov GV, *et al.* [Efficiency and safety of chemotherapy regimen with SQ109 in those suffering from multiple drug-resistant tuberculosis.] *Tuberkulez i Bolezni Lëgkih* 2018; 96: 6–18.

86. Kling A, Lukat P, Almeida DV, *et al.* Antibiotics targeting DnaN for tuberculosis therapy using novel griselimycins. *Science* 2015; 348: 1106–1112.

87. Working Group on New TB Drugs. CPZEN-45. www.newtbdrugs.org/pipeline/compound/cpzen-45 Date last accessed: May 28, 2018. Date last updated: 2016.

88. Ishizaki Y, Hayashi C, Inoue K, *et al.* Inhibition of the first step in synthesis of the mycobacterial cell wall core, catalyzed by the GlcNAc-1-phosphate transferase WecA, by the novel caprazamycin derivative CPZEN-45. *J Biol Chem* 2013; 288: 30309–30319.

89. Salomon JJ, Galeron P, Schulte N, *et al.* Biopharmaceutical *in vitro* characterization of CPZEN-45, a drug candidate for inhalation therapy of tuberculosis. *Ther Deliv* 2013; 4: 915–923.

90. Krieger D, Vesenbeckh S, Schönfeld N, *et al.* Mefloquine as a potential drug against multidrug resistant tuberculosis. *Eur Respir J* 2015; 46: 1503–1505.

91. Rodrigues-Junior VS, Villela AD, Goncalves RS, *et al.* Mefloquine and its oxazolidine derivative compound are active against drug-resistant *Mycobacterium tuberculosis* strains and in a murine model of tuberculosis infection. *Int J Antimicrob Agents* 2016; 48: 203–207.

92. Alsaad N, Wilffert B, van Altena R, *et al.* Potential antimicrobial agents for the treatment of multidrug-resistant tuberculosis. *Eur Respir J* 2014; 43: 884–897.

93. Working Group on New TB Drugs. www.newtbdrugs.org Date last accessed: May 28, 2018.

94. Caminero JA, Scardigli A, van der Werf T, *et al.* Treatment of drug-susceptible and drug-resistant tuberculosis. *In*: Migliori GB, Bothamley G, Duarte R, *et al.*, eds. Tuberculosis (ERS Monograph). Sheffield, European Respiratory Society, 2018; pp. 152–178.

95. Ahmad Khan F, Salim MAH, du Cros P, *et al.* Effectiveness and safety of standardised shorter regimens for multidrug-resistant tuberculosis: individual patient data and aggregate data meta-analyses. *Eur Respir J* 2017; 50: 1700061.

96. Medical Research Council Clinical Trials Unit. Preliminary results from STREAM trial provide insight into shorter treatment for multidrug-resistant tuberculosis. www.ctu.mrc.ac.uk/news/2017/preliminary_results_from_stream_trial_provide_insight_into_shorter_treatment_for_multidrug_resistant_tuberculosis Date last accessed: May 10, 2018. Date last updated: October 13, 2017.

97. Conradie F, Diacon A, Everitt D, *et al.* The NIX-tuberculosis trial of pretomanid, bedaquiline, and linezolid to treat XDR-tuberculosis. *In*: Conference on Retroviruses and Opportunistic Infections, Boston, MA, February 13–16, 2017; abstract 80LB.

98. Tadolini M, Lingtsang RD, Tiberi S, *et al.* First case of extensively drug-resistant tuberculosis treated with both delamanid and bedaquiline. *Eur Resp J* 2016; 48: 935–938.

99. Ferlazzo G, Mohr E, Laxmeshwar C, *et al.* Early safety and efficacy of the combination of bedaquiline and delamanid for the treatment of patients with drug-resistant tuberculosis in Armenia, India, and South Africa: a retrospective cohort study. *Lancet Infect Dis* 2018; 18: 536–544.

100. Pontali E, Sotgiu G, Tiberi S, *et al.* Cardiac safety of bedaquiline: a systematic and critical analysis of the evidence. *Eur Resp J* 2017; 50: 1701462.
101. Matteelli A, D'Ambrosio L, Centis R, *et al.* Compassionate and optimum use of new tuberculosis drugs. *Lancet Infect Dis*; 15: 1131–1132.

Disclosures: S. Borisov reports receiving personal fees from Infectex LLC.

Acknowledgements: The paper is part of the operational research plan of the WHO Collaborating Centre for Tuberculosis and Lung Diseases, Tradate, ITA-80, 2017–2020-GBM/RC/LD.

https://doi.org/10.1183/2312508X.10021517

Chapter 12

Adverse anti-tuberculosis drug events and their management

José A. Caminero[1,2], Paula Lasserra[3,4], Alberto Piubello[2,5] and Rupak Singla[6]

It is currently possible to cure TB, but multiple drugs are required over a long term, and both of these factors produce adverse drug reactions (ADRs). ADRs can be caused by all anti-TB drugs but are much more frequent with second-line drugs. Fortunately, most anti-TB ADRs are mild or moderate and do not always require removal of the offending drug. However, some ADRs can be severe or potentially life-threatening, requiring urgent clinical interventions, including removal of the suspected drug(s). Early detection and adequate management of ADRs is essential for a good TB treatment outcome. This chapter reviews the majority of the possible ADRs to anti-TB drugs. In addition, practical recommendations to identify the possible drug(s) involved in the different reactions and the most adequate management in each situation are outlined.

Cite as: Caminero JA, Lasserra P, Piubello A, et al. Adverse anti-tuberculosis drug events and their management. In: Migliori GB, Bothamley G, Duarte R, et al., eds. Tuberculosis (ERS Monograph). Sheffield, European Respiratory Society, 2018; pp. 205–227 [https://doi.org/10.1183/2312508X.10021617].

🐦 @ERSpublications
All anti-TB drugs can produce adverse drug reactions, most of them mild or moderate. Early detection and adequate management of these adverse reactions is essential for a good TB treatment outcome. http://ow.ly/cfVQ30lqCfE

A ll anti-TB drugs can produce some adverse drug reactions (ADRs) or adverse events. The difference between ADRs and adverse events is described in table 1 [1]. Most first-line anti-TB drugs are well tolerated by most patients. However, this is not the case for many of the second-line drugs. ADRs/adverse events can lead to abandonment or irregularity of treatment, thus contributing to increased morbidity, reduced quality of life, treatment failure, death and the risk of amplification of resistance [2]. All this aggravates transmission of the disease [2–5]. Comorbidities are common among TB patients, and such patients are prone to a higher risk of ADRs and adverse events. Therefore, careful monitoring and counselling are the basis of patient adherence, especially in these populations [6].

[1]Dept of Pneumology, University Hospital of Gran Canaria "Dr Negrín", Las Palmas de Gran Canaria, Spain. [2]International Union against Tuberculosis and Lung Disease (The Union), Paris, France. [3]National Tuberculosis Control Program, Montevideo, Uruguay. [4]School of Medicine, Universidad de la República Oriental del Uruguay, Montevideo, Uruguay. [5]Damien Foundation, Niamey, Niger. [6]National Institute of Tuberculosis and Respiratory Diseases, New Delhi, India.

Correspondence: José A. Caminero, Dept of Pneumology, University Hospital of Gran Canaria "Dr Negrín", Barranco de la Ballena s/n, 35010 Las Palmas de Gran Canaria, Spain. E-mail: jcamlun@gobiernodecanarias.org

Table 1. Glossary of basic terms for active anti-TB drug-safety monitoring and management

Term	Description
Active TB drug-safety monitoring and management (aDSM)	The active and systematic, clinical and laboratory assessment of patients on treatment with new anti-TB drugs, novel MDR-TB regimens or XDR-TB regimens to detect, manage and report suspected or confirmed drug toxicities. While all detected adverse events need to be managed, the core package of aDSM requires the reporting of serious adverse events only
Adverse drug reaction	A response to an anti-TB medicine that is noxious and unintended, and which occurs at doses normally used in humans
Adverse event	Any untoward medical occurrence that presents in a TB patient during treatment with a pharmaceutical product, but which does not necessarily have a causal relationship with this treatment
Serious adverse event	An adverse event that leads to death or a life-threatening experience, to hospitalisation or prolongation of hospitalisation, to persistent or significant disability, or to a congenital anomaly. Serious adverse events that do not immediately result in one of these outcomes but that require an intervention to prevent them from happening are included

Reproduced and modified from [1] with permission.

The WHO has emphasised the importance of detection, assessment, management and prevention of ADRs during anti-TB treatment [7]. The incidence of ADRs is generally obtained from the medical records, and thus relies entirely on clinician documentation. A South African study showed that ADRs were reported much more frequently in patient interviews than in medical records [3, 8]. This indicates a major drawback of pharmacovigilance, as it can lead to an inaccurate representation of actual outcomes [3].

Early detection and adequate management of ADRs and adverse events is essential in the treatment of TB, especially because anti-TB drug resistance is increasing globally. This chapter reviews the most frequently occurring ADRs and adverse events to anti-TB drugs, and the most appropriate management.

Prevalence of adverse drug reactions

The most common ADRs associated with first-line drugs are gastrointestinal, cutaneous and, less frequently, hepatic. Studies have reported that 25–60% of patients had at least one type of reaction. Most of these were mild and either self-limiting or responded to simple supportive treatment. Only 10% of patients required treatment interruption for 1 week or longer, and one or more drugs had to be terminated in 8% of the patients [3, 9, 10].

ADRs are more frequent with the use of second-line drugs and may produce obstacles in the management of MDR-TB patients. Wide variations, ranging from 10.7% to 70.4%, in the occurrence of ADRs leading to a change of treatment have been reported [3, 11–15].

https://doi.org/10.1183/2312508X.10021617

Data collected from initial five DOTS-Plus sites showed that, among 818 patients enrolled on MDR-TB treatment, 30% required removal of the suspected drug(s) from the regimen due to adverse events, but only 2% of patients stopped treatment [11].

A recent meta-analysis of the effectiveness and safety of standardised shorter MDR-TB regimens included 796 individuals across five studies. In four studies, grade 3 or 4 ADRs occurred in 55 out of 304 participants (18.1%). Overall, 669 out of 796 participants (83.0%) were treated successfully [3, 14]. The most frequently observed ADRs were ototoxicity, gastrointestinal disturbances, arthralgia, hepatitis and dermatological effects. TRÉBUCQ et al. [15] reported 10.7% adverse reactions and 81.6% treatment success among 1006 patients who received a shorter MDR-TB regimen in South Africa. These studies showed that ADRs are manageable in the treatment of MDR-TB, even in resource-limited settings, and may not compromise the success rates.

A detailed list of the common ADRs/adverse events to anti-TB drugs, their clinical presentation, the responsible drugs and their management are shown in table 2.

Risk factors for adverse drug reactions

The frequency and severity of ADRs varies with different drugs and regimens, comorbidities and host factors, such as ethnic and racial variations [17–19]. A list of the risk factors likely to cause ADRs and adverse events is shown in table 3 [20, 21].

In people living with HIV, a 2-fold higher relative risk of ADRs has been reported. Hepatotoxicity is a well-recognised ADR of a combination of anti-TB drugs and ART [22–25]. Hepatitis B and C also increase the risk of hepatotoxicity [23]. Coinfection with both hepatitis C and HIV can aggravate the risk of hepatotoxicity more than 14-fold [26].

Pharmacovigilance

Pharmacovigilance is the science related to the detection, assessment, understanding and prevention of adverse effects from any drug(s). Pharmacovigilance aims to get the best outcome from treatment with medicines and to improve health-related quality of life [3, 27]. The WHO released its first implementation manual for pharmacovigilance of anti-TB drugs in 2012 [27]. Three years later, the WHO Global TB Programme coordinated with key technical and funding agencies to discuss the implementation of active pharmacovigilance and proper management of ADRs when introducing new anti-TB medicines or novel MDR-TB regimens [1].

Grading of adverse events

The Division of AIDS Table for Grading the Severity of Adult and Pediatric Adverse Events, version 2.1, consists of parameters and adverse events, with severity grading guidance (table 4). This is designed for safety data reporting to maintain accuracy and consistency in the evaluation of adverse events [28]. The advice in table 4 should be followed in the evaluation of adverse events and possible interventions.

Table 2. Clinical presentation, possible responsible drugs and management of adverse drug events

Clinical presentation	Responsible drugs	Treatment/management
Gastrointestinal disorders		
Nausea and vomiting	Pto/**Eto**, **PAS**, H, R, E, Z, Cfz, Bdq	1) Rehydration (with oral rehydration solution). 2) Take a light meal before taking the medication. 3) Metoclopramide 10–20 mg 30 min before drug intake. 4) If vomiting persists, take ondansetron 2–8 mg 30 min before drug intake. 5) Divide Pto/Eto dose into morning and evening doses if DOT is ensured (dose-dependent effect; most patients tolerate the higher dose better in the evening). 6) For patients concerned about possible nausea, take diazepam 5 mg 30 min before taking the medication.
Gastritis	**Pto/Eto**, **PAS**	1) Take a light meal before taking the medication. 2) FQ absorption is reduced by drugs containing cations such as magnesium and aluminium (and sucralfate) (high reduction), iron (moderate reduction) or calcium and zinc (and multivitamins) (low reduction). 3) Omeprazole 20–40 mg in the evening (or 2 h before or 3 h after taking the medication).
Diarrhoea	**PAS**, Pto/Eto	1) Encourage patient to tolerate mild diarrhoea. 2) Encourage fluid intake. 3) Treat noncomplicated diarrhoea (no blood in the stools and with no fever) with loperamide 4 mg followed by 2 mg after each bowel movement up to a maximum of 10 mg in 24 h. 4) Check the potassium level and hydration status in case of severe diarrhoea.
Hepatotoxicity from first-line anti-TB drugs	**Z, H, R**	These drugs are identified liver risk factors. 1) If ALT/AST is more than five times the ULN, or ALT/AST is more than three times the ULN and there are hepatitis symptoms or jaundice (bilirubin >3 mg·dL^{-1}), then potentially hepatotoxic medications should be stopped immediately and the patient evaluated promptly. Assess the transaminases every week. After they return to less than two times the ULN, rifampicin may be restarted with E. After 3–7 days, H may be re-introduced, with subsequent rechecking of ALT (see text for detailed plan for re-introduction of anti-TB drugs). 2) If symptoms recur or ALT increases, the last drug added should be stopped; replace it with another if this is an essential drug.

Continued

https://doi.org/10.1183/2312508X.10021617

Table 2. Continued

Clinical presentation	Responsible drugs	Treatment/management
		3) If the patient had prolonged or severe hepatotoxicity, but tolerates R and H, a re-challenge with Z may be hazardous. In this circumstance, Z may be permanently discontinued, with treatment extended to 9 months. 4) Monitor transaminase levels monthly.
Hepatotoxicity from second-line anti-TB drugs	Pto/Eto, Bdq, PAS, Lzd, FQs (very rarely)	These drugs are identified liver risk factors. 1) If ALT/AST is five or less times the ULN and there is no jaundice, continue treatment, and treat nausea and vomiting. 2) If ALT/AST is more than five times the ULN and/or there is jaundice (bilirubin >3 mg·dL^{-1}), stop all drugs and assess transaminases every week; if they return to less than two times the ULN, re-introduce the last hepatotoxic drugs (Km, E, Mfx, Cfz) and check the transaminases. Then re-introduce hepatotoxic drugs in this order: Pto/Eto, H and Z, and monitor transaminases every 3 days. Check the values of the transaminases after the introduction of each drug. 3) If the re-introduction leads to the return of the signs of hepatotoxicity, remove the culprit drug from the treatment and replace it with another if this is an essential drug. 4) Monitor transaminase levels monthly.
Kidney disorders Nephrotoxicity	**Km, Am, Cm, Cs, E**, Z	1) Close monitoring of creatinine (and electrolytes) every week or every 2 weeks. 2) Adequate hydration. 3) If creatinine clearance is <90 mL·min^{-1}, treat with Km two to three times weekly at 12–15 mg·kg^{-1}, and E and Z, three times weekly. 4) If creatinine clearance is <60 mL·min^{-1} despite the dose reduction to two to three times weekly, stop the injectable drug and replace it with Lzd, E and Z three times weekly. 5) If Lzd is contraindicated, consider Bdq.
Electrolyte imbalances: hypokalaemia (K$^+$ <3.5 mEq·L^{-1}) and hypomagnesaemia (Mg^{2+} <1.5 mEq·L^{-1})	**Cm, Km, Am**	1) Encourage dietary intake of potassium (e.g. bananas, oranges, tomatoes, chocolate). 2) Check for signs of dehydration among patients with vomiting and diarrhoea; start oral or intravenous rehydration. 3) For supplementation of potassium, use oral slow-release tablets of potassium chloride 1200–3600 mg daily in two or three divided doses (600 mg=8 mEq).

Continued

Table 2. Continued

Clinical presentation	Responsible drugs	Treatment/management
		4) In the case of severe hypokalaemia, treat with KCl *i.v.* at 10 mEq·h^{-1} (10 mEq of KCl will raise the serum potassium by 0.1 mEq·L^{-1}). 5) If the potassium level is low, check the magnesium (if this is not possible, consider empirical treatment with magnesium in all cases of hypokalaemia with magnesium gluconate at 1000 mg twice daily). 6) Use spironolactone 25 mg daily in refractory cases. 7) Check ECG for risk of QT prolongation Note that: • Hypokalaemia may be refractory if the concurrent hypomagnesaemia is not corrected • The risk is higher if the intensive phase is prolonged • Electrolyte disturbances are reversible on discontinuation of the injectable drug (although this might last weeks or months)
Neurological disorders		
Peripheral neuropathy	**Lzd, Cs, H, FQs, Km, Pto/Eto, E**	1) Pyridoxine 100–200 mg/day (maximum 100 mg daily in pregnant women). 2) Amitriptyline 25–50 mg in the evening (maximum dose 150 mg daily in three doses). 3) Carbamazepine 100–400 mg twice daily (follow-up and monitoring of transaminases required). 4) Eto, Cs or FQ doses could be reduced; TDM is required to ensure an adequate drug level for efficacy.
Optic neuritis	**Lzd, E**	1) Immediate discontinuation of Lzd and/or E and consult ophthalmologist.
Seizures	**Cs, H, FQs**	1) Discontinue Cs, which is the most suspect medication. 2) Always check creatinine levels among patients with sudden onset of seizures; compromised renal functions may cause increased serum concentrations of Cs. 3) Begin anticonvulsive treatment (*e.g.* carbamazepine, phenytoin or valproic acid). 4) Replace Cs with Pto/Eto (or PAS) if not previously used in a failed regimen.
Osteoarticular disorders		
Arthralgia	**Z, FQs, Bdq**	1) Prescribe NSAIDs: ibuprofen 600 mg three times daily. 2) Give rest to the joint. 3) Symptoms of arthralgia generally diminish with time and without any intervention.
Tendinitis (Achilles tendon)	**FQs (all)**	1) Prescribe NSAIDs: ibuprofen 600 mg three times daily in case of tendinitis.

Continued

https://doi.org/10.1183/2312508X.10021617

Table 2. Continued

Clinical presentation	Responsible drugs	Treatment/management
		2) Give rest to the joint. 3) Tendon rupture is more probable among patients with DM and among the elderly but is usually an uncommon occurrence. 4) If significant inflammation persists, discontinue FQ use and replace with Bdq.
Dermatological disorders		
Pruritus, itchiness, skin rashes and allergic reactions	**All**	1) Generally resolve spontaneously in the first few weeks. 2) In the case of dryness of the skin, use moisturising cream. 3) Prescribe antihistamines (diphenhydramine 25–50 mg or cetirizine 5–10 mg before taking drugs). 4) Corticosteroid ointments may be used. 5) Prednisolone in low doses (10–20 mg daily) if there is no improvement. 6) Identify and discontinue the drug in question only in cases of serious adverse events (*e.g.* Stevens–Johnson syndrome and Lyell's syndrome). See text for further details.
Thyroid disorders		
Hypothyroidism	**Pto/Eto+PAS**, Pto/Eto, PAS	Initiate treatment if TSH level is more than 1.5 to two times the ULN. 1) Levothyroxine 100–150 µg daily for adults; 75–100 µg daily for young adults; 50 µg daily for elderly people; 25 µg in case of serious cardiovascular disease. 2) Re-assess TSH levels after 1–2 months and adjust the levothyroxine dosage accordingly.
Metabolic disorders		
Hypoglycaemia and hyperglycaemia	**Gfx, Mfx**	1) Treat hypoglycaemia and hyperglycaemia as needed. 2) Stop gatifloxacin, replace with moxifloxacin and monitor glycaemia. Note that: • These disorders are reversible at the end of treatment • Good glucose control is important during treatment
Lactic acidosis[#]	**Lzd**	1) Stop Lzd and replace the drug with another drug with similar anti-TB characteristics (*i.e.* imipenem or meropenem+clavulanic acid). 2) Monitor with a blood test (arterial or venous).
Haematological disorders	**Lzd**	1) Discontinue Lzd immediately in the case of severe medullary aplasia (grade 3) of the white or red blood cells or platelets. 2) Consider a blood transfusion in cases of severe anaemia. 3) Consider possible causes of haematological disorders unrelated to Lzd.

Continued

Table 2. Continued

Clinical presentation	Responsible drugs	Treatment/management
		4) Can consider a reduction in Lzd dosage (300 mg daily or 600 mg three times weekly instead of 600 mg daily) in case the aplasia resolves and monitor with complete blood counts.
Psychiatric disorders		
Depression	**Cs, H, FQs**	1) Assess psychological and socioeconomic conditions as they could be a common cause. 2) Discontinue Cs, which is the most likely drug causing depression. 3) Always check creatinine levels in patients with sudden onset of depression; impaired renal functions can raise serum Cs concentrations. 4) If moderate or severe symptoms persist, initiate antidepressant treatment with fluoxetine, amitriptyline or similar drugs. Do not administer these in conjunction with Lzd (risk of serotonin syndrome). 5) Replace Cs with Pto/Eto (or PAS) if not previously used in a failed drug regimen.
Psychosis	**Cs**, H, FQs	1) Discontinue Cs, which is the most likely responsible drug. 2) Always check creatinine levels in patients with sudden onset of psychosis; impaired renal function can raise serum CS concentrations. 3) If moderate or severe symptoms persist, initiate antipsychotic treatment with haloperidol. 4) Replace Cs with Pto/Eto (or PAS) if not previously used in a failed regimen.
Cardiac disorders		
QTc interval prolongation	**FQs** (Mfx prolongs QTc more than Lfx and Gfx), **Bdq**, Dlm, Cfz	1) Repeat ECG and confirm QTc prolongation. 2) Check for: another QTc-prolonging medication, a history of TdP, congenital long-QT syndrome, hypothyroidism, bradyarrhythmias, uncompensated heart failure and electrolyte levels. 3) Take note of conditions such as: use of aminoglycoside or capreomycin (nephrotoxic and electrolyte wasting associated), medications that cause electrolyte wasting (i.e. diuretics) or other sources of potassium loss (i.e. vomiting, diarrhoea). 4) Check potassium, magnesium and calcium levels and maintain normal electrolyte levels. 5) If QTc <500 ms, continue Mfx or Bdq or Dlm and perform ECG once weekly. 6) If QTc $\geqslant$500 ms, temporarily hold all drugs prolonging QT and replace Mfx with high-dose Lfx later on.

Continued

https://doi.org/10.1183/2312508X.10021617

Table 2. Continued

Clinical presentation	Responsible drugs	Treatment/management
		7) If QTc is still $\geqslant$500 ms, consider discontinuing Cfz.
		8) If QTc is still $\geqslant$500 ms, consider discontinuing Bdq and/or Dlm.
Ototoxicity Hearing loss	**Km, Am, Cm**	Caution: continuing SLIDs despite hearing loss almost invariably results in irreversible deafness.
		1) If there is deterioration of hearing loss at month 2 ($\geqslant$grade 1), replace Km with Lzd and/or Bdq.
		2) If there is grade 1 or more hearing loss already at month 0, consider the use of Lzd (or Bdq) instead of Km.
		3) If Lzd is contraindicated, consider Bdq.
		4) Avoid furosemide, which increases drug toxicity.
		5) Hearing aids should be used if hearing loss is grade 2 or 3, if there is ototoxicity at treatment completion.

Drugs shown in bold are more strongly associated with the adverse effect. Pto: protionamide; Eto: ethionamide; H: isoniazid; R: rifampicin; E: ethambutol; Z. pyrazinamide; Cfz: clofazimine; Bdq: bedaquiline; DOT: directly observed therapy; FQ: fluoroquinolone: ALT: alanine aminotransferase; AST: aspartate aminotransferase; ULN: upper limit of normal; Lzd: linezolid; Km: kanamycin; Mfx: moxifloxacin; Am: amikacin, Cm: capreomycin; Cs: cycloserine; NSAID: nonsteroidal anti-inflammatory drug; Gfx: gatifloxacin; Dlm: delamanid; Lfx: levofloxacin; QTc: corrected QT interval; TdP: torsade de pointe. [#]: lactic acidosis is caused by a build-up of lactate in the body, which results in an excessively low pH in the blood, resulting in mitochondrial toxicity; symptoms include abdominal pain, nausea, vomiting, rapid deep breathing and general weakness. Reproduced and modified from [16] with permission.

Serious adverse events, which are either life-threatening or could cause permanent damage (degrees 3 and 4), can be managed by an experienced clinician who can identify the drug responsible for adverse event. In managing an adverse event, altering the dosage of the suspected drug(s) and using ancillary drugs should be tried before stopping the suspected causative drug(s).

Common adverse events: monitoring and management

The clinical presentation of the following ADRS, the drug(s) likely to be responsible and their treatment and management are summarised in table 2.

Hepatotoxicity

Hepatotoxicity is the most common adverse event of anti-TB treatment that leads to the interruption of therapy. In general, DILI accounts for 7% of reported drug adverse effects,

Table 3. Risk factors for adverse drug events (ADRs) and adverse events with anti-TB drugs

Advanced age
Malnutrition
Pregnancy and lactation
Alcoholism
Liver failure
Chronic renal failure
HIV infection
Disseminated and advanced TB
Allergy/atopy
Anaemia
DM
Family history of ADRs
Patients receiving intermittent treatment
Patients receiving medication for other disorders, in addition to anti-TB drugs

Reproduced and modified from [20] with permission.

2% of jaundice in hospitals and ~30% of fulminant liver failure [29]. The risk of DILI across diverse studies ranges from 5% to 33% [25].

DILI is a clinical diagnosis of exclusion. Other causes of liver injury, such as acute viral hepatitis, should be ruled out. The time of onset of acute liver injury ranges from weeks to months of starting a drug. The strongest confirmation of the diagnosis of DILI is re-challenging with the suspected offending agent leading to a >2-fold serum alanine aminotransferase (ALT) elevation, and discontinuation leading to a fall in ALT levels [30]. An increase in serum ALT is more specific for hepatocellular injury than an increase in

Table 4. Estimating severity grade for clinical adverse events not identified in the Division of AIDS grading table

Grade 1	Grade 2	Grade 3	Grade 4	Grade 5
Mild symptoms causing no or minimal interference with usual social and functional activities with intervention not indicated	Moderate symptoms causing greater than minimal interference with usual social and functional activities with medical intervention indicated, including ancillary drugs (see text)	Severe symptoms causing inability to perform usual social and functional activities with intervention or hospitalisation indicated	Potentially life-threatening symptoms causing inability to perform basic self-care functions with intervention indicated to prevent permanent impairment, persistent disability or death	All deaths related to an adverse event

Reproduced and modified from [28] with permission.

 https://doi.org/10.1183/2312508X.10021617

aspartate aminotransferase (AST), which can be due to abnormalities in the muscle, heart or kidney [31].

Although there are different definitions of hepatitis, the most accepted one is that recommended by the WHO [28], where hepatitis can be considered when one or more of the following three criteria are present during treatment: 1) ALT or AST five or more times the upper limit of normal (ULN); 2) ALT or AST three times the ULN with clinical manifestation; and/or 3) ALT or AST three or more times the ULN with a concomitant increase in bilirubin of ⩾1.5 times.

Drug-induced liver injury during anti-tuberculosis treatment

Metabolic idiosyncratic reactions appear to be responsible for most DILI from first-line anti-TB medications and fluoroquinolones. Isoniazid-associated hepatotoxicity occurs generally within weeks to months rather than the days to weeks of onset seen with hypersensitivity reactions. Unlike a classical hypersensitivity reaction, isoniazid re-challenge does not always elicit a rapid recurrence of hepatotoxicity [32]. The regression of isoniazid hepatotoxicity usually takes weeks, and recovery is complete in most patients after discontinuation of isoniazid. The severity of isoniazid-related hepatitis has been reported to increase with alcohol consumption [33] and with increasing age, with higher mortality in those >50 years [32].

Isoniazid inhibits the activity of several cytochrome P450 2E and 2C enzymes, potentially increasing the plasma concentrations of other potentially hepatotoxic drugs, such as phenytoin and carbamazepine [34].

In severe hepatotoxicity, patients may either be asymptomatic or manifest constitutional symptoms, which can last from days to weeks. Nausea, vomiting and abdominal pain are seen in 50–75% of patients with severe illness [25]. Overt jaundice, dark-coloured urine and clay-coloured stools are late signs of clinical worsening. Coagulopathy, hypoalbuminaemia and hypoglycaemia signify life-threatening hepatic dysfunction [25].

Rifampicin and rifapentine may occasionally cause dose-dependent interference with bilirubin uptake, resulting in subclinical unconjugated hyperbilirubinaemia or jaundice without hepatocellular damage. This may be transient and occurs early in treatment [35].

Rifampicin can occasionally cause hepatocellular injury and potentiate hepatotoxicity of other anti-TB medications. Rarely, hepatocellular injury appears to be a hypersensitivity reaction, and may be more common with large, intermittent dosages [35]. Intermittent dosages of rifampicin may also rarely lead to renal dysfunction, haemolytic anaemia or "flu-like syndrome" [36].

Idiosyncratic hypersensitivity reactions to rifampicin manifest as anorexia, nausea, vomiting, malaise, fever, mildly elevated ALT and elevated bilirubin, and usually occur in the first month of treatment initiation [35].

Pyrazinamide is probably the most hepatotoxic first-line anti-TB drug. This hepatotoxicity can be caused by two mechanisms: idiosyncratic and dose dependent. The hepatotoxicity of pyrazinamide increases with higher dosages. The half-life of pyrazinamide is longer than that of isoniazid and rifampicin; in patients with pre-existing hepatic disease, it may be increased to 15 h, requiring intermittent dosing in patients with renal insufficiency [37].

Drug-induced liver injury with second-line anti-tuberculosis agents

Generally, fluoroquinolones can be used safely in designing a new regimen when serious hepatitis has been generated by other anti-TB drugs [38]. Moxifloxacin is metabolised in part by the liver, whereas others (gatifloxacin, levofloxacin and ofloxacin) are largely excreted unchanged by the kidneys. Reversible transaminase elevation among the fluoroquinolones may occur in 2–3% of cases, and severe hepatocellular injury and cholestasis have been reported to occur in <1% of all fluoroquinolone recipients [38]. The mechanism of fluoroquinolone hepatotoxicity is believed to be a hypersensitivity reaction, often manifested by eosinophilia [25, 39].

In terms of other second-line anti-TB drugs, hepatotoxicity has been recognised to occur in ~2% of patients treated with ethionamide or prothionamide, and in 0.3% of patients treated with PAS [40, 41]. Cycloserine does not appear to be associated with hepatotoxicity but should be used with caution in patients at risk for alcohol-withdrawal seizures [42].

New anti-TB drugs (bedaquiline and delamanid) and new repurposed drugs (linezolid and clofazimine) do not usually cause hepatitis, although all of them have the potential to cause hepatitis [43]. Other first-line anti-TB drugs, such as ethambutol and streptomycin, and SLIDs are excreted by the kidneys and are not considered to be hepatotoxic [20, 21].

Management of drug-induced hepatitis

When DILI develops, the anti-TB treatment should be withheld until all biochemical markers of liver injury have returned to normal levels or when the ALT level is less than two times the ULN with resolution of hepatitis symptoms. This may take 2–4 weeks. If hepatitis develops when the patient has improved and has become smear negative, it is not necessary to give any anti-TB drugs, and recovery can be awaited. However, if the hepatitis develops in the initial stage of treatment, or when the patient is very sick, and the patient is smear positive, the patient should be initiated on an optimal "hepatitis-free" regimen during this period of recovery. This "hepatitis-free" regimen should include ethambutol, streptomycin or SLDIs, a fluoroquinolone and, if necessary, cycloserine [20, 21].

No evidence-based guidelines for re-introduction of anti-TB drugs after recovery of hepatitis are available, because of the lack of prospective RCTs. A study by Sharma *et al.* [44], which compared three predefined anti-TB drug re-introduction regimens in patients without liver risk factors, provided evidence of safety of introducing all three potentially hepatotoxic drugs (isoniazid, rifampicin and pyrazinamide) together. Overall, 89% of patients had successful re-introduction without recurrence. Even increased severity of the first episode of DILI was not associated with an increased risk of recurrence [44]. However, a study by Tahaoglu *et al.* [45], which included patients with liver risk factors, showed a higher recurrence rate of hepatotoxicity with re-introduction of a full-dose regimen including pyrazinamide than with gradual re-introduction of a regimen without pyrazinamide [45]. The first study revealed pre-treatment serum albumin levels to be an important predictor of a second recurrence of DILI [44].

Regarding the sequence of re-introduction of first-line drugs after an episode of hepatitis, and considering good bactericidal and sterilising activity, rifampicin should be introduced first [46]. Treatment with rifampicin, together with any other anti-TB drugs, can cure most TB patients with 9 months of therapy. Ideally, all the anti-TB drugs should be re-introduced by increasing the dose gradually until the recommended dose is tolerated.

https://doi.org/10.1183/2312508X.10021617

However, ethambutol can be restarted with the recommended dose from the first day because of its renal metabolism.

On day 1 of re-introduction, ethambutol should be given at full dose with rifampicin at a low dose of 100 mg. On day 2, the dose of rifampicin can be increased to 200 mg, and to 300 mg on day 3, and LFTs should be repeated. If LFTs show no worsening, rifampicin can be increased to 400 mg on day 4, to 500 mg on day 5 and to 600 mg on day 6, and LFTs should be repeated. If LFTs are favourable after this re-introduction of ethambutol with rifampicin, isoniazid can be added, depending on the severity of the hepatitis. If the onset of hepatitis was severe, isoniazid should not be re-introduced because the combination of ethambutol and rifampicin with any other effective drug, such as a fluoroquinolone, has the potential to cure all types of TB disease. If isoniazid is to be re-introduced, it should also be done gradually, with 50 mg on day 1, 100 mg on day 2 and 150 mg on day 3. LFTs should then be repeated. If the LFTs are favourable, 200 mg can be given on day 4, 250 mg on day 5 and 300 mg on day 6 [20, 21]. If ethambutol plus rifampicin plus isoniazid has been re-introduced without causing hepatitis, it may not be necessary to add pyrazinamide. A regimen with 2–3 months of ethambutol plus rifampicin plus isoniazid followed by 6–7 months of rifampicin plus isoniazid can cure practically all TB patients. Additionally, pyrazinamide is the most hepatotoxic first-line anti-TB drug [20, 21]. Once the drugs have been introduced, the levels of transaminases should be monitored on a monthly basis. If the re-introduction of drugs leads to a recurrence of the signs of hepatotoxicity, the culprit drug should be removed from the treatment and replaced with another drug.

Among the second-line drugs, ethionamide/prothionamide, PAS, linezolid and bedaquiline can also cause hepatitis, and very rarely the fluoroquinolones. Once hepatitis has been produced by these second-line drugs, re-challenge can be justified with core drugs (*e.g.* linezolid, bedaquiline and fluoroquinolones), but may not be justified with companion drugs (*e.g.* ethionamide/prothionamide and PAS), because companion drugs can usually be substituted by other drugs, or can even be removed, without compromising the efficacy of the regimen.

QT interval prolongation

The QT interval is an ECG measure that quantifies the flow of ion currents across the cell membrane of ventricular myocytes, which occurs through specialized protein channels. When these channels malfunction, they can disrupt normal cardiac rhythms and place a patient at risk of developing fatal cardiac arrhythmias [47]. Figure 1 shows a diagram of one ECG period or one heartbeat, while figure 2 shows a sample printout of the corrected QT interval (QTc) by Fridericia (QTcF or QTcFrid).

Many drugs have the potential to cause QT interval prolongation, with a risk of causing fatal arrhythmias. These drugs include fluoroquinolones (moxifloxacin more than levofloxacin and gatifloxacin), clofazimine, bedaquiline and delamanid. The risk of QTc prolongation with the fluoroquinolones is higher when there are electrolyte abnormalities and when other QTc-prolonging medications are used [49]. In addition, all macrolides have been shown to be associated with QTc prolongation and the development of torsade de pointe [50]. These drugs need close monitoring, especially when being used with other QT-prolonging drugs or in patients with a raised QT interval.

QT prolongation can be congenital, associated with abnormalities in potassium or sodium channels, or an acquired disorder. Risk factors for an acquired disorder are: female sex, the

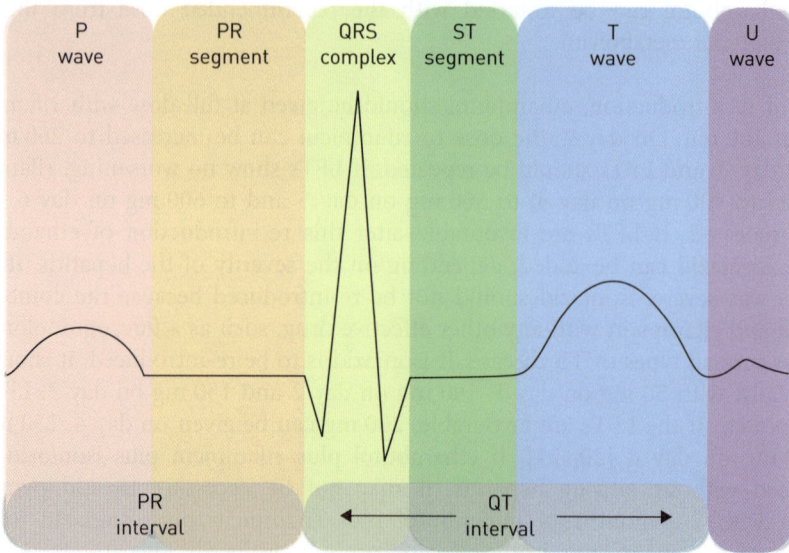

Figure 1. Diagram of one ECG period or one heartbeat. Reproduced and modified from [48] with permission.

elderly, cardiac pathologies (*e.g.* hypertrophy, heart failure, ischaemia), a slow heart rate, electrolytes imbalance (hypokalaemia, hypomagnesaemia or hypocalcaemia), some diseases (TB has been associated with this) and hundreds of medications that have been shown to prolong the QTc interval, such as antiemetics (metoclopramide and ondansetron at high dose), antipsychotics (haloperidol), antidepressants, antimalarials, diuretics (furosemide and thiazides) and anti-TB drugs [47].

Most patients with QTc prolongation are asymptomatic and the abnormality is only noted on routine ECG monitoring, but some patients may develop dizziness or light-headedness, or have episodes of syncope or near-syncope. These symptoms should prompt a thorough clinical assessment of a patient. If the patient develops torsade de pointe, they may succumb to sudden cardiac death, and hence emergency treatment is needed [47].

Because nearly all MDR-TB patients are receiving at least one QTc-prolonging drug, those who present suggestive symptoms should be hospitalised for intensive monitoring. Stopping bedaquiline and other QTc-prolonging medications should be considered if the

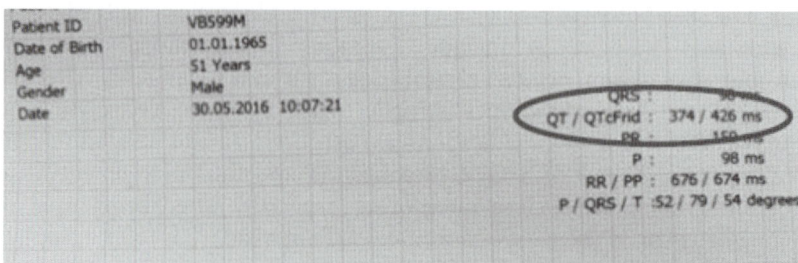

Figure 2. Sample printout showing the corrected QT interval by Fredericia (QTcFrid). Reproduced from [48] with permission.

https://doi.org/10.1183/2312508X.10021617

patient develops clinically significant ventricular arrhythmia or a QTc of >500 ms on multiple ECGs [48].

The QT interval is measured on a standard 12-lead ECG on leads II or V2 or V3 when it is longest, and with aVR and aVL leads where the U wave is absent, by assessing the interval from the beginning of the QRS complex to the end of the T wave. The QT interval is inversely proportional to heart rate, and needs correction for the same. There are several methods for correcting the QT interval; the most reliable are the Fridericia and the Framingham formulae [51–53]. A study by VISKIN et al. [54] showed that most physicians (60%), including many nonarrhythmia expert cardiologists (50%), cannot accurately calculate a QTc and cannot correctly determine whether the QT is normal or prolonged.

Two recently approved anti-TB drugs, bedaquiline and delamanid, have the potential to prolong the QTc interval and may be part of regimens including drugs with the same potential effect, such as fluoroquinolones, clofazimine, pretomanid, delamanid and azithromycin [47].

An evaluation of published studies highlighted the limited information provided on the cardiac safety of bedaquiline [55]. A systematic search showed that bedaquiline is a relatively well-tolerated drug, as its discontinuation occurred in only 3.4% and 0.6% of patients due to adverse events and QTc prolongation, respectively. Nevertheless, no complacency can be allowed, and strict ECG monitoring remains mandatory [55].

If QTc-prolonging medications are discontinued for cardiotoxicity, it is important that monitoring continues even after the agent is stopped. This is especially true for bedaquiline, which has a terminal elimination half-life of 5.5 months and should be monitored frequently to confirm that the QTc has returned to baseline. If necessary, the patient could be re-challenged with bedaquiline once all other potential QTc-prolonging conditions have been addressed, but this should only be done in extreme cases [56].

The risk of QTc prolongation is increased in persons taking delamanid who have low albumin levels, and this is another compelling reason to ensure that nutritional support is provided to individuals with DR-TB, especially those taking delamanid [57].

Recent data show that the use of bedaquiline and delamanid in combination appears to be safe [58].

Dermatological reactions

Self-limiting flushing and/or itching of the skin, usually on the face and the scalp with or without a rash, may occur within 2–3 h after drug ingestion, especially with rifampicin or pyrazinamide [3, 59].

A full range of cutaneous hypersensitivity reactions may occur with any anti-TB medication. The Division of AIDS Adverse Experience Reporting System (DAERS) has classified rash into different grades: mild (localised rash), moderate (diffuse rash or target lesions), severe (diffuse rash and vesicles or limited number of bullae or superficial ulcerations of mucous membrane limited to one site) and potentially life-threatening (extensive or generalised bullous lesions or ulceration of mucous membrane involving two or more distinct mucosal sites or Stevens–Johnson syndrome or toxic epidermal necrolysis) [28].

Acute allergic reactions have been classified into different grades based on the type of rash and the intervention required: mild (localised urticarial with no medical intervention indicated), moderate (localised urticaria with intervention indicated or mild angioedema with no intervention indicated), severe (generalised urticaria or angioedema with intervention indicated or symptoms of mild bronchospasm) and potentially life-threatening (acute anaphylaxis or life-threatening bronchospasm or laryngeal oedema) [28].

For moderate and severe reactions, anti-TB drugs should be stopped. After the skin rash subsides, re-challenging with core drugs (rifampicin, isoniazid, fluoroquinolones and linezolid) should be done sequentially and gradually every 1–3 days under close observation. Almost always, it is not justified to try re-challenging with companion drugs (ethambutol, ethionamide/prothionamide, cycloserine or PAS) because of the severity of the ADR and the secondary role of these drugs. This should preferably be done in order of increasing risk of hypersensitivity (isoniazid and rifampicin in the case of first-line drugs) [59]. If a reaction occurs during drug re-challenge and the causative drug cannot readily be replaced or discontinued, drug desensitisation may be considered, except in patients with severe skin reactions or reactions involving the mouth or mucous membranes [3, 59, 60]. Desensitisation should be carried out in a hospital or clinical area with the ability to monitor and respond to possible anaphylaxis and with microbiological monitoring, because rapid emergence of drug resistance has been reported during desensitisation [3, 60, 61].

Gastrointestinal reactions

Gastritis, nausea and vomiting occur commonly with anti-TB drugs, especially PAS and thionamides. Nevertheless, acute or chronic medical/surgical problems, such as hepatotoxicity, should be ruled out. In females of reproductive age, pregnancy should also be ruled out [3, 18, 62]. Diarrhoea, although encountered less frequently than nausea and vomiting, is also commonly associated with PAS and thionamides, and other anti-TB drugs may also be responsible [62]. Recent unusual food or drug intake and associated symptoms should also be examined to exclude alternative causes or other acute or chronic medical/ surgical problems [3].

Nephrotoxicity

Nephrotoxicity is a known complication of the injectable drugs, including both capreomycin and aminoglycosides. Kanamycin and amikacin are more nephrotoxic than streptomycin [3, 62]. Ethambutol and cycloserine are metabolised mainly in the kidneys, and for this reason they can produce renal impairment and should be used with caution in patients with renal insufficiency.

The risk factors identified for nephrotoxicity include old age, underlying renal impairment, a high blood concentration (especially trough levels) of injectable drugs, prolonged use of injectable drugs, concurrent use of other nephrotoxic drugs or loop diuretics, hypotension, dehydration and liver disease [3, 62]. In the presence of such risk factors, pre-treatment screening and serial monitoring of serum creatinine and potassium are indicated [62, 63].

https://doi.org/10.1183/2312508X.10021617

In patients with reduced creatinine clearance or those undergoing haemodialysis, no change in the dosing of isoniazid and rifampicin is necessary, as they are metabolised mainly through the hepatic route. However, in these situations, dose adjustment is required for ethambutol and pyrazinamide [3, 17, 18].

Because of an increased risk of nephrotoxicity and ototoxicity, injectable drugs should be avoided in patients with renal impairment. However, if their use is necessary, the dose and/or the interval between dosing should be adjusted initially, and subsequent modification should be done as per TDM [3, 17, 18]. Among the newer/repurposed drugs, bedaquiline, delamanid, linezolid and clofazimine do not require any dose adjustment in renal impairment.

Neurotoxicity

Peripheral neuropathy has been associated with isoniazid, ethionamide, cycloserine, linezolid and, rarely, fluoroquinolones and ethambutol [3, 59, 62]. Neuropathy with most anti-TB drugs, except linezolid, can usually be prevented with pyridoxine prophylaxis, especially in patients with DM, alcoholism, HIV infection, hypothyroidism, pregnancy or poor nutrition, and in those with inadequate dietary intake of pyridoxine [3, 59, 60, 62].

Neuropathy is usually diagnosed clinically. The patient complains of a prickling, tingling or burning sensation in the fingers and/or toes in a symmetrical stocking and glove distribution. This may be followed by sensory loss, absent ankle reflexes, weakness of dorsiflexion of the toes, centripetal progression with involvement of the fingers and hands, and unsteadiness of gait due to proprioceptive loss. In these situations, aggravating factors or alternative causes should be excluded [3, 59, 60, 62].

Ototoxicity

Vestibular and auditory toxicity have been associated with aminoglycosides and capreomycin, especially with increasing age, pre-existing hearing loss, coexistent use of ototoxic drugs (e.g. thiazide diuretics), high serum drug concentrations, prior aminoglycoside use and high accumulative dose [3, 62]. Streptomycin causes mostly vestibular toxicity, while capreomycin is more toxic to the cochlea [64].

Vestibular toxicity may present as vertigo, incoordination, unsteadiness, dizziness, tinnitus and nausea. Auditory toxicity with hearing loss could also be associated with vestibular toxicity. Rarely, cycloserine, fluoroquinolones, ethionamide, isoniazid or linezolid may also cause similar symptoms, and need to be carefully excluded as a cause [3, 60, 62, 65]. Drug-induced vestibular toxicity is generally irreversible and is linked to the destruction of basal hairy cells of the reticular membrane of the cochlea. These cells do not regenerate. Injectable drugs should be stopped if tinnitus and unsteadiness develop due to vestibular toxicity [17–19, 60].

Some degree of hearing loss occurs in nearly all patients treated for DR-TB. Auditory toxicity usually affects higher frequencies at an early stage. Frequencies between 500 and 4000 Hz are considered to be those of a normal conversation. Higher frequencies (4000–8000 Hz) are the first to be affected, while the frequencies of the human voice come next. Hearing loss becomes perceptible for patients at a frequency of <4000 Hz when it reaches

25–30 dB [64, 66]. When patients mention hearing loss, there is already a severe degree of loss. Serial audiograms may help to detect ototoxicity early and monitor patients at risk [18, 63, 67]. Extended audiometry analysing higher frequencies (12 000–20 000 Hz) allows the detection of early ototoxicity. Patients with hearing loss beyond 8000 Hz should be evaluated on an individual basis. To decrease the risk of hearing loss, injectable drugs may be switched to three times per week. Therefore, if auditory toxicity develops, injectable drugs should be stopped and replaced by other drugs [67].

Ophthalmic toxicity

Ethambutol is associated with optic neuritis, especially at doses >15 mg daily, when used over 2 months, in elderly patients and in those with renal insufficiency. In renal insufficiency, if ethambutol cannot be avoided, suitable adjustment of the dose/dosing interval should be made [17–19, 60]. In a meta-analysis by EZER et al. [68], some visual impairment was observed in 22.5 per 1000 persons receiving standard doses of ethambutol for up to 9 months, with permanent impairment in 2.3 per 1000 persons treated. The majority of episodes were reversible, and resolution of impairment occurred after an average of 3 months [3, 68].

Ocular toxicity can be caused by linezolid (toxic ocular neuropathy, often nonreversible), isoniazid, ethionamide, rifabutin (reversible panuveitis) and clofazimine (bullseye pigmentary maculopathy and generalised retinal degeneration) [60, 69]. Special attention should be paid to possible toxic ocular neuropathy when linezolid is used. Optic neuritis typically presents with blurred vision, scotoma and/or red/green colour blindness. Early detection can be achieved through proper patient education, together with baseline testing and monthly monitoring of visual acuity and colour discrimination [60]. Nutritional deficiency, especially of B-complex vitamins and folate, should be evaluated and corrected. When optic neuritis is suspected, the drug(s) likely to have caused this reaction (ethambutol and linezolid) should be removed.

Central nervous system toxicity

Cycloserine, thionamides, isoniazid and fluoroquinolones are known to cause central nervous system toxicity [3, 62]. Patients should be cautioned about symptoms such as headache, concentration problems, irritability, mild mood changes, insomnia and agitation, as well as drowsiness, peripheral neuropathy and convulsions. Central nervous system toxicity commonly occurs early in the treatment but typically becomes less problematic after the initial weeks of therapy [3, 60].

In isoniazid-induced depression, withdrawal of the drug usually leads to rapid recovery [3, 60]. Antidepressants may be tried in patients with more severe depression, although these drugs may be contraindicated when the patient is taking linezolid.

Neuropsychiatric reactions to cycloserine are common, especially with higher doses or concomitant alcohol use. These reactions may include excitement, anxiety, aggression, confusion, depression, suicidal ideation and psychosis [62]. Psychiatric assessment should be done for neuropsychiatric symptoms, especially in patients with a history of seizures or psychiatric problems [3, 18, 60]. Psychosocial support and clinical assessment should be

https://doi.org/10.1183/2312508X.10021617

considered, and other possible aetiologies or contributing factors (including drug interactions) should be carefully excluded [18, 60].

Miscellaneous adverse reactions

Haematological toxicity

A diverse range of haematological reactions can follow the administration of anti-TB drugs. Most of these are rare, with the exception of the haematological abnormalities associated with thioacetazone [3, 70].

Immune-mediated thrombocytopenic purpura and haemolytic anaemia have been associated with rifamycins, especially with intermittent use at high doses. For major haematological toxicities such as rifamycin-associated thrombocytopenic purpura and haemolytic anaemia, the offending drug should be stopped promptly and not used again [3, 60, 62]. Dose-dependent bone marrow toxicity is very common with the prolonged use of linezolid at the conventional dosage (600 mg twice daily), common with an attenuated dosage (600–800 mg once daily) [30] and uncommon with a highly attenuated dosage (300 mg once daily) [71]. For mild linezolid-associated haematological toxicity, dose reduction under close monitoring should be tried, after carefully balancing the benefits and risks [71]. Pyridoxine-responsive sideroblastic anaemia can be prevented and treated with pyridoxine [3]. For isolated and asymptomatic eosinophilia, in the absence of other associated hypersensitivity reactions, it is often possible to continue treatment with close monitoring [3].

Influenza-like syndrome

An immune-mediated influenza-like syndrome has been associated with the use of rifamycins, especially with intermittent therapy at a high dose [62]. The syndrome usually presents after 3–6 months of intermittent therapy with fever, headache and bone pain 1–2 h after drug administration, and generally resolves within 12 h. Besides symptomatic treatment, switching from intermittent therapy to daily dosing may reduce the frequency and severity of symptoms [3, 62].

Arthralgia

Arthralgia presenting with mild pain and tenderness of joints has been associated with pyrazinamide, fluoroquinolones, ethambutol and isoniazid in decreasing frequency [3, 59, 62]. Gout syndrome may occur with pyrazinamide and rarely with ethambutol. Uric acid levels may be elevated in these patients. However, raised uric acid levels should, in general, not be a reason to interrupt treatment [3, 59, 60, 62].

Tendinitis and tendon rupture have been reported with fluoroquinolone use, especially in older patients, patients with DM or chronic renal failure, those receiving corticosteroids and those undertaking new physical activities [3, 60].

Hypothyroidism

Hypothyroidism may develop with either PAS or ethionamide. When both drugs are used, a high incidence of hypothyroidism has been observed, ranging from 10% to 50% of patients [18, 72, 73]. As the symptoms can be subtle, it is recommended that patients are screened for hypothyroidism by measurement of serum thyroid-stimulating hormone (TSH). In areas where iodine-deficiency goitres are endemic, early screening may be

Table 5. Ancillary drugs used in the management of adverse drug reactions

Therapeutic class	Drug(s)
Antidepressants	Amitriptyline
Antidiarrhoeals	Loperamide
Antiemetics	Metoclopramide (or metopimazine) and ondansetron
Antihistamines	Cetirizine
Antiulcer drugs	Cimetidine (or ranitidine) and omeprazole
Corticosteroids	Prednisolone and hydrocortisone
Nonsteroidal anti-inflammatory drugs	Acetylsalicylic acid and ibuprofen
Vitamins and mineral supplements	Pyridoxine (vitamin B6), potassium and magnesium

indicated, with iodine treatment where necessary [3, 73]. If the TSH level rises to 1.5–2.6 times the ULN, thyroid hormone replacement should be instituted, with adjustment as necessary to return the TSH level to the normal range. Thyroid hormone replacement can usually be stopped when TB treatment is complete [3, 60].

Ancillary drugs in the management of adverse drug reactions

Grade 1 adverse events need only be noted in the patient's card, whereas grade 2 adverse events require medical intervention with ancillary drugs, the most frequently used of which are shown in table 5. These drugs should be stocked and available at all times in TB treatment units where patients with DR-TB are being treated.

Recording and reporting of anti-tuberculosis adverse drug reactions

All adverse events should be recorded in the patient's card and in a database by type, degree and month of appearance. The database should be updated with an annual analysis of each patient cohort.

Severe adverse events (grades 3 and 4) should be notified to the relevant authorities using national adverse events reporting forms.

Conclusion

As TB treatment requires long-term treatment with several drugs, each with its own set of potentially adverse reactions, the early detection and adequate management of these reactions is essential for successful treatment of TB. As these drugs may produce a wide range of adverse reactions involving various systems, it is imperative to ensure the availability of and coordination with medical experts of the respective specialties for proper management of these toxicities. Ancillary drugs required for the treatment of these reactions should also be made available. Taking all of these factors into account will go a long way in maximising patient compliance, leading to good outcomes.

Severe adverse events, which are either life-threatening or could cause permanent damage (degrees 3 and 4), should be managed by an experienced clinician who will identify the

https://doi.org/10.1183/2312508X.10021617

drug responsible, reduce the dosage or discontinue its use, and replace it with an equivalent drug if the drug needs to be definitively discontinued.

References

1. WHO. Active Tuberculosis Drug-safety Monitoring and Management (aDSM). Framework for Implementation. WHO/HTM/TB/2015.28. Geneva, WHO, 2015. www.who.int/tb/publications/aDSM/en/
2. Tupasi T, Garfin AMCG, Mangan JM, *et al.* Multidrug-resistant tuberculosis patients' views of interventions to reduce treatment loss to follow-up. *Int J Tuberc Lung Dis* 2017; 21: 23–31.
3. Leung CC, Daley CL, Rieder HL, *et al.* Management of adverse drug events in TB therapy. *In:* Lange C, Migliori GB, eds. Tuberculosis (ERS Monograph). Sheffield, European Respiratory Society, 2012; pp. 167–193.
4. Chang KC, Leung CC, Tam CM. Risk factors for defaulting from anti-tuberculosis treatment under directly observed treatment in Hong Kong. *Int J Tuberc Lung Dis* 2004; 8: 1492–1498.
5. Tekle B, Mariam DH, Ali A. Defaulting from DOTS and its determinants in three districts of Arsi Zone in Ethiopia. *Int J Tuberc Lung Dis* 2002; 6: 573–579.
6. Mori T, Leung CC. Tuberculosis in the global aging population. *Infect Dis Clin North Am* 2010; 24: 751–768.
7. Pal S N, Lienhardt C, Olsson S, *et al.* Enhancing patient safety: new WHO guidance on pharmacovigilance in tuberculosis care. *Eur Respir J* 2012; 40: Suppl. 56, P2875.
8. Kelly AM, Smith B, Luo Z, *et al.* Discordance between patient and clinician reports of adverse reactions to MDR-TB treatment. *Int J Tuberc Lung Dis* 2016; 20: 442–447.
9. British Thoracic Association. A controlled trial of 6 months' chemotherapy in pulmonary tuberculosis. Final report: results during the 36 months after the end of chemotherapy and beyond. *Br J Dis Chest* 1984; 78: 330–336.
10. Hong Kong Chest Service/British Medical Research Council. Controlled trial of 4 three-times-weekly regimens and a daily regimen all given for 6 months for pulmonary tuberculosis. Second report: the results up to 24 months. *Tubercle* 1982; 63: 89–98.
11. Nathanson E, Gupta R, Huamani P, *et al.* Adverse events in the treatment of multidrug-resistant tuberculosis: results from the DOTS-Plus initiative. *Int J Tuberc Lung Dis* 2004; 8: 1382–1384.
12. Törün T, Güngör G, Ozmen I, *et al.* Side effects associated with the treatment of multidrug-resistant tuberculosis. *Int J Tuberc Lung Dis* 2005; 9: 1373–1377.
13. Wu S, Zhang Y, Sun F, *et al.* Adverse events associated with the treatment of multidrug-resistant tuberculosis: a systematic review and meta-analysis. *Am J Ther* 2016; 23: e521–e530.
14. Ahmad Khan F, Salim MAH, du Cros P, *et al.* Effectiveness and safety of standardised shorter regimens for multidrug-resistant tuberculosis: individual patient data and aggregate data meta-analyses. *Eur Respir J* 2017; 27: 1700061.
15. Trébucq A, Schwoebel V, Kashongwe Z, *et al.* Treatment outcome with a short multidrug-resistant tuberculosis regimen in nine African countries. *Int J Tuberc Lung Dis* 2018; 11: 17–25.
16. Daley CL, Caminero JA. Management of multidrug-resistant tuberculosis. *Sem Respir Crit Care Med* 2018; 39: 310–324.
17. WHO. Guidelines for Treatment of Tuberculosis. Document WHO/HTM/TB/2009.420. 4th Edn. Geneva, WHO, 2010. www.who.int/tb/publications/2010/9789241547833/en/
18. WHO. Guidelines for Treatment of Drug-susceptible Tuberculosis and Patient Care (2017 Update). Document WHO/HTM/TB/2017.05. Geneva, WHO, 2017. www.who.int/tb/publications/2017/dstb_guidance_2017/en/
19. WHO. Treatment of Drug-resistant TB: Resources 2016 Update, October 2016 revision. Document WHO/HTM/TB/2016.04. Geneva, WHO, 2016. www.who.int/tb/areas-of-work/drug-resistant-tb/treatment/resources/en/
20. Farga V, Caminero JA. Tuberculosis. Santiago, Mediterráneo, 2011.
21. Caminero JA. A Tuberculosis Guide for Specialist Physicians. Paris, IUATLD 2003.
22. Breen RA, Miller RF, Gorsuch T, *et al.* Adverse events and treatment interruption in tuberculosis patients with and without HIV co-infection. *Thorax* 2006; 61: 791–794.
23. Marks DJ, Dheda K, Dawson R, *et al.* Burden of antituberculosis and antiretroviral drug-induced liver injury at a secondary hospital in South Africa. *S Afr Med J* 2012; 102: 506–511.
24. Schutz C, Ismail Z, Proxenos C. Burden of antituberculosis and antiretroviral drug-induced liver injury at a secondary hospital in South Africa. *S Afr Med J* 2012; 102: 506–511.
25. Saukkonen JJ, Cohn DL, Jasmer RM, *et al.* An official ATS statement: hepatotoxicity of antituberculosis therapy. *Am J Respir Crit Care Med* 2006; 174: 935–952.
26. Ungo JR, Jones D, Ashkin D, *et al.* Antituberculosis drug-induced hepatotoxicity: the role of hepatitis C virus and the human immunodeficiency virus. *Am J Respir Crit Care Med* 1998; 157: 1871–1876.
27. WHO. A Practical Handbook on the Pharmacovigilance of Medicines Used in the Treatment of Tuberculosis. Enhancing the Safety of the TB patient. Geneva, Switzerland, 2012. www.who.int/medicines/publications/pharmacovigilance_tb/en/

28. Division of AIDS, National Institute of Allergy and Infectious Diseases. Division of AIDS (DAIDS) Table for Grading the Severity of Adult and Pediatric Adverse Events. Corrected version 2.1. Bethesda, US Department of Health and Human Services, National Institutes of Health, 2017. https://rsc.tech-res.com/docs/default-source/safety/daidsgradingcorrecetedv21.pdf

29. Larrey D. Epidemiology and individual susceptibility to adverse drug reactions affecting the liver. *Semin Liver Dis* 2002; 22: 145–155.

30. Bénichou C. Criteria for drug-induced liver disorder: report of an international consensus meeting. *J Hepatol* 1990; 11: 272–276.

31. Dufour DR, Lott JA, Nolte FS, *et al.* Diagnosis and monitoring of hepatic injury: I. Performance characteristics of laboratory tests. *Clin Chem* 2000; 46: 2027–2049.

32. Mitchell JR, Zimmerman HJ, Ishak KG, *et al.* Isoniazid liver injury: clinical spectrum, pathology, and probable pathogenesis. *Ann Intern Med* 1976; 84: 181–192.

33. Kopanoff DE, Snider DE, Johnson M. Isoniazid related hepatitis: a U.S. Public Health Service cooperative surveillance study. *Am Rev Respir Dis* 1979; 117: 991–1001.

34. Desta Z, Soukhova NV, Flockhart DA. Inhibition of cytochrome P450 (CYP450) isoforms by isoniazid: potent inhibition of CYP2C19 and CYP3A. *Antimicrob Agents Chemother* 2001; 45: 382–392.

35. Grosset J, Leventis S. Adverse effects of rifampin. *Rev Infect Dis* 1983; 5: Suppl. 3, S440–S446.

36. Martinez E, Collazos J, Mayo J. Hypersensitivity reactions to rifampin. *Medicine* 1999; 78: 361–369.

37. Lacroix C, Tranvouez JL, Phan HT, *et al.* Pharmacokinetics of pyrazinamide and its metabolites in patients with hepatic cirrhotic insufficiency. *Arzneimittelforschung* 1990; 40: 76–79.

38. Bertino J Jr, Fish D. The safety profile of the fluoroquinolones. *Clin Ther* 2000; 22: 798–817.

39. Coleman CI, Spencer JV, Chung JO, *et al.* Possible gatifloxacin-induced fulminant hepatic failure. *Ann Pharmacother* 2002; 36: 1162–1167.

40. British Thoracic Association. A comparison of the toxicity of prothionamide and ethionamide: a report from the research committee of the British Tuberculosis Association. *Tubercle* 1968; 49: 125–135.

41. Rossouw JE, Saunders J. Hepatic complications of antituberculous therapy. *QJM* 1975; 44: 1–16.

42. Blumberg HM, Burman WJ, Chaisson RE, *et al.* American Thoracic Society/Centers for Disease Control and Prevention/Infectious Diseases Society of America: treatment of tuberculosis. *Am J Respir Crit Care Med* 2003; 167: 603–662.

43. DR-TB STAT. Treatment of Drug-Resistant TB with New and Re-Purposed Medications: a Field Guide. Cleveland, DR-TB STAT, 2018.

44. Sharma SK, Singla R, Sarda P, *et al.* Safety of 3 different reintroduction regimens of antituberculosis drugs after development of antituberculosis treatment-induced hepatotoxicity. *Clin Infect Dis* 2010; 50: 833–839.

45. Tahaoğlu K, Ataç G, Sevim T, *et al.* The management of anti-tuberculosis drug-induced hepatotoxicity. *Int J Tuberc Lung Dis* 2001; 5: 65–69.

46. Caminero JA, Alberto Matteelli A, Lange C. Treatment of TB. *In*: Lange C, Migliori GB, eds. Tuberculosis (ERS Monograph). Sheffield, European Respiratory Society, 2012; pp. 154–166.

47. Harausz E, Cox H, Rich M, *et al.* QTc prolongation and treatment of multidrug-resistant tuberculosis. *Int J Tuberc Lung Dis* 2015; 119: 385–391.

48. USAID/KNCV Tuberculosis Foundation/Challenge TB. Guidance on Requirements for QTc Measurement in ECG Monitoring When Introducing New Drugs and Shorter Regimens for the Treatment of Drug-Resistant Tuberculosis. USAID/Challenge TB/KNCV Tuberculosis Foundation, 2017. https://www.challengetb.org/publications/tools/pmdt/Guidance_on_ECG_monitoring_in_NDR.pd

49. Falagas ME, Rafailidis PI, Rosmarakis ES. Arrhythmias associated with fluoroquinolone therapy. *Int J Antimicrob Agents* 2007; 29: 374–379.

50. Abu-Gharbieh E, Vasina V, Poluzzi E, *et al.* Antibacterial macrolides: a drug class with a complex pharmacological profile. *Pharmacol Res* 2004; 50: 211–222.

51. Vandenberk B, Vandael E, Robyns T, *et al.* Which QT correction formulae to use for QT monitoring? *J Am Hear Assoc* 2016; 5: e003264.

52. Goldenberg I, Moss AJ, Zareba W. QT interval: how to measure it and what is "normal". *J Cardiovasc Electrophysiol* 2006; 17: 333–336.

53. Indik JH, Pearson EC, Fried K, *et al.* Bazett and Fridericia QT correction formulas interfere with measurement of drug-induced changes in QT interval. *Hear Rhythm* 2006; 3: 1003–1007.

54. Viskin S, Rosovski U, Sands AJ, *et al.* Inaccurate electrocardiographic interpretation of long QT: the majority of physicians cannot recognize a long QT when they see one. *Hear Rhythm* 2005; 2: 569–576.

55. Pontali E, Sotgiu G, Tiberi S, *et al.* Cardiac safety of bedaquiline: a systematic and critical analysis of the evidence. *Eur Respir J* 2017; 50: 1701462.

56. CDC. Provisional CDC guidelines for the use and safety monitoring of bedaquiline fumarate (Sirturo) for the treatment of multidrug-resistant tuberculosis. *MMWR Recomm Rep* 2013; 62: 1–12.

57. Potter JL, Capstick T, Ricketts WM, *et al.* A UK-based resource to support the monitoring and safe use of anti-tuberculosis drugs and second-line treatment of multidrug-resistant tuberculosis. *TB Drug Monographs* 2015; 2015: 90–96.

https://doi.org/10.1183/2312508X.10021617

58. Ferlazzo G, Mohr E, Laxmeshwar C, *et al.* Early safety and efficacy of the combination of bedaquiline and delamanid for the treatment of patients with drug-resistant tuberculosis in Armenia, India, and South Africa: a retrospective cohort study. *Lancet Infect Dis* 2018; 18: 536–544.

59. Girling DJ. Adverse effects of antituberculosis drugs. *Drugs* 1982; 23: 56–74.

60. Francis J. Curry National Tuberculosis Center and California Department of Public Health. Drug-resistant Tuberculosis: a Survival Guide for Clinicians. 2nd Edn. Oakland, Francis J. Curry National Tuberculosis Center and California Department of Public Health, 2008. www.tn.gov/content/dam/tn/health/documents/tuberculosis_guidelines/TB_FJCSurvivalGuide.pdf

61. Horne NW, Grant IWB. Development of drug resistance to isoniazid during desensitization: a report of two cases. *Tubercle* 1963; 44: 180–182.

62. Philadelphia Tuberculosis Control Program. Guidelines for the Management of Adverse Drug Effects of Antimycobacterial Agents. Philadelphia, Lawrence Flick Memorial Tuberculosis Clinic, Philadelphia Tuberculosis Control Program, 1998.

63. Begg EJ, Barclay ML. Aminoglycosides – 50 years on. *Br J Clin Pharmacol* 1995; 39: 597–603.

64. de Jager P, van Altena R. Hearing loss and nephrotoxicity in long-term aminoglycoside treatment in patients with tuberculosis. *Int J Tuberc Lung Dis* 2002; 6: 622–627.

65. Selimoglu E. Aminoglycoside-induced ototoxicity. *Curr Pharm Des* 2007; 13: 119–126.

66. Brummett RE, Fox KE. Aminoglycoside-induced hearing loss in humans. *Antimicrob Agents Chemother* 1989; 33: 797–800.

67. Duggal P, Sarkar M. Audiologic monitoring of multi-drug resistant tuberculosis patients on aminoglycoside treatment with long term follow-up. *BMC Ear Nose Throat Disord* 2007; 7: 1–7.

68. Ezer N, Benedetti A, Darvish-Zargar M, *et al.* Incidence of ethambutol-related visual impairment during treatment of active tuberculosis. *Int J Tuberc Lung Dis* 2013; 17: 447–455.

69. Tang S, Yao L, Hao X, *et al.* Efficacy, safety and tolerability of linezolid for the treatment of XDR-TB: a study in China. *Eur Respir J* 2015; 45: 161–170.

70. Holdiness MR. A review of blood dyscrasias induced by the antituberculosis drugs. *Tubercule* 1987; 68: 301–309.

71. Koh WJ, Kwon OJ, Gwak H, *et al.* Daily 300 mg dose of linezolid for the treatment of intractable multidrug-resistant and extensively drug-resistant tuberculosis. *J Antimicrob Chemother* 2009; 64: 388–391.

72. Satti H, Mafukidze A, Jooste PL, *et al.* High rate of hypothyroidism among patients treated for multidrug-resistant tuberculosis in Lesotho. *Int J Tuberc Lung Dis* 2012; 16: 468–472.

73. Thee S, Zöllner EW, Willemse M, *et al.* Abnormal thyroid function tests in children on ethionamide treatment. *Int J Tuberc Lung Dis* 2011; 15: 1191–1193.

Disclosures: None declared.

Chapter 13

Surgery as a treatment

Anne Olland[1,2], Pierre-Emmanuel Falcoz[1,2], Sophie Guinard[1,2],
Joseph Seitlinger[1,2] and Gilbert Massard[1,2]

To date, well conducted chemotherapy will cure up to 85% of all pulmonary TB cases. In this vast majority of patients, surgery will be limited to a diagnostic tool. Video-assisted thoracic surgery and other elective mini-invasive approaches (mediastinoscopy) will help biopsy small lung nodules and/or diseased lymph nodes. But, in the case of MDR-/XDR-TB patients, anatomical lung resections (lobectomy and pneumonectomy) will help eradicate tuberculous cavitations still hosting mycobacterias, despite well-conducted chemotherapy. The strategy for lung resection in MDR-/XDR-TB patients will be determined by a multidisciplinary team taking into account the medical history of the patient, comorbidities, the recent history and evolution of the TB under appropriate chemotherapy, and a complete pre-operative work up of the patient, including nutritional status, and respiratory and cardiovascular functional status. High rates of favourable outcomes (over 90%) have been described provided surgery was applied during the first year of newly diagnosed MDR-/XDR-TB. In the meantime, reporting results of collapse therapy (pneumothorax/pneumoperitoneum) during the first year of a newly diagnosed destructive TB, studies demonstrate clinical recovery in 93.9% of patients. Surgery provides excellent results for curing MDR-/XDR-TB insisting on the need for performing surgery following the actual guidelines, and during the first year of TB diagnose without neglecting the true efficiency of collapse therapy despite its old-fashioned appearance.

Cite as: Olland A, Falcoz P-E, Guinard S, et al. Surgery as a treatment. In: Migliori GB, Bothamley G, Duarte R, et al, eds. Tuberculosis (ERS Monograph). Sheffield, European Respiratory Society, 2018; pp. 228–233 [https://doi.org/10.1183/2312508X.10021717].

🐦 @ERSpublications
To date surgery still has an important role to play, especially in MDR-/XDR-TB patients. Anatomical resections of destroyed lung or tuberculous cavitation will act in a multidisciplinary approach combined to pre- and post-operative chemotherapy. http://ow.ly/cfVQ30lqCfE

Before the era of anti-TB drugs, surgery was the only treatment available for respiratory TB; it initially relied on the different variants of collapse therapy including intrapleural pneumothorax, extrapleural pneumothorax, extraperiosteal plombage and thoracoplasty [1–4].

[1]Thoracic Surgery Dept, University Hospital Strasbourg, Strasbourg, France. [2]INSERM (French National Institute of Health and Medical Research), UMR 1260, Regenerative Nanomedicine (RNM), FMTS, Strasbourg, France.

Correspondence: Gilbert Massard, Hôpitaux Universitaires de Strasbourg, Thoracic Surgery Dept, Nouvel Hôpital Civil, 1 place de l'Hôpital, Strasbourg 67000, France. E-mail: gilbert.massard@chru-strasbourg.fr

https://doi.org/10.1183/2312508X.10021717

Nowadays, with the exception of MDR-TB and XDR-TB, well-conducted TB chemotherapy will cure up to 85% of all sputum-positive patients. In these patients, the role of surgery will be limited to a diagnostic purpose [5]. Indeed, surgery will objectively help for diagnostic purposes when dealing with a high suspicion of TB, but will also correct the diagnose to TB when considering pulmonary nodules detected during thoracic imaging.

Surgery still has a place of choice for treating post-TB sequalae and MDR-/XDR-TB [2, 3, 6, 7].

Surgical diagnosis of tuberculosis

In the era of low-dose computed tomography and video-assisted thoracic surgery (VATS), incidental TB may arise from large cohorts of patients undergoing screening for lung cancer [8, 9]. At the time of surgery, TB is not yet the indication for surgery, only the nodule represents a target in high-risk patients for bronchogenic carcinoma. In only a few cases will the nodule eventually turn out to be TB, and so performing explorative surgical resection for a lung nodule should not neglect the hypothesis for TB, even if scarce [8, 9].

Besides incidental surgery for TB, surgery may also be the choice for a definitive diagnosis of TB. Mediastinoscopy or VATS surgery for highly suspicious lymph nodes or lung nodules have an excellent diagnostic yield [9].

Surgery for multidrug-resistant/extensively drug-resistant tuberculosis

Epidemiology

The practise and experience in surgery for the treatment of TB will be highly dependent on the incidence of TB in a given geographical region. Nowadays, surgery for TB is commonly performed in countries with a high incidence of TB. In the meantime, in countries with a low incidence of TB, the practise of surgery in that indication will be concentrated in a few highly specialised centres.

Exploring the data from a nationwide French prospective database, RIVERA et al. [10] showed 5975 pneumonectomies were performed over a 10-year period (January 2003 to June 2013). Amongst them, 321 pneumonectomies had been performed for benign disease and of these 48 (15%) had been performed to treat TB. On the contrary, in countries with a high incidence of TB, surgeons may present with an individual performance of nearly 5600 surgical procedures with curative intent for the treatment of TB [4]. In South Africa, ALEXANDER et al. [11] reported 60 surgical cases for curative treatment of TB in a single institution over a 1-year study period (2012–2013).

Indications

Historically, surgery was the first efficient treatment for TB. HASTINGS and STORKS [1] performed the first cavernostomy in 1844. In the modern era, well-conducted chemotherapy offers a successful treatment to most TB cases with no need for further surgery except for diagnostic purposes.

However, when addressing MDR-/XDR-TB, surgery will be most helpful to eradicate parenchymal cavitations hosting *Mycobacterium tuberculosis* persisting under well-conducted chemotherapy [7, 12]. Only a few procedures are dedicated to emergency cases (6%) while most of the procedures are planned elective surgery for MDR-/XDR-TB (94%) [13]. Anatomical resections (lobectomy or pneumonectomy) are the preferred type of resection to avoid opening the tuberculous cavitation and spilling bacterial load into the pleura. In various published series, operative morbidity and mortality range from 8% to 29% and up to 12.5%, respectively [4]. In their meta-analysis, MARRONE et al. [14] published up to 92% and 87% on short- and long-term successful outcomes, respectively. Surgery achieved a 2.2-fold increase in the success of treating MDR-/XDR-TB in comparison to chemotherapy alone [12]. The profile of the operable candidate is a patient with MDR-TB, in whom we may prognose a high risk of relapse or recurrence once chemotherapy is stopped and with localised disease amenable to complete surgical resection. Surgery is performed once sufficient chemotherapy has been administered to diminish the initial burden of bacterial load and favour the bronchial stump healing. Surgery should be discussed in the following cases: 1) MDR-TB after 18–24 months of anti-TB chemotherapy combining multiple drugs, negative smears and culture; 2) persistence of TB excretion despite an intensive course of anti-TB chemotherapy; and 3) lack of radiological improvement of TB sequelae or drug resistance in sputum-positive patients [7, 12]. The WHO has established a comprehensive list of indications for surgery when dealing with DR-TB: the document should not be considered as a recommendation but as a consensus of expert opinions [15]. Nevertheless, the authors insist on the right timing to perform surgery according not only to the medical treatment but also the need for accurate pre-operative work-up including functional respiratory status of the patient but also nutritional status. Contra-indications for surgery would be: bilateral extensive cavitary lesions, impaired pulmonary function test, pulmonary–heart failure III–IV (functional classification of the New York Heart Association), body mass index up to 40–50% of the normal range, severe comorbidities such as decompensation in diabetes, hepatic or renal impairment, and active bronchial TB [15].

Recent recommendations advocate a prior minimal 3 months of well-conducted anti-TB chemotherapy followed by surgery. Then, following surgery, a further 12–24 months of chemotherapy are recommended by the same guidelines [16, 17]. Surgery should only be performed by experienced surgeons in centres with expertise in the field. The decision making for surgery should rely on a multidisciplinary team, taking into account the medical history of the patient, comorbidities, recent history and evolution of the TB under appropriate chemotherapy, and a complete pre-operative work-up of the patient including nutritional status, and respiratory and cardiovascular functional status [16, 17].

These guidelines rely on expert opinions and observational studies. While performing their meta-analysis, MARRONE et al. [14] were able to demonstrate the true benefit of surgery for patients but they could not firmly demonstrate the benefit of the consecutive chemotherapy/surgery/chemotherapy sequence in comparison to chemotherapy alone. The authors advocated performing randomised comparative studies to definitively validate the alternated sequence of chemotherapy and surgery. Nevertheless, demonstrating a 2.2-fold increase in the rate of successful treatment when undergoing the sequence of chemotherapy alternated with surgery, one could actually question the ethical legitimacy of performing a randomised comparison of chemotherapy alone *versus* chemotherapy alternated with surgery. More recently, GILLER et al. [4] reported their experience with over 5500 surgical procedures with curative intent for MDR-/XDR-TB. All procedures were performed following the actual

https://doi.org/10.1183/2312508X.10021717

guidelines of preparing the patients with well-conducted chemotherapy initiated at least 3 months prior to surgery; the latter chemotherapy would be prolonged in the post-operative period. Surgery was based on all means of anatomical lung resection with or without thoracoplasty according to the initial destructive lesion [4]. The success rate reached 93% in MDR patients and 92.1% in XDR patients based on immediate and long-term achievements. Reviewing worldwide publications, especially from countries submitted to the same epidemiological pressure of MDR-/XDR-TB, the authors reported high rates of favourable outcomes in recent patient series provided surgery was applied during the first year of newly diagnosed MDR-/XDR-TB. In the meantime, reporting results of collapse therapy (pneumothorax/pneumoperitoneum) during the first year of newly diagnosed destructive TB, authors demonstrated clinical recovery in 93.9% of their patients [4]. Quite logically, GILLER et al. [4] concluded that surgery provides excellent results for curing MDR-/XDR-TB, insisting on the need for performing surgery following the actual guidelines and during the first year of TB diagnose without neglecting the true efficiency of collapse therapy despite its old-fashioned appearance.

In a more recent meta-analysis, HARRIS et al. [18] demonstrated a better outcome of treatment when combining surgery to chemotherapy in MDR-TB patients in comparison to chemotherapy alone. Furthermore, patients with partial lung resection had the better outcome while those who had to undergo pneumonectomy did not differ from those not undergoing surgery. Partial lung resection would give the best results when patients experienced culture conversion from chemotherapy first. Nevertheless, when grading the quality of evidence of their own study, the authors determined very low evidence for their conclusions. Patients fit for surgery and undergoing surgery were compared to all others including patients with a theoretical indication but who were unfit for surgery. Moreover, no study reported the results of surgery in HIV-immunosuppressed MDR-TB patients. In the end, the authors emphasised the need for better constructed studies when assessing the benefits of surgery, and better reporting of results [18].

According to KEMPKER et al. [19], less than 10% of MDR-/XDR-TB patients will receive adequate treatment in accordance with the international guidelines. Surgery should not be neglected. Surgery will help control dangerous conveying-resistant TB populations by enabling at least cessation of bacterial excretion. This epidemiological benefit will add to the individual benefit to patients [19].

In conclusion, to date, the role of surgery in mycobacterial pulmonary disease is usually limited to medically refractory localised disease, but the challenges of MDR- and XDR-TB may re-expand the role of surgery for these diseases, including collapse therapy.

Surgery for post-tuberculosis sequelae

Post-TB sequelae can be divided into two different features: either related to TB and its physiopathology or, more frequently, related to the surgical therapy proposed for TB, classically collapse therapy but more recently anatomical resections. TB itself will determine two different types of elementary lesions either involving the lung parenchyma or involving the lymph nodes. Lung lesions present as bronchiectasis, fibrostenosis or cavitation. Lymph node lesions are characterised as broncholithiasis. These elementary lesions may also combine and achieve chronic suppurative disease leading to completely destroyed lungs as broncholithiasis may erode the bronchus until haemoptysis and/or lung infection.

Lung lesions, especially parenchymal cavitation, may be further complicated by fungal infection, with aspergilloma being the most frequent. Furthermore, broncho-oeosophagal fistula may arise by erosive broncholithiasis [6].

In almost all cases, surgery is to be discussed once these lesions are revealed by symptoms. Only in the particular case of aspergilloma has preventive surgery been recommended: surgical outcomes are marked by a decreased mortality and morbidity rate when surgery is performed in asymptomatic patients [18]. On the contrary, emergency surgery in symptomatic patients presenting with acute haemoptysis is described as substantial mortality and morbidity. In the setting of post-TB sequelae, adjuvant TB chemotherapy may be indicated either because of persistent bacilli or granuloma in the surgical specimen, or because the patient was not compliant with the initial regimen. When performing surgery for post-TB sequelae, some general rules have to be respected. The lung in TB patients undergoes fibrotic changes which interfere with adequate re-expansion after partial resection; the surgeon should keep in mind that immediate or deferred thoracoplasty may be required. Anatomical lung resection, preferably lobectomy, should be preferred to prevent spilling of the pleura. Bronchial fistula is a classic complication; the hilar dissection should be performed carefully and should preserve bronchial blood supply to support proper bronchial healing. In case pneumonectomy needs to be performed for a destroyed lung, careful covering of the bronchial stump is mandatory. Last but not least, at each surgical step starting with adhesiolysis, meticulous haemostasis is required to lower the risk of post-operative bleeding [6]. Despite these cautions, one may end up with the classical complications described previously; thus, thoracoplasty, re-covering of the bronchial stump, pleurostomy with repeated dressings or vacuum-assisted therapy will be the remaining solutions.

The usual complication of therapeutic pneumothorax is an exudate blowing the residual space of pneumothorax or the extra pleural pocket. This exudate may be sterile, infected with nonspecific flora or present as reactivated tuberculous empyema. Exceptional cases of haematoma in patients on blood thinning treatment have been reported. The best option in these patients is a decortication. Although the underlying lung has low functional value, it will act as a "prosthesis" filling the pleural space, which is the main condition to heal empyema. Long-term complications of extraperiosteal plombage are exceptional, because most of the patients underwent routine removal of the material. Complications include infection of the plombage space and migration of the material. Treatment consists of removal of all plombage material followed by a thoracoplasty achieved by excision of the devitalised ribs surrounding the plombage space [2, 3].

References

1. Hastings J, Storks R. A Case of Tuberculosis Excavation of the Left Lung Treated by Perforation of the Cavity Through the Walls of the Chest. London, Wilson and Ogilvy, 1844.
2. Massard G, Rougé C, Ameur S, et al. Decortication is a valuable option for late empyema after collapse therapy. Ann Thorac Surg 1995; 60: 888–895.
3. Massard G, Thomas P, Barsotti P, et al. Long-term complications of extraperiosteal plombage. Ann Thorac Surg 1997; 64: 220–224.
4. Giller DB, Giller BD, Giller GV, et al. Treatment of pulmonary tuberculosis: past and present. Eur J CardioThorac Surg 2018; 53: 967–972.
5. Sotgiu G, Migliori GB. Pulmonary tuberculosis. In: Palange P, Simonds A, eds. ERS Handbook of Respiratory Medicine. Sheffield, European Respiratory Society, 2013; pp. 229–240.
6. Massard G, Olland A, Santelmo N, et al. Surgery for the sequelae of post-primary tuberculosis 2012; 22: 287–300.

https://doi.org/10.1183/2312508X.10021717

7.   Weyant M, Mitchell J. Multidrug-resistant pulmonary tuberculosis: surgical challenges. *Thorac Surg Clin* 2012; 22: 271–276.

8.   McWilliams A, Tammemagi MC, Mayo JR, *et al.* Probability of cancer in pulmonary nodules detected on first screening CT. *N Engl J Med* 2013; 369: 910–919.

9.   Kim HJ, Kim DK, Kim YW, *et al.* Outcome of incidentally detected airway nodules. *Eur Respir J* 2016; 47: 1510–1517.

10. Rivera C, Arame A, Pricopi C, *et al.* Pneumonectomy for benign disease: indications and postoperative outcomes, a nationwide study. *Eur J Cardiothorac Surg* 2015; 48: 435–440.

11. Alexander GR, Biccard B. A retrospective review comparing treatment outcomes of adjuvant lung resection for drug-resistant tuberculosis in patients with and without human immunodeficiency virus co-infection. *Eur J Cardiothorac Surg* 2016; 49: 823–828.

12. Yablonski P, Cordosi I, Sokolovitch E, *et al.* Surgical treatment of pulmonary tuberculosis. *In:* Rohde G, Subotic D, eds. ERS Monograph. Sheffield, European Respiratory Society, 2013; pp. 20–36.

13. Hosaka N, Kameko M, Nishimura H, *et al.* Prevalence of tuberculosis in small pulmonary nodules obtained by video-assisted thoracoscopic surgery. *Respir Med* 2006; 100: 238–243.

14. Marrone MT, Venkataramanan V, Goodman M, *et al.* Surgical interventions for drug resistant tuberculosis: a systematic review and meta-analysis. *Int J Tuberc Lung Dis* 2013; 17: 6–16.

15. World Health Organization. The role of surgery in the treatment of pulmonary TB and multidrug- and extensively drug-resistant TB. Geneva, WHO, 2014.

16. World Health Organization. WHO treatment guidelines for drug-resistant tuberculosis 2016 update. Geneva, WHO, 2016.

17. American Thoracic Society, CDC, Infectious Diseases Society of America. Treatment of tuberculosis. *MMWR* 2003; 52: 1–77.

18. Harris RC, Khan MS, Martin LJ, *et al.* The effect of surgery on the outcome of treatment for multidrug-resistant tuberculosis: a systematic review and meta-analysis. *BMC Infect Dis* 2016; 16: 262.

19. Kempker RR, Vashakidze S, Solomonia N, *et al.* Surgical treatment of drug resistant tuberculosis. *Lancet Infect Dis* 2012; 12: 157–166.

Disclosures: None declared.

	Chapter 14

Challenges in childhood tuberculosis

H. Simon Schaaf[1], Ben J. Marais[2], Isabel Carvalho[3] and
James A. Seddon[1,4]

TB in children has been the invisible part of the global TB epidemic; however, it is responsible for high morbidity and mortality, especially in TB-endemic settings where most children remain undiagnosed and untreated. Added to this are the challenges of diagnosing DR-TB in children. In the face of these diagnostic challenges, it is even more important to prioritise prevention efforts. TB in children is mainly paucibacillary, which means that fewer drugs and/or shorter treatment regimens may be used, but severe forms of TB such as tuberculous meningitis need special consideration. In general, outcomes of both drug-susceptible and drug-resistant disease in children are good if diagnosed early and treated appropriately, but challenges remain regarding optimal drug dosing, availability of child-friendly formulations and child-appropriate regimens. HIV infection is decreasing due to prevention of mother-to-child transmission roll-out, but antiretroviral and anti-TB drug–drug interactions remain a challenge. Optimal prevention strategies, diagnostic tools, treatment regimens and practical operational issues remain key research questions.

Cite as: Schaaf HS, Marais BJ, Carvalho I, *et al*. Challenges in childhood tuberculosis. *In*: Migliori GB, Bothamley G, Duarte R, *et al.*, eds. Tuberculosis (ERS Monograph). Sheffield, European Respiratory Society, 2018; pp. 234–262 [https://doi.org/10.1183/2312508X.10021817].

@ERSpublications
TB in children is often missed, leading to severe disease and death. Treatment outcomes are good if TB is diagnosed early and treated appropriately, but improvements in prevention and diagnosis, as well as treatment of drug-resistant disease, are needed. http://ow.ly/cfVQ30lqCfE

A major challenge for childhood TB has been the "invisibility" of the disease burden in resource-limited TB-endemic areas. In these settings TB is traditionally diagnosed by sputum smear microscopy, which excludes young children from diagnostic access as they are unable to expectorate sputum and, even if respiratory samples are collected, smear microscopy is insensitive in children with paucibacillary disease. In addition, young children

---

[1]Desmond Tutu TB Centre, Dept of Paediatrics and Child Health, Faculty of Medicine and Health Sciences, Stellenbosch University, Cape Town, South Africa. [2]Marie Bashir Institute for Infectious Diseases and Biosecurity and The Children's Hospital at Westmead, School of Child and Adolescent Health, University of Sydney, Sydney, Australia. [3]Dept of Paediatrics, Hospital Centre Vila Nova de Gaia, Vila Nova de Gaia, Portugal. [4]Centre for International Child Health, Imperial College London, London, UK.

Correspondence: H. Simon Schaaf, Desmond Tutu TB Centre, Dept of Paediatrics and Child Health, Faculty of Medicine and Health Sciences, Stellenbosch University, PO Box 241, Cape Town, 8000, South Africa. E-mail: hss@sun.ac.za

Copyright ©ERS 2018. Print ISBN: 978-1-84984-099-6. Online ISBN: 978-1-84984-100-9. Print ISSN: 2312-508X. Online ISSN: 2312-5098.

were not considered important from an epidemic control perspective as they rarely transmit disease. However, it is estimated that 1 million children (aged <15 years) develop TB disease every year [1], and it is increasingly recognised that adolescents also contribute significantly to the overall TB burden and transmission within communities. A recent modelling exercise estimated that 1.8 million young people (aged between 10 and <25 years) develop TB each year [2]. Only a third of children with TB receive appropriate treatment and approximately 250 000 children die of TB each year; 96% without treatment and almost all <5 years of age [1, 3]. Given poor diagnostic access in most TB-endemic areas, most child TB deaths are not recorded as such, but are included in mortality figures for pneumonia, meningitis and malnutrition [4]. Recent estimates are that TB is a global "top 10" cause of mortality in those <5 years of age, emphasising its importance as a preventable cause of death in children, irrespective of their contribution to transmission and epidemic spread.

Natural history of infection and disease in children

Children become infected with *Mycobacterium tuberculosis* following exposure to an infectious TB source case, usually within the immediate or extended household. TB infection is traditionally defined as having no clinical symptoms or signs of disease and a normal chest radiograph, but with evidence of immunological sensitisation to *M. tuberculosis* through a positive TST or IGRA. It is estimated that nearly 70 million children (aged <15 years) worldwide have TB infection [5]. From this silent reservoir, each year some children will develop TB disease, defined as clinical, radiological and/or microbiological evidence of disease [6]. Young children (aged <5 years) are at high risk of disease progression, with the risk reaching a nadir in the pre-adolescent age group, before rising again through adolescence and into adulthood [7]. Conditions that impair immunity, such as HIV infection [8], malnutrition [9] or the use of immunosuppressive drugs [10], also increase the risk of disease progression.

Challenges of diagnosis

Types of tuberculosis disease in children

Intrathoracic disease
During primary infection young children develop a parenchymal (Ghon) focus with spread *via* the lymphatics to the intrathoracic lymph nodes. Lymph node disease is mainly paucibacillary, but may cause local complications such as airway compression with hyperinflation of a lobe or lung (partial large airway obstruction) or collapse (complete large airway obstruction), or may rupture into a bronchus causing lobar or bronchopneumonic spread. Parenchymal lesions may be contained or uncontained (often with breakdown causing cavities) or may break into blood vessels causing disseminated spread (miliary TB). A switch in disease phenotype to adult-type disease with lung cavities occurs in adolescent children with the onset of puberty [11, 12].

Bacteriological confirmation can be challenging in younger children (aged <5 years) due to the difficulty in obtaining suitable specimens and the paucibacillary nature of uncomplicated lymph node disease, with culture confirmation rarely exceeding 30–40% [13, 14]. However, adolescents and children older than ~8 years of age may develop adult-type PTB and can expectorate, and sputum smear microscopy or Xpert MTB/RIF is commonly positive in this age group [13]. Adolescents also pose a transmission risk to household and/or school contacts [15].

Extrathoracic disease

ETTB, including severe and disseminated forms (meningitis and miliary TB), is more common in infants and toddlers who have less effective T-cell responses [16, 17]. Peripheral lymphadenitis is the most common form of ETTB, but is fairly easy to diagnose and rarely has severe consequences [18]. Other severe forms of ETTB are abdominal and osteoarticular TB (50% of which is spinal TB). The main challenge of these ETTB forms is early diagnosis, as subtle initial symptoms and signs are often missed. Treatment of central nervous system (CNS) and osteoarticular TB also presents special challenges, related to optimal drug choice (due to differences in penetration), drug dose, treatment duration, additional drug use (*e.g.* steroids) and ancillary measures such as surgical intervention [19].

Diagnosis: a constellation of symptoms, signs and special investigations

There is no single, sensitive test to diagnose TB in children. Diagnosing TB in a child can be compared to putting together a puzzle: the more pieces (of evidence) are found, the clearer the picture (diagnosis) becomes (figure 1). This could also be seen as putting together a constellation of symptoms, signs and special investigations to come to a final decision of TB or not TB.

Two main scenarios may lead the clinician to consider TB in a child: active contact tracing or passive case finding. Obtaining a thorough history of persistent symptoms such as non-remitting cough (figure 2), ongoing fever, decreased playfulness and loss of weight (or failure to gain weight) is important [20], although younger children in particular may present with acute onset of symptoms [21]. Symptoms and signs are often nonspecific, and may mimic other common childhood diseases [22], but can be helpful if accurately characterised [23].

Taking a detailed history of recent (in the past year) TB contact is essential but challenging as source cases may not be household members and/or may still be undiagnosed [24, 25]. It is also important to know about possible drug-resistant disease in the likely source case.

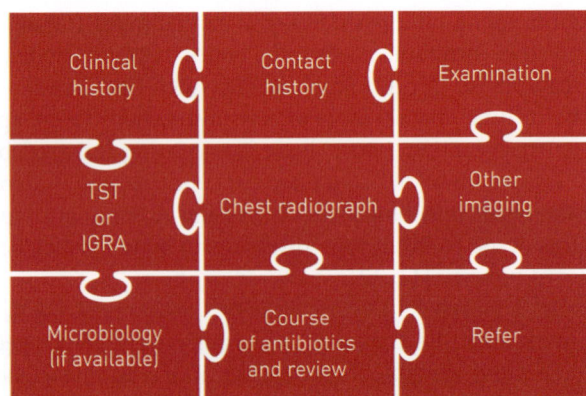

Figure 1. Diagnosing TB in a child can be compared to putting together a puzzle: the more pieces (of evidence) are found, the clearer the picture (diagnosis) becomes.

https://doi.org/10.1183/2312508X.10021817

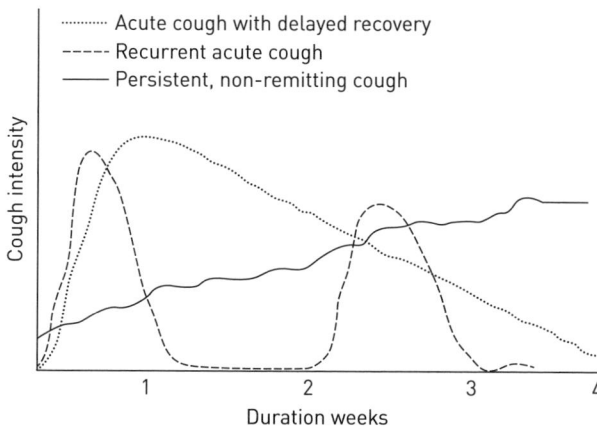

Figure 2. "Chronic cough" patterns in children. Progressive TB disease is typically associated with a persistent, non-remitting cough. Reproduced and modified from [23] with permission.

Infection and disease risk relates to the infectiousness of the source case, the intensity and duration of TB exposure, the child's age and immune/nutritional status, as well as the preventive measures taken, such as BCG immunisation and preventive therapy. Even a short occasional exposure to an infectious TB case could lead to infection and disease [26].

A specific challenge is the early diagnosis of tuberculous meningitis, which is the most serious form of TB in children. Initial symptoms and signs are nonspecific, such as decreased activity, failure to thrive or loss of weight (often documented in a growth chart), occasional vomiting, low-grade fever and sleepiness. Older children may complain of headache. Unless a detailed history of recent TB contact and subtle symptoms/signs are obtained, this early stage of tuberculous meningitis, when complete cure is possible, will be missed and only once the child presents with overt neurological symptoms, and likely permanent sequelae, will the diagnosis be considered [27, 28].

Tuberculosis immunological tests

Two types of test are available for identifying previous immunological sensitisation to *M. tuberculosis*: TSTs (mainly the Mantoux method) and IGRAs (including QuantiFERON TB-Gold Plus (Qiagen, Hilden, Germany) and T-SPOT.TB (Oxford Immunotec, Abingdon, UK)). These tests can be used as one piece of the puzzle when evaluating a symptomatic child for TB disease or to determine the likelihood that a well child has TB infection and consequently would benefit from TB infection treatment. In general, the tests provide the same information, although the IGRAs have an advantage in terms of specificity, not being influenced by *Mycobacterium bovis* BCG and NTM infections [29]. However, both tests fail to differentiate TB infection from disease and are not sufficiently sensitive to be used as "rule-out" tests. Other limitations to consider include the "conversion window", since it takes up to 3 months to render these tests positive after infection; both tests may also be false negative in young infants or those with immunosuppression, severe malnutrition and even in severe TB disease. In addition, re-infection cannot be evaluated by these tests. Given the high percentage of false-negative or false-positive results, the results of these tests should be interpreted with caution [30].

Radiology

Chest radiography

Chest radiography is the most widely performed investigation, but although certain features such as lymphadenopathy with/without airway compression, a miliary picture or parenchymal opacification with cavities may point towards TB, there are no pathognomonic chest radiographic features of TB [13, 21]. The challenges with chest radiography are to get good quality chest radiographs and to have experienced clinicians interpret these chest radiographs [31, 32]. Despite this, both inter- and intrareader variability in chest radiograph interpretation remains high [33]. Teaching clinicians to use a systematic approach and a standardised form may improve chest radiograph reading ability [31], and use of a follow-up chest radiograph when interpretation is uncertain is often helpful. Automated chest radiograph reading has demonstrated promise in adult TB screening [34, 35] and studies to develop computer-based interpretation of child chest radiographs are ongoing, but radiological TB disease manifestations in children are typically more variable and less specific than in adults [36].

Ultrasound

An ultrasound scan is useful in identifying pleural and pericardial effusions, and may guide diagnostic taps of these effusions. Ultrasound can be useful in identifying intra-abdominal lymph nodes and splenic lesions [37]. There is emerging expertise using ultrasound to identify intrathoracic lymph nodes [38].

Chest computed tomography

Chest computed tomography (CT) plays an important role in selected cases, confirming intrathoracic lymph node involvement, large airway compression due to lymphadenopathy and finding typical parenchymal lesions [39]. Chest CT availability is limited in TB-endemic areas and it is used mainly for complicated cases, while in well-resourced countries it is often used in children with possible intrathoracic TB [40, 41]. The challenge is to determine the exact role and added value of chest CT in children, since it is difficult to differentiate recent TB infection from early TB disease in asymptomatic children and the treatment implications of this distinction are unclear [42]. The high radiation dose associated with chest CT is particularly problematic in children.

^{18}F-fluorodeoxyglucose-positron emission tomography/CT

^{18}F-fluorodeoxyglucose-positron emission tomography (FDG-PET)/CT is a new imaging tool to detect a spectrum of manifestations in patients with TB. FDG-PET/CT has demonstrated promising results in diagnosing TB early, assessing extrathoracic disease extension and assessing response to therapy [43]. Given the cost and limited availability of the test, it is generally reserved for problematic cases where other diagnostic modalities are uninformative.

Imaging for extrathoracic tuberculosis

The challenge with ETTB is finding the optimal imaging technique to assist in diagnosis, as well as assessment of complications and prognosis. Plain radiography is of value in osteoarticular TB; ultrasound is mostly available and is effective in assessing pericardial effusions and abdominal TB. CT scans have excellent spatial resolution and are widely used for CNS TB as well as in abdominal and osteoarticular TB, but CT is associated with high radiation exposure [44]. Magnetic resonance imaging (MRI) is preferred for assessing CNS and spinal TB, since it has no radiation exposure and detects early diffusion restriction,

https://doi.org/10.1183/2312508X.10021817

as well as posterior fossa and spinal lesions, with greater accuracy than CT [39]. High TB burden areas often have limited access to these imaging modalities.

Bacteriological confirmation of tuberculosis the elusive gold standard

The challenges of bacteriological confirmation of TB disease in children are multiple, including low bacillary load, difficulty obtaining suitable specimens, transporting low-yield specimens, inadequate laboratory infrastructure and insensitive bacteriological tests. Bacterial confirmation should be sought using all available specimens and laboratory facilities, and is especially important for children who have suspected DR-TB, HIV infection, complicated or severe TB disease (in whom the yield is highest), an uncertain diagnosis, or have been treated previously [6].

Obtaining suitable specimens

Advantages and disadvantages of different specimens are summarised in table 1. In the case of ETTB, obtaining respiratory specimens is still of value even if chest radiography is normal, since the lungs remain the original "port of entry" of infection in most cases. The challenge of bacteriological confirmation often lies in obtaining a minimum of two good quality specimens before starting TB treatment (although treatment in probable tuberculous meningitis should start immediately), as well as in proper preparation and rapid specimen transport [45], although the availability of laboratory facilities, equipment and trained staff is a major challenge in many settings [46].

Tests for bacteriological confirmation

Smear microscopy for acid-fast bacilli

Sputum smear microscopy for acid-fast bacilli (AFB) remains a valuable investigation even in children, but has very low yield (usually <15%) in this age group; however, older children with adult-type cavitary disease may have yields similar to adult PTB cases [47, 48]. Positive AFB results do not differentiate MTBC from NTM or DR-TB from drug-susceptible (DS)-TB.

Culture confirmation of Mycobacterium tuberculosis and phenotypic drug-susceptibility testing

Mycobacterial culture remains the reference standard for bacterial confirmation. Liquid culture methods have improved time to positivity and sensitivity compared with solid medium cultures, but performing both culture methods (liquid and solid) is often preferred. Phenotypic DST is only possible if a positive mycobacterial culture is obtained.

Nucleic acid amplification tests

New PCR-based molecular tests allow rapid detection and identification of MTBC, either directly from clinical samples or from cultured isolates, with genotypic DST guiding appropriate patient management [49]. We focus our discussion on Xpert MTB/RIF and the line probe assays (LPAs).

Xpert MTB/RIF and Xpert MTB/RIF Ultra

Xpert MTB/RIF (Cepheid, Sunnyvale, CA, USA) performs MTBC detection and genotypic DST for rifampicin in <2 h. The WHO recommends Xpert MTB/RIF as a replacement for AFB smear microscopy in all children [50]. Although the sensitivity of Xpert MTB/RIF compared with culture in children with presumed intrathoracic TB is only ~70% [51], it is

Table 1. Diagnostic options in children with a brief summary of the advantages and disadvantages

Diagnostic approach	Advantages	Disadvantages
Clinical		
History	Easy to undertake and no cost	Requires training; poor sensitivity and specificity
Examination	Easy to undertake and no cost	Requires training and appropriate environment
Scoring systems	Allow risk assessment without requiring clinical expertise	Not validated
Radiology		
Chest radiography	Relatively inexpensive and available	Often of poor quality and few features pathognomonic for TB; interpretation highly variable
Chest CT	Expensive; not widely available; large radiation dose	Demonstrates intrathoracic lymph nodes with greater clarity than chest radiography
Chest MRI	Very expensive; not commonly available; often requires general anaesthetic in young children	No radiation; excellent definition for soft tissues
PET/CT	Very high radiation dose; rarely available	Provides insight into location and metabolic activity of lesions
Ultrasound scan	No radiation; portable; good for visualisation of fluid and consolidation	Poor visualisation through air-filled structures; requires training; subjective
Microbiology: sampling		
Expectorated sputum	Easy and cheap; acceptable	Not possible in children under ~6 years; infection control risk needs to be considered
Gastric aspirate	Easy and cheap to perform	Requires equipment; needs to be performed early in the morning after an overnight fast; invasive; not accepted in some communities
Induced sputum	Can be performed as an outpatient and at any time of day on any age of child	Requires equipment and monitoring; invasive
Nasopharyngeal aspirate	Can be performed as an outpatient and at any time of day on any age of child	Requires equipment; invasive; not well tolerated in older children
FNAB	Easy to perform and can be done as an outpatient under local anaesthetic; good yield	Can be distressing
Tissue biopsy	Often gives definitive diagnosis	Usually requires general anaesthetic; invasive
EBUS	Allows sampling at site of disease in lungs; high yield	Requires expensive equipment and training
Body fluids (e.g. CSF, pleural fluid, pericardial fluid or ascites)	Allows evaluation of microbiology as well as other tests (e.g. biochemistry, etc.)	Low yield; invasive
Microbiology: laboratory		
Smear	Easy and quick to perform, cheap	Low sensitivity
Xpert MTB/RIF (Ultra)	Better sensitivity than smear; results within 2 h and provides information on drug resistance	Expensive; needs servicing; requires power supply and information technology capability

Continued

https://doi.org/10.1183/2312508X.10021817

Table 1. Continued

Diagnostic approach	Advantages	Disadvantages
MODS assay	Cheap and robust; provides information on drug resistance	Takes days for results; kits not widely available
LPA	Provides information on DST to multiple drugs and for multiple mutations	Requires laboratory infrastructure and training, for children; rarely possible to perform directly on clinical specimens
Solid culture	Relatively cheap; easy to use	Takes weeks for results; requires laboratory infrastructure and training
Liquid culture	More sensitive than all other investigations to detect *Mycobacterium tuberculosis* and drug resistance	Takes weeks for results; requires laboratory infrastructure; expensive
WGS	Provides information on multiple genes associated with resistance; permits evaluation of relatedness of strains for epidemiological surveillance	Still unclear correlation between genotype and phenotypic resistance; for children rarely possible to perform directly on clinical specimens
Immunological tests		
TST	Cheap and relatively easy to use	Requires two visits; imperfect sensitivity especially in young children and children living with HIV; specificity impaired by BCG and NTM
IGRA	Improved specificity; only requires one visit	Expensive and requires laboratory infrastructure; imperfect sensitivity, especially in young children and children living with HIV
Host RNA biomarkers	Could assist in the diagnosis of TB disease in children who are microbiologically unconfirmed	Still at experimental stage; likely to be very expensive for a number of years

CT: computed tomography; MRI: magnetic resonance imaging; PET: positron emission tomography; FNAB: fine needle aspiration biopsy; EBUS: endobronchial ultrasound; CSF: cerebrospinal fluid; MODS: microscopic observation drug susceptibility; LPA: line probe assay; WGS: whole-genome sequencing.

much better than smear microscopy in settings where culture is not available. The new Xpert MTB/RIF Ultra has improved sensitivity [52], but further evaluation of "trace" results, often with rifampicin DST indeterminate/unsuccessful, is required, although the WHO recommends treating children with Xpert MTB/RIF Ultra "trace" results as TB [53].

Line probe assays
LPAs are endorsed by the WHO for both first-line (isoniazid and rifampicin) and second-line (fluoroquinolones and SLIDs) DST [54, 55]. An LPA assay such as GenoType MTBDR*plus* (Hain Lifescience, Nehren, Germany) identifies common mutations in the *rpoB* or *katG* genes, or the *inhA* promoter region. Low-level isoniazid resistance and coresistance with ethionamide occurs with *inhA* promoter region mutations [56]. Phenotypic (culture-based) DST for isoniazid needs to be done if the LPA shows only rifampicin resistance, as up to 15% of isoniazid resistance may be conferred by mutations

that are not assessed by the LPA. GenoType MTBDR*sl* (Hain Lifescience) identifies >80% of resistance to SLIDs and fluoroquinolones, but additional phenotypic DST is recommended as LPA sensitivity is variable [54]. Rapid and accurate DST is essential for optimal individualised treatment of MDR/XDR-TB. Genotypic methods rapidly identify drug resistance, but combined phenotypic and genotypic testing usually provides complimentary information [57].

Whole-genome sequencing

LPAs only screen for common resistance-determining mutations, whereas phenotypic DST is slow and expensive. Whole-genome sequencing (WGS) enables the screening of all known resistance-associated loci while also providing opportunities to characterise new mutations and deletion events associated with drug resistance, as well as identifying the *M. tuberculosis* strain type and potential transmission pathways [58]. More than 100 single genetic loci have been associated with drug resistance and there are many other mutations that may collectively contribute to drug resistance. A complete library of resistance-determining mutations could negate the need for phenotypic DST. Although the cost and feasibility of WGS are rapidly improving, it still relies on a positive mycobacterial culture, which is a major rate-limiting and implementation barrier in patients with paucibacillary disease [59, 60].

Biopsies and histopathology

Histopathology and cytology on surgical or fine needle aspirate biopsies (FNABs) remain important methods for diagnosing TB. FNAB is a simple and safe procedure that can be done in limited resource settings, and allows histopathological and bacteriological confirmation [61]. Histology or cytology cannot differentiate TB from NTM or other granulomatous diseases; however, the presence of caseating granulomas with giant cells is highly suggestive of TB. Finding AFB is variable, and depends on the bacillary load of the specimen and the type of material [62]. Xpert MTB/RIF and/or mycobacterial culture provide bacteriological confirmation and usually have an excellent yield on these specimens [63].

HIV testing

Routine HIV testing is recommended in all children with presumed TB, especially in high HIV prevalence areas or risk groups. HIV-infected children are more likely to have other comorbidities, many of which may present similar to TB. The further challenge is to determine the optimal ART regimen and decide on timing of treatment initiation, if not already on ART [64].

Additional investigations

Finding a reliable sputum-independent test remains the "holy grail" of child TB diagnostics. Unfortunately, the urinary lipoarabinomannan assay has poor sensitivity and specificity in children [65]. Many biomarker studies are ongoing, such as those on host transcriptional signatures, metabolomics markers and host or pathogen micro-RNAs, of which some show promise [66, 67] but none are yet available for clinical use [68].

https://doi.org/10.1183/2312508X.10021817

Bronchoscopy and transbronchial biopsy

Bronchoscopy plays an important role in complicated intrathoracic TB cases, but expertise and equipment to perform bronchoscopy are limited [69]. If available, it may confirm nodal airway compression, and obtain bronchoalveolar lavage specimens and biopsies of intraluminal granulomatous tissue or hilar lymph nodes. It is also useful to exclude causes other than TB and for procedures that may re-establish airway patency [70]. Endobronchial ultrasound-guided transbronchial needle aspiration biopsy is safe and when combined with standard bronchoscopy significantly increases the diagnostic yield in patients of suspicious PTB with lymphadenopathy [71, 72].

When to consider drug-resistant tuberculosis

DR-TB should be presumed in children with TB who have close contact with an infectious DR-TB source case; it should further be considered in child contacts of source cases who are treatment failures, re-treatment cases or who have recently died from TB. Possible DR-TB should be considered if a child is not responding to first-line therapy despite good adherence and if a previously treated child develops recurrent TB, in which case disease relapse should be differentiated from re-infection if at all possible. The prompt diagnosis of DR-TB allows early appropriate treatment, which increases cure rates and reduces mortality. When DR-TB is suspected, every effort should be made to obtain specimens for bacteriological confirmation and DST, preferably before starting any TB treatment [6, 46].

Challenges in treatment

Treatment regimens are usually presented as a number (months) and a string of letters referring to specific drugs (as defined in table 2), with a forward slash separating the intensive phase of treatment from the continuation phase.

Treatment of drug-susceptible tuberculosis

Current standard three-drug (2HRZ/4HR) or four-drug (2HRZE/4HR) regimens for the treatment of DS-TB are effective in most forms of TB if diagnosed in a timely manner and if treatment adherence is good. The recommended paediatric drug doses were adjusted by the WHO after reviewing existing pharmacokinetic data in children (table 2). However, data to guide optimal treatment regimens in CNS and osteoarticular TB, as well as nonsevere types of TB, remain a challenge.

Central nervous system and osteoarticular tuberculosis
The WHO currently recommends a 12-month antituberculous regimen of 2HRZE/10HR for both CNS TB and osteoarticular (mainly spinal) TB [6]. Observational cohorts of children with tuberculous meningitis have shown good outcomes (mortality of <5%) with a regimen of 6–9HRZEto, continuing all four drugs for the full treatment duration [78]. The need for more effective regimens for treating CNS TB and good outcomes of the shorter regimen in South Africa has led to two ongoing RCTs in tuberculous meningitis evaluating a 6-month regimen of isoniazid/pyrazinamide plus high-dose rifampicin and levofloxacin compared with the 12-month WHO regimen [79, 80]. However, the main challenge with the management of tuberculous meningitis remains earlier diagnosis and prevention of the vascular and immune complications of the disease. Tumour necrosis factor-α inhibitors

Table 2. TB drugs used in children for drug-susceptible and drug-resistant disease

	Dose	Important adverse events	Future developments
First-line drugs			
Pyrazinamide (Z)	30–40 mg·kg^{-1}·day^{-1}	Arthritis/arthralgia, hepatitis, skin rashes	Optimal dosing in particular subpopulations, *e.g.* neonates
Ethambutol (E)	15–25 mg·kg^{-1}·day^{-1}	Optic neuritis	Risk–benefit of using higher doses
Isoniazid (H)	7–15 mg·kg^{-1}·day^{-1} (neonates only 10 mg·kg^{-1}·day^{-1}); high dose 15–20 mg·kg^{-1}·day^{-1}	Hepatitis, peripheral neuropathy	Investigate possible interaction with cycloserine/ terizidone (decreased concentration of isoniazid) [73]
Rifampicin (R)	10–20 mg·kg^{-1}·day^{-1}	Hepatitis, discolouration of secretions	Higher doses currently investigated, up to 50 mg·kg^{-1}·day^{-1}
Rifapentine (Rpt)	Preventive therapy: children ⩾2 years: weight-banded dosing once weekly (>10–14 kg: 300 mg per dose; >14–25 kg: 450 mg per dose; >25–32 kg: 600 mg per dose; >32–50 kg: 750 mg per dose; >50 kg: 900 mg per dose)	Hepatitis, discolouration of secretions, gastrointestinal disturbance	Pharmacokinetic data for children <2 years
Rifabutin (Rfb)	Dose not established in children; 5 mg·kg^{-1} daily to 3 times a week has been used (maximum 300 mg)	Uveitis, myelosuppression	Needs further evaluation
Fluoroquinolones			
Levofloxacin (Lfx)	15–20 mg·kg^{-1}·day^{-1}	Sleep disturbance, gastrointestinal disturbance, arthralgia/arthritis, raised intracranial pressure	Modelling data suggest higher doses but variation in pharmacokinetic data with different formulations [74]
Moxifloxacin (Mfx)	10–15 mg·kg^{-1}·day^{-1}	As levofloxacin with QTc prolongation	Pharmacokinetic data in young infants needed
Gatifloxacin (Gfx)	Not used in children	As levofloxacin with QTc prolongation and glucose metabolism disturbance	No further development planned
SLIDs			
Amikacin[#] (Am)	15–20 mg·kg^{-1} *i.m.* or *i.v.* injection daily	Ototoxicity (irreversible), nephrotoxicity	Higher doses only if TDM is available

Continued

https://doi.org/10.1183/2312508X.10021817

Table 2. Continued

	Dose	Important adverse events	Future developments
Kanamycin (Km)	15–20 mg·kg^{-1} *i.m.* injection daily	As amikacin	Higher doses only with TDM
Capreomycin (Cm)	15–20 mg·kg^{-1} *i.m.* injection daily	As amikacin	Higher doses only with TDM
Other second-line agents			
Ethionamide (Eto)/ prothionamide (Pto)	15–20 mg·kg^{-1}·day^{-1}	Gastrointestinal disturbance, metallic taste, hypothyroidism	
Cycloserine (Cs)/ terizidone (Trd)	15–20 mg·kg^{-1}·day^{-1}	Neurological and psychological effects	Pharmacokinetic studies in children ongoing
Linezolid (Lzd)	Children <10 years: 10 mg·kg^{-1} per dose every 12 h; children >10 years: 300–600 mg daily according to weight at ±10–15 mg·kg^{-1} once daily	Diarrhoea, headache, nausea, myelosuppression, peripheral neuritis, optic neuritis, lactic acidosis, pancreatitis	Pharmacokinetic studies in TB ongoing: initial data show good exposures with recommended doses [75]
Clofazimine (Cfz)	2–5 mg·kg^{-1}·day^{-1}; because of current 50 or 100 mg gel capsule formulations, alternate-day dosing may be necessary in young children	Skin discolouration, abdominal pain, QTc prolongation	No pharmacokinetic studies in children planned
PAS	150–200 mg·kg^{-1} daily as single or divided dose	Gastrointestinal intolerance, hypothyroidism, hepatitis	Pharmacokinetic studies indicated; tolerance with single daily dose good according to experience
Imipenem (Ipm)– cilastatin	Not used in children	Gastrointestinal intolerance, hypersensitivity reactions, seizures, liver and renal dysfunction	
Meropenem (Mpm)	20–40 mg·kg^{-1} every 8 h (*i.v.*)	As imipenem	
Amoxicillin– clavulanate (Amx–Clv)	80 mg·kg^{-1}·day^{-1} in divided doses of amoxicillin component; always combine with a carbapenem (not effective on its own)	As imipenem	
Novel agents			
Bedaquiline (Bdq)	>12 years and >30 kg body weight: adult dose of 400 mg daily×2 weeks followed by 200 mg Monday/Wednesday/ Friday×24 weeks; data on dose in younger children not yet available	Headache, nausea, liver dysfunction, QTc prolongation	Dose-finding and safety studies ongoing; studies on combining bedaquiline and delamanid still to be done

Continued

Table 2. Continued

	Dose	Important adverse events	Future developments
Delamanid (Dlm)	>12 years and >35 kg: 100 mg twice daily; 6–12 years and 20–34 kg: 50 mg·kg^{-1} twice daily; data in younger children not yet available	Nausea, vomiting, dizziness, paraesthesia, anxiety, QTc prolongation	Dose-finding and safety studies ongoing
Pretomanid (Ptm)	No data in children		Dose-finding and safety studies planned
Sutezolid	No data in children		Paediatric dose-finding and safety studies should be performed [76]
SQ109	No data in children		Paediatric dose-finding and safety studies should be performed

QTc: corrected QT interval; *i.v.*: intravenous; *i.m.*: intramuscular. [#]: can be given with lidocaine to reduce pain of *i.m.* injections [77].

such as thalidomide and infliximab have been used to effectively manage pseudo-abscesses and tuberculomas causing critical intracranial compression despite optimal TB treatment and steroids [81]. Very little data are forthcoming regarding the drug management of spinal TB, but 12-month treatment seems to remain the norm [6]. In our own experience we continue the intensive phase for a minimum of 4 months, but we often reduce the total duration to 9 months with good outcomes.

Nonsevere tuberculosis
The majority of TB in children is nonsevere paucibacillary disease, especially if diagnosed during active contact tracing. Although recent RCTs in adults were unable to identify effective shorter course regimens [82], children with nonsevere TB are far more likely to benefit from shorter treatment courses [83]. The SHINE trial is currently recruiting children with nonsevere TB to compare a 4-month course (2HRZ(E)/2HR) *versus* the standard 6-month course [84].

Optimal dosing of first-line drugs
The first 2 years of life, especially during the neonatal period and infancy, is a time of major changes in metabolism and body composition that may influence drug metabolism. A pharmacokinetic study of isoniazid in low-birthweight infants found that all infants exceeded the 2 h target of 3 mg·L^{-1} using a 10 mg·kg^{-1} daily dose [85]. In contrast, two rifampicin suspensions gave maximum concentrations far below the 2 h concentration target of 8–24 mg·L^{-1} using WHO-recommended doses of 10–20 mg·kg^{-1} daily [86]. Therefore, isoniazid should not be overdosed in pre-term neonates and rifampicin suspensions should preferably not be used. The early bactericidal activity of rifampicin

https://doi.org/10.1183/2312508X.10021817

increases linearly with dose beyond the current maximum dose of 600 mg daily [87]. Doses of up to 35 mg·kg^{-1} daily have not been associated with increased short-term hepatotoxicity in adults [88] and similar doses are currently being evaluated in children (OptiRIF Kids) [89]. These studies may lead to recommendations of higher rifampicin dosing, especially with severe forms of TB such as CNS TB where penetration is poor and rifampicin may play an important role.

Treatment of drug-resistant tuberculosis

Isoniazid-monoresistant tuberculosis treatment

Confirmation of isoniazid-monoresistant (HMR)-TB remains a challenge, since Xpert MTB/RIF only detects rifampicin resistance and even LPAs may miss up to 15% of isoniazid resistance as they only test for *katG* and *inhA* mutations. Optimal treatment of HMR-TB cases is important to prevent amplification of drug resistance, which is a particular concern in those with high bacillary loads. A recent individual patient data meta-analysis of HMR-TB treatment showed reasonable outcomes with 6(H)RZE, but outcome was optimised if a fluoroquinolone was added [90].

Rifampicin-resistant, isoniazid-susceptible tuberculosis

A clear distinction is needed between rifampicin-resistant, isoniazid-susceptible TB and Xpert-positive RR-TB; the latter should be considered as MDR unless isoniazid susceptibility is phenotypically confirmed. Rifampicin-resistant, isoniazid-susceptible *M. tuberculosis* strains are mostly susceptible to other first- and second-line TB drugs [91], and therefore a regimen of four or five effective drugs can usually be compiled without necessarily adding an injectable agent. The current WHO-recommended shorter regimen [92] for pulmonary rifampicin-monoresistant (RMR)-TB cases could be used in children with confirmed RMR-TB (phenotypic isoniazid susceptible) even without the use of the injectable agent, as all other drugs in the regimen would still be effective, including isoniazid at the normal dose. The duration of treatment should be at least 9 months. In case of additional drug resistance apart from isoniazid, a regimen of at least four or five effective drugs should be used as for MDR-TB. The shorter WHO RMR/MDR-TB regimen could still be used if there is no resistance to the fluoroquinolones or SLIDs.

Multidrug-resistant/extensively drug-resistant tuberculosis

Adult treatment regimens should be at least as effective in children as in adults and therefore similar regimens, including the WHO shorter MDR regimen of 9–12 months, may be used [92]. In those with additional resistance to second-line drugs, individualised MDR-TB treatment regimens should be constructed as shown in figure 3. Currently recommended doses are summarised in table 2. A number of considerations/challenges are listed in table 3.

Anti-tuberculosis and antiretroviral therapy drug–drug interactions

Combining these drug groups is often a challenge. Known drug–drug interactions (DDIs) are summarised in table 4.

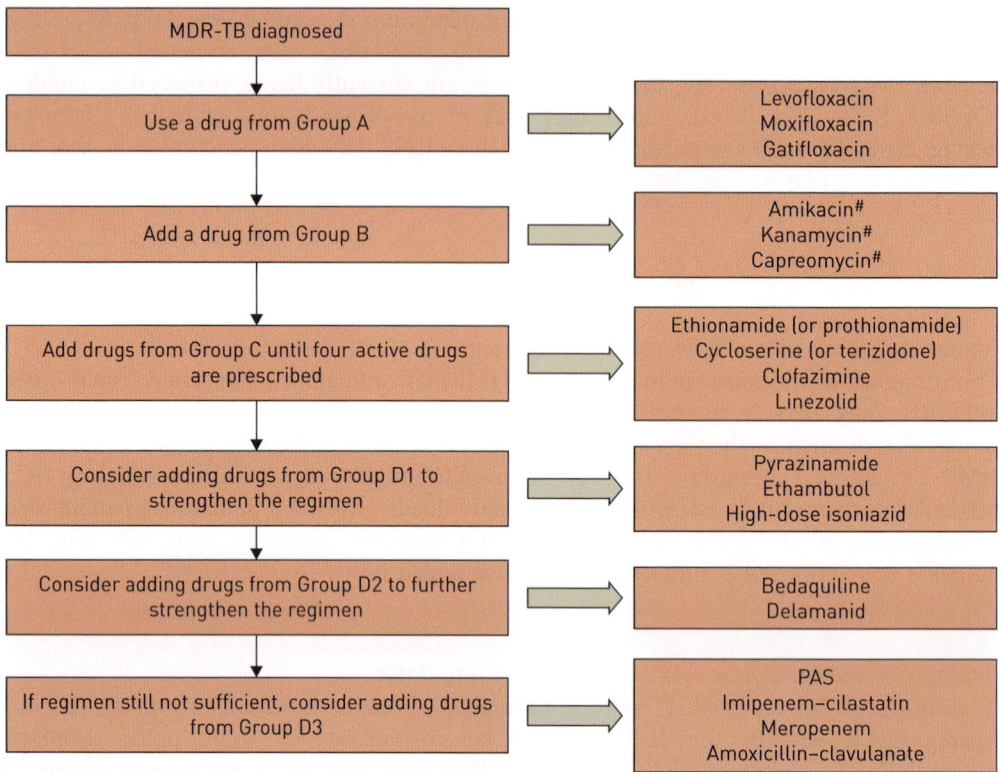

Figure 3. Constructing an effective regimen for MDR- or XDR-TB entails adding drugs from different WHO MDR-TB drug groups until a minimum of four active drugs are included. #: a recent development in the management of DR-TB in children is to replace the injectable agent with either PAS, delamanid or bedaquiline depending on availability and the age of the child (see dosing in table 2) [93]. Reproduced and modified from [94] with permission.

Challenges in prevention

Reducing transmission within the community

At a population level, early diagnosis and effective treatment of highly infectious TB cases is important to terminate ongoing transmission and protect children [114]. However, as demonstrated by the DOTS strategy, an exclusive focus on adults with sputum smear-positive TB ignores the burden of preventable and treatable TB disease in children [115]. Using traditional passive case finding, most TB cases experience significant diagnostic delay and have already infected most of their close contacts by the time they receive treatment. Diagnostic delay is influenced by a multitude of health system and health-seeking behaviour factors that are often difficult to address. This triggered a shift in emphasis to active case finding, as demonstrated by the "FAST" strategy for the early detection of DR-TB, which is comprised of three components: 1) Find cases Actively by cough surveillance and rapid molecular testing, 2) Separate safely, and 3) Treat effectively [116]. Active case finding among high-risk individuals, such as close TB contacts, facilitates early diagnosis and is crucial to protect children.

Nosocomial transmission is a major challenge, as demonstrated in South Africa where transmitted XDR-TB resulted in high mortality among HIV-infected patients and

Table 3. Challenges and proposed solutions in the management of DR-TB

Challenges and considerations	Proposed solutions
Nonsevere or paucibacillary disease	Can be treated for shorter duration compared with adults with cavitating PTB. It may also be possible to treat such children without an injectable agent as long as there are at least three or four effective drugs in the regimen [92, 95].
ETTB, especially central nervous system and miliary TB	These types of disease require careful consideration of drugs that penetrate the blood–brain barrier. Second-line drugs with good cerebrospinal fluid penetration are ethionamide, the fluoroquinolones, linezolid and cycloserine.
Pharmacokinetics and safety of second-line drugs in children	Ongoing pharmacokinetic studies in children are guiding suggested changes in dosing of second-line drugs. SLIDs cause hearing loss in 25% of children treated and efforts should be made to eliminate or minimise their use [96]. The use of N-acetylcysteine may reduce hearing loss in those treated with SLIDs and requires further investigation [97].
New and repurposed drugs	These drugs are rapidly changing the management of MDR/XDR-TB. Although the repurposed drugs, such as the fluoroquinolones, clofazimine and linezolid, are already extensively used in DR-TB management, data on their pharmacokinetics and safety with prolonged use in children are limited. Some guidance has been provided on their use [98, 99]. New drugs such as bedaquiline, delamanid and pretomanid still await paediatric studies to determine both dose and safety [100], which seriously hampers effective and safe treatment of children.
Child-friendly drug formulations	Infants and children with low bodyweight almost universally have had to use tablets formulated for adults. Child-friendly formulations permit the prevention of cutting and crushing of adult tablets to dose children, which leads to over- or underdosing of drugs, increased adverse effects, uncertain bioavailability and poor palatability. The development of palatable, dispersible, smaller milligram-size tablets for children can be achieved, but it remains challenging to get these properly and continuously manufactured, approved, and distributed to where these are needed most [100, 101].
Anti-TB and ART in HIV-infected children	The combined use of TB and ART remains a challenge of high pill burdens, DDIs, immune reconstitution inflammatory syndrome and similar drug-related adverse effects [100]. Continuously changing MDR-TB regimens create challenges determining relevant DDIs.
Adherence to treatment	Adherence to treatment remains challenging due to a variety of factors including adverse effects, palatability of drugs, having a reliable caregiver or treatment supporter, socioeconomic factors, distance from clinics, stubbornness of toddlers and teenagers, peer pressure/stigma, and many other factors. These issues need to be addressed early and repeatedly by the healthcare workers in a supporting, nonjudgemental way, as the aim is to build trust and assist all patients to complete an effective course of treatment.

Continued

Table 3. Continued	
Challenges and considerations	**Proposed solutions**
Drug adverse effects and drug tolerability	Adverse effects due to the second-line drugs are common and can be graded according to severity [102], but additional knowledge is required to determine which drug causes what adverse effect in a particular patient [103, 104]. In children, the permanent discontinuation of TB drugs is uncommon, except for hearing loss induced by SLIDs. Sometimes drugs need to be interrupted or doses adapted for nonserious adverse effects such as nausea caused by prothionamide/ethionamide or skin discolouration with clofazimine. In general it is better for the clinician to assist patients in finding an acceptable regimen than to risk nonadherence. Any regimen adjustment should take into account the patient's treatment response. If good, then an offending drug could be replaced with an effective alternative drug, but if treatment response is poor or uncertain, then a full treatment review should be performed without adding or changing a single drug at a time.

DDI: drug–drug interaction.

healthcare workers in a rural hospital [117]. Infection control in the healthcare setting requires close attention to administrative measures such as cough triage and effective respiratory isolation of infectious patients. Separation of potentially infectious patients (*e.g.* coughing adults) and vulnerable young children has particular relevance, and is rarely implemented in primary or secondary care settings in TB-endemic areas [118].

Vaccination and comorbidity

The classic strategy to reduce disease vulnerability at the population level is through vaccination. *M. bovis* BCG is an attenuated live vaccine with multiple beneficial effects, including protection against disseminated forms of TB in infants and young children. Continued at-birth BCG vaccination is crucial in TB-endemic areas, since it provides limited, but important, protection against severe forms of TB, including DS-TB and DR-TB [119]. Unfortunately, BCG offers limited protection against adult forms of disease and has not demonstrated any discernible epidemic impact [120]. Enhanced vaccines that could potentially replace BCG are in advanced stages of development, but a superior BCG replacement is unlikely in the near future [121].

Unlike TB, classic vaccine-preventable diseases such as smallpox or measles have a high "attack rate" and disease usually leads to lifelong acquired immunity. With *M. tuberculosis*, >90% of immune-competent individuals never develop TB disease following infection, which demonstrates the importance of immune immaturity associated with young age and comorbidities such as HIV infection, DM, malnutrition and other poverty-related factors, which increases individual risk and reduces "community-level herd immunity" [122]. The protective effect of ART is well documented, and provides a strong case in point that the

https://doi.org/10.1183/2312508X.10021817

Table 4. Possible drug–drug interactions (DDIs) between anti-TB drugs and antiretroviral drugs

Anti-TB drug	Antiretroviral drug	DDIs
Rifampicin [105, 106]	Lopinavir/ritonavir and other protease inhibitors	Protease inhibitor concentrations decreased by >75%. Need adapted dosing. With lopinavir/ritonavir, superboosting ritonavir to the same level as lopinavir in children is required.
Rifampicin [105]	Nucleoside reverse transcriptase inhibitor: zidovudine	47% decrease in zidovudine AUC.
Rifampicin [105]	Non-nucleoside reverse transcriptase inhibitors: nevirapine, efavirenz and etravirine	Nevirapine decreased by 20–58%. Switch to efavirenz preferred. Infants on prevention of mother-to-child transmission programmes could have low nevirapine concentration if on rifampicin. Efavirenz and etravirine decreased by 15–30%. No dose adaptation required.
Rifampicin [105, 107]	Integrase strand transfer inhibitors: raltegravir and dolutegravir	In adults, significant decrease in exposure requiring doubling the twice daily dose for raltegravir and twice daily instead of once daily dose for dolutegravir.
Rifabutin (only DDIs of note) [105, 108]	Efavirenz	Reduces rifabutin exposure by 38%. Rifampicin preferred rifamycin with efavirenz.
Rifabutin [105]	Protease inhibitors	Increase rifabutin AUC by 55–473%: lopinavir/ritonavir increases rifabutin and metabolite AUC by 473%; darunavir/ritonavir increases rifabutin AUC by 55%. Even with reduced doses, high adverse effects (uveitis and neutropenia) were seen in a small study. Rifabutin NOT recommended.
Rifapentine [109, 110]	Integrase strand transfer inhibitors: raltegravir and dolutegravir	Studies in healthy adult volunteers showed raltegravir to be safe and no significant change in exposure, while dolutegravir AUC decreased by 46% with rifapentine/isoniazid and had serious toxicities.
High-dose isoniazid, ethionamide, ethambutol, pyrazinamide, amikacin and terizidone [111]	Lopinavir/ritonavir	No significant effect on lopinavir/ritonavir.

Continued

Table 4. Continued

Anti-TB drug	Antiretroviral drug	DDIs
Bedaquiline (and its M2 metabolite) [100, 112]	Lopinavir/ritonavir (boosted protease inhibitor)	Increase in bedaquiline exposure due to reduced clearance; however, no increased toxicity as M2 metabolite lowered.
Bedaquiline (and its M2 metabolite) [100]	Nevirapine	No significant interaction.
Bedaquiline [100]	Efavirenz	About 50% reduction in bedaquiline exposure when chronically coadministered with efavirenz.
Delamanid [113]	Efavirenz, nevirapine, tenofovir and boosted protease inhibitor	No relevant DDIs with any antiretrorvirals, as no induction or inhibition of the cytochrome CYP450 system.
Pretomanid (PA824) [100]	Efavirenz	Cytochrome CYP3A minor metabolic pathway for PA824. Reduces PA824 exposure by 35%.
Pretomanid (PA824) [100]	Lopinavir/ritonavir (boosted protease inhibitor)	Cytochrome CYP3A minor metabolic pathway for PA824. Reduces PA824 exposure by 17%.
Clofazimine [100]		No known DDIs with antiretrorvirals, but studies lacking.
Linezolid [100]	Antiretroviral drugs	No known DDIs, but possible increase risk of mitochondrial optic neuropathies with nucleotide reverse transcriptase inhibitors.
Fluoroquinolones [100]		No known DDIs with antiretrorvirals.

AUC: area under the concentration–time curve.

prevention and optimal management of chronic diseases protect against TB, including DR-TB. In children, the prevention of vertical HIV infection and early initiation of ART in those who do become infected drastically improves child survival and reduces the risk of TB disease [8].

Preventive therapy

Estimates suggest that nearly 2 billion people have TB infection [123]. TB infection treatment aims to reduce the reservoir of infection from which future cases will arise and is a key component of the WHO End TB Strategy [124]. An important additional aim is to protect vulnerable young children against rapid disease progression following documented TB exposure/infection. The rationale to provide preventive therapy to vulnerable young children is even stronger in settings where diagnostic access is limited and TB is a major contributor to mortality in those <5 years of age. However, despite the strong theoretical

https://doi.org/10.1183/2312508X.10021817

rationale and proven benefit of preventive therapy, this is rarely implemented in TB-endemic areas [125]. This major policy practice gap requires urgent attention to reduce the paediatric TB disease burden in settings with poor epidemic control and should be a major focus of the upcoming United Nations (UN) General Assembly resolution on TB [126]. It should be recognised that preventive therapy may only provide transient protection in settings with uncontrolled transmission, given the high likelihood of re-infection. In settings with low re-infection risk the protection provided by preventive therapy should be long lived. As a public health intervention, large-scale community-wide TB infection treatment would be most effective if transmission is controlled at the same time through active case finding: a truly durable effect can be achieved when all TB infection and active disease is eliminated at the same time [127].

Several effective regimens are available to treat DS-TB infection (table 5). Daily rifampicin for 4 months (4R) or 3 months of isoniazid/rifampicin (3HR) has demonstrated equivalent protection to 9 months of isoniazid (9H), with improved treatment adherence and fewer adverse effects [128–131]. In children, 3HR is a highly desirable regimen given that child-friendly dispersible combination tablets are now widely available *via* the Global Drug Facility. 12 doses of weekly isoniazid/rifapentine (3HP) has also been shown to be equivalent to 9H [132], and can be used in children as young as 2 years of age and among people living with HIV. While US CDC guidelines now recommend 3HP as the preferred regimen, rifapentine has limited availability outside the USA, and its efficacy and safety have not been established in children aged <2 years [133]. Among people living with HIV who are on ART, DDIs especially with the rifamycins should be taken into consideration (table 4).

In isoniazid-resistant, rifampicin-susceptible TB contacts 4R and in rifampicin-resistant, isoniazid-susceptible contacts 6–9H should be adequate as preventive therapy. For MDR-TB contacts the evidence is mounting that secondary disease could be prevented [134, 135]. A number of observational studies suggest efficacy and safety of a fluoroquinolone-based 6–12-month preventive therapy regimen for MDR-TB contacts [136–139]. The most recent WHO guidelines indicate that preventive therapy should be considered in high-risk household contacts of patients with MDR-TB, based on individualised risk–benefit assessment [129]. In an expert consensus Policy Brief the provision of MDR-TB prophylaxis to all high-risk contacts, including children aged <5 years and immunocompromised individuals, is recommended using a fluoroquinolone alone (moxifloxacin or levofloxacin) for 6 months or a fluoroquinolone combined with another agent to which the source case's isolate is susceptible, such as ethambutol or ethionamide [134]. Two RCTs comparing levofloxacin to placebo are ongoing (TB-CHAMP and VQUIN) [100]. A single-drug preventive therapy regimen has the advantage of lower cost, less risk of adverse effects and better adherence. Currently there is no suggested effective regimen for MDR-TB contacts with additional fluoroquinolone resistance; however, a delamanid *versus* isoniazid preventive study is planned which would treat all MDR-TB contacts, including those with additional resistance (PHOENIx) [100]. In the absence of preventive therapy these children need to be observed for 1–2 years to exclude disease development.

Preventive therapy in newborn infants
Neonates born to mothers with a recent prenatal or post-natal diagnosis of TB are at high risk of infection and progression to TB disease [140, 141]. Post-natal infection may also occur through contact with other infectious source cases [141]. Risk of TB infection and

Table 5. Options for the treatment of LTBI in children exposed to drug-susceptible TB and MDR-TB[#]

Drug regimens (in order of preference)	Benefits	Limitations
DS-TB exposure		
3HP (12 weekly doses)	Highly feasible, low toxicity, only 12 doses required; endorsed by the CDC and WHO	Not advised in children <2 years; no pharmacokinetic/safety data available; limited rifapentine availability outside the USA; no child-friendly preparations
3HR (daily dosing)	Child-friendly water-dispersible fixed-dose combination tablets available via the Global Drug Facility; endorsed by the UK (NICE guidelines), WHO and Canadian TB standards	DDI should be considered when using rifampicin in children on ART
4R (daily dosing)	Limited risk of hepatotoxicity; endorsed by the WHO and Canadian TB standards	DDI should be considered when using rifampicin in children on ART
6–9H (daily dosing)	Strong historical data demonstrating efficacy and safety in children; endorsed by the WHO, CDC, NICE and Canadian TB standards	Poor implementation and persistent practice policy gaps despite years of promotion; suboptimal treatment adherence given prolonged course of treatment
MDR-TB exposure		
6 Lfx/Mfx (daily dosing)	Simple single-drug intervention; well tolerated	Not yet endorsed by the WHO, advises individualised management (ongoing studies); may not be equally effective in all locations; risk of drug resistance amplification if active disease not ruled out
At least two drugs, based on DST profile of source case	Generic approach that can be applied to a range of drug resistance profiles	Not yet endorsed by the WHO, advises individualised management; carefully consider potential risks and benefits

DS-TB: drug-susceptible TB; DDI: drug–drug interaction; NICE: National Institute for Health and Care Excellence. See table 2 for drug abbreviations. [#]: resistant to isoniazid and rifampicin.

disease is further increased if mothers are infected with HIV [142]. Preventive therapy should be provided in all TB-exposed infants after exclusion of active disease, considering that disease would be primarily abdominal with placental transmission and pulmonary with aspiration of infected vaginal secretions or post-partum inhalation, with high risk of disease dissemination. In DS-TB contacts, preventive therapy with 6–9H, 3HR or 4R should be started as soon as TB disease has been excluded. The dose of isoniazid should not exceed 10 mg·kg^{-1} daily in neonates [85]. DDIs with concomitant ART should be considered. In MDR-TB contacts, a fluoroquinolone with or without another effective drug should be used for prevention. Currently there is no effective preventive therapy for pre- or XDR-TB exposure. In these cases infants should preferably be separated from any infectious source case or, if not possible, effective infectious control measures implemented. BCG is usually withheld until preventive therapy is completed.

https://doi.org/10.1183/2312508X.10021817

Addressing the barriers to preventive therapy

Barriers to the uptake of this evidence-based intervention are multiple [125, 126]. Health system managers require evidence of population-scale impact in a modern setting, and are reluctant to implement a strategy that lacks international consensus and is not effectively monitored. Prescribers in many settings express reluctance to prescribe TB infection treatment, since they fear it will facilitate the development of drug resistance and are worried about potential adverse effects in someone who is otherwise healthy. People with TB infection are often reluctant themselves to commit to a prolonged course of treatment for something that does not affect their quality of life or perception of risk.

Way forward

The greatest positive impact would likely be achieved by better implementation of preventive therapy strategies, which requires a strong emphasis on family-centred care to enhance entry and retention within the cascade of care. Other key priorities for operational research and implementation include integration of child TB into routine maternal and child health services, HIV care, and nutrition programmes, since children with TB are unlikely to present to the TB programme. This would require better training and empowerment of front-line healthcare workers to screen TB contacts for active disease using simple symptom-based approaches, provide preventive therapy as appropriate and to refer children for further evaluation. Table 6 provides a summary of TB research priorities identified by the Stop TB Partnership Child and Adolescent TB Working Group and summarised by the Treatment Action Group.

The UN High-Level Meeting on TB in September 2018 represented an unprecedented opportunity to strengthen the commitment of countries to the WHO End TB Strategy. Countries have been challenged to increase child TB awareness, identify their own solutions and to meet the following targets [144]: 1) by 2019, all states to have established an Inter-Ministry Task Force and developed a funded action plan to address childhood TB comprehensively across maternal, child and adolescent populations; 2) by 2022, 100% of children at high risk of TB (2.4 million TB-exposed children aged <5 years per year) to receive preventive therapy; and 3) by 2022, 90% of children with TB (900 000) and MDR-TB (28 800) are diagnosed each year and put on appropriate treatment.

Conclusion

Childhood TB still faces many challenges. However, the implementation of available, established, evidence-based interventions would have the greatest impact. These include active contact tracing of infectious TB cases, followed by screening of contacts for TB disease and then starting high-risk child contacts, without TB disease, on effective preventive therapy. Furthermore, it is important to always consider the diagnosis of TB disease in children, especially in young children presenting with lung infection, meningitis or symptoms and signs consistent with other forms of ETTB. If TB is missed, it can lead to severe morbidity and death. More sensitive diagnostic tools will be a great advantage, but even with existing diagnostic tools many more children could be diagnosed by carefully assembling the different pieces of the puzzle. It is important to emphasise that although many developments are ongoing for the treatment of TB infection and disease, effective

Table 6. Overview of paediatric TB research priorities[#]

Epidemiology	Describe and monitor the burden of TB infection and disease (including DR-TB) and treatment outcomes among children and adolescents at the national level
	Describe and monitor the burden of TB infection and disease (including DR-TB), socioeconomic impact and treatment issues for children and adolescents living with HIV
	Describe the occurrence of residual morbidity after cure or treatment completion (both in HIV-negative and -positive children and adolescents), including long-term adverse effects and socioeconomic impacts of TB treatment
	Evaluate completeness of routine recording and reporting of childhood TB along the care cascade, including how to strengthen and standardise reporting of child contact management and the provision of preventive therapy
Basic science (fundamental research)	Characterise the immune response to TB infection and disease in children, considering variability by age, nutritional status, coinfections, disease phenotype, as well as mycobacterial and host genotype
	Through multicentre longitudinal paediatric cohort studies, support the discovery, evaluation and validation of novel biomarkers (including those that can: accurately distinguish children with TB disease from those presenting with similar symptoms; distinguish between infection and disease; predict risk of disease progression among children with TB infection; and be used to assess response to treatment and vaccine efficacy) among children with a broad spectrum of disease presentations
	Other basic science priorities are included within the relevant following entries
Prevention	Conduct pharmacokinetic and safety studies of new preventive drug regimens in children to inform optimal dosing, including for children coinfected with HIV
	Evaluate shorter and simplified drug treatment regimens for TB infection in children, including those that can be used to prevent TB among contacts of DR-TB
	Develop a vaccine to be given to neonates (with and without HIV exposure), children or adolescents that improves on the safety and efficacy of BCG
Diagnosis	Identify, evaluate and validate host biomarkers derived from paediatric populations as potential novel tests for TB infection, TB disease, risk of disease progression and response to treatment in children
	Identify novel assays that meet criteria to be used as a highly sensitive "rule-out" screening test (requiring noninvasive samples and for use at the point of care)
	Identify, evaluate and validate novel pathogen-associated biomarkers in paediatric populations as potential novel diagnostic tests for active TB (e.g. DNA, mRNA expression profiles, micro-RNA, next-generation lipoarabinomannan-based assays)
	Optimise the current microbiological reference standard by: improving and harmonising specimen collection; supporting laboratory research to optimise specimen processing to optimise diagnostic yield using current assays; and improving phenotypic and genotypic DST on paediatric clinical specimens
	Harmonise collection, processing and storage of well-characterised biorepository specimens, support their maintenance and improve collaborative efforts to allow testing of novel assays on larger, harmonised specimen banks

Continued

https://doi.org/10.1183/2312508X.10021817

	Table 6. Continued

Treatment
Conduct timely pharmacokinetic and safety studies of new TB medications in children to inform optimal dosing, including for children coinfected with HIV

Ensure adolescent inclusion in late-stage clinical trials of new TB drugs, regimens and treatment strategies

Evaluate treatment shortening and simplification strategies, including those that reduce treatment-related toxicities for children with TB, including DR-TB

Evaluate regimens to improve treatment outcomes, including residual morbidities caused by TB and certain TB treatments, and reduce treatment duration among children with the most severe forms of TB, including tuberculous meningitis

Operational research
Determine the most appropriate and cost-effective service delivery models for children of all ages (0–18 years) among the maternal and child health continuum of care

Evaluate programme integration strategies for paediatric TB, including with HIV, maternal, neonatal and child health, nutrition, and other relevant programmes

Assess health system needs, including human resources and cost, for scaling up evidence-based interventions and programme integration for TB prevention and treatment at the national level

Identify pragmatic and scalable decentralised community-based strategies (e.g. family-centred models) for TB screening and provision of preventive therapy and TB treatment to enhance early entry and retention in the cascade of care

Conduct qualitative research to better understand facilitators of and barriers to provision of preventive therapy, diagnostic access, treatment adherence and effective management for families affected by TB

Conduct social research to better understand the impacts of stigma and TB on education among school-aged children and adolescents

Determine efficient and reliable systems for specimen collection, transport and laboratory evaluation, especially important for following up children with smear-negative, paucibacillary specimens

#: research priorities identified by the Stop TB Partnership Child and Adolescent TB Working Group and summarised by the Treatment Action Group towards: improved prevention, diagnosis and management of children and adolescents affected by TB; a vaccine with better and lasting protective efficacy; accurate, non-sputum-based point-of-care diagnostics tests; and shorter, safer and more child-friendly regimens for TB prevention and treatment. Reproduced and modified from [143] with permission.

therapy is available for the vast majority of children with both DS-TB and DR-TB, if diagnostic and treatment access can be secured.

References

1. World Health Organization. Global Tuberculosis Report 2016. Geneva, WHO, 2017.
2. Snow KJ, Sismanidis C, Denholm J, et al. The incidence of tuberculosis among adolescents and young adults: a global estimate. Eur Respir J 2018; 51: 1702352.
3. Dodd PJ, Yuen CM, Sismanidis C, et al. The global burden of tuberculosis mortality in children: a mathematical modelling study. Lancet Glob Health 2017; 5: e898–e906.

4. Graham SM, Sismanidis C, Menzies HJ, *et al.* Importance of tuberculosis control to address child survival. *Lancet* 2014; 383: 1605–1607.

5. Dodd PJ, Sismanidis C, Seddon JA. Global burden of drug-resistant tuberculosis in children: a mathematical modelling study. *Lancet Infect Dis* 2016; 16: 1193–1201.

6. World Health Organization. Guidance for National Tuberculosis Programmes on the Management of Tuberculosis in Children. 2nd Edn. Geneva, WHO, 2014.

7. Marais BJ, Gie RP, Schaaf HS, *et al.* The natural history of childhood intra-thoracic tuberculosis: a critical review of literature from the pre-chemotherapy era. *Int J Tuberc Lung Dis* 2004; 8: 392–402.

8. Dodd PJ, Prendergast AJ, Beecroft C, *et al.* The impact of HIV and antiretroviral therapy on TB risk in children: a systematic review and meta-analysis. *Thorax* 2017; 72: 559–575.

9. Jaganath D, Mupere E. Childhood tuberculosis and malnutrition. *J Infect Dis* 2012; 206: 1809–1815.

10. Horsburgh CR Jr, Rubin EJ. Latent tuberculosis infection in the United States. *N Engl J Med* 2011; 364: 1441–1448.

11. Perez-Velez CM, Marais BJ. Tuberculosis in children. *N Engl J Med* 2012; 367: 348–361.

12. Donald PR, Marais BJ, Barry CE 3rd. Age and the epidemiology and pathogenesis of tuberculosis. *Lancet* 2010; 375: 1852–1854.

13. Hertting O, Shingadia D. Childhood TB: when to think of it and what to do when you do. *J Infect* 2014; 68: Suppl. 1, S151–S154.

14. Marais BJ, Hesseling AC, Gie RP, *et al.* The bacteriologic yield in children with intrathoracic tuberculosis. *Clin Infect Dis* 2006; 42: e69–e71.

15. Steppacher A, Scheer I, Relly C, *et al.* Unrecognized pediatric adult-type tuberculosis puts school contacts at risk. *Pediatr Infect Dis J* 2014; 33: 325–328.

16. Marais BJ, Gie RP, Schaaf HS, *et al.* The spectrum of disease in children treated for tuberculosis in a highly endemic area. *Int J Tuberc Lung Dis* 2006; 10: 732–738.

17. Bang ND, Caws M, Truc TT, *et al.* Clinical presentations, diagnosis, mortality and prognostic markers of tuberculous meningitis in Vietnamese children: a prospective descriptive study. *BMC Infect Dis* 2016; 16: 573.

18. Marais BJ, Wright CA, Schaaf HS, *et al.* Tuberculous lymphadenitis as a cause of persistent cervical lymphadenopathy in children from a tuberculosis-endemic area. *Pediatr Infect Dis J* 2006; 25: 142–146.

19. Schaaf HS, Garcia-Prats AJ. Diagnosis of the most common forms of extrathoracic tuberculosis in children. *In:* Starke JR, Donald PR, eds. Handbook of Child and Adolescent Tuberculosis. New York, Oxford University Press, 2016; pp. 177–199.

20. Marais BJ, Gie RP, Hesseling AC, *et al.* A refined symptom-based approach to diagnose pulmonary tuberculosis in children. *Pediatrics* 2006; 118: e1350–e1359.

21. Marais BJ, Schaaf HS. Tuberculosis in children. *Cold Spring Harb Perspect Med* 2014; 4: a017855.

22. Mandal N, Anand PK, Gautam S, *et al.* Diagnosis and treatment of paediatric tuberculosis: an insight review. *Crit Rev Microbiol* 2017; 43: 466–480.

23. Marais BJ, Gie RP, Obihara CC, *et al.* Well defined symptoms are of value in the diagnosis of childhood pulmonary tuberculosis. *Arch Dis Child* 2005; 90: 1162–1165.

24. Schaaf HS, Donald PR, Scott F. Maternal chest radiography as supporting evidence for the diagnosis of tuberculosis in childhood. *J Trop Pediatr* 1991; 37: 223–225.

25. Schaaf HS, Michaelis IA, Richardson M, *et al.* Adult-to-child transmission of tuberculosis: household or community contact? *Int J Tuberc Lung Dis* 2003; 7: 426–431.

26. Luzzati R, Migliori GB, Zignol M, *et al.* Children under 5 years are at risk for tuberculosis after occasional contact with highly contagious patients: outbreak from a smear-positive healthcare worker. *Eur Respir J* 2017; 50: 1701414.

27. Solomons R, Grantham M, Marais BJ, *et al.* IMCI indicators of childhood TBM at primary health care level in the Western Cape Province of South Africa. *Int J Tuberc Lung Dis* 2016; 20: 1309–1313.

28. Philip N, William T, John DV. Diagnosis of tuberculous meningitis: challenges and promises. *Malays J Pathol* 2015; 37: 1–9.

29. Mandalakas AM, Kirchner HL, Walzl G, *et al.* Optimizing the detection of recent tuberculosis infection in children in a high tuberculosis-HIV burden setting. *Am J Respir Crit Care Med* 2015; 191: 820–830.

30. European Centre for Disease Prevention and Control, Stockholm, Sweden. Use of Interferon-gamma Release Assays in Support of TB Diagnosis. Stockholm, ECDC, 2011.

31. Seddon JA, Padayachee T, Du Plessis AM, *et al.* Teaching chest X-ray reading for child tuberculosis suspects. *Int J Tuberc Lung Dis* 2014; 18: 763–769.

32. Graham SM. Chest radiography for diagnosis of tuberculosis in children: a problem of interpretation. *Int J Tuberc Lung Dis* 2014; 18: 757.

33. Swingler GH, du Toit G, Andronikou S, *et al.* Diagnostic accuracy of chest radiography in detecting mediastinal lymphadenopathy in suspected pulmonary tuberculosis. *Arch Dis Child* 2005; 90: 1153–1156.

34. Muyoyeta M, Maduskar P, Moyo M, *et al.* The sensitivity and specificity of using a computer aided diagnosis program for automatically scoring chest X-rays of presumptive TB patients compared with Xpert MTB/RIF in Lusaka Zambia. *PLoS One* 2014; 9: e93757.

https://doi.org/10.1183/2312508X.10021817

35. Melendez J, Hogeweg L, Sanchez CI, *et al.* Accuracy of an automated system for tuberculosis detection on chest radiographs in high-risk screening. *Int J Tuberc Lung Dis* 2018; 22: 567–571.

36. Palmer M, Walters E, Hesseling AC, *et al.* Atypical radiological patterns in children with bacteriologically confirmed pulmonary tuberculosis. *Int J Tuberc Lung Dis* 2016; 20: Suppl. 1, S296–S297.

37. Belard S, Heuvelings CC, Banderker E, *et al.* Utility of point-of-care ultrasound in children with pulmonary tuberculosis. *Pediatr Infect Dis J* 2018; 37: 637–642.

38. Pool KL, Heuvelings CC, Belard S, *et al.* Technical aspects of mediastinal ultrasound for pediatric pulmonary tuberculosis. *Pediatr Radiol* 2017; 47: 1839–1848.

39. Andronikou S, Wieselthaler N. Imaging for tuberculosis in children. *In:* Schaaf HS, Zumla A, eds. Tuberculosis: A Comprehensive Clinical Reference. London, Saunders, 2009; pp. 216–226.

40. Concepcion NDP, Laya BF, Andronikou S, *et al.* Standardized radiographic interpretation of thoracic tuberculosis in children. *Pediatr Radiol* 2017; 47: 1237–1248.

41. Ziemele B, Ranka R, Ozere I. Pediatric and adolescent tuberculosis in Latvia, 2011–2014: case detection, diagnosis and treatment. *Int J Tuberc Lung Dis* 2017; 21: 637–645.

42. Gomez-Pastrana D, Carceller-Blanchard A. Debe realizarse una tomografia computarizada toracica a los ninos con infeccion tuberculosa sin enfermedad aparente? [Should pulmonary computed tomography be performed in children with tuberculosis infection without apparent disease?] *An Pediatr* 2007; 67: 585–593.

43. Agarwal KK, Behera A, Kumar R, *et al.* ^{18}F-Fluorodeoxyglucose-positron emission tomography/computed tomography in tuberculosis: spectrum of manifestations. *Indian J Nucl Med* 2017; 32: 316–321.

44. Joshi AR, Basantani AS, Patel TC. Role of CT and MRI in abdominal tuberculosis. *Curr Radiol Rep* 2014; 2: 66.

45. Roya-Pabon CL, Perez-Velez CM. Tuberculosis exposure, infection and disease in children: a systematic diagnostic approach. *Pneumonia* 2016; 8: 23.

46. Schaaf HS, Garcia-Prats AJ. Multidrug-resistant tuberculosis in children: recent developments in diagnosis, treatment and prevention. *Curr Pediatr Rep* 2016; 4: 53–62.

47. Ramos JM, Perez-Butragueno M, Tisiano G, *et al.* Evaluation of Ziehl–Neelsen smear for diagnosis of pulmonary tuberculosis in childhood in a rural hospital in Ethiopia. *Int J Mycobacteriol* 2013; 2: 171–173.

48. Marais BJ, Gie RP, Hesseling AH, *et al.* Adult-type pulmonary tuberculosis in children 10–14 years of age. *Pediatr Infect Dis J* 2005; 24: 743–744.

49. Slim-Saidi L, Mehiri-Zeghal E, Ghariani A, *et al.* Nouvelles methodes de diagnostic de la tuberculose. [New methods of diagnosis in tuberculosis.] *Rev Pneumol Clin* 2015; 71: 110–121.

50. World Health Organization. Automated Real-time Nucleic Acid Amplification Technology for Rapid and Simultaneous Detection of Tuberculosis and Rifampicin Resistance: Xpert MTB/RIF System: Policy Statement. Geneva, WHO, 2011.

51. Detjen AK, DiNardo AR, Leyden J, *et al.* Xpert MTB/RIF assay for the diagnosis of pulmonary tuberculosis in children: a systematic review and meta-analysis. *Lancet Respir Med* 2015; 3: 451–461.

52. Nicol MP, Workman L, Prins M, *et al.* Accuracy of Xpert MTB/RIF Ultra for the diagnosis of pulmonary tuberculosis in children. *Pediatr Infect Dis J* 2018; 37: e261–e263.

53. World Health Organization. WHO Meeting Report of a Technical Expert Consultation: Non-inferiority Analysis of Xpert MTF/RIF Ultra Compared to Xpert MTB/RIF. Geneva, WHO, 2017.

54. World Health Organization. The Use of Molecular Line Probe Assays for the Detection of Resistance to Second-line Anti-tuberculosis Drugs: Policy Guidance. Geneva, WHO, 2016.

55. World Health Organization. The Use of Molecular Line Probe Assays for the Detection of Resistance to Isoniazid and Rifampicin: Policy Update. Geneva, WHO, 2016.

56. Schaaf HS, Victor TC, Venter A, *et al.* Ethionamide cross- and co-resistance in children with isoniazid-resistant tuberculosis. *Int J Tuberc Lung Dis* 2009; 13: 1355–1359.

57. Schon T, Miotto P, Koser CU, *et al. Mycobacterium tuberculosis* drug-resistance testing: challenges, recent developments and perspectives. *Clin Microbiol Infect* 2017; 23: 154–160.

58. Martinez E, Holmes N, Jelfs P, *et al.* Genome sequencing reveals novel deletions associated with secondary resistance to pyrazinamide in MDR *Mycobacterium tuberculosis. J Antimicrob Chemother* 2015; 70: 2511–2514.

59. Zhang Y, Yew WW. Mechanisms of drug resistance in *Mycobacterium tuberculosis*: update 2015. *Int J Tuberc Lung Dis* 2015; 19: 1276–1289.

60. Walker TM, Kohl TA, Omar SV, *et al.* Whole-genome sequencing for prediction of *Mycobacterium tuberculosis* drug susceptibility and resistance: a retrospective cohort study. *Lancet Infect Dis* 2015; 15: 1193–1202.

61. Wright CA, Warren RM, Marais BJ. Fine needle aspiration biopsy: an undervalued diagnostic modality in paediatric mycobacterial disease. *Int J Tuberc Lung Dis* 2009; 13: 1467–1475.

62. Ahmed HG, Nassar AS, Ginawi I. Screening for tuberculosis and its histological pattern in patients with enlarged lymph node. *Pathol Res Int* 2011; 2011: 417635.

63. Coetzee L, Nicol MP, Jacobson R, *et al.* Rapid diagnosis of pediatric mycobacterial lymphadenitis using fine needle aspiration biopsy. *Pediatr Infect Dis J* 2014; 33: 893–896.

64. Venturini E, Turkova A, Chiappini E, *et al.* Tuberculosis and HIV co-infection in children. *BMC Infect Dis* 2014; 14: Suppl. 1, S5.

65. Nicol MP, Allen V, Workman L, *et al.* Urine lipoarabinomannan testing for diagnosis of pulmonary tuberculosis in children: a prospective study. *Lancet Glob Health* 2014; 2: e278–e284.

66. Anderson ST, Kaforou M, Brent AJ, *et al.* Diagnosis of childhood tuberculosis and host RNA expression in Africa. *N Engl J Med* 2014; 370: 1712–1723.

67. Portevin D, Moukambi F, Clowes P, *et al.* Assessment of the novel T-cell activation marker-tuberculosis assay for diagnosis of active tuberculosis in children: a prospective proof-of-concept study. *Lancet Infect Dis* 2014; 14: 931–938.

68. Walzl G, McNerney R, du Plessis N, *et al.* Tuberculosis: advances and challenges in development of new diagnostics and biomarkers. *Lancet Infect Dis* 2018; 18: e199–e210.

69. Goussard P, Gie RP. The need for bronchoscopic services for children in low and middle-income countries. *Expert Rev Respir Med* 2016; 10: 477–479.

70. Goussard P, Gie RP, Kling S, *et al.* Bronchoscopic assessment of airway involvement in children presenting with clinically significant airway obstruction due to tuberculosis. *Pediatr Pulmonol* 2013; 48: 1000–1007.

71. Dhooria S, Aggarwal AN, Gupta D, *et al.* Utility and safety of endoscopic ultrasound with bronchoscope-guided fine-needle aspiration in mediastinal lymph node sampling: systematic review and meta-analysis. *Respir Care* 2015; 60: 1040–1050.

72. Goussard P, Gie RP, Kling S, *et al.* The diagnostic value and safety of transbronchial needle aspiration biopsy in children with mediastinal lymphadenopathy. *Pediatr Pulmonol* 2010; 45: 1173–1179.

73. No author. Cycloserine. *Tuberculosis* 2008; 88: 100–101.

74. Denti P, Garcia-Prats AJ, Draper HR, *et al.* Levofloxacin population pharmacokinetics in South African children treated for multidrug-resistant tuberculosis. *Antimicrob Agents Chemother* 2018; 62: e01521-17.

75. Schaaf HS. Current status of drugs used in treatment of MDR-TB in children. 2018. https://bc.lung.ca/sites/default/files/5%20-%20Simon%20Schaaf.pdf Date last accessed: June 11, 2018.

76. Nachman S, Ahmed A, Amanullah F, *et al.* Towards early inclusion of children in tuberculosis drugs trials: a consensus statement. *Lancet Infect Dis* 2015; 15: 711–720.

77. Garcia-Prats AJ, Rose PC, Draper HR, *et al.* Effect of co-administration of lidocaine on the pain and pharmacokinetics of intramuscular amikacin in children with multidrug-resistant tuberculosis: a randomized crossover trial. *Pediatr Infect Dis J* 2018; in press [http://dx.doi.org/10.1097/INF.0000000000001983].

78. van Toorn R, Schaaf HS, Laubscher JA, *et al.* Short intensified treatment in children with drug-susceptible tuberculous meningitis. *Pediatr Infect Dis J* 2014; 33: 248–252.

79. ClinicalTrials.gov. Optimizing treatment to improve TBM outcomes in children (TBM-KIDS). 2017. https://clinicaltrials.gov/ct2/show/NCT02958709 Date last accessed: June 11, 2018.

80. McKenna L. Momentum in the pediatric tuberculosis treatment pipeline. 2015. http://i-base.info/htb/28481 Date last accessed: June 11, 2018.

81. van Toorn R, du Plessis AM, Schaaf HS, *et al.* Clinicoradiologic response of neurologic tuberculous mass lesions in children treated with thalidomide. *Pediatr Infect Dis J* 2015; 34: 214–218.

82. Lanoix JP, Chaisson RE, Nuermberger EL. Shortening tuberculosis treatment with fluoroquinolones: lost in translation? *Clin Infect Dis* 2016; 62: 484–490.

83. Wiseman CA, Gie RP, Starke JR, *et al.* A proposed comprehensive classification of tuberculosis disease severity in children. *Pediatr Infect Dis J* 2012; 31: 347–352.

84. ISRCTN Registry. SHINE study: shorter treatment for minimal TB in children. 2015. www.isrctn.com/ISRCTN63579542 Date last accessed: June 11, 2018.

85. Bekker A, Schaaf HS, Seifart HI, *et al.* Pharmacokinetics of isoniazid in low-birth-weight and premature infants. *Antimicrob Agents Chemother* 2014; 58: 2229–2234.

86. Bekker A, Schaaf HS, Draper HR, *et al.* Pharmacokinetics of rifampin, isoniazid, pyrazinamide, and ethambutol in infants dosed according to revised WHO-recommended treatment guidelines. *Antimicrob Agents Chemother* 2016; 60: 2171–2179.

87. Diacon AH, Patientia RF, Venter A, *et al.* Early bactericidal activity of high-dose rifampin in patients with pulmonary tuberculosis evidenced by positive sputum smears. *Antimicrob Agents Chemother* 2007; 51: 2994–2996.

88. Boeree MJ, Diacon AH, Dawson R, *et al.* A dose-ranging trial to optimize the dose of rifampin in the treatment of tuberculosis. *Am J Respir Crit Care Med* 2015; 191: 1058–1065.

89. Hesseling AC. TB scientific committee update: 2017. 2017. http://impaactnetwork.org/DocFiles/2017AnnualMtg/presentations/tb/AHesseling_IMPAACT%20TBSC%20Update%2020170530.pdf Date last accessed: June 11, 2018.

90. Fregonese F, Ahuja SD, Akkerman OW, *et al.* Comparison of different treatments for isoniazid-resistant tuberculosis: an individual patient data meta-analysis. *Lancet Respir Med* 2018; 6: 265–275.

91. Kurbatova EV, Cavanaugh JS, Shah NS, *et al.* Rifampicin-resistant *Mycobacterium tuberculosis*: susceptibility to isoniazid and other anti-tuberculosis drugs. *Int J Tuberc Lung Dis* 2012; 16: 355–357.

92. World Health Organization. WHO Treatment Guidelines for Drug-resistant Tuberculosis 2106 Update. Geneva, WHO, 2016.

https://doi.org/10.1183/2312508X.10021817

93. World Health Organization. Rapid Communication: Key Changes to Treatment of Multidrug- and Rifampicin-resistant Tuberculosis (MDR/RR-TB). Geneva, WHO, 2018.

94. Seddon JA, Schaaf HS. Drug-resistant tuberculosis and advances in the treatment of childhood tuberculosis. *Pneumonia* 2016; 8: 20.

95. Seddon JA, Hesseling AC, Godfrey-Faussett P, *et al.* High treatment success in children treated for multidrug-resistant tuberculosis: an observational cohort study. *Thorax* 2014; 69: 458–464.

96. Seddon JA, Thee S, Jacobs K, *et al.* Hearing loss in children treated for multidrug-resistant tuberculosis. *J Infect* 2013; 66: 320–329.

97. Kranzer K, Elamin WF, Cox H, *et al.* A systematic review and meta-analysis of the efficacy and safety of *N*-acetylcysteine in preventing aminoglycoside-induced ototoxicity: implications for the treatment of multidrug-resistant TB. *Thorax* 2015; 70: 1070–1077.

98. Harausz EP, Garcia-Prats AJ, Seddon JA, *et al.* New and repurposed drugs for pediatric multidrug-resistant tuberculosis. Practice-based recommendations. *Am J Respir Crit Care Med* 2017; 195: 1300–1310.

99. Tadolini M, Garcia-Prats AJ, D'Ambrosio L, *et al.* Compassionate use of new drugs in children and adolescents with multidrug-resistant and extensively drug-resistant tuberculosis: early experiences and challenges. *Eur Respir J* 2016; 48: 938–943.

100. Schaaf HS, Garcia-Prats AJ, McKenna L, *et al.* Challenges of using new and repurposed drugs for the treatment of multidrug-resistant tuberculosis in children. *Expert Rev Clin Pharmacol* 2018; 11: 233–244.

101. Taneja R, Garcia-Prats AJ, Furin J, *et al.* Paediatric formulations of second-line anti-tuberculosis medications: challenges and considerations. *Int J Tuberc Lung Dis* 2015; 19: Suppl. 1, 61–68.

102. National Institute of Allergy and Infectious Diseases. Division of AIDS (DAIDS) table for grading the severity of adult and pediatric adverse events. Version 2.1. 2017. https://rsc.tech-res.com/docs/default-source/safety/daids-ae-grading-table-mar2017.pdf Date last accessed: June 11, 2018.

103. Schaaf HS, Thee S, van der Laan L, *et al.* Adverse effects of oral second-line antituberculosis drugs in children. *Expert Opin Drug Saf* 2016; 15: 1369–1381.

104. Garcia-Prats AJ, Schaaf HS, Hesseling AC. The safety and tolerability of the second-line injectable antituberculosis drugs in children. *Expert Opin Drug Saf* 2016; 15: 1491–1500.

105. Sahasrabudhe V, Zhu T, Vaz A, *et al.* Drug metabolism and drug interactions: potential application to antituberculosis drugs. *J Infect Dis* 2015; 211: Suppl. 3, S107–S114.

106. Rabie H, Decloedt EH, Garcia-Prats AJ, *et al.* Antiretroviral treatment in HIV-infected children who require a rifamycin-containing regimen for tuberculosis. *Expert Opin Pharmacother* 2017; 18: 589–598.

107. Burger DM. Drug–drug interactions with raltegravir. *Eur J Med Res* 2009; 14: Suppl. 3, 17–21.

108. Regazzi M, Carvalho AC, Villani P, *et al.* Treatment optimization in patients co-infected with HIV and *Mycobacterium tuberculosis* infections: focus on drug–drug interactions with rifamycins. *Clin Pharmacokinet* 2014; 53: 489–507.

109. Weiner M, Egelund EF, Engle M, *et al.* Pharmacokinetic interaction of rifapentine and raltegravir in healthy volunteers. *J Antimicrob Chemother* 2014; 69: 1079–1085.

110. Brooks KM, George JM, Pau AK, *et al.* Cytokine-mediated systemic adverse drug reactions in a drug–drug interaction study of dolutegravir with once-weekly isoniazid and rifapentine. *Clin Infect Dis* 2018; 67: 193–201.

111. van der Laan LE, Garcia-Prats AJ, Schaaf HS, *et al.* Pharmacokinetics and drug–drug interactions of lopinavir–ritonavir administered with first- and second-line antituberculosis drugs in HIV-infected children treated for multidrug-resistant tuberculosis. *Antimicrob Agents Chemother* 2018; 62: e00420-17.

112. Brill MJ, Svensson EM, Pandie M, *et al.* Confirming model-predicted pharmacokinetic interactions between bedaquiline and lopinavir/ritonavir or nevirapine in patients with HIV and drug-resistant tuberculosis. *Int J Antimicrob Agents* 2017; 49: 212–217.

113. Mallikaarjun S, Wells C, Petersen C, *et al.* Delamanid coadministered with antiretroviral drugs or antituberculosis drugs shows no clinically relevant drug–drug interactions in healthy subjects. *Antimicrob Agents Chemother* 2016; 60: 5976–5985.

114. Fox GJ, Schaaf HS, Mandalakas A, *et al.* Preventing the spread of multidrug-resistant tuberculosis and protecting contacts of infectious cases. *Clin Microbiol Infect* 2017; 23: 147–153.

115. Marais BJ, Hesseling AC, Gie RP, *et al.* The burden of childhood tuberculosis and the accuracy of community-based surveillance data. *Int J Tuberc Lung Dis* 2006; 10: 259–263.

116. Barrera E, Livchits V, Nardell E. F-A-S-T: a refocused, intensified, administrative tuberculosis transmission control strategy. *Int J Tuberc Lung Dis* 2015; 19: 381–384.

117. Gandhi NR, Weissman D, Moodley P, *et al.* Nosocomial transmission of extensively drug-resistant tuberculosis in a rural hospital in South Africa. *J Infect Dis* 2013; 207: 9–17.

118. Heyns L, Gie RP, Goussard P, *et al.* Nosocomial transmission of *Mycobacterium tuberculosis* in kangaroo mother care units: a risk in tuberculosis-endemic areas. *Acta Paediatr* 2006; 95: 535–539.

119. Marais BJ, Seddon JA, Detjen AK, *et al.* Interrupted BCG vaccination is a major threat to global child health. *Lancet Respir Med* 2016; 4: 251–253.

120. Moliva JI, Turner J, Torrelles JB. Prospects in *Mycobacterium bovis* Bacille Calmette et Guerin (BCG) vaccine diversity and delivery: why does BCG fail to protect against tuberculosis? *Vaccine* 2015; 33: 5035–5041.

121. Fletcher HA, Schrager L. TB vaccine development and the End TB Strategy: importance and current status. *Trans R Soc Trop Med Hyg* 2016; 110: 212–218.

122. Marais BJ, Tadolini M, Zignol M, *et al.* Paediatric tuberculosis in Europe: lessons from Denmark and inclusive strategies to consider. *Eur Respir J* 2014; 43: 678–684.

123. Houben RM, Dodd PJ. The global burden of latent tuberculosis infection: a re-estimation using mathematical modelling. *PLoS Med* 2016; 13: e1002152.

124. Rangaka MX, Cavalcante SC, Marais BJ, *et al.* Controlling the seedbeds of tuberculosis: diagnosis and treatment of tuberculosis infection. *Lancet* 2015; 386: 2344–2353.

125. Szkwarko D, Hirsch-Moverman Y, Du Plessis L, *et al.* Child contact management in high tuberculosis burden countries: a mixed-methods systematic review. *PLoS One* 2017; 12: e0182185.

126. Hill PC, Rutherford ME, Audas R, *et al.* Closing the policy-practice gap in the management of child contacts of tuberculosis cases in developing countries. *PLoS Med* 2011; 8: e1001105.

127. Fox GJ, Dobler CC, Marais BJ, *et al.* Preventive therapy for latent tuberculosis infection – the promise and the challenges. *Int J Infect Dis* 2017; 56: 68–76.

128. World Health Organization. Guidelines on the Management of Latent Tuberculosis Infection. Geneva, WHO, 2015.

129. World Health Organization. Latent Tuberculosis Infection: Updated and Consolidated Guidelines for Programmatic Management. Geneva, WHO, 2018.

130. Cruz AT, Starke JR. Completion rate and safety of tuberculosis infection treatment with shorter regimens. *Pediatrics* 2018; 141: e20172838.

131. Ena J, Valls V. Short-course therapy with rifampin plus isoniazid, compared with standard therapy with isoniazid, for latent tuberculosis infection: a meta-analysis. *Clin Infect Dis* 2005; 40: 670–676.

132. Villarino ME, Scott NA, Weis SE, *et al.* Treatment for preventing tuberculosis in children and adolescents: a randomized clinical trial of a 3-month, 12–dose regimen of a combination of rifapentine and isoniazid. *JAMA Pediatr* 2015; 169: 247–255.

133. Centers For Disease Control and Prevention. Treatment regimens for latent TB infection (LTBI). 2018. www.cdc.gov/tb/topic/treatment/ltbi.htm Date last accessed: June 11, 2018. 2017.

134. Seddon JA, Fred D, Amanullah F, *et al.* Post-exposure Management of Multidrug-resistant Tuberculosis Contacts: Evidence-based Recommendations: Policy Brief. Dubai, Harvard Medical School Centre for Global Health Delivery–Dubai, 2015.

135. Byrne AL, Fox GJ, Marais BJ. Better than a pound of cure: preventing the development of multidrug-resistant tuberculosis. *Future Microbiol* 2018; 13: 577–588.

136. Bamrah S, Brostrom R, Dorina F, *et al.* Treatment for LTBI in contacts of MDR-TB patients, Federated States of Micronesia, 2009–2012. *Int J Tuberc Lung Dis* 2014; 18: 912–918.

137. Seddon JA, Hesseling AC, Finlayson H, *et al.* Preventive therapy for child contacts of multidrug-resistant tuberculosis: a prospective cohort study. *Clin Infect Dis* 2013; 57: 1676–1684.

138. Adler-Shohet FC, Low J, Carson M, *et al.* Management of latent tuberculosis infection in child contacts of multidrug-resistant tuberculosis. *Pediatr Infect Dis J* 2014; 33: 664–666.

139. Marks SM, Mase SR, Morris SB. Systematic review, meta-analysis, and cost-effectiveness of treatment of latent tuberculosis to reduce progression to multidrug-resistant tuberculosis. *Clin Infect Dis* 2017; 64: 1670–1677.

140. Schaaf HS, Collins A, Bekker A, *et al.* Tuberculosis at extremes of age. *Respirology* 2010; 15: 747–763.

141. Bekker A, Du Preez K, Schaaf HS, *et al.* High tuberculosis exposure among neonates in a high tuberculosis and human immunodeficiency virus burden setting. *Int J Tuberc Lung Dis* 2012; 16: 1040–1046.

142. Adhikari M, Jeena P, Bobat R, *et al.* HIV-associated tuberculosis in the newborn and young infant. *Int J Pediatr* 2011; 2011: 354208.

143. Treatment Action Group. Research priorities for paediatric tuberculosis. 2018. www.treatmentactiongroup.org/sites/default/files/pediatric_tb_research_priorities_9_24.pdf Date last accessed: October 6, 2018.

144. Detjen AK, McKenna L, Graham SM, *et al.* The upcoming UN general assembly resolution on tuberculosis must also benefit children. *Lancet Glob Health* 2018; 6: e485–e486.

Disclosures: H.S. Schaaf's institute, Stellenbosch University (Cape Town, South Africa), receives a per-patient grant from Otsuka Pharmaceutica for pharmacokinetic and safety studies of delamanid in children; H.S. Schaaf is a co-investigator but receives no financial or other benefits. H.S. Schaaf reports receiving grants from IMPAACT P1108 for pharmacokinetic studies of bedaquiline in children at Stellenbosch University; H.S. Schaaf is an investigator on this study but has received no financial or other support.

https://doi.org/10.1183/2312508X.10021817

Chapter 15

Pregnancy and the elderly

Alice Repossi[1] and Graham Bothamley ⓘ[2,3,4]

TB in both pregnancy and the elderly may occur more frequently and with more EPTB than in the general population, possibly due to immunological changes relevant to these conditions. They both share complexities in the difficulty of clinical diagnosis, related to the nature of nonspecific symptoms in TB disease. New molecular tests are especially helpful in diagnosing paucibacillary disease. Treatment of TB disease in pregnancy is complicated by adverse effects, especially of second-line drugs, affecting both mother and fetus, and in the elderly by a high rate of DILI with increasing age. Screening for TB has been suggested in both populations as part of the plan to eliminate TB. Treatment of LTBI is possible in both populations, but clinicians are concerned by adverse effects, which may be less than they fear.

Cite as: Repossi A, Bothamley G. Pregnancy and the elderly. *In:* Migliori GB, Bothamley G, Duarte R, *et al.*, eds. Tuberculosis (ERS Monograph). Sheffield, European Respiratory Society, 2018; pp. 263–275 [https://doi.org/10.1183/2312508X.10021917].

🐦 @ERSpublications
Screening for TB in high-risk groups during pregnancy and in the elderly can avoid delay in diagnosis. Treatment requires closer supervision but improves the outlook for all, including friends and family. http://ow.ly/cfVQ30lqCfE

Treatment of TB in pregnancy and in the elderly, as well as in children and in those with comorbidities, illustrates why TB is more difficult to manage than most other respiratory infections. Symptoms in these groups are especially difficult to distinguish from many other diagnoses. The laboratory diagnosis is complicated by the more frequent occurrence of EPTB, and immunological tests are also affected. Chest radiographs (CXRs) are frequently atypical. Treatment will affect both mother and fetus during pregnancy, and even standard treatment is met with more adverse effects in the elderly. Social determinants are an important factor, both in the outcome of pregnancy and in the elderly, and obscure the epidemiology of TB in these populations.

This chapter is written with the aim of guiding the physician towards evidence-based decisions and of removing some of the fears that surround the management of TB in pregnancy and in the elderly.

[1]Respiratory Unit, ASST Lodi, Lodi, Italy. [2]Homerton University Hospital, London, UK. [3]Blizard Institute, Barts and The London School of Medicine and Dentistry, Queen Mary University of London, London, UK. [4]London School of Hygiene and Tropical Medicine, London, UK.

Correspondence: Graham Bothamley, Dept of Respiratory Medicine, Homerton University Hospital, London E9 6SR, UK. E-mail: g.bothamley@nhs.net

Tuberculosis and pregnancy

Risk of tuberculosis in pregnancy

TB most commonly affects those aged 20–35 years, and these are the very years when women are most likely to become pregnant [1]. An estimated 216 500 pregnant women develop TB each year [2]. In the USA, the rate of TB in pregnancy is steady, and particularly affects racial and ethnic groups associated with lower incomes and social deprivation [3, 4]. A cohort study of 192 801 pregnancies in the UK suggested that the rate of TB was higher during pregnancy (15.4 per 100 000, 22 cases) or in the 6 months post-partum (22 cases) compared with women in the same age cohort who were not pregnant or post-partum by the same criteria (9.4 per 100 000, 133 cases), a significant difference assuming that those with a higher risk of TB did not have more pregnancies [5]. Starting with TB as the diagnosis, a TBnet cross-sectional survey observed 224 pregnancies in 15 217 TB patients (1.5%), at a rate expected from the birth rate for the clinic populations [6]. TB was diagnosed most frequently post-partum, suggesting that investigations such as a CXR should not be delayed until the child is born if TB disease is considered [4, 5].

In middle- and low-income countries, TB is the leading cause of maternal mortality, especially in those with HIV coinfection [2]. Even in high-income countries, HIV/TB coinfection is associated with significant mortality and a poor outcome of pregnancy [4, 7].

Clinical aspects

TB symptoms can occur in normal pregnancy and include general malaise, fatigue, sweating and cough due to reflux [8]. EPTB, which is itself more difficult to detect, is also more common in pregnancy [9].

Sputum examination and CXRs are the most important investigations in the diagnostic approach in pregnant women. Concern about radiation safety in pregnancy limited the use of CXRs in the past, but shielding the abdomen with a lead apron and the lower doses of radiation that are now needed to obtain a CXR mean that radiation exposure to the fetus is now considered negligible [10]. In addition to standard sputum smears and culture, the WHO recommends the use of the Xpert MTB/RIF nucleic acid amplification test (Cepheid, Sunnyvale, CA, USA), as a first-line diagnostic test, in view of its benefit in smear-negative, culture-positive PTB [11, 12]. This test has shown 80% sensitivity among gynaecology and obstetrics patients in Zambia [13], although with a lower sensitivity (43%) in women with HIV coinfection in Kenya (largely related to the effect of prior probability on a diagnostic test) [14]. In EPTB, a CXR can be useful for identifying miliary and pleural TB. Lymph node TB can be diagnosed by needle aspiration and mycobacteriological examination. Tuberculous meningitis presents with symptoms that recommend cerebrospinal fluid sampling, where the standard tests (protein, glucose, microscopy, culture and sensitivities, mycobacterial culture and cytology) will help identify TB. If concern about TB is high, then use of the Xpert MTB/RIF test or even an IGRA on the sample can be helpful [15, 16].

Immunological tests for tuberculosis in pregnancy

Pregnancy does not appear to alter the performance of the TST [17]. Longitudinal studies have shown that the TST did not change throughout pregnancy but raised the possibility

https://doi.org/10.1183/2312508X.10021917

that tests based on lymphocyte proliferation might be affected [18]. However, longitudinal studies using the QuantiFERON-TB Gold in-tube test (Qiagen, Hilden, Germany) in India showed that the IGRA was in fact more likely to be positive than the TST ($\geqslant$10 mm), but although levels of IFN-γ fell, none was reduced below the cut-off value for a positive result [19]. In low-incidence settings, these tests do not appear to be altered by pregnancy [20]. Mitogen responses using the QuantiFERON-TB Gold Plus test were lower as pregnancy proceeded, but the differences in the number of indeterminate tests did not attain significance, except in those with HIV coinfection [21]. The diagnosis of EPTB can often be difficult. These data suggest that the use of either the TST or an IGRA can be used not only for screening but also in a diagnostic setting where further investigations can then be justified on the basis of a positive test for TB. If the immunological tests are negative, the clinical circumstances may support further investigation. For example, if the patient is ill, then miliary TB can be considered, but if the symptoms are nonspecific, then factors such as contact with TB disease, previous residence in a country with a high TB incidence and/ or membership of a high-risk group (*e.g.* HIV coinfection, alcohol excess, homeless) can justify further consideration of TB disease.

Effect of HIV infection in pregnancy in relation to tuberculosis

HIV infection is associated with reduced resistance to TB infection and an increased likelihood of TB disease in those with a positive TST or IGRA result, especially in those with a CD4$^+$ count of <200 μL^{-1} (discussed in another chapter in this *Monograph* [22]). Although symptom screening was thought to be useful in people living with HIV (PLHIV) [23] and had a high negative predictive value [24], studies in pregnant women showed a poor sensitivity (reviewed in [9]). In PLHIV, in whom pregnancy was considered a contraindication to a CXR, testing a single sputum sample with Xpert MTB/RIF gave a significantly better yield and without which 70% of TB cases in pregnancy would have been missed [25].

Immunological tests are problematic in PLHIV. A cut-off value of 5 mm for TST is routinely used, considering that tuberculin responses may be smaller or absent [26]. Some have considered the T-SPOT. *TB* test (Oxford Immunotech, Abingdon, UK) superior to the QuantiFERON-TB tests in that the former will standardise the number of cells tested [27]. However, mitogen responses are poorer, both in late pregnancy and in those with a CD4$^+$ count of <200 μL^{-1}, making indeterminate results more likely [28]. Thus, a positive test in PLHIV recommends further investigation for TB disease and consideration of preventative treatment, but a negative test is less helpful.

Screening for latent tuberculosis infection and preventative treatment

A systematic review of LTBI in pregnancy in HIV-negative women revealed a prevalence of 14–48% in the USA, with a positive TST varying with ethnicity [18]. The CDC recommend LTBI screening only for high-risk women, *i.e.* those with known or suspected TB contacts, injection drug use, HIV or other immunosuppression, foreign birth or residence in congregate settings in countries with a low TB burden [24]. Uptake of TB screening in pregnancy varied with ethnicity/social circumstances in New York but was considered an effective intervention [29].

https://doi.org/10.1183/2312508X.10021917

The WHO has recommended isoniazid preventative treatment therapy for all HIV-infected individuals, including pregnant women, irrespective of TST status in settings where TST implementation may be impractical [30]. In a setting with high TB incidence (India), this strategy seemed to be cost-effective and likely to result in greater health benefits than TST-driven strategies [31]. In a low-incidence setting (Japan), again cost-effectiveness was demonstrated [32]. Isoniazid is safe in pregnancy and is not teratogenic [33]. The WHO guideline group recommend 6 months of preventative treatment with isoniazid, noting the interactions of other preventative treatments with ART [28]. Chemoprophylaxis, to prevent infection with TB, over a period of 36 months in PLHIV in Botswana was examined in HIV-infected women who experienced pregnancy during the course of therapy, and also showed no adverse pregnancy outcomes compared with a control group [34].

The antenatal clinic may be the first contact of women with the local healthcare system. Screening for both TB and LTBI in those with an HIV infection is valuable, and other high-risk groups, as noted above, may also benefit [9].

Treatment of tuberculosis in pregnancy

Standard treatment for drug-sensitive TB is considered safe in pregnancy and is recommended by the WHO [35]. As with all patients, measurement of liver function before the start of treatment is standard, and if abnormal, appropriate management is undertaken (discussed elsewhere in this *Monograph* [36, 37]).

Anecdotal reports indicate that second-line drugs can be used in MDR-TB and pregnancy, but are small in number [38]. Apart from deafness due to aminoglycosides, evidence of adverse effects is limited by sample size such that risk estimates have wide confidence intervals. Table 1 shows drugs used in the management of MDR-TB and pregnancy and their possible adverse effects [39].

Management of these patients involves a multidisciplinary approach; treatment regimens and the duration of therapy need to be individualised in accordance with the susceptibility pattern of the infecting strain (discussed elsewhere in this *Monograph* [36]).

Outcome of pregnancy

Ectopic tubal pregnancy is associated with genital TB: in India, in a group of 17 adolescents with acute presentation of ectopic pregnancy, six out of 17 had genital TB compared with one out of 20 in the control group [40].

One of the earlier and largest studies to date (542 pregnant women with TB compared with 133826 pregnant women without TB) suggested that toxaemia, vaginal bleeding and fetal death between 16 and 28 weeks was associated with TB [41]. Smaller studies have also suggested a poorer outcome of pregnancy if there is concurrent TB. However, none has corrected for the population with TB, itself associated with unemployment, social deprivation, and more rarely HIV, alcohol and drug addiction, and imprisonment, all of which are themselves associated with a poorer outcome in pregnancy [42, 43].

Maternal TB disease is associated with poorer neonatal outcomes, but again these may represent the result of social deprivation and other factors that are associated with a higher

https://doi.org/10.1183/2312508X.10021917

Table 1. Drugs used in the management of MDR-TB and pregnancy

Drug	FDA classification[#]	Comments
Aminoglycosides: amikacin, kanamycin, streptomycin	D	Deafness in up to 17% of children
Bedaquiline	B	Provisional CDC guidelines
Capreomycin	C	Some reports indicate safe
Clofazimine	C	(Use in leprosy not contraindicated)
Cycloserine/terizidone	C	Animal models and anecdotal human studies have not shown toxicity
Delaminid	Not approved	Not recommended
Ethambutol	B	Considered safe in pregnancy
Fluoroquinolones	C	Arthropathy in puppies and adverse events with norfloxacin Levofloxacin at high doses leads to fetal weight loss and mortality in rats No teratogenicity observed in human subjects
Linezolid	C	High doses in animals associated with fetal toxicity and teratogenicity
Meropenem with co-amoxiclav	B	Limited data
PAS	C	Animal models and anecdotal human studies have not shown toxicity
Pyrazinamide	C	Lack of controlled data (always used in conjunction with other drugs); WHO recommended
Thionamides	C	Possible congenital defects

[#]: A: no risk in controlled human studies; B: no risk in other studies (safe in animals and no human studies), or animal studies have shown an adverse effect but controlled human studies have failed to demonstrate a risk; C: risk not ruled out; animal studies indicate possible risk and there are no adequate and well-controlled human studies: potential benefits may warrant use of drug in pregnancy; D: positive evidence of risk but potential benefits may warrant use in pregnancy despite potential risks. Data from [39].

risk of TB [44]. As long as the mother has received at least 2 weeks of treatment for drug-sensitive TB, isolation of the baby is not required. Disseminated TB in the mother can cause congenital TB in the infant, but this is a rare condition [45]. Neonatal TB is most commonly due to inhalation of tubercle bacilli (discussed in another chapter in this *Monograph* [46]). Early diagnosis and treatment ensure that the best possible outcome of TB in pregnancy can be attained by both mother and infant.

Tuberculosis in the elderly

As TB has become better controlled and treated, its epidemiology has shown a reduction in incidence in the 20–35-year-old age group and a relatively higher incidence in those >65 years, perhaps related to previous lifetime exposures [1, 47]. Difficulty in making the diagnosis of TB in the elderly and the potential for transmission, both within nursing homes and from grandparent to grandchildren, are important concerns. The pathogenesis of re-activation may also usefully be explored within this population and may provide clues as to how to mitigate the problem of LTBI and prevent re-activation.

Epidemiology

The prevalence ratio for bacteriologically confirmed TB increases with age in most countries by comparison with the 15–24-year-old age group, although the incidence is highest in the 15–44-year-old age range for all areas except the Western Pacific and countries such as China and Bangladesh where the elderly predominate [2]. However, regional estimates by the WHO differ from case notifications, with higher incidences in those >65 years in the eastern Mediterranean Region and several high-burden countries, notably Cambodia, Pakistan, Papua New Guinea and Thailand [2]. In a community-based project for active TB case finding, 26% were in those >65 years compared with 13% presenting to healthcare facilities [48]. The failure of notification in the elderly has been interpreted as a failure to seek healthcare but also as reduced access to healthcare for social or economic reasons.

Due to the fall in incidence and prevalence of TB over the last 65 years, the rates of TB in the elderly may reflect their lifetime exposure rather than the current incidence. However, the rate of notifications should fall according to the general trend, but appears instead to increase in those >80 years of age (figure 1). The disability-adjusted life years lost due to TB in those >65 years ranges from 8.2% of the total TB population in Europe to 18.7% in East and Central Asia [50].

Recent infection remains a problem, even in this age group. Residents of nursing homes can become infected by an index case and develop PTB (see later) [51, 52]. The incidence of TB in the elderly is also affected by comorbidities, notably DM, chronic renal impairment and smoking.

Immunological changes with ageing and re-activation

Immunological memory is fundamental to ensure that infections do not recur and vaccination works. In response to a pathogen, there is rapid proliferation of immune cells

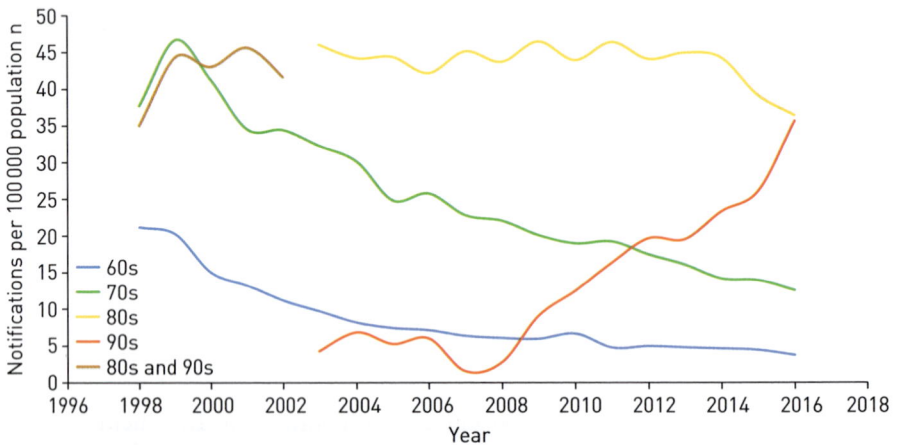

Figure 1. Difference between notification rates of TB in Japan compared with previous decades. The national rate of decline from 1998 to 2016 was 4.5% per year and is reflected in the comparisons between decades for people in their 60s and 70s. However, compared with TB notifications for those aged 70–80 years, there was no decline for those aged 80–90 years and a rise in notifications for those aged ⩾90 years compared with those aged 80–90 years. Data from [49].

https://doi.org/10.1183/2312508X.10021917

associated with both cellular and antibody-mediated immunity. At the end of infection, these cells are cleared by apoptosis, and memory cells remain that can respond more quickly to the same pathogen. Immunosenescence includes a decline in immune parameters, both innate and adaptive responses, and a more inflammatory reaction to pathogens [53]. Increasing age is associated with re-activation of latent and self-healed TB [54]. Studies in immunosenescence have highlighted changes in pattern recognition receptors (Toll-like receptors for DNA, lipopolysaccharides and lipoproteins; nucleotide-binding oligomerisation domain-like receptors (NOD-like receptors); and retinoic acid-inducible gene I-like receptors that sense intracellular RNA), dysfunctional mitochondria, defective autophagy, inflamma-somes, dysbiosis in the gut microbiome and the senescence-associated secretory phenotype in response to reactive oxygen species [55]. Both $CD4^+$ and $CD8^+$ T-cell functions are poorer with ageing, perhaps related to problems with cell division as well as poorer cytokine secretion [56, 57]. Re-activation of TB with tumour necrosis factor inhibitors and HIV/TB coinfection with low $CD4^+$ counts share many clinical features with TB in the elderly (discussed elsewhere in this *Monograph* [22, 58, 59]).

Tuberculin reactivity has been shown to decline with age [60]. The IFN-γ responses also show a waning response [61].

Clinical diagnosis and the spectrum of tuberculosis

Diagnosis of TB in the elderly is thought to be more difficult [62]. Symptoms do not differ compared with younger patients (cough, weight loss, night sweats and haemoptysis all at similar frequencies) [63–65], although others have reported lesser symptoms in the elderly [66]. However, comorbidities with similar symptoms are commoner in the elderly and include congestive cardiac failure, COPD, DM and malignancy. Contact with TB in the past is often remembered, but the effect of stigma means that only direct questioning will bring this to light. Time spent in concentration camps or in areas of starvation, such as the Netherlands during the Second World War, make TB more likely.

As with younger patients, anaemia, a normal neutrophil count, occasional lymphopenia and an erythrocyte sedimentation rate of >90 mm·h^{-1} are associated with TB. A low serum sodium may indicate inappropriate secretion of antidiuretic hormone. Albumin tends to be low with an increase in globulin fraction. LFTs are frequently abnormal, and this may be due to disseminated TB as much as to any other underlying disorder [67].

However, a positive sputum smear is less common in PTB with increasing age [61, 68–70]. EPTB is more common, often with features of primary TB [60]. Thus, the ratio of TB disease similar to primary TB compared with post-primary disease appears to increase from ~45 years of age (figure 2).

Atypical radiographic appearances

PTB in older persons tends to show a different distribution compared with that in younger adults [61]. Only 7% of 93 patients showed a purely apical appearance, whereas infection in the apical segments of the lower lobes was more common, cavities were rarer and a pleural reaction was common. This is similar to the pattern seen in females and in those with DM or an alcohol problem [71], although with less cavitation [72]. There may also be evidence of self-healed disease with apical scarring. Miliary TB is also

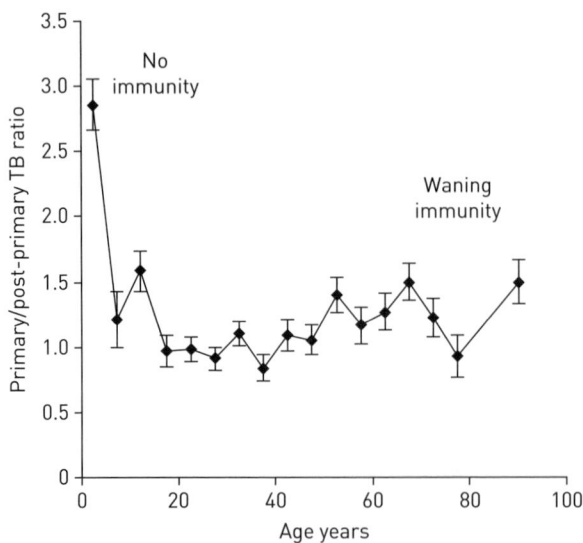

Figure 2. Ratio of primary/post-primary forms of TB with age. Data are from notifications at the Homerton University Hospital, London, UK, from 1995 to 2000. Error bars were calculated using the fact that simple random sampling bias approaches the square root of the number of individuals.

more common and is consistent with the elderly immune response being less active and more like that in subjects with no previous immunological experience of TB (primary disease) [73].

Problems with tuberculosis treatment in the elderly

DILI increases with age [74, 75]. Three unselected series of patients treated for LTBI with isoniazid showed an overall incidence of hepatitis of 0.1% (n=3788) [76], 0.3% (n=3788) [77] and 0.56% (n=3377) [78], all increasing with age, the last showing a rate of 4.4 per 1000 patients for 25–34-year-olds, rising to 20.83 for those $\geqslant$50 years. Rates of DILI were higher in treatment of TB (4.8% of 13 359 patients <60 years and 23% of 1192 patients aged $\geqslant$60 years) [79]. A recent evaluation from the REMoxTB (Rapid evaluation of moxifloxacin in tuberculosis) trial indicated that 21% (eight out of 31) of those aged >55 years had an alanine aminotransferase/aspartate transaminase ratio that was more than three times the upper limit of normal [80].

Ethambutol is excreted by the kidney. A low glomerular filtration rate (GFR) of <30 mL·min^{-1} has a poor prognosis in the treatment of TB [81]. In the elderly, the dose should be reduced according to the estimated GFR, but also the time between doses increased to ensure that high levels of the drug do not persist [82].

Older individuals are likely to have several comorbidities and to be taking a large number of drugs [83]. The interaction between the anticoagulant warfarin and rifampicin is especially problematic, and either heparin or a non-vitamin K oral anticoagulant are considerably safer. Other important interactions include statins, analgesics such as celecoxib, losartan, oral antidiabetic medications, steroids, calcium channel blockers and theophyllines, to name a few. When prescribing TB treatment, especially in the elderly, always ask about other

https://doi.org/10.1183/2312508X.10021917

medications and change doses according to known effects on cytochrome P450 metabolism. Preventative treatment with isoniazid is, therefore, likely to be better tolerated in view of the many interactions of rifamycin-containing regimens. The standard regimen for treatment of active disease is still to be preferred, as the increase in DILI is attributable to isoniazid rather than other component drugs. If a problem arises, moxifloxacin can replace isoniazid [84], but tendinitis is more common in the elderly, who are also more likely to be taking other medications that prolong the corrected QT interval. The use of the regimen of rifampicin and ethambutol for 12 months with initial pyrazinamide for 2 months (2RZE/10RE) may therefore be used should problems arise [85].

Treatment outcomes for TB have been reported to be poorer in the elderly [61, 86]. Sputum smear conversion after the intensive phase of treatment in a Nigerian population was poorer in those >60 years (18 out of 76, 23.7%) compared with the younger group (169 out of 853, 19.8%) [67]. However, in this study, poorer outcomes were also associated with a rural location and private care; only EPTB and HIV coinfection were significant predictors of a poorer outcome in the elderly. WHO outcome reporting does not distinguish among deaths due to TB, deaths where TB contributed and deaths unrelated to TB [87]. Thus, outcomes in the elderly should be corrected for the likelihood of death related to age.

Nursing homes: screening and outbreaks

An outbreak of TB in a nursing home in the USA that was followed from 1972 to 1981 prompted a series of studies throughout Arkansas to investigate its incidence and the value of preventative therapy [88]. Tuberculin conversion was observed within 30 months of arrival in a nursing home in 8.8%, with a 5% conversion rate per year if a case of TB had been notified within the last 3 years, and was still 3.5% per annum with no recognised case [48]. TB disease occurred in 79 out of 370 (2.4%) of those untreated with isoniazid compared with one out of 534 (0.2%) individuals treated with isoniazid. Screening of 227 nursing homes (~53 000 individuals) with the TST revealed 2135 with a positive test who were then treated with isoniazid preventative therapy [48]. Hepatotoxicity was observed in 84 (4.4%), and other drug intolerances prevented completion of treatment in another 116 (6.0%). The risk/benefit ratio was favourable for those who had shown tuberculin conversion (negative to >12 mm) since taking up residence in the nursing home, but not for those who had a positive tuberculin reaction of unknown duration.

Screening for TB in nursing homes continues to occur in the USA, and outbreaks in Italy, Taiwan, Russia and Japan have been reported in the literature within the last decade using screening with IGRAs and molecular typing of the isolated strains [89–93]. However, currently, in most areas, screening only occurs following an outbreak of TB.

The elderly and tuberculosis elimination

A population-based survey of tuberculin reactivity and subsequent TB disease suggested that re-activation was more likely in those >50 years of age (uncorrected for previous lifetime TB exposure) [94]. However, age-related cohorts from Norway, the USA, Hong Kong, England and Wales, and Japan all showed a decline in TB incidence [95–98]. Looking at the 12-year follow-up of 33 146 contacts, after the high incidence of TB in those <20 years, TB rates remained steady until a steady increase in those from 40 years of age to those >60 years [99]. In a review of medical and nursing students, TB disease was 79% less likely in those who had a positive tuberculin response than in those who were tuberculin negative [100]. Together with the previous section, this suggests that recent tuberculin converters and those with a previously positive tuberculin response who have come into contact with a new case of TB should be given preferential preventative treatment, in order to prevent intergenerational spread of TB.

Conclusion

Immunological changes with pregnancy and ageing may affect the likelihood of active TB. More importantly, antenatal care may be the first opportunity to screen for TB in at-risk populations, while elimination of TB may be contingent on considering preventative treatment in the elderly after recent infection in tuberculin converters or in those with a documented positive response in the past where screening reveals a now-negative reaction.

References

1. WHO. Global Tuberculosis Report 2017. Geneva, WHO, 2017. http://www.who.int/tb/publications/global_report/gtbr2017_main_text.pdf
2. Sugarman J, Colvin C, Moran AC, et al. Tuberculosis in pregnancy: an estimate of the global burden of disease. Lancet Glob Health 2014; 2: e710–e716.
3. Salemi JL, Salihu HM. The prevalence of active tuberculosis infection among pregnant women is not increasing in the United States. Am J Obstet Gynecol 2017; 217: 490–491.
4. Dennis EM, Hao Y, Tamambang M, et al. Tuberculosis during pregnancy in the United States: racial/ethnic disparities in pregnancy complications and in-hospital death. PLoS One 2018; 13: e0194836.
5. Zenner D, Kruijshaar ME, Andrews N, et al. Risk of tuberculosis in pregnancy: a national, primary care-based cohort and self-controlled case series study. Am J Respir Crit Care Med 2012; 185: 779–784.
6. Bothamley GH, Ehlers C, Salonka I, et al. Pregnancy in patients with tuberculosis: a TBNET cross-sectional survey. BMC Pregnancy Childbirth 2016; 16: 304.
7. Zenner D, Abubakar I, Conti S, et al. Impact of TB on the survival of people living with HIV infection in England, Wales and Northern Ireland. Thorax 2015; 70: 566–573.
8. Bothamley GH. Management of TB during pregnancy, especially in high-risk communities. Expert Rev Obstet Gynecol 2009; 4: 555–563.
9. Bothamley GH. Screening for tuberculosis in pregnancy. Expert Rev Obstet Gynecol 2012; 7: 387–395.
10. Repossi AC, Bothamley GH. Tuberculosis and pregnancy: an updated systematic review. Pulm Res Respir Med Open J 2015; 2: 63–68.
11. WHO. Automated Real-time Nucleic Acid Amplification Technology for Rapid and Simultaneous Detection of Tuberculosis and Rifampicin Resistance: Xpert MTB/RIF System. Policy Statement. Geneva, WHO, 2011. www.who.int/tb/publications/tb-amplificationtechnology-statement/en/
12. WHO. Xpert MTB/RIF Implementation Manual. Technical and Operational "How-to": Practical Considerations. Geneva, WHO, 2014. www.who.int/tb/publications/xpert_implem_manual/en/
13. Bates M, Ahmed Y, Chilukutu L, et al. Use of the Xpert MTB/RIF assay for diagnosing pulmonary tuberculosis comorbidity and multidrug-resistant TB in obstetrics and gynaecology inpatient wards at the University Teaching Hospital, Lusaka. Zambia Trop Med Int Health 2013; 18: 1134–1140.
14. LaCourse SM, Cranmer LM, Matemo D, et al. Tuberculosis case finding in HIV-infected pregnant women in Kenya reveals poor performance of symptom screening and rapid diagnostic tests. J Acquir Immune Defic Syndr 2016; 71: 219–227.
15. Cresswell FV, Bangdiwale AS, Bahr NC, et al. Can improved diagnostics reduce mortality from tuberculous meningitis? Findings from a 6.5 year cohort in Uganda. Wellcome Open Res 2018; 3: 64.
16. Yu J, Wang ZJ, Chen LH, et al. Diagnostic accuracy of interferon-gamma release assays for tuberculous meningitis: a meta-analysis. Int J Tuberc Lung Dis 2016; 20: 494–499.
17. Present PA, Comstock GW. Tuberculin sensitivity in pregnancy. Am Rev Respir Dis 1975; 112: 413–416.
18. Covelli HD, Wilson RT. Immunologic and medical consideration in tuberculin-sensitized pregnant patients. Am J Obstet Gynecol 1978; 132: 256–259.

https://doi.org/10.1183/2312508X.10021917

19. Mathad JS, Bhosale R, Sangar V, *et al.* Pregnancy differentially impacts performance of latent tuberculosis diagnostics in a high-burden setting. *PLoS One* 2014; 9: e92308.
20. Malhamé I, Cormier M, Sugarman J, *et al.* Latent tuberculosis in pregnancy: a systematic review. *PLoS One* 2016; 11: e0154825.
21. König Walles J, Tesfaye F, Jansson M, *et al.* Performance of QuantiFERON-TB Gold Plus for detection of latent tuberculosis infection in pregnant women living in a tuberculosis- and HIV-endemic setting. *PLoS One* 2018; 13: e0193589.
22. Magis-Escurra C, Carvalho ACC, Kritski AL, *et al.* Comorbidities. *In:* Migliori GB, Bothamley G, Duarte R, *et al.*, eds. Tuberculosis (ERS Monograph). Sheffield, European Respiratory Society, 2018; pp. 276–290.
23. Getahun H, Sculier D, Sismanidis C, *et al.* Prevention, diagnosis, and treatment of tuberculosis in children and mothers: evidence for action for maternal, neonatal, and child health services. *J Infect Dis* 2012; 205: Suppl., S216–S227.
24. Gupta A, Chandrasekhar A, Gupta N, *et al.* Symptom screening among HIV-infected pregnant women is acceptable and has a high negative predictive value for active tuberculosis. *Clin Infect Dis* 2011; 53: 1015–1018.
25. Modi S, Cavanaugh JS, Shiraishi RW, *et al.* Performance of clinical screening algorithms for tuberculosis intensified case finding among people living with HIV in Western Kenya. *PLoS One* 2016; 11: e0167685.
26. American Thoracic Society. Targeted tuberculin testing and treatment of latent tuberculosis infection. *Am J Respir Crit Care Med* 2000; 161: S221–S247.
27. Overton K, Varma R, Post JJ. Comparison of interferon-γ release assays and the tuberculin skin test for the diagnosis of tuberculosis in human immunodeficiency virus: a systematic review. *Tuberc Respir Dis* 2018; 81: 59–72.
28. LaCourse SM, Cranmer LM, Matemo D, *et al.* Effect of pregnancy on interferon gamma release assay and tuberculin skin test detection of latent TB infection among HIV-infected women in a high burden setting. *J Acquir Immunodefic Syndr* 2017; 75: 128–138.
29. Schwartz N, Wagner SA, Keeler SM, *et al.* Universal TB screening in pregnancy. *Am J Perinatol* 2009; 26: 447–451.
30. WHO. Latent Tuberculosis Infection: Updated and Consolidated Guidelines for Programmatic Management. Geneva, WHO, 2018. www.who.int/tb/publications/2018/latent-tuberculosis-infection/en/
31. Kapoor S, Gupta A, Shah M. Cost-effectiveness of isoniazid preventive therapy for HIV-infected pregnant women in India. *Int J Tuberc Ling Dis* 2016; 20: 85–92.
32. Kowada A. Cost effectiveness of interferon-γ release assay for TB screening of HIV positive pregnant women in low TB incidence countries. *J Infect* 2014; 68: 32–42.
33. Bothamley G. Drug treatment for tuberculosis: safety considerations. *Drug Saf* 2001; 24: 553–565.
34. Taylor AW, Mosimaneotsile B, Mathebula U, *et al.* Pregnancy outcomes in HIV-infected women receiving long-term isoniazid prophylaxis for tuberculosis and antiretroviral therapy. *Infect Dis Obstet Gynecol* 2013; 2013: 195637.
35. WHO. Treatment of Tuberculosis: Guidelines. 4th Edn. Geneva, WHO, 2011. www.who.int/tb/publications/2010/9789241547833/en/
36. Caminero JA, Scardigli A, van der Werf T, *et al.* Treatment of drug-susceptible and drug-resistant tuberculosis. *In:* Migliori GB, Bothamley G, Duarte R, *et al.*, eds. Tuberculosis (ERS Monograph). Sheffield, European Respiratory Society, 2018; pp. 152–178.
37. Caminero JA, Lasserra P, Piubello A, *et al.* Adverse anti-tuberculosis drug events and their management. *In:* Migliori GB, Bothamley G, Duarte R, *et al.*, eds. Tuberculosis (ERS Monograph). Sheffield, European Respiratory Society, 2018; pp. 205–227.
38. Palacios E, Dallman R, Muñoz M, *et al.* Drug-resistant tuberculosis and pregnancy: treatment outcomes of 38 cases in Lima, Peru. *Clin Infect Dis* 2009; 48: 1413–1419.
39. Curry International Tuberculosis Center and California Department of Public Health. Drug-resistant Tuberculosis: a Survival Guide for Clinicians. 3rd Edn. California, Curry International Tuberculosis Center and California Department of Public Health, 2016.
40. Banerjee A, Prateek S, Malik S, *et al.* Genital tuberculosis in adolescent girls from low socioeconomic status with acute ectopic pregnancy presenting at a tertiary care hospital in urban Northern India: are we missing an opportunity to treat? *Arch Gynecol Obstet* 2012; 286: 1477–1482.
41. Bjerkedal T, Bahna SL, Lehman EH. Course and outcome of pregnancy in women with pulmonary tuberculosis. *Scand J Respir Dis* 1975; 56: 245–250.
42. Fernandez D, Salami I, Davis J, *et al.* HIV-TB coinfection among 57 million pregnant women, obstetric complications, alcohol use, drug abuse, and depression. *J Pregnancy* 2018; 2018: 5896901.
43. Sobhy S, Babiker Z, Zamora J, *et al.* Maternal and perinatal mortality and morbidity associated with tuberculosis during pregnancy and the postpartum period: a systematic review and meta-analysis. *BJOG* 2017; 124: 727–733.
44. LaCourse SM, Greene SA, Dawson-Hahn EE, *et al.* Risk of adverse outcomes associated with maternal tuberculosis in a low burden setting: a population-based retrospective cohort study. *Infect Dis Obstet Gynecol* 2016; 2016: 6413713.
45. Chang CW, Wu PW, Yeh CH, *et al.* Congenital tuberculosis: case report and review of the literature. *Paediatr Int Child Health* 2017; 19: 1–4.

46.   Schaaf HS, Marais BJ, Carvalho I, et al. Challenges in childhood tuberculosis. In: Migliori GB, Bothamley G, Duarte R, et al., eds. Tuberculosis (ERS Monograph). Sheffield, European Respiratory Society, 2018; pp. 234–262.

47.   Powell KE, Farer LS. The rising age of the tuberculosis patient: a sign of success and failure. J Infect Dis 1980; 142: 946–948.

48.   Lorent N, Choun K, Thai S, et al. Community-based active tuberculosis case finding in poor urban settlements of Phnom Penh, Cambodia: a feasible and effective strategy. PLoS One 2014; 9: e92754.

49.   Tuberculosis Surveillance Center. Statistics of TB. www.jata.or.jp/rit/ekigaku/en/statistics-of-tb/ Date last accessed: September 12, 2018. Date last updated: April, 2018.

50.   Institute for Health Metrics and Evaluation. Global burden of disease. www.healthdata.org/gbd Date last accessed: September 11, 2018. Date last updated: 2018.

51.   Stead WW, Lofgren JP, Warren E, et al. Tuberculosis as an endemic and nosocomial infection among the elderly in nursing homes. N Engl J Med 1985; 312: 1483–1487.

52.   Advisory Committee for Elimination of Tuberculosis. Prevention and control of tuberculosis in facilities providing long-term care to the elderly. MMWR Recomm Rep 1990; 39: 7–20.

53.   Fulop T, Larbi A, Dupuis G, et al. Immunosenescence and inflamm-aging as two sides of the same coin: friends or foes. Front Immunol 2018; 8:1960.

54.   McIntosh R, Thatcher N. Pulmonary tuberculosis in the elderly: a different disease? Thorax 1990; 45: 912–913.

55.   Montgomery RR, Shaw AC. Paradoxical changes in innate immunity in aging: recent progress and new directions. J Leukoc Biol 2015; 98: 937–943.

56.   Haynes I, Eaton SM, Burns EM, et al. CD4 T cell memory derived from young naïve cells functions well into old age, but memory generated from aged naïve cells functions poorly. Proc Natl Acad Sci U S A 2003; 100: 15053–15058.

57.   Buchholz VR, Neuenbahn M, Busch DH. CD8+ T cell differentiation in the aging immune system: until the last clone standing. Curr Opin Immunol 2011; 23: 1–6.

58.   Barreira-Silva P, Torrado E, Nebenzahl-Guimaraes H, et al. Aetiopathogenesis, immunology and microbiology. In: Migliori GB, Bothamley G, Duarte R, et al., eds. Tuberculosis (ERS Monograph). Sheffield, European Respiratory Society, 2018; pp. 62–82.

59.   Rendon A, Goletti D, Matteelli A, et al. Diagnosis and treatment of latent tuberculosis infection. In: Migliori GB, Bothamley G, Duarte R, et al., eds. Tuberculosis (ERS Monograph). Sheffield, European Respiratory Society, 2018; pp. 381–398.

60.   Roberts-Thomson IC, Whittingham S, Youngchaivyud U, et al. Ageing, immune response and mortality. Lancet 1974; 2: 368–370.

61.   Mori T, Haeda N, Higuchi K, et al. Waning of the specific interferon-gamma response after years of tuberculosis infection. Int J Tuberc Lung Dis 2007; 11: 102105.

62.   Fulton JD, McCallion J. Tuberculosis – diagnostic difficulty in the elderly. J Clin Exp Gerontol 1987; 9: 303–311.

63.   Morris CDW. Pulmonary tuberculosis in the elderly: a different disease? Thorax 1990; 45: 912–913.

64.   Pérez-Guzman C, Vargas MH, Torres-Cruz A, et al. Does aging modify pulmonary tuberculosis? A meta-analytical review. Chest 1999; 116: 961–967.

65.   Velayutham BRV, Nair D, Chandrasekaran V, et al. Profile and response to anti-tuberculosis treatment among elderly tuberculosis patients treated under the TB control programme in South India. PLoS One 2014; 9: e88045.

66.   Yew WW, Yoshiyama T, Leung CC, et al. Epidemiological, clinical and mechanistic perspectives of tuberculosis in older people. Respirology 2018; 23: 567–575.

67.   Morris CDW. The radiography, haematology and biochemistry of pulmonary tuberculosis in the aged. Q J Med 1989; 71: 529–535.

68.   Cruz-Hervert LP, García-García I, Ferreyra-Reyes I, et al. Tuberculosis in ageing: high rates, complex diagnosis and poor clinical outcomes. Age Ageing 2012; 41: 488–495.

69.   Wang CS, Chen HC, Yang CJ, et al. The impact of age on the demographic, clinical radiographic characteristics and treatment outcomes of pulmonary tuberculosis patients in Taiwan. Infection 2008; 236: 335–340.

70.   Hauer B, Brodhiun B, Altmann D, et al. Tuberculosis in the elderly in Germany. Eur Respir J 2011; 38: 467–470.

71.   Aktou S, Yorgancioglu A, Çirak K, et al. Clinical spectrum of pulmonary and pleural tuberculosis: a report of 5,480 cases. Eur Respir J 1996; 9: 2031–2035.

72.   Pérez-Guzman C, Torres-Cruz A, Villerreal-Verlade H, et al. Progressive age-related changes in pulmonary tuberculosis images and the effect of diabetes. Am J Respir Crit Care Med 2000; 162: 1738–1740.

73.   Korzeniewska-Kosella M, Krysl J, Muller N, et al. Tuberculosis in young adults and the elderly. A prospective comparison study. Chest 1994; 106: 28–32.

74.   Comstock GW, Edwards PQ. The competing risks of tuberculosis and hepatitis for adult tuberculin reactors. Am Rev Respir Dis 1975; 111: 573–577.

75.   Saukonnen JJ, Cohn DL, Jasmer RM, et al. An Official ATS statement: hepatotoxicity of antituberculosis therapy. Am J Respir Crit Care Med 2006; 174: 935–952.

76.   LoBue PA, Moser KS. Use of isoniazid for latent tuberculosis infection in a public health clinic. Am J Respir Crit Care Med 2003; 168: 443–447.

https://doi.org/10.1183/2312508X.10021917

77.   Nolan CM, Goldberg SV, Buskin SE. Hepatotoxicity associated with isoniazid preventive therapy: a 7-year survey from a public health tuberculosis clinic. *JAMA* 1999; 281: 1014–1018.

78.   Fountain FF, Tolley E, Chrisman CR, *et al.* Isoniazid hepatotoxicity associated with treatment of latent tuberculosis infection: a 7-year evaluation from a public health tuberculosis clinic. *Chest* 2005; 128: 116–123.

79.   Hosford JD, von Fricken ME, Lauzado M, *et al.* Hepatotoxicity from antituberculous therapy in the elderly: a systematic review. *Tuberculosis* 2015; 95: 112–122.

80.   Tweed CD, Wills GH, Crook AM, *et al.* Liver toxicity associated with tuberculosis chemotherapy in the REMoxTB study. *BMC Med* 2018; 16: 46.

81.   Igari H, Imasawa T, Noguchi N, *et al.* Advanced stage of chronic kidney disease is risk of poor treatment outcome for smear-positive pulmonary tuberculosis. *J Infect Chemother* 2015; 21: 559–563.

82.   Launay-Vacher V, Izzedine H, Deray G. Pharmacokinetic considerations in the treatment of tuberculosis in patients with renal failure. *Clin Pharmacokinet* 2005; 44: 221–235.

83.   Spinewine A, Schmader KE, Barber N, *et al.* Appropriate prescribing in elderly people: how well can it be measured and optimised? *Lancet* 2007; 370: 173–184.

84.   Gillespie SH, Crook AM, McHugh TD, *et al.* Four-month moxifloxacin-based regimens for drug-sensitive tuberculosis. *N Engl J Med* 2014; 371: 1577–1587.

85.   Stagg HR, Harris RJ, Hatherall HA, *et al.* What are the most efficacious treatment regimens for isoniazid-resistant tuberculosis? A systematic review and network meta-analysis. *Thorax* 2016; 71: 940–949.

86.   Oshi DC, Oshi SN, Alobu I, *et al.* Profile and treatment outcomes of tuberculosis in the elderly in southeastern Nigeria, 2011–12. *PLos One* 2014; 9: e111910.

87.   WHO. Definitions and Reporting Framework for Tuberculosis: 2013 Revision. Document WHO/HTM/TB/2013.2. Geneva, WHO, 2013. www.who.int/tb/publications/definitions/en/

88.   Narain JP, Lofgren JP, Warren E, *et al.* Epidemic tuberculosis in a nursing home: a retrospective cohort study. *J Am Geriatr Soc* 1985; 33: 258–263.

89.   Reddy D, Walker J, White LF, *et al.* Latent tuberculosis infection testing practices in long-term care facilities, Boston, Massachusetts. *J Am Geriatr Soc* 2017; 65: 1145–1151.

90.   Ferrara G, Losi M, D'Amico R, *et al.* Interferon-γ-release assays detect recent tuberculosis re-infection in elderly contacts. *Int J Immunopathol Pharmacol* 2009; 22: 669–677.

91.   Lai CC, Hsieh YC, Yeh YP, *et al.* A pulmonary tuberculosis outbreak in a long-term care facility. *Epidemiol Infect* 2016; 144: 1455–1462.

92.   Antusheva E, Mironuk O, Tarasova I, *et al.* Outbreak of tuberculosis in a closed setting: views on transmission based on results from molecular and conventional methods. *J Hosp Infect* 2016; 93: 187–190.

93.   Iwamoto S, Yano S, Nishikawa E, *et al.* An outbreak of pulmonary tuberculosis due to definite exogenous reinfection among elderly individuals in welfare facilities. *Kekkaku* 2016; 91: 451–455.

94.   Horsburgh CR Jr, O'Donnell M, Chamblee S, *et al.* Revisiting rates of reactivation tuberculosis: a population-based approach. *Am J Respir Crit Care Med* 2010; 182: 420–425.

95.   Wiker HG, Mustafa T, Bjune GA, *et al.* Evidence for waning of latency in a cohort study of tuberculosis. *BMC Infect Dis* 2010; 10: 37.

96.   Comstock GW. Frost revisited: the modern epidemiology of tuberculosis. *Am J Epidemiol* 1975; 101: 363–382.

97.   Tocque K, Bellis MA, Tam CM, *et al.* Long-term trends in tuberculosis: comparison of age-cohort data between Hong Kong and England and Wales. *Am J Respir Crit Care Med* 1998; 158: 484–488.

98.   Tuberculosis Surveillance Center. Tuberculosis in Japan: Annual Report – 2017. Tokyo, Department of Epidemiology and Clinical Research, Research Institute of Tuberculosis, 2017. www.jata.or.jp/english/dl/pdf/TB_in_Japan_2017.pdf

99.   Moran-Mendoza O, Marion SA, Elwood K, *et al.* Risk factors for developing tuberculosis: a 12-year follow-up of contacts of tuberculosis cases. *Int J Tuberc Lung Dis* 2010; 14: 1112–1119.

100.   Andrews JR, Noubary F, Walensky RP, *et al.* Risk of progression to active tuberculosis following re-infection with *Mycobacterium tuberculosis*. *Clin Infect Dis* 2012; 54: 784–791.

Disclosures: None declared.

Chapter 16

Comorbidities

Cecile Magis-Escurra[1], Anna Cristina C. Carvalho[2], Afrânio L. Kritski[3] and Enrico Girardi[4]

In this chapter, we provide practical treatment advice for physicians to treat patients with TB and different comorbidities (HIV, diabetes, renal failure and liver cirrhosis), and TB patients post-solid organ transplant, based on the recommendations of different (inter)national guidelines, publications and expert opinions.

Cite as: Magis-Escurra C, Carvalho ACC, Kritski AL, *et al.* Comorbidities. *In:* Migliori GB, Bothamley G, Duarte R, *et al.*, eds. Tuberculosis (ERS Monograph). Sheffield, European Respiratory Society, 2018; pp. 276–290 [https://doi.org/10.1183/2312508X.10022017].

Comorbidities and TB treatment do not always get along. Important drug–drug interactions, immunological problems and higher relapse rates cause trouble, especially in the case of HIV-TB, diabetes, renal failure, liver cirrhosis and post transplant. http://ow.ly/cfVQ30lqCfE

Although TB treatment follows national guidelines and the WHO treatment guidelines, caring for a TB patient always implies conducting a thorough assessment of conditions that could affect treatment response or outcome. Comorbidities, psychosocial factors and substance abuse all increase the risk of developing active TB but also influence final treatment outcome. For that reason, each patient needs an individual plan of care including assessment of and referrals for treatment for other illnesses. Clinicians should establish close cooperation between a specialist of the specific comorbidity, a specialist in the management of TB and a hospital pharmacist and consider the option of TDM to provide the appropriate, individualised dose to each patient. Comorbidities such as diabetes, HIV, hepatic and renal dysfunction, and mental disorders may sometimes force clinicians to alter their TB drug selection or to prolong treatment. After solid organ transplantation the role of the hospital pharmacist is even more prominent due to important drug–drug interactions between TB drugs and drugs used to prevent organ transplant rejection.

In this chapter we provide treatment advice for patients with TB and different comorbidities and TB patients post-solid organ transplant (SOT), based on the recommendations of different (inter)national guidelines, publications and expert opinions.

---

[1]Radboud University Medical Centre-TB expert centre Dekkerswald, Dept of Respiratory Diseases, Nijmegen-Groesbeek, The Netherlands. [2]Oswaldo Cruz Institute (IOC), Laboratory of Innovations in Therapies, Education and Bioproducts, (LITEB), Fiocruz, Rio de Janeiro, Brazil. [3]Federal University of Rio de Janeiro, TB Academic Program Medical School, Rio de Janeiro, Brazil. [4]National Institute for Infectious Diseases L. Spallanzani, Rome, Italy.

Correspondence: Cecile Magis-Escurra, Radboud UMC-Dekkerswald, Pulmonology, Nijmeegsebaan 31, Nijmegen, Gelderland, 6561KE, The Netherlands E-mail: cecile.magis-escurra@radboudumc.nl

Copyright ©ERS 2018. Print ISBN: 978-1-84984-099-6. Online ISBN: 978-1-84984-100-9. Print ISSN: 2312-508X. Online ISSN: 2312-5098.

https://doi.org/10.1183/2312508X.10022017

Tuberculosis treatment in patients with HIV infection

HIV infection represents the main risk factor for LTBI reactivation and progressive disease after infection with *Mycobacterium tuberculosis*. Individuals with TB–HIV co-infection have a 29 times higher risk of active TB than HIV-negative patients, with a mean annual risk of developing TB of 10% [1, 2]. For HIV-positive patients with active TB, the standard anti-TB therapy is a 6-month daily regimen, consisting of an intensive phase of 2 months of isoniazide, rifampicin, pyrazinamide, and ethambutol followed by a continuation phase of 4 months of isoniazide and rifampicin [3]. Some authors recommend the extension of the continuation phase with rifampicin and isoniazid from 4 to 7 months for HIV-positive patients not on concomitant ART, but the level of evidence is low [4]. Intermittent regimens should not be used in HIV-positive patients [3], mainly in the intensive phase (first 2 months) [4], or should be used with much caution in the three times per week schedule [5] due to the higher risk of failure, relapse and rifamycin resistance. Malabsorption of anti-TB drugs in HIV-positive patients has been described, leading to sub-therapeutic plasma levels, thus increasing the risk of therapeutic failure and emergence of resistant *M. tuberculosis* strains. For this reason, TDM of anti-TB drugs, in particular for rifampicin, has been recommended by some authors [6, 7]. In HIV-positive patients on isoniazide, pyridoxine $25–50$ mg·day^{-1} has been recommended due to increased risk of neuropathy [3, 5, 8].

Concomitant ART in HIV-positive individuals with TB is highly recommended. Patients who are already using antiretrovirals (ARV) at the time of TB diagnosis should have their regimen reassessed, considering the possibility of pharmacokinetic interaction of some ARV with rifampicin (tables 1 and 2) [9, 10]. The most optimal time to initiate ART for newly diagnosed HIV co-infected TB patients has been evaluated in multiple clinical trials

Table 1. ART considerations when treating TB disease with rifamycins

Consideration	Rationale/comments
TAF is not recommended with any rifamycin-containing regimen	Rifamycins may significantly reduce TAF exposure
If rifampin is used:	
EFV can be used without dosage adjustment	Rifampin has a less significant effect on EFV concentration than on other NNRTIs, PIs and INSTIs
If RAL is used, increase RAL dose to 800 mg twice daily	Rifampin is a strong inducer of CYP3A4 and UGT1A1 enzymes, causing significant decrease in concentrations of PIs, INSTIs and RPV
Use DTG at 50 mg twice daily only in patients without selected INSTI mutations (refer to product label)	
If using a PI-based regimen, rifabutin should be used in place of rifampin in the TB regimen	Rifabutin is a less potent inducer and is an option for patients receiving non-EFV-based regimens

TAF: tenofovir alafenamide; EFV: efavirenz; RAL: raltegravir; DTG: dolutegravir; INSTI: integrase strand transfer inhibitor; PI: protease inhibitor; NNRTI: non-nucleoside reverse transcriptase inhibitor; RPV: rilpivirine. Data from [10].

Table 2. ART considerations when treating DR-TB disease

Consideration	Rationale/comments
If aminoglycosides are used: Concomitant use of TDF may increase nephrotoxicity	TAF, a novel prodrug of tenofovir, is less nephrotoxic than TDF
If ethionamide or PAS is used: Concomitant use with NVP and some PIs may increase hepatotoxicity	EFV and NVP are not recommended and TPV/r is contraindicated in patients with hepatic insufficiency (Child–Pugh class B or C)
If linezolid is used: Concomitant use of ZDV increases the risk of myelosuppression	
If bedaquiline is used: If used with a PI-based regimen, more intensive monitoring of cardiac drug toxicity is recommended	Concomitant use of bedaquiline and PIs has been associated with an increase in the AUC of bedaquiline, particularly with LPV/r
Association with EFV and ETR should be avoided	EFV and ETR induce decrease on bedaquiline concentration
Association with NVP and integrase strand transfer inhibitors does not require dose adjustment	Antiretroviral exposure was not affected by delamanid
If delamanid is used: No clinically significant drug–drug interactions between delamanid and TDF, EFV and LPV/r	

TDF: tenofovir disoproxil fumarate; NVP: nevirapine; PI: protease inhibitor; ZDV: zidovudine; EFV: efavirenz; ETR: etravirine; LPV/r: lopinavir/ritonavir; TAF: tenofovir alafenamide; TPV/r: tipranavir/ritonavir. Data from [10].

[11–13]. The start of ART is now recommended within 8 weeks of initiation of anti-TB therapy for all TB–HIV co-infected patients, regardless of their CD4+ cell count [3, 10], since it is associated with reduction in overall mortality. This effect is particularly relevant in patients with a CD4+ cell count <50 cells·mm^{-3}, where reduction in the rate of new AIDS-defining illness and death was observed with early ART initiation [11, 12]. Therefore, patients with CD4+ cell counts <50 cells·mm^{-3} should initiate ART within the first 2 weeks of TB treatment, except in cases of TB meningitis due to the higher risk of severe paradoxical reactions in these patients [4, 14].

The concomitant use of ARV and anti-TB drugs, in particular rifampicin, leads to the possibility of drug–drug interactions. Rifampicin induces the activity of the cytochrome P-450 CYP3A complex, particularly the CYP3A and CYP2C subfamilies, P-glycoprotein and uridine diphosphate glucuronosyltransferase (UGT) 1A1 enzymes, reducing ARV exposure and leading to sub-therapeutic ARV levels, which is associated with incomplete viral suppression and resistance to these drugs [10, 15, 16].

Rifabutin is a weaker inducer, the relative potency as inducers is as follows: rifampicin=1; rifapentine=0.85; and rifabutin=0.40 [16]. Rifabutin is the preferred rifamycin to use in patients on a protease inhibitor (PI)-based ARV regimen as it has a substantially lower risk of drug interactions with PIs in respect to rifampicin and no dose adjustment is required for PIs. However, rifabutin concentration may increase by the concomitant use of PIs, thus enhancing the risk of drug-induced side-effects (mainly uveitis). Rifabutin 150 mg once

https://doi.org/10.1183/2312508X.10022017

daily or 300 mg three times a week are the regimens usually recommended when the drug is used with PIs [10]. As rifampicin is a potent inducer of UGT1A1 enzyme, decreased concentrations of raltegravir and dolutegravir, mainly metabolised by UGT1A1 isozymes, are anticipated when these drugs are given in combination with rifampicin [10, 16].

However, the use of efavirenz with rifampicin was associated with good virologic, immunologic and clinical outcomes in several studies. In addition, increasing the dose of efavirenz from 600 to 800 mg when used with rifampicin in patients weighing >50 kg is generally not required [10, 17–19]. Rifampicin remains the most potent TB drug widely in use today; therefore, despite the issues related to pharmacokinetics interaction of rifampicin with ARV, rifampicin should be maintained in the TB treatment regimen, with the exception of cases of M. tuberculosis resistant to the drug or serious side-effects [9]. Table 1 presents the main considerations to be identified when treating patients on anti-TB therapy with ARV.

Immune reconstitution inflammatory syndrome (IRIS), an exacerbated immune response in patients who present immune recovery upon initiation of ART, may complicate clinical management of TB–HIV patients. IRIS is classified into two forms: paradoxical or unmasking. Paradoxical IRIS refers to clinical and/or radiological findings of recurrent, new or worsening symptoms and signs of TB. In unmasking TB–IRIS, patients who have unrecognised TB at the start of ART may present with a particularly accelerated and inflammatory presentation of TB disease in the first weeks of ART. Patients may present with fever accompanied by clinical worsening of pulmonary findings or the appearance of new lesions, as well as lymph node enlargement. After thorough investigation to exclude resistance to TB drugs or other opportunistic infections, management of IRIS is based on the combined use of TB treatment and anti-inflammatory drugs, including corticosteroids for the most severe cases [20–22].

MDR-/XDR-TB in HIV-positive patients was associated with higher mortality in some studies [23, 24], while in others a higher mortality was observed only in HIV-positive individuals without ART or in older patients [25]. HIV-positive MDR-/XDR-TB patients on ART have a lower risk of death and are more likely to be cured [26, 27]. Therefore, rapid diagnosis and timely initiation of ART, usually within 2–8 weeks after starting MDR-/XDR-TB treatment, regardless of CD4+ cell count, become even more important for HIV-positive patients with suspected MDR-/XDR-TB [28].

The regimen for DR-TB has been based on the WHO principles [28], with particular attention to the overlap of drug toxicities; HIV-positive patients may also be eligible for a shorter MDR-TB regimen [29]. Caution is advised when co-administering drugs with similar and potentially additive toxicities, for instance: tenofovir and aminoglycosides (nephrotoxicity), non-nucleoside reverse transcriptase inhibitors, in particular nevirapine, and some PIs with ethionamide and PAS (hepatotoxicity) or zidovudine with linezolid (myelosuppression) [10, 20]. Results based on an interim cohort analysis suggest that the use of bedaquiline is safe regardless of HIV status [30]. However, the use of bedaquiline with PIs, in particular with lopinavir/ritonavir, has been associated with an increase in the AUC of bedaquiline, therefore careful monitoring of cardiac drug toxicity is recommended [10, 31]. The use of nevirapine seems to be safer, as well as integrase strand transfer inhibitors, and does not require dose adjustment but the association with efavirenz and etravirine should be avoided, since these drugs induce a decrease on bedaquiline concentration [10, 29, 32]. With regard to delamanid, MALLIKAARJUN et al. [33] described no clinically significant drug–drug interactions between delamanid and selected antiretroviral agents (tenofovir, efavirenz, lopinavir and ritonavir) (table 2).

Tuberculosis treatment in patients with diabetes mellitus

Individuals with DM have a two to three times higher risk of developing active TB when compared to people without DM [34, 35]. The population attributable fraction of DM as a risk factor for TB is higher than 12% in all WHO regions, except in Africa and the Western Pacific regions [36]. DM accounted for almost 11% of global TB deaths among HIV-negative individuals in 2015 [37].

The innate immune response to *M. tuberculosis* is impaired in diabetics and is followed by hyper-reactive adaptive immune responses [38]. An efficient immune response in TB reflects a balance between protective and damaging immune activation; DM could push this balance toward the damage activation response [39–41].

TB symptoms in patients with DM appear to be more frequent and severe [42], which may reflect their generally more advanced age [43, 44]. Chest radiographs often present multiple cavities, bilateral pulmonary involvement and lymph node enlargement, besides "atypical" findings of lower lobe lesions especially in patients with poor glycaemic control [45–48]. The presence of atypical findings may delay the diagnosis of TB in patients with DM since these radiologic aspects may mimic community pneumonia or neoplasia.

Most guidelines still recommend the same duration of treatment for TB patients with and without DM [49–51]. To date, there is no consensus regarding the best anti-TB regimen and glycaemic control for patients with DM despite an increased severity of the disease and worse final outcomes [47, 52]. Optimal glycaemic control in diabetics is associated with faster bacteriological sputum conversion, a higher rate of successful treatment and a lower risk of recurrence [53, 54]. DM may lead to low plasma concentrations of anti-TB drugs, and therefore TDM was recommended by some authors [6, 55, 56]. As TDM is not yet widely available many physicians pragmatically extend therapy to 9 months when treatment response is suboptimal to prevent relapse [57]. Mortality was higher in the presence of other comorbidities. In a cohort study in South Korea, the association between diabetes and smoking increased the risk of TB-related deaths by almost six times during the first year of follow-up [58].

TB treatment leads to increased toxicity in patients with DM; peripheral neuropathy due to isoniazid and ocular neuropathy due to ethambutol [49, 59]. Another important aspect of treatment in DM is the possibility of drug–drug interactions, especially with rifampicin. Rifampicin is a potent hepatic enzyme inducer and increases the hepatic metabolism of sulphonyl urea derivatives, lowering their plasma levels. No effect of rifampicin is known on the exposure of glucagon-like peptide-1 receptor agonists and only a slight effect on dipeptidyl peptidase-4 inhibitors [60]. Although not metabolised by the P450 enzymes system, metformin may have its hypoglycaemic effect increased by rifampicin, enhancing the expression of organic cation transporter and hepatic uptake of metformin [59–61]. As insulin is not metabolised, no pharmacokinetic interactions with anti-TB drugs occur [59]. For that reason, the use of insulin in the beginning of TB treatment to achieve faster bacteriological sputum conversion and prevent drug–drug interactions is recommended by NIAZI *et al.* [62].

https://doi.org/10.1183/2312508X.10022017

Screening for DM in TB patients is currently widely recommended [51], although the best approach has not yet been defined and there is no evaluation of the clinical impact of this recommendation. Some programmes recommend the assessment of glycaemia by fasting blood glucose or glycated haemoglobin at the start of TB treatment, but time intervals for re-testing are still unclear [34, 51]. However, once the test has been performed at initiation of TB treatment, it should be repeated during or at the end of treatment, especially considering that the inflammatory response secondary to TB may be a cause of transient hyperglycaemia due to insulin resistance [59].

Screening for TB/LTBI in diabetics remains a subject of debate as a variable prevalence has been found (from 1.7% to 36%) according to TB burden in different countries [34], and there is a lack of evidence regarding the risk-benefit ratio of LTBI testing and treatment of patients with DM. Systematic testing for LTBI is not recommended for people with DM, except when these patients are in other risk categories for evaluation of LTBI [63].

Tuberculosis treatment in patients with chronic renal impairment

Advanced chronic renal impairment is associated with functional abnormalities of neutrophils, reduced T- and B-cell function and compromised monocyte and natural killer cell function leading to immunodeficiency. Low levels of 25-hydroxyvitamin D also endanger immunity. The relative risk of developing active TB is high in patients with chronic renal impairment or on haemodialysis and even higher for renal transplant recipients (further attenuation of immunity by immunosuppressive therapy) [64]. Due to this acquired immunodeficiency state, active TB may present atypically and therefore be difficult to diagnose in patients with chronic renal impairment.

Chronic renal disease is classified in different stages [65]. Stage 1: normal creatinine clearance but urinary tract abnormality, for example, polycystic kidney structural abnormality. Stage 2: creatinine clearance 60–90 mL·min^{-1}. Stage 3: creatinine clearance 30–60 mL·min^{-1}. Stage 4: creatinine clearance 15–30 mL·min^{-1}. Stage 5: creatinine clearance <15 mL·min^{-1} with(out) dialysis.

Before starting TB treatment it is important to assess the severity of the impairment (stage 1–5) and establish a close cooperation between a renal physician and a specialist in the management of TB [8]. Any patient with active TB, either pulmonary or non-pulmonary, should receive standard chemotherapy agents and for the standard duration [8]. Rifampicin is cleared hepatically and can be used safely in patients with renal disease. Interstitial nephritis may occur incidentally and may lead to further worsening of creatinine clearance. This side-effect can be managed with steroids in close collaboration with a renal physician. Isoniazid, also metabolised by the liver, is used safely although increased incidence of neurotoxic side-effects occur, especially in slow acetylators and haemodialysis patients. Although never adapted to international guidelines [8, 65], a higher dose of pyridoxine (100 mg) was recommended for the first time in 1993 to prevent this side-effect [66, 67]. Pyrazinamid is metabolised hepatically but the metabolites are mainly excreted by the kidneys. In case of advanced renal disease, metabolites may accumulate leading to toxic levels of uric acid causing gout. Dosing intervals should therefore be increased to three times weekly for patients with stage 4 and 5 renal disease. Ethambutol is fully cleared *via* the kidneys. Only in stages 1–3 can it be used safely in a daily dose of 10–15 mg·kg^{-1}. For patients with stages 4 and 5, dosing intervals of ethambutol should be increased (three times per week). As soon as drug susceptibility tests show normal results, ethambutol is stopped. To avoid premature drug removal pyrazinamid and ethambutol are given immediately after haemodialysis. This provides an opportunity to observe drug intake to ensure adherence. With this strategy there is a small risk of elevated drug levels between dialysis sessions. Clinicians should therefore consider the option of TDM to provide appropriate and individualised dose. Expected drug interactions after renal transplantation may be evaluated with TDM as well (table 3).

Mycobacterial infection in peritoneal dialysis patients often poses diagnostic challenges (diagnostic delay >6 weeks) and carries a high mortality rate (differing in the literature from 15% to 30%). Clinicians should have a high index of suspicion for mycobacterial peritonitis in peritoneal dialysis patients with features of peritonitis who do not respond promptly to conventional anti-microbial agents. The most common symptoms are fever, abdominal pain, and cloudy dialysate with a predominance of polymorphonuclear cells. A smear for acid-fast bacilli or a culture is positive in most cases. Whether the peritoneal dialysis catheter should be removed during mycobacterial peritonitis needs further investigation [68]. TB treatment is started with four drugs (rifampicin, isoniazid, pyrazinamide and a fluoroquinolone (instead of ethambutol)) on a daily basis. Unpublished data (C. Peloquin, College of Pharmacy, University of Florida, Gainesville, FL, USA) suggests that ethambutol is poorly cleared by peritoneal dialysis. Also, in peritoneal dialysis the option of TDM should be considered as rifampicin dialysis fluid levels were low due to its high molecular weight, high protein-binding capacity and lipid solubility [69]. High-dose pyridoxine (100 mg) should be given to avoid isoniazid-induced neurotoxicity.

Tuberculosis treatment in patients with chronic liver disease

Chronic liver disease involves progressive destruction and regeneration of the liver parenchyma leading to fibrosis and cirrhosis. The incidence of TB is increased in patients

Table 3. Recommendation for the use of anti-TB drugs in chronic renal disease

Drug	Stage 1–3	Stage 4–5	Haemodialysis	Peritoneal dialysis	Post-transplant
Rifampicin	Normal daily dose	Normal daily dose	Normal daily dose	Normal daily dose, consider TDM	Normal, daily dose (evaluate with TDM important drug interactions with immunosuppressants)
Isoniazid[#]	Normal daily dose, normal pyridoxine dose	Normal daily dose, use 100 mg pyridoxine	Normal daily dose, use 100 mg pyridoxine	Normal daily dose, use 100 mg pyridoxine	Normal daily dose, normal pyridoxine dose
Pyrazinamid[#]	Normal daily dose	Normal dose, 3 times per week	Normal dose, 3 times per week		Normal daily dose
Ethambutol[#]	Normal daily dose	Normal dose, 3 times per week	Normal dose, 3 times per week		Normal daily dose

[#]: TDM is recommended to prevent toxicity and use optimal dosages.

https://doi.org/10.1183/2312508X.10022017

with chronic liver diseases, more so in those with decompensated disease, probably because of cirrhosis-associated immune dysfunction syndrome, and case fatality rates are high [70]. Presentation of TB in many cases is atypical, with a greater incidence of extrapulmonary and disseminated disease with atypical clinical symptoms [71]. Multiple conditions are associated causing chronic liver disease (viral hepatitis, alcohol and drugs, metabolic disorders, autoimmune diseases and right heart failure). Advancing chronic liver disease may lead to portal hypertension, synthetic dysfunction, encephalopathy, hepatopulmonary syndrome, hepatorenal syndrome and hepatocellular carcinoma. A patient with decompensated liver cirrhosis may present with drowsiness, hyperventilation, asterixis, jaundice, ascites, peripheral oedema and bruising. Liver biochemistry can be normal depending on the severity of the cirrhosis. In most cases there is at least a slight elevation in the serum alkaline phosphatase and serum aminotransferases. The best indicator of liver function is serum albumin. In decompensated cirrhosis serum electrolytes and haematology may be deranged. Biochemical findings to classify cirrhosis (Child–Pugh classification as an indicator for severity and survival) are bilirubin, international normalised ratio and albumin level besides possible findings of hepatic encephalopathy and ascites. The Child–Pugh score is defined as follows: class A (score 5–6), class B (score 7–9) and class C (score 10–15, most severe form with a poor 2-year survival of only 35%).

Although handling and clearance of anti-TB-drugs is expected to be altered in patients with chronic liver disease, insufficient evidence exists as to whether the hepatic impairment increases the risk of hepatotoxicity [72–75].

Hepatotoxicity for anti-TB drug results are unpredictable and still not completely understood [76]. Most drugs show idiosyncratic mechanisms leading to reactive metabolites which are thought to result *via* genetic or acquired polymorphisms in cytochrome P450 enzymes, acetylator status or other metabolic pathway(s). If hepatotoxicity develops in a patient with liver cirrhosis, particularly decompensated cirrhosis, the risk of severe liver failure is markedly increased [71, 77].

Globally there is no consensus on the drugs to be given for different stages of liver injury [71], although the WHO treatment guidelines [78] mention that the more unstable or severe the liver disease is (according to Child–Pugh score), the fewer hepatotoxic anti-TB drugs should be used. Overall, clinical judgment combined with close biochemical monitoring remains the mainstay in this setting. Starting treatment in patients with advanced or unstable liver disease is preferably done clinically in a TB expert centre or at least under close supervision of a TB expert. In 2012, a recommendation was published for the use of anti-TB drugs according to the Child–Pugh score. A combination of this advice [77] and the WHO recommendations [78] resulted in the recommendations showed in table 1. According to the Dutch National Clinical TB Consultants, rifampicin can be administered safely to a patient with class C cirrhosis of the liver, provided that the patient is hospitalised in the first weeks of treatment. Clinicians should also consider the option of TDM to provide an appropriate, individualised dose to each patient (table 4).

Tuberculosis and solid organ transplantation

Persons undergoing SOT have a risk of developing TB which is 20–70 times higher than in the general population [79, 80], although the cumulative incidence of this condition varies

Table 4. Recommendations for the use of anti-TB-drugs in chronic liver disease

Child-Pugh score	Liver disease	Treatment	Remarks
Class A (5–6)	Stable	Use of two potentially hepatotoxic drugs, likely to be well tolerated; avoid pyrazinamide	Prolong therapy to 9 months when pyrazinamid is not used
Class B (7–9)	Advanced	Use a regimen with only one potentially hepatotoxic drug; rifampicin is preferred above isoniazide; pyrazinamid should not be used	Prolong therapy to 9 months when pyrazinamid is not used. Prolong therapy to 18–24 months when rifampicin is not used
Class C (10–15)	Very advanced	Rifampicin can be safely used in a clinical setting[#] In case of liver failure, use an (initial) regimen with no potentially hepatotoxic drugs; ethambutol, fluoroquinolones, aminoglycosides and other second-line oral drugs can be used	Prolong therapy to 9 months when pyrazinamid is not used. Prolong therapy to 18–24 months when rifampicin is not used

[#]: expert opinion Dutch National TB consultants.

considerably among different geographical areas depending on the background TB incidence rates [79]. Immune suppression due to the condition which led to transplant, for example chronic renal failure, as well as the use of an immunosuppressant agent are the primary cause of the increased susceptibility to TB in SOT recipients, and different mechanisms may be involved in the development of active TB in these patients (figure 1) [81].

It is generally assumed that most of the TB cases in SOT recipients are due to reactivation of LTBI, favoured by immune suppression [81]. These cases could be prevented, at least partly, by screening and treatment of LTBI in SOT candidates [82], as detailed in the chapter by RENDON *et al.* [83] in this issue of the *Monograph*. A minority of cases can be due to rapid progression to overt disease of a newly acquired infection, in some cases because of exposure to infectious cases in hospital settings. For example, a nosocomial outbreak of TB that involved 10 renal transplant patients occurred in a hospital unit in the USA, and the source case for this outbreak was a patient who had post-transplant exposure to an infectious TB patient at another hospital [84]. Donor-derived TB, *i.e.* active disease in SOT recipients due to reactivation of LTBI or less frequently presence of active infection in the donor graft, has also been documented but appears to be rare. In a recently published review of more than 2000 cases of post-transplant TB, only 20 cases could be classified as caused by donor-derived infection [85]. However, there is a concern that these cases may become more frequent even in low-incidence countries with the increasing proportion of donors originating from high-incidence countries, and recommendations have been issued that stress the importance of carefully evaluating the infectious risk of the donor of ruling out active TB [86]. Most donor-derived TB cases are in lung recipients. Finally, patients with active TB may undergo transplantation. Patients with TB may develop acute hepatic

https://doi.org/10.1183/2312508X.10022017

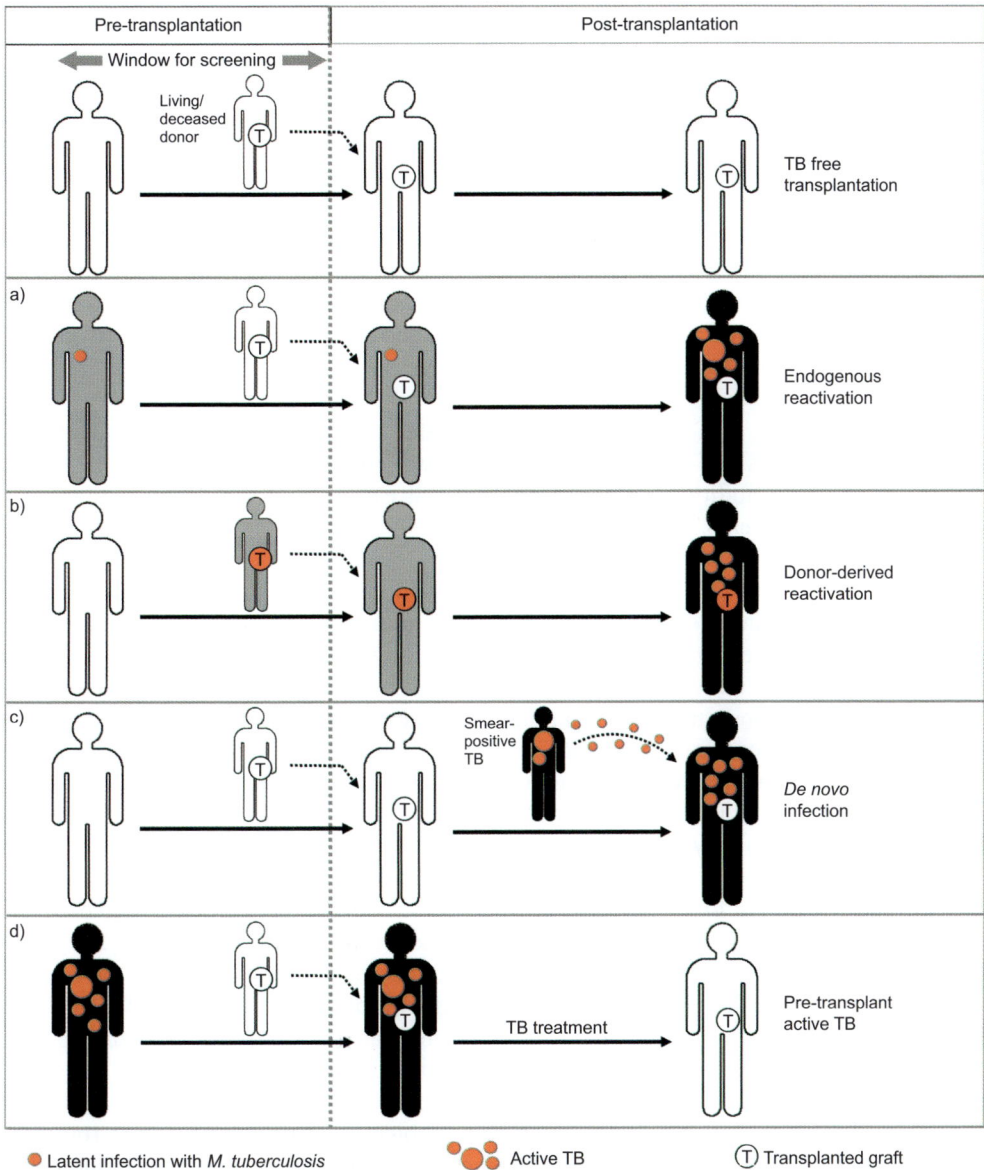

Figure 1. The risk of TB in transplant candidates and recipients: a Tuberculosis Network European Trials Group consensus statement. The four different scenarios for infection with *Mycobacterium tuberculosis* in the transplant setting. a) Endogenous reactivation due to LTBI in the candidate recipient. b) Donor-derived reactivation due to LTBI in a living or deceased donor. c) *De novo* exposure and infection post-transplantation. d) When a patient with active TB urgently requires a transplant (*i.e.* urgent liver transplantation). White, grey and black figures represent uninfected individuals, individuals with LTBI, and individuals with active TB, respectively. Reproduced from [81] with permission.

failure requiring liver transplantation because of hepatotoxic effects of anti-TB drugs or they may have unrecognised TB at the time of transplantation [87]. Time from transplant to diagnosis of TB varies in different studies, however, most of the cases usually present within the first year after transplant, while the presentation of TB in renal transplant recipients tend to be more delayed with a median of 18 months or more after transplantation [79, 81, 85]. In contrast, donor-derived TB tends to present much earlier, a median of 3 months after transplantation [79, 85].

Clinical manifestation of TB in SOT recipients tends to be more severe compared to immune-competent hosts. Approximately half of cases present with pulmonary manifestation, and one-fifth have extrapulmonary localisation and one-third may have disseminated disease [80, 81]. Among pulmonary cases, presence of cavitations is relatively uncommon. Other radiographic manifestations including interstitial and military patterns, and focal infiltrates and pleural effusions have been described. General symptoms of TB such as fever, night sweats and weight loss have been reported with varying frequency. Mortality of SOT patients with TB as high as 40% has been reported, and the majority of deaths in these patients appears to be directly attributable to TB.

Treatment of TB in SOT recipients is complicated by the pharmacologic interaction between anti-TB drugs and immunosuppressant drugs and by the increased risk of toxicity of anti-TB drugs. In addition, some uncertainty still exists about the optimal duration of treatment in these patients.

Rifamycins are potent inducers of cytochrome P450 3A4 (CYP3A4). Administration of rifampin and rifabutin to SOT recipients results in increased clearance and a reduced plasma level of calcineurin inhibitors (cyclosporine and tacrolimus) and mTOR inhibitor (rapamycin/sirolimus), and also of mycophenolate and corticosteroids used for the induction and maintenance of post-transplant immunosuppression [88]. In spite of this, the use of a standard rifampicin-containing 6-month treatment regimen is generally recommended for most SOT recipients, with frequent monitoring of plasma level of immunosuppressant drugs. Doses of cyclosporine, tacrolimus and sirolimus may in fact need to be increased two- to five-fold [80]. Rifabutin may be used as an alternative to rifampicin, given its reduced potency as a CYP3A4 inducer. Some physicians use a rifamycin-free regimen in individuals with localised and less severe forms, without central nervous system, pericardial or osteoarticular involvement. This regimen is based on the use of isoniazid and ethambutol for 18 months, with the addition of pyrazinamide for the first 2 months [81]. Moxifloxacin may be regarded as an alternative to rifampin. However, it should be noted that clinical experience with rifampicin-free regimens in SOT recipients is limited, and no evidence is available of an increased risk of SOT rejection in clinical practice with the use of rifamycins [89].

Hepatotoxicity due to anti-TB drugs is a major problem, in particular for liver transplant recipients, and requires strict monitoring. In fact, in these patients, isoniazid-induced liver damage may be particularly frequent, and it may pose significant additional problems for the differential diagnosis with rejection-related hepatitis [79].

The clinical usefulness of extending standard treatment beyond 6 months is still the subject of debate. A 7-month continuation phase is recommended for PTB patients with cavitation or with a sputum culture which is positive for *M. tuberculosis* after the first 2 months of treatment, and some experts suggest a continuation phase of 7–10 months in patients with central nervous system involvement. Based on data suggesting increased mortality, some experts suggest extending the total duration of TB treatment to at least 9 months for all SOT recipients to reduce mortality [49, 90].

Finally, paradoxical reactions and IRIS as described above in patients with co-infection of HIV–TB, also frequently complicate the course of TB treatment in SOT recipients.

 https://doi.org/10.1183/2312508X.10022017

Recently, IRIS has been described in nine (14%) out of 64 patients with post-transplant TB, a median of 47 days after the initiation of anti-TB treatment [87]. IRIS is more common in liver transplant recipients and no association was documented with reduction in immune suppression or dosage of specific immune-suppressant drugs. Mortality at 1 year after diagnosis was 33.3% in patients with IRIS compared to 17.2% in those without IRIS.

References

1. Allen S, Batungwanayo J, Kerlikowske K, *et al.* Two-year incidence of tuberculosis in cohorts of HIV-infected and uninfected urban Rwandan women. *Am Rev Respir Dis* 1992; 146: 1439–1444.
2. World Health Organization. WHO Policy on Collaborative TB/HIV Activities: Guidelines for National Programmes and Other Stakeholders. Geneva, WHO, 2012.
3. World Health Organization. Guidelines for treatment of drug-susceptible tuberculosis and patient care. 2017 update. Geneva, WHO, 2017.
4. Sotgiu G, Nahid P, Loddenkemper R, *et al.* The ERS-endorsed official ATS/CDC/IDSA clinical practice guidelines on treatment of drug-susceptible tuberculosis. *Eur Respir J* 2016; 48: 963–971.
5. Nahid P, Dorman SE, Alipanah N, *et al.* Executive Summary: Official American Thoracic Society/Centers for Disease Control and Prevention/Infectious Diseases Society of America Clinical Practice Guidelines: Treatment of Drug-Susceptible Tuberculosis. *Clin Infect Dis* 2016; 63: 853–867.
6. Magis-Escurra C, Anthony RM, van der Zanden AGM, *et al.* Pound foolish and penny wise – when will dosing of rifampicin be optimised? *Lancet Respir Med* 2018; 6: e11–e12.
7. Daskapan A, de Lange WC, Akkerman OW, *et al.* The role of therapeutic drug monitoring in individualised drug dosage and exposure measurement in tuberculosis and HIV co-infection. *Eur Respir J* 2015; 45: 569–571.
8. National Institute for Health and Care Excellence. Tuberculosis. NICE Guideline 33. www.nice.org.uk/guidance/ng33 Date last updated: May 2016; date last accessed: June 2018.
9. WHO, PEPFAR, UNAIDS, The Global Fund. A guide to monitoring and evaluation for collaborative TB/HIV activities. 2015 revision Geneva, WHO, 2015.
10. AIDSinfo. Guidelines for the Use of Antiretroviral Agents in HIV-1-Infected Adults and Adolescents. https://aidsinfo.nih.gov/contentfiles/lvguidelines/adultandadolescentgl.pdf Date last updated: May 30, 2018; date last accessed: June 2018.
11. Abdool Karim SS, Naidoo K, Grobler A, *et al.* Integration of antiretroviral therapy with tuberculosis treatment. *N Engl J Med* 2011; 365: 1492–1501.
12. Havlir DV, Kendall MA, Ive P, *et al.* Timing of antiretroviral therapy for HIV-1 infection and tuberculosis. *N Engl J Med* 2011; 365: 1482–1491.
13. Blanc FX, Sok T, Laureillard D, *et al.* Earlier *versus* later start of antiretroviral therapy in HIV-infected adults with tuberculosis. *N Engl J Med* 2011; 365: 1471–1481.
14. Torok ME, Yen NT, Chau TT, *et al.* Timing of initiation of antiretroviral therapy in human immunodeficiency virus (HIV) – associated tuberculous meningitis. *Clin Infect Dis* 2011; 52: 1374–1383.
15. Wenning LA, Hanley WD, Brainard DM, *et al.* Effect of rifampin, a potent inducer of drug-metabolizing enzymes, on the pharmacokinetics of raltegravir. *Antimicrob Agents Chemother* 2009; 53: 2852–2856.
16. Regazzi M, Carvalho AC, Villani P, *et al.* Treatment optimization in patients co-infected with HIV and *Mycobacterium tuberculosis* infections: focus on drug-drug interactions with rifamycins. *Clin Pharmacokinet* 2014; 53: 489–507.
17. Atwine D, Bonnet M, Taburet AM. Pharmacokinetics of efavirenz in patients on antituberculosis treatment in high human immunodeficiency virus and tuberculosis burden countries: a systematic review. *Br J Clin Pharmacol* 2018; 84: 1641–1658.
18. Manosuthi W, Kiertiburanakul S, Sungkanuparph S, *et al.* Efavirenz 600 mg/day *versus* efavirenz 800 mg/day in HIV-infected patients with tuberculosis receiving rifampicin: 48 weeks results. *AIDS* 2006; 20: 131–132.
19. Friedland G, Khoo S, Jack C, *et al.* Administration of efavirenz (600 mg/day) with rifampicin results in highly variable levels but excellent clinical outcomes in patients treated for tuberculosis and HIV. *J Antimicrob Chemother* 2006; 58: 1299–1302.
20. Tiberi S, Carvalho AC, Sulis G, *et al.* The cursed duet today: tuberculosis and HIV-coinfection. *Presse Med* 2017; 46: e23–e39.
21. Lai RP, Nakiwala JK, Meintjes G, *et al.* The immunopathogenesis of the HIV tuberculosis immune reconstitution inflammatory syndrome. *Eur J Immunol* 2013; 43: 1995–2002.
22. Meintjes G, Lawn SD, Scano F, *et al.* Tuberculosis-associated immune reconstitution inflammatory syndrome: case definitions for use in resource-limited settings. *Lancet Infect Dis* 2008; 8: 516–523.

23. Gandhi NR, Moll A, Sturm AW, et al. Extensively drug-resistant tuberculosis as a cause of death in patients co-infected with tuberculosis and HIV in a rural area of South Africa. Lancet 2006; 368: 1575–1580.

24. Gandhi NR, Shah NS, Andrews JR, et al. HIV coinfection in multidrug- and extensively drug-resistant tuberculosis results in high early mortality. Am J Respir Crit Care Med 2010; 181: 80–86.

25. Bastard M, Sanchez-Padilla E, du Cros P, et al. Outcomes of HIV-infected versus HIV-non-infected patients treated for drug-resistance tuberculosis: multicenter cohort study. PLoS One 2018; 13: e0193491.

26. Lange C, Abubakar I, Alffenaar JW, et al. Management of patients with multidrug-resistant/extensively drug-resistant tuberculosis in Europe: a TBNET consensus statement. Eur Respir J 2014; 44: 23–63.

27. Brust JCM, Shah NS, Mlisana K, et al. Improved survival and cure rates with concurrent treatment for multidrug-resistant tuberculosis-human immunodeficiency virus coinfection in South Africa. Clin Infect Dis 2018; 66: 1246–1253.

28. World Health Organization. WHO Treatment Guidelines for Drug-Resistant Tuberculosis, 2016 update. Geneva, WHO, 2016.

29. Dheda K, Gumbo T, Maartens G, et al. The epidemiology, pathogenesis, transmission, diagnosis, and management of multidrug-resistant, extensively drug-resistant, and incurable tuberculosis. Lancet Respir Med 2017; in press https://doi.org/10.1016/S2213-2600(17)30079-6.

30. Ndjeka N, Conradie F, Schnippel K, et al. Treatment of drug-resistant tuberculosis with bedaquiline in a high HIV prevalence setting: an interim cohort analysis. Int J Tuberc Lung Dis 2015; 19: 979–985.

31. Svensson EM, Dooley KE, Karlsson MO. Impact of lopinavir-ritonavir or nevirapine on bedaquiline exposures and potential implications for patients with tuberculosis-HIV coinfection. Antimicrob Agents Chemother 2014; 58: 6406–6412.

32. Svensson EM, Aweeka F, Park JG, et al. Model-based estimates of the effects of efavirenz on bedaquiline pharmacokinetics and suggested dose adjustments for patients coinfected with HIV and tuberculosis. Antimicrob Agents Chemother 2013; 57: 2780–2787.

33. Mallikaarjun S, Wells C, Petersen C, et al. Delamanid coadministered with antiretroviral drugs or antituberculosis drugs shows no clinically relevant drug-drug interactions in healthy subjects. Antimicrob Agents Chemother 2016; 60: 5976–5985.

34. Jeon CY, Harries AD, Baker MA, et al. Bi-directional screening for tuberculosis and diabetes: a systematic review. Trop Med Int Health 2010; 15: 1300–1314.

35. Leung CC, Lam TH, Chan WM, et al. Diabetic control and risk of tuberculosis: a cohort study. Am J Epidemiol 2008; 167: 1486–1494.

36. Creswell J, Raviglione M, Ottmani S, et al. Tuberculosis and noncommunicable diseases: neglected links and missed opportunities. Eur Respir J 2011; 37: 1269–1282.

37. GBD Tuberculosis Collaborators. The global burden of tuberculosis: results from the Global Burden of Disease Study 2015. Lancet Infect Dis 2018; 18: 261–284.

38. Kumar Nathella P, Babu S. Influence of diabetes mellitus on immunity to human tuberculosis. Immunology 2017; 152: 13–24.

39. Kumar NP, Sridhar R, Banurekha VV, et al. Type 2 diabetes mellitus coincident with pulmonary tuberculosis is associated with heightened systemic type 1, type 17, and other proinflammatory cytokines. Ann Am Thorac Soc 2013; 10: 441–449.

40. Kumar NP, Sridhar R, Banurekha VV, et al. Expansion of pathogen-specific T-helper 1 and T-helper 17 cells in pulmonary tuberculosis with coincident type 2 diabetes mellitus. J Infect Dis 2013; 208: 739–748.

41. Martinez N, Kornfeld H. Diabetes and immunity to tuberculosis. Eur J Immunol 2014; 44: 617–626.

42. Gil-Santana L, Almeida-Junior JL, Oliveira CA, et al. Diabetes is associated with worse clinical presentation in tuberculosis patients from Brazil: a retrospective cohort study. PLoS One 2016; 11: e0146876.

43. Al-Tawfiq JA, Saadeh BM. Radiographic manifestations of culture-positive pulmonary tuberculosis: cavitary or non-cavitary? Int J Tuberc Lung Dis 2009; 13: 367–370.

44. Perez-Guzman C, Torres-Cruz A, Villarreal-Velarde H, et al. Progressive age-related changes in pulmonary tuberculosis images and the effect of diabetes. Am J Respir Crit Care Med 2000; 162: 1738–1740.

45. Dooley KE, Chaisson RE. Tuberculosis and diabetes mellitus: convergence of two epidemics. Lancet Infect Dis 2009; 9: 737–746.

46. Perez-Guzman C, Torres-Cruz A, Villarreal-Velarde H, et al. Atypical radiological images of pulmonary tuberculosis in 192 diabetic patients: a comparative study. Int J Tuberc Lung Dis 2001; 5: 455–461.

47. Jimenez-Corona ME, Cruz-Hervert LP, Garcia-Garcia L, et al. Association of diabetes and tuberculosis: impact on treatment and post-treatment outcomes. Thorax 2013; 68: 214–220.

48. Huangfu P, Pearson F, Ugarte-Gil C, et al. Diabetes and poor tuberculosis treatment outcomes: issues and implications in data interpretation and analysis. Int J Tuberc Lung Dis 2017; 21: 1214–1219.

49. Nahid P, Dorman SE, Alipanah N, et al. Official American Thoracic Society/Centers for Disease Control and Prevention/Infectious Diseases Society of America Clinical Practice Guidelines: Treatment of Drug-Susceptible Tuberculosis. Clin Infect Dis 2016; 63: e147–e195.

https://doi.org/10.1183/2312508X.10022017

50. Tuberculosis Coalition for Technical Assistance. International standard for tuberculosis care. The Hauge, Tuberculosis Coalition for Technical Assistance, 2006.

51. World Health Organization. Collaborative framework for care and control of tuberculosis and diabetes. Geneva, WHO, 2011.

52. Baker MA, Harries AD, Jeon CY, et al. The impact of diabetes on tuberculosis treatment outcomes: a systematic review. BMC Med 2011; 9: 81.

53. Jorgensen ME, Faurholt-Jepsen D. Is there an effect of glucose lowering treatment on incidence and prognosis of tuberculosis? A systematic review. Curr Diab Rep 2014; 14: 505.

54. Shewade HD, Jeyashree K, Mahajan P, et al. Effect of glycemic control and type of diabetes treatment on unsuccessful TB treatment outcomes among people with TB-diabetes: a systematic review. PLoS One 2017; 12: e0186697.

55. van der Burgt EP, Sturkenboom MG, Bolhuis MS, et al. End TB with precision treatment! Eur Respir J 2016; 47: 680–682.

56. Srivastava S, Pasipanodya JG, Meek C, et al. Multidrug-resistant tuberculosis not due to noncompliance but to between-patient pharmacokinetic variability. J Infect Dis 2011; 204: 1951–1959.

57. Wang JY, Lee MC, Shu CC, et al. Optimal duration of anti-TB treatment in patients with diabetes: nine or six months? Chest 2015; 147: 520–528.

58. Reed GW, Choi H, Lee SY, et al. Impact of diabetes and smoking on mortality in tuberculosis. PLoS One 2013; 8: e58044.

59. Riza AL, Pearson F, Ugarte-Gil C, et al. Clinical management of concurrent diabetes and tuberculosis and the implications for patient services. Lancet Diabetes Endocrinol 2014; 2: 740–753.

60. Tornio A, Niemi M, Neuvonen PJ, et al. Drug interactions with oral antidiabetic agents: pharmacokinetic mechanisms and clinical implications. Trends Pharmacol Sci 2012; 33: 312–322.

61. Sun H, Scott DO. Impact of genetic polymorphisms of cytochrome P450 2 C (CYP2C) enzymes on the drug metabolism and design of antidiabetics. Chem Biol Interact 2011; 194: 159–167.

62. Niazi AK, Kalra S. Diabetes and tuberculosis: a review of the role of optimal glycemic control. J Diabetes Metab Disord 2012; 11: 28.

63. World Health Organization. Latent tuberculosis infection: updated and consolidated guidelines for programmatic management. Geneva, WHO, 2018.

64. Lemesch S, Ribitsch W, Schilcher G, et al. Mode of renal replacement therapy determines endotoxemia and neutrophil dysfunction in chronic kidney disease. Sci Rep 2016; 6: 34534.

65. Milburn H, Ashman N, Davies P, et al. Guidelines for the prevention and management of Mycobacterium tuberculosis infection and disease in adult patients with chronic kidney disease. Thorax 2010; 65: 557–570.

66. Siskind MS, Thienemann D, Kirlin L. Isoniazid-induced neurotoxicity in chronic dialysis patients: report of three cases and a review of the literature. Nephron 1993; 64: 303–306.

67. Constantinescu SM, Buysschaert B, Haufroid V, et al. Chronic dialysis, NAT2 polymorphisms, and the risk of isoniazid-induced encephalopathy – case report and literature review. BMC Nephrol 2017; 18: 282.

68. Li PK, Szeto CC, Piraino B, et al. Peritoneal dialysis-related infections recommendations: 2010 update. Perit Dial Int 2010; 30: 393–423.

69. Ahn C, Oh KH, Kim K, et al. Effect of peritoneal dialysis on plasma and peritoneal fluid concentrations of isoniazid, pyrazinamide, and rifampin. Perit Dial Int 2003; 23: 362–367.

70. Bonnel AR, Bunchorntavakul C, Reddy KR. Immune dysfunction and infections in patients with cirrhosis. Clin Gastroenterol Hepatol 2011; 9: 727–738.

71. Kumar N, Kedarisetty CK, Kumar S, et al. Antitubercular therapy in patients with cirrhosis: challenges and options. World J Gastroenterol 2014; 20: 5760–5772.

72. Singanayagam A, Sridhar S, Dhariwal J, et al. A comparison between two strategies for monitoring hepatic function during antituberculous therapy. Am J Respir Crit Care Med 2012; 185: 653–659.

73. Saukkonen JJ, Powell K, Jereb JA. Monitoring for tuberculosis drug hepatotoxicity: moving from opinion to evidence. Am J Respir Crit Care Med 2012; 185: 598–599.

74. Chang TE, Huang YS, Chang CH, et al. The susceptibility of anti-tuberculosis drug-induced liver injury and chronic hepatitis C infection: a systematic review and meta-analysis. J Chin Med Assoc 2018; 81: 111–118.

75. Shin HJ, Lee HS, Kim YI, et al. Hepatotoxicity of anti-tuberculosis chemotherapy in patients with liver cirrhosis. Int J Tuberc Lung Dis 2014; 18: 347–351.

76. Saukkonen JJ, Cohn DL, Jasmer RM, et al. An official ATS statement: hepatotoxicity of antituberculosis therapy. Am J Respir Crit Care Med 2006; 174: 935–952.

77. Dhiman RK, Saraswat VA, Rajekar H, et al. A guide to the management of tuberculosis in patients with chronic liver disease. J Clin Exp Hepatol 2012; 2: 260–270.

78. World Health Organization. Treatment of tuberculosis guidelines. Fourth edition. Geneva, WHO, 2010.

79. Singh N, Paterson DL. Mycobacterium tuberculosis infection in solid-organ transplant recipients: impact and implications for management. Clin Infect Dis 1998; 27: 1266–1277.

80. Subramanian A, Dorman S, Practice ASTIDCo. *Mycobacterium tuberculosis* in solid organ transplant recipients. *Am J Transplant* 2009; 9: Suppl. 4, S57–S62.

81. Bumbacea D, Arend SM, Eyuboglu F, *et al.* The risk of tuberculosis in transplant candidates and recipients: a TBNET consensus statement. *Eur Respir J* 2012; 40: 990–1013.

82. Getahun H, Matteelli A, Abubakar I, *et al.* Management of latent *Mycobacterium tuberculosis* infection: WHO guidelines for low tuberculosis burden countries. *Eur Respir J* 2015; 46: 1563–1576.

83. Rendon A, Goletti D, Matteelli A. Diagnosis and treatment of latent tuberculosis infection. *In:* Migliori GB, Bothamley G, Duarte R, *et al.*, eds. Tuberculosis (ERS Monograph). Sheffield, European Respiratory Society, 2018; pp. 381–398.

84. Jereb JA, Burwen DR, Dooley SW, *et al.* Nosocomial outbreak of tuberculosis in a renal transplant unit: application of a new technique for restriction fragment length polymorphism analysis of *Mycobacterium tuberculosis* isolates. *J Infect Dis* 1993; 168: 1219–1224.

85. Abad CLR, Razonable RR. *Mycobacterium tuberculosis* after solid organ transplantation: a review of more than 2000 cases. *Clin Transplant* 2018; 32: e13259.

86. Morris MI, Daly JS, Blumberg E, *et al.* Diagnosis and management of tuberculosis in transplant donors: a donor-derived infections consensus conference report. *Am J Transplant* 2012; 12: 2288–2300.

87. Sun HY, Munoz P, Torre-Cisneros J, *et al. Mycobacterium tuberculosis*-associated immune reconstitution syndrome in solid-organ transplant recipients. *Transplantation* 2013; 95: 1173–1181.

88. Trofe-Clark J, Lemonovich TL, AST Infectious Diseases Community of Practice. Interactions between anti-infective agents and immunosuppressants in solid organ transplantation. *Am J Transplant* 2013; 13: Suppl. 4, 318–326.

89. Canet E, Dantal J, Blancho G, *et al.* Tuberculosis following kidney transplantation: clinical features and outcome. A French multicentre experience in the last 20 years. *Nephrol Dial Transplant* 2011; 26: 3773–3778.

90. Aguado JM, Herrero JA, Gavalda J, *et al.* Clinical presentation and outcome of tuberculosis in kidney, liver, and heart transplant recipients in Spain. Spanish Transplantation Infection Study Group, GESITRA. *Transplantation* 1997; 63: 1278–1286.

Disclosures: E. Girardi reports receiving the following, outside the submitted work: personal fees from Otsuka, Gilead, Mylan and Jannsen; grants from Mylan.

 https://doi.org/10.1183/2312508X.10022017

Chapter 17

Access and adherence to prevention and care for hard-to-reach groups

Kerri Viney[1,2], Tom Wingfield ![ORCID][1,3,4,5], Liga Kuksa[6,7] and Knut Lönnroth[1]

In this chapter, we discuss two key concepts of TB prevention and care: access and adherence. We discuss these in the context of "hard-to-reach" groups, defined as groups of people who are under-represented or underserved. By definition, these groups may experience particular difficulties in accessing TB care (including preventative, diagnostic and care services) and remaining in care once it has been accessed. As TB often affects hard-to-reach groups, healthcare services should be designed with such groups in mind, aiming for equitable and affordable access to people-centred TB care. We also describe barriers to healthcare access and adherence, and provide some solutions to overcoming these barriers, based on current evidence. Ensuring that access and adherence are addressed, with the most disadvantaged groups in mind, is a necessary step towards achieving the ambitious goals of the WHO End TB Strategy and SDGs, which aim to eliminate TB by 2030.

Cite as: Viney K, Wingfield T, Kuksa L, *et al*. Access and adherence to prevention and care for hard-to-reach groups. *In:* Migliori GB, Bothamley G, Duarte R, *et al*., eds. Tuberculosis (ERS Monograph). Sheffield, European Respiratory Society, 2018; pp. 291–307 [https://doi.org/10.1183/2312508X.10022117].

@ERSpublications
People in hard-to-reach groups experience difficulties in accessing and adhering to TB care, but these difficulties can be overcome with people-centred healthcare. http://ow. ly/cfVQ30lqCfE

In this chapter, we provide definitions of access, adherence and hard to reach, and outline proven strategies to promote access to care and adherence to treatment. Ensuring good health outcomes and limiting TB transmission within hard-to-reach groups can prove challenging, as, by definition, they may experience difficulties in accessing care, and if they do access it, they may experience difficulties remaining in it. As TB has the potential to be

[1]Dept of Public Health Sciences, Karolinska Institutet, Centre of Global Health, Widerströmska Huset, Stockholm, Sweden. [2]Research School of Population Health, National Centre of Epidemiology and Population Health, Dept of Global Health, Australian National University, Canberra, Australia. [3]Dept of Clinical Infection, Microbiology and Immunology, Institute of Infection and Global Health, University of Liverpool, Liverpool, UK. [4]Tropical and Infectious Diseases Unit, Royal Liverpool University and Broadgreen Hospitals NHS Trust, Liverpool, UK. [5]LIV-TB Collaboration, Depts of Clinical Science and Health Systems Group, Liverpool School of Tropical Medicine, Liverpool, UK. [6]MDR TB Dept, Riga East University Hospital, Tuberculosis and Lung Disease Clinic, Riga, Latvia. [7]Riga Stradins University, Infectology and Dermatology Board, Riga, Latvia.

Correspondence: Kerri Viney, Dept of Public Health Sciences, Karolinska Institutet, Centre of Global Health, Widerströmska Huset, Tomtebodavägen 18 A, 171 77 Stockholm, Sweden. E-mail: kerri.viney@ki.se

a debilitating or lethal condition, with long-term clinical, social and economic sequelae, there are significant benefits to individuals if they are diagnosed soon after the onset of signs and symptoms, and if they can access and remain in care that is high quality and low cost. The WHO End TB Strategy highlights the need for patient-centred care and the necessity to devise policies that guarantee access and adherence to prevention and care, especially for hard-to-reach groups [1]. It also emphasises the vital role of research in defining how access and adherence barriers can be overcome [1].

Definitions of access and adherence to healthcare

Healthcare access

Healthcare access has been described as "the timely use of personal health services to achieve the best health outcomes" [2]. Such access is commonly understood to have three key dimensions: physical accessibility, financial affordability and acceptability (expanded in table 1), all of which have been described as being underpinned by equity [3]. In contrast, universal health coverage (UHC), which is explained later in this chapter, is achieved as people obtain the healthcare they need without financial hardship [4]. Both access and UHC are of particular relevance to TB prevention, treatment and care, as TB diagnosis usually involves accessing a healthcare facility multiple times, and the duration of current TB treatment is between 6 and 24 months. Moreover, people with TB may have complicating factors, including side-effects, physical disability, comorbidities (such as HIV or DM), stigma, social problems and mental illness [5]. These can result in the need to repeatedly access other health and/or social services where available.

Adherence to treatment

Adherence to treatment has been defined as "the extent to which the patient's history of therapeutic drug-taking coincides with the prescribed treatment" [6, 7]. In relation to TB, this corresponds to a patient remaining in care throughout the intended treatment duration and taking all prescribed medicines regularly and without missed doses. Adherence can be measured using outcome-oriented definitions (e.g. treatment success rate) or, less

Table 1. The three dimensions of healthcare access

Physical accessibility	The availability of good health services within reasonable reach of those who need them, with opening hours, appointment systems and other aspects of service organisation and delivery that allow people to obtain the services when they need them.
Financial affordability	A measure of people's ability to pay for services without financial hardship. It takes into account not only the cost of the health services but also indirect and opportunity costs (e.g. the costs of transportation to and from facilities and of taking time off work). Affordability is influenced by the wider health financing system and by household income.
Acceptability	People's willingness to seek services. Acceptability is low when patients perceive services to be ineffective or when social and cultural factors such as language or the age, sex, ethnicity or religion of the health provider discourage them from seeking services.

Reproduced and modified from [3] with permission.

https://doi.org/10.1183/2312508X.10022117

commonly, process-oriented definitions (*e.g.* intermediate indicators, such as appointment keeping or pill counts) [6]. While it is important to know how much treatment a patient has had to determine the likelihood of cure, the labels of "adherent" and "nonadherent" may not be helpful when discussing individual patients. For example, labelling a patient as nonadherent may give the impression that TB treatment interruptions are the patient's fault, whereas the barriers may actually relate to the healthcare service itself (*i.e.* "delivery side") or other factors outside the patient's control. Defining and minimising these barriers is a component of people-centred TB care.

Hard-to-reach groups for prevention and care

Definition of hard-to-reach

In order to elaborate further on access and adherence to TB prevention and care for hard-to-reach groups, it is essential to first define what is meant by the term "hard to reach", including in the context of TB. There are many synonyms in the literature that have been used interchangeably with hard to reach, such as hidden populations, vulnerable, fragile, socially excluded, disengaged, marginalised, refusers, disadvantaged, non- or reluctant users, high risk or at risk, multiple/complex needs, minority groups and less likely to access [8–10].

Definitions of what constitutes a hard-to-reach group have been variable, lacking in consensus and inconsistently applied. Indeed, the term hard to reach has been criticised for potentially stigmatising certain people and implying that the issue or problem lies within the group itself rather than in society or society's approach towards that group [11]. For example, a family in which there is incomplete uptake of routine immunisations or poor school attendance may be labelled as hard to reach when it is actually the immunisation service or education system being offered that is hard for the family to either accept or engage with [12]. Furthermore, a unifying definition of hard-to-reach groups is difficult to realise, given the vast heterogeneity both across different settings and within hard-to-reach groups (*e.g.* not all people who belong to a hard-to-reach group are hard to reach, and some who are classified as belonging to a certain high-risk group may not associate with others within that group) [9, 13].

Nevertheless, for the purposes of this chapter, hard to reach will be the term used throughout because it is the most widely used and understood term in the scientific (*e.g.* studies and trials) and grey (*e.g.* policy statements and reports) literature [14]. Broadly, a hard-to-reach group is a group within society that is under-represented and underserved [15]. Such groups include but are not limited to: ethnic or language minority groups, sexual minority communities, migrants and asylum seekers, community sex workers, disabled people, young people, the elderly, certain sexes or gender identities (*e.g.* being female or transgender), the homeless, those incarcerated or previously incarcerated, people with low education and/or low literacy levels, people with alcohol and/or drug addiction, people with low socioeconomic status, and those who for other reasons lack agency or capacity to engage [9, 16]. With respect to TB, a hard-to-reach group refers to a group of people who are underserved by existing TB services, resulting in limited, inequitable access and adherence to TB prevention and care. It is worth noting that many of the social determinants and risk factors that identify people as belonging to a hard-to-reach group overlap across such groups (*e.g.* perceived or actual stigma, low socioeconomic status and/or education levels). Those explored here are intended to provide the reader with an overview from which to stimulate further reading.

Hard-to-reach groups

Migrants

Migrants include asylum seekers, refugees, and those from language and ethnic minorities. The Oxford English Dictionary (www.oed.com/) defines a migrant as "a person who moves from one place to another, especially in order to find work or better living conditions". Clearly, there is wide heterogeneity in the backgrounds of migrants (*e.g.* country of origin, cultural practices, TB burden), their socioeconomic status and their reasons for migration (*e.g.* seeking asylum, employment, other reasons). This heterogeneity makes it difficult to accurately describe the plethora of barriers to accessing and engaging with TB prevention and care that migrants may face, without making generalisations [13]. Nevertheless, taking into account this limitation, the barriers faced can be broadly divided into individual, community and system (*e.g.* health or social care systems) barriers.

At an individual level, migrants may initially have limited ability to speak, write or understand the language of the country to which they have moved [17]. Moreover, those seeking asylum due to war, violence or persecution in their country of origin may have concomitant psychological and social trauma [14]. Social upheaval may also be persistent in the country to which they have relocated, due to, for example, regular changes to the location of housing while seeking leave to remain.

At a community level, there may be fear, stigma, misperceptions and lack of knowledge related to TB. For example, research with Somali migrants has shown a persistent misperception that TB can be inherited, which can lead to feelings of shame and guilt for families [18]. Moreover, lack of engagement with TB clinical care and prevention teams can sometimes reflect a broader fear of engagement with public services as a whole, due to concerns about perceived or actual risk of deportation [19]. It must be noted that lack of engagement with healthcare services may also occur in ethnic minority groups who are not migrants, due to disenfranchisement, cultural practices or other reasons [20]. Examples include poor coverage of HIV testing in people of Afro-Caribbean origin born in England [21] or delayed presentation to healthcare services among Roma people with symptoms of TB [22].

At a systems level, TB-related services, such as clinics and social or housing support, may not meet the needs of migrant populations. Common barriers perceived by migrants include: opening hours and location of services that make it difficult to attend (especially in relation to work or care of dependents); a lack of continuity of health personnel creating difficulty in developing a rapport and trust, which can be made worse by a lack of cultural understanding from health staff; and lack of translators or education materials to support education and knowledge about TB [8, 13, 23, 24].

Prisoners and inmates

There are a number of overlapping issues relating to TB prevention and care in prisoners and inmates. Diagnostic, treatment and prevention services may be limited in prisons, and there may be discontinuity in prescriptions of TB medication (*e.g.* TB treatment or chemoprophylaxis), either from community to prison or vice versa [17]. Lack of

https://doi.org/10.1183/2312508X.10022117

communication and a level of mistrust between prison populations and services such as healthcare and law enforcement may also negatively influence prisoners' or ex-prisoners' health-seeking behaviour and healthcare access, especially when receiving care is contingent on the presentation of valid identification and/or home address documents [25, 26].

Prison populations have been found to have high rates of drug misuse (including injecting drug use and opioid addiction) and coinfection (*e.g.* TB and HIV or hepatitis C), which can influence the efficacy and outcomes of TB treatment and prevention regimens, including through co-medications and adverse events [14, 27]. More specifically, in those with immune compromise secondary to HIV, clinical features of TB coinfection may be atypical or misdiagnosed as other HIV-related opportunistic infections, and microbiological confirmation of TB may be less likely [28]. Prisoners are often not able to access timely healthcare and diagnoses due to legal issues, but more often due to poor infrastructure and lack of funding.

The homeless

Rates of incident TB in homeless populations are much higher than general rates among nonhomeless adults in the same settings [29]. The reasons behind this are complex, relating to overlapping social determinants of both TB disease and adverse TB treatment outcomes, such as a high prevalence of HIV, poor nutrition, assortative mixing [30–33], poor living conditions [31], mental illness, and high rates of alcohol and drug addiction [34, 35].

In addition to the above, homeless people may have difficulties accessing healthcare services due to a lack of knowledge of the services available, restricted opening hours, competing health priorities (*e.g.* patients who receive daily opioid substitutes may consider these a priority over a TB clinic appointment), no available transport or funding for transport to and from healthcare facilities, and perceived or actual stigma from healthcare professionals [17, 36].

Other hard-to-reach groups

While it is beyond the scope of this chapter to provide an in-depth exploration of all hard-to-reach groups, it is worthwhile briefly mentioning some of these groups and the barriers to accessing TB care and prevention they face, many of which overlap.

Sex workers

Male and female sex workers in diverse settings have been found to have high HIV prevalence, which increases the likelihood of developing TB [37–39]. In addition, similar to homeless and prisoner groups, high rates of drug addiction and mental health issues have been reported in this group, all of which can contribute to chaotic lifestyles, poor nutrition and difficulties accessing healthcare [40, 41]. Sex workers may have poor access to TB care for a range of reasons including the perception that they may be reported to the criminal justice system if they access healthcare.

Sexual minorities and transgender people

Certain sexual minorities, including men who have sex with men, are at higher risk of HIV than the general population [28]. Transgender people, particularly transgender women, are also at higher risk of HIV [42, 43]. Both sexual minority groups and transgender people also face perceived and actual stigma, which can reduce their engagement with multiple systems including employment and healthcare services [44, 45].

The elderly

There are a multitude of reasons that can account for barriers to accessing TB care and prevention among the elderly. They may be less well informed regarding available healthcare services (especially in those who are not computer literate or who do not have access to online services), are more likely to have comorbidities and other health and social needs, and may be isolated and lacking social capital [46, 47]. Moreover, in studies comparing older and younger TB patients, older patients have been shown to have a higher likelihood of diagnostic delay and diagnostic uncertainty (*e.g.* misdiagnosed as carcinoma or persistent pneumonia), adverse reactions to TB treatment or preventative therapy, and loss to follow-up or death on treatment [46, 47].

Rural or limited geographical access

Geographical location of available services may be a limiting factor for access and adherence, such as people who live in rural communities, in communities with no road access or in mountainous areas [48, 49]. This situation is compounded when services are not decentralised and do not offer home visits, outreach services or alternatives to healthcare worker-led DOTS [48, 49]. People with TB symptoms and their households who face geographical barriers to accessing TB care may also choose to attend local traditional healers or allied healthcare services prior to seeking care from more distant (and costly) formal healthcare providers [50].

Low socioeconomic position/poverty

While the association between poverty and TB infection and disease is clear, much research is still required to disentangle the upstream and downstream determinants along the causal pathway. Poverty is, by its very nature, multidimensional, incorporating factors such as financial position, social capital, educational and literacy level, overall health and wellbeing, and living standards [51]. Many of these factors are strongly collinear and intertwined (*e.g.* low income is associated with a low education level, which is associated with increased likelihood of alcohol or drug addiction and malnutrition), making it impossible to evaluate them in isolation [52]. Healthcare providers and policy makers should consider these co-relationships of poverty in their assessment of whether a TB patient or exposed household member belongs to a hard-to-reach group.

Barriers to accessing health and care, and remaining in care

In addition to the barriers listed above, there are many "delivery-side" reasons why patients in hard-to-reach groups may not access TB diagnostic and care services, or complete TB treatment. These include an inadequate drug supply, a large daily drug intake, the costs of TB care, distance to a health facility and rigid health facility practices such as facility-based DOT (directly observed therapy). A lack of integrated care may lead patients to abandon treatment. Side-effects and mismanagement of these are other reasons for nonadherence. Table 2 outlines some of the key barriers to accessing healthcare, at the individual or household, community and health system levels.

Initiatives and interventions to improve access to healthcare

A number of initiatives and interventions can improve access to TB care for hard-to-reach groups. These range from national policies, such as UHC, to tailored health system interventions, such as incentives and enablers. Some of these interventions will lie outside

https://doi.org/10.1183/2312508X.10022117

Table 2. Barriers to accessing healthcare services at the individual/household, community and health system levels

Individual/household	Community	Health system
Low socioeconomic position/ poverty	Stigma (perceived and actual)	Lack of cultural sensitivity
Mental illness	Misperceptions and myths (e.g. TB is hereditary)	Language (including jargon) used to educate and inform
Rural/isolated	Lack of social capital and cohesion	Language (including jargon) and literacy level of written or other educational and informative materials
Intra-family social difficulties (including domestic violence and unstable relationships)	Distrust of services and systems offered	
Low educational or literacy level	Disempowered and disenfranchised	Lack of knowledge or understanding about social or clinical condition by service or practitioners
Language difficulties	Lack of knowledge and understanding relating to certain health conditions	Lack of linkage of social and healthcare
Disabilities or comorbidities	Lack of interaction or dialogue between service providers and community	Stigmatising or disempowering behaviour
Mental illness	Lack of ownership of services offered	Timing, location, waiting times, setting, resources, infrastructure, staff turnover and quality of services provided
Voluntary isolation from services and systems (including prisoners or high-crime environment, refugees and asylum seekers, sex workers and travellers)	Health beliefs and cultural practices	
	Alternative informal health services prioritised within the community (including faith or traditional healers)	Lack of engagement with communities (including outreach and community participation/stakeholders)
Alcohol or drug misuse and addiction	Lack of agency or advocacy within the community to represent those requiring health services	Lack of visibility in community
Previous substandard experience of service use		Lack of political or systemic will to meet the needs of hard-to-reach groups
		Budget constraints

Information from [8] and [53].

the health sector, such as broader socioeconomic and poverty reduction policies that aim to prevent poverty and socioeconomic disparities, those that provide access to social benefits in times of sickness and unemployment, and housing initiatives.

Universal health coverage

UHC aims to provide high-quality healthcare services to those who need them at an affordable cost. It is a key target of SDG-3 (which also includes a target about TB). Target 3.8 of SDG-3 is to achieve UHC "including financial risk protection, access to quality essential healthcare services and access to safe, effective, quality and affordable essential medicines and vaccines for all" [4]. The UHC mantra of "leave no one behind" suggests that data on UHC should be disaggregated by age, sex, income level, ethnicity, migration status and disability status, allowing a full description of access to healthcare by hard-to-reach groups [4]. The latest WHO report on UHC describes how coverage of essential health services has increased by 20% since 2000; however, approximately half of the world's 7.3 billion people still do not have access to full coverage with essential health services [4]. This is particularly important for low-income countries, with sub-Saharan Africa having the lowest regional UHC service index globally (with an index of 42 out of 100) [4]. It is also important for hard-to-reach groups for TB (including in high-income countries where UHC may still be incomplete), such as migrants and the homeless, who may not have full healthcare access due to legal or other bureaucratic issues [54, 55].

TB care is an important component of UHC. TB effective treatment coverage is one of 16 tracer indicators used to measure the UHC index, and combines two indicators commonly used in global TB reporting, the case detection rate and the treatment success rate, to estimate the proportion of TB cases that are detected and successfully treated [4]. This is important because the financial burden of TB care is relatively greater in low-income countries with poorer access to UHC [56]. Of the few published studies on UHC and TB, the focus has been on service gaps and barriers to care, and suggested potential improvements to move healthcare services towards achieving UHC [57–59].

Social protection

While UHC is necessary, it may not be sufficient to protect TB patients from the high social, emotional and financial costs of TB care. For example, a study in Burkina Faso highlighted that, even when health system user fees are removed, TB care is not free and that three-quarters of TB patients faced catastrophic health expenditure, with health system and health policy inadequacies responsible for almost half of these costs [59]. In addition, while financial mechanisms to compensate TB patients in times of illness may be a key component of UHC, some have large gaps, leaving patients uncovered or still significantly out of pocket [60, 61].

In recognition of the economic burden faced by TB-affected families, the WHO End TB Strategy includes a high-level global indicator on the costs of TB care: that zero TB-affected families should face catastrophic costs associated with TB care. The operational definition of "catastrophic costs as a result of TB" refers to medical and nonmedical out-of-pocket payments and indirect costs exceeding a given threshold (e.g. 20%) of a household's income [1]. The barrier of high costs for accessing and engaging with TB care have been well documented historically and also by recent national TB patient cost surveys [62–64]. Such TB-related direct and indirect costs limit healthcare access, increase the risk of poor TB treatment outcomes, exacerbate poverty and contribute to ongoing TB transmission [65].

Therefore, UHC, while essential, may not be sufficient for effective and equitable access to TB services. Adjunctive social protection interventions that prevent or mitigate other financial risks associated with TB, including income losses and nonmedical expenditures such as on transport and food, are also essential [65]. Social protection is defined as "the set of policies and programmes designed to reduce and prevent poverty and vulnerability throughout the life cycle" and includes "benefits for children and families, maternity, unemployment, employment injury, sickness, old age, disability, survivors, as well as health protection" [66].

UHC focuses on the health system and the provision of accessible, affordable and high-quality care, creating a "pull" for people to access healthcare services. However, other factors may continue to drive people away from TB services, such as the nonmedical costs of care, income loss, stigma, and healthcare worker perceptions and behaviours. Social protection interventions may complement UHC by providing access to broader social welfare and poverty reduction schemes, compensation for nonmedical costs including income loss and access to a wider range of services including psychosocial support, a much-needed component of TB care. These social protection interventions can include a range of initiatives and interventions, such as decentralised TB care, social health insurance, policies that minimise hospitalisation, sickness insurance, and the provision of cash transfers, enablers, incentives, food packages and transport vouchers. A number of these also promote adherence. Figure 1 outlines the three dimensions of UHC with the added dimension of social protection, highlighting the potential additive effect that social protection interventions may have in improving access to TB care. In recognition of this, pillar 1 of the WHO End TB Strategy focuses on integrated patient-centred care and prevention, and explicitly states that "all patients should receive educational, emotional and economic support to enable them to complete the diagnostic process and full course of required treatment" [1]. This is also elaborated in the 2017 update of the WHO TB treatment guidelines for treatment of drug-susceptible TB and patient care, in which a number of patient care and support interventions are recommended [67].

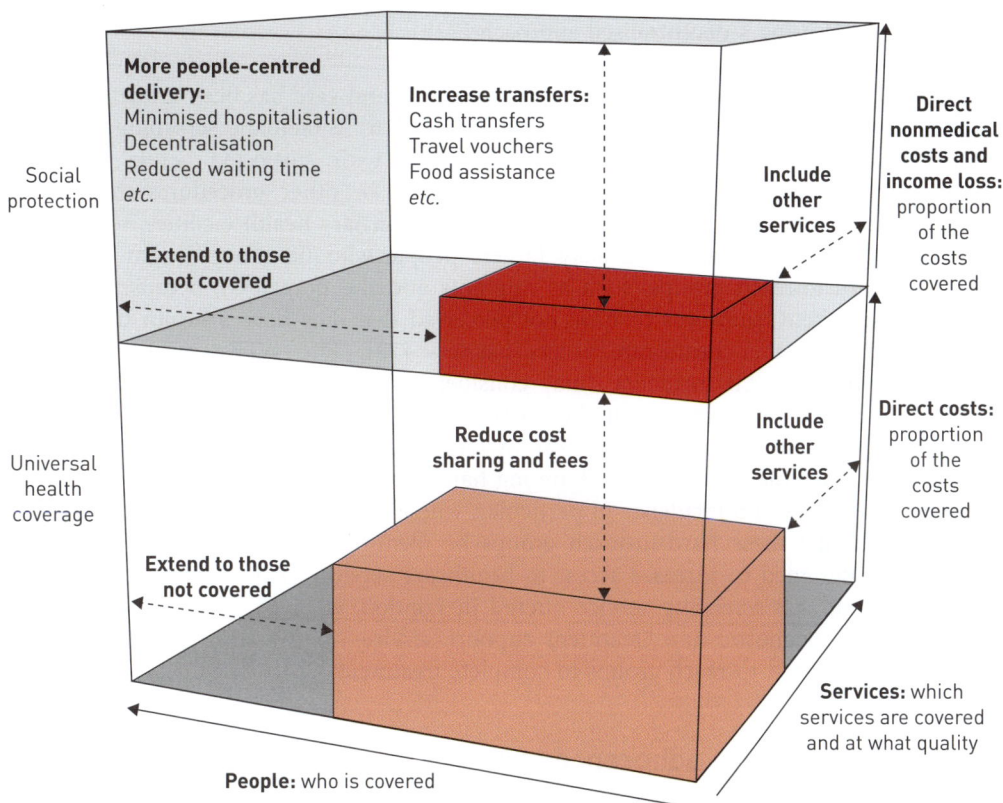

Figure 1. The three dimensions of universal health coverage, with the added dimension of financial risk protection against nonmedical costs. Elements in red are nonmedical costs and additional interventions within healthcare and beyond to provide financial protection. Reproduced and modified from [65] with permission.

Decentralisation and screening

Two tangible ways that access to TB care can be improved are decentralised healthcare and systematic screening for TB. Both interventions aim to bring TB services closer to people with presumptive TB, so that some of the traditional access barriers, such as distance, transport and cost, are overcome. A decentralised healthcare system with diagnosis available at lower levels of the healthcare system has been found to be associated with improved access, lower costs and better treatment outcomes [68]. For example, in China, WEI et al. [68] compared access to TB care in areas of China that had decentralised TB care in township hospitals with other areas where persons with presumptive TB were referred to county TB dispensaries. They found that in the decentralised group, patients spent less money on travel and treatment, had improved TB treatment outcomes, and reported a higher quality of care, and there were increased TB case notification rates. These findings have been reinforced by studies in South Africa where improved rates of treatment initiation, shorter times to culture conversion and a reduced time to treatment initiation were reported [69, 70]. Similarly, in Ethiopia, health extension workers (trained community health workers who provide essential health services to the community) involved in sputum collection and TB treatment improved case detection and TB treatment success rates, possibly attributed to improved service access [71]. Decentralised diagnosis and care may be even more important for patients with MDR-TB who face lengthy treatment. A recent systematic review concluded that treatment success was more likely among patients with MDR-TB treated using a decentralised approach [72].

Accessing hard-to-reach populations with TB diagnosis and care has been a focus of active TB case finding or systematic screening programmes [73]. Systematic screening for TB is defined as "the systematic identification of people with suspected active TB, in a predetermined target group, using tests, examinations or other procedures that can be applied rapidly" [73], and is often provided outside of tertiary health facilities, serving as a proxy for decentralised care. It usually targets people who have not sought healthcare (including hard-to-reach groups, such as migrants and the homeless), because they have not recognised their symptoms or have not perceived that they have a health problem, or have experienced other healthcare access barriers [73]. The WHO recommends that countries with a low TB incidence "may consider systematic screening for active TB in migrants, either before migration, at the point of arrival or after arrival", with subsequent referral to a TB programme, if needed [73]. Systematic screening may be particularly useful when the TB epidemic is concentrated among hard-to-reach groups, such as the homeless. In countries with low TB incidence in particular, where this may be the case, the WHO has recommended that these hard-to-reach groups be identified and described, with specific interventions designed to increase access to healthcare services [74]. Examples include the "Find and Treat" TB screening service offered in London, whereby a specialised outreach team takes TB diagnostic and treatment support services to the streets of London and offers support to hard-to-reach groups to complete treatment [36].

Measures to improve adherence to care

Types of support to promote adherence

Many TB programmes are already providing adherence-enhancing interventions, such as close supervision or DOTS, tailored case management, health education, psycho-emotional

https://doi.org/10.1183/2312508X.10022117

counselling, nutritional support, and financial incentives and enablers [75–77]. A summary of some of these interventions is summarised in table 3. Patient support, DOTS and patient education may be considered the corner stones of adherence support. However, a number of additional interventions are also useful, including psycho-social and economic interventions.

Integrated or combined psycho-emotional and/or socioeconomic interventions

The meta-analysis by VAN HOORN et al. [75] showed that psycho-emotional support, socioeconomic support, and combined psycho-emotional and socioeconomic support improved TB treatment outcomes in a variety of settings (including low-, medium- and high-income countries). They also showed that there was a tendency towards better TB treatment outcomes in the psycho-emotional support or combined support groups compared with socioeconomic support alone [75]. However, there was much heterogeneity in the data, which limited the ability of the authors to make firm conclusions about the impact of these interventions on adherence, nor did the review specifically examine subpopulations or hard-to-reach groups.

A more recent meta-analysis by MÜLLER et al. [78] published in 2018 examined the impact of DOTS, financial incentives, and patient education and counselling on TB treatment

Table 3. Types of psycho-emotional and socioeconomic support for TB-affected households

Type of support	Specific interventions
Psycho-emotional	Cognitive behavioural therapy/psychotherapy Psychologist/psychiatrist referral and evaluation Group therapy Stigma reduction
Social	Information, education Mutual support groups Formation of civil society groups Community mobilisation Community councils Women's groups
Economic/financial	Conditional cash transfers Unconditional cash transfers In-kind support Microcredit Microfinance/microloans Back-to-work schemes Disability and sickness insurance
Food	Food baskets Nutritional supplements Food vouchers Subsidised hot meals/canteen Patient collectives
Other/integrated	Vocational training Pooled health insurance and social protection Community cooperatives Social protection Rights-based approaches mHealth interventions (e.g. video-observed therapy) plus incentives

outcomes and loss to follow-up rates. It found a significant increase in cure rates with DOTS (18% increase) and patient education and counselling (16% increase) but not with financial incentives [78]. Loss to follow-up rates were significantly decreased by DOTS (49%), financial incentives (26%), and patient education and counselling (13%) [78]. The review did not focus specifically on hard-to-reach groups.

In 32 impoverished shantytown communities in Lima, Peru, the Innovation for Health and Development (IFHAD) implemented the Innovative Socioeconomic Interventions Against TB (ISIAT) project, which evaluated a panel of psychosocial and economic support for TB-affected households [52]. The most acceptable and successful elements of ISIAT were combined into a standardised intervention that consisted of integrated social support (household visits and participatory community meetings) and economic support (conditional cash transfers), evaluated during the Household-Randomised Controlled Evaluation of a Socioeconomic Intervention to Prevent TB (HRESIPT) [20]. HRESIPT showed that patients offered the intervention were more likely to achieve treatment success, and their contacts were more likely to initiate preventative therapy [19]. In addition, their household was less likely to incur catastrophic costs [51]. The intervention has since been simplified with greater involvement of TB civil society and peer support, and is being assessed in the Community Randomised Evaluation of a Socioeconomic Intervention to Prevent TB (CRESIPT) trial.

Other complex interventions have been trialled including a cluster-RCT from Senegal, which showed that patient counselling alongside decentralised treatment, patient choice of DOTS supporter and enhanced healthcare supervision improved TB treatment success and reduced loss to follow-up [74].

Education and counselling

Two systematic reviews have focused on TB treatment and preventative therapy for LTBI. The systematic review by M'IMUNYA et al. [79] of patient education and counselling to promote adherence to TB treatment showed mixed results. Nurse-led counselling about TB prevention by phone and home visits improved LTBI preventative therapy completion in children [80], and counselling improved LTBI preventative therapy completion rates among prisoners (although completion rates were low overall) [81]. However, peer counselling for adolescents showed no effect on TB treatment completion rates [82]. The review concluded that counselling may improve completion of TB treatment and preventative LTBI therapy, but that this was setting dependent and constrained by limited, low-quality evidence [79].

A cluster-RCT in Ethiopia evaluated the impact of psychological counselling (focusing on reducing anxiety and depression) and adherence education on adherence to MDR-TB medication in 698 patients with MDR-TB. The findings showed that patients with MDR-TB who received the intervention were less likely (adjusted OR 0.3, 95% CI 0.2–0.5) to have poor adherence than controls [83]. These results complement findings from a nonrandomised before/after evaluation, from Kazhakstan of psychosocial support for people with MDR-TB, which suggested reduced loss to follow-up rates [84].

Economic interventions

A systematic review by LUTGE et al. [85] showed that, in studies focusing on general rather than hard-to-reach populations, there was no evidence that food [86] or shop vouchers [85] improved long-term TB treatment outcomes (although the study involving shop vouchers was limited by the low fidelity to the intervention). In high-risk groups including homeless people, drug users [87–89] and prisoners [81, 90], one-off incentives increased access to preventative therapy services, with more clinic visits reported. The authors suggested that cash was more effective than noncash incentives, immediate cash was more effective than cash delayed until the end of treatment, and more cash was preferable to less [85]. The review concluded that there was reasonable evidence for improvements in short-term outcomes on LTBI therapy (*e.g.* adherence), but it was difficult to conclude about their impact on long-term TB treatment outcomes (*e.g.* TB treatment success with prolonged cure and no recurrence).

In Brazil, adherence rates have been positively impacted in regions in which patients have had support from a TB multidisciplinary team in a reference unit [91], and Brazil's Bolsa Família social welfare programme has been associated with improved TB treatment outcomes and reduced incidence [92, 93]. More broadly, cross-country ecological comparisons have shown an association between higher spending on social protection (including pooled health and disability insurance and UHC) as a proportion of gross domestic product and lower TB rates. However, such studies do not indicate causality and so must be interpreted cautiously.

The role of mHealth

mHealth is the support of existing, overstretched medical and public health practice through the use of mobile phones, tablets, video observation and device-facilitated direct monitoring (*e.g.* through embedded sensors) or indirect monitoring [94]. mHealth has been recommended by the WHO as a useful tool to improve health outcomes, including, for example, electronic reminders and monitoring, which have been shown to improve adherence for HIV [95–97]. With regard to TB, a cluster-RCT in China showed that audio-reminders from electronic pill boxes improved TB treatment adherence medication, while text messages had no impact [98]. In South India, a nonrandomised study found that voice reminders were the most locally appropriate medication reminders, increasing treatment success, whereas text messages excluded the elderly and illiterate [99]. The exclusion of these hard-to-reach groups was mirrored by a study from Peru, which found that access to mobile phones among patients with TB was insufficient, and was rarest in the poorest patients who were least likely to achieve TB treatment success [100]. Consequently, the authors recommended that mHealth programmes should provide phones or related technology to all participants/recipients to ensure equity.

Conclusion

Access and adherence are two key issues for TB prevention and care. They are particularly important for hard-to-reach groups in which the TB epidemic is often concentrated. TB services should be designed to provide equitable and affordable access for hard-to-reach groups. Despite advances in the development of new diagnostic tests, shorter treatment regimens and the potential future development of a more effective vaccine, access and adherence will remain as two key issues that will impede achievement of the WHO End TB Strategy goals and SDG targets unless they are adequately addressed. A number of interventions have been proven to improve access to healthcare and promote adherence, and these should be tailored to the context. These will be important interventions to promote patient-centred TB care and achieve the ambitious goal of ending TB as a public health problem by 2030.

References

1.	WHO. Implementing the End TB Strategy: the Essentials. Geneva, WHO, 2015. www.who.int/tb/publications/2015/The_Essentials_to_End_TB/en/

2.	Institute of Medicine Committee on Monitoring Access to Personal Health Care Services. Access to Health Care in America. Washington, National Academies Press (US), 1993.

3.	Evans D, Hsu J, Boerma T. Universal health coverage and universal access. *Bull World Health Organ* 2013; 91: 546–546A.

4.	WHO. Tracking Universal Health Coverage: 2017 Global Monitoring Report. Geneva, WHO, 2017. www.who.int/healthinfo/universal_health_coverage/report/2017/en/

5.	Lönnroth K, Castro KG, Chakaya JM, *et al.* Tuberculosis control and elimination 2010–50: cure, care, and social development. *Lancet* 2010; 375: 1814–1829.

6.	WHO. Adherence to Long-term Therapies: Evidence for Action. Geneva, WHO, 2003. www.who.int/chp/knowledge/publications/adherence_report/en/

7.	Urquhart J. Patient non-compliance with drug regimens: measurement, clinical correlates, economic impact. *Eur Heart J* 1996; 17: Suppl. A, 8–15.

8.	Boag-Munroe G, Evangelou M. From hard to reach to how to reach: a systematic review of the literature on hard-to-reach families. *Res Pap Educ* 2012; 27: 209–239.

9.	Flanagan SM, Hancock B. 'Reaching the hard to reach' – lessons learned from the VCS (Voluntary and Community Sector). A qualitative study. *BMC Health Serv Res* 2010; 10: 92.

10.	Benoit C, Jansson M, Millar A, *et al.* Community-academic research on hard-to-reach populations: benefits and challenges. *Qual Health Res* 2005; 15: 263–282.

11.	Coe C, Gibson A, Spencer N, *et al.* Sure start: voices of the 'hard-to-reach'. *Child Care Health Dev* 2008; 34: 447–453.

12.	Crozier G, Davies J. Hard to reach parents or hard to reach schools? A discussion of home-school relations, with particular reference to Bangladeshi and Pakistani parents. *Br Educ Res J* 2007; 33: 295–313.

13.	de Vries SG, Cremers AL, Heuvelings CC, *et al.* Barriers and facilitators to the uptake of tuberculosis diagnostic and treatment services by hard-to-reach populations in countries of low and medium tuberculosis incidence: a systematic review of qualitative literature. *Lancet Infect Dis* 2017; 17: e128–e143.

14.	Heuvelings CC, de Vries SG, Greve PF, *et al.* Effectiveness of interventions for diagnosis and treatment of tuberculosis in hard-to-reach populations in countries of low and medium tuberculosis incidence: a systematic review. *Lancet Infect Dis* 2017; 17: e144–e158.

15.	Eltis.org. Definition of hard-to-reach group. Glossary of Sustainable Urban Mobility Plans (SUMP). www.eltis.org/glossary/hard-reach-group Date last accessed: August 28, 2018. Date last updated: November 12, 2015.

16.	Brackertz N. Who is Hard to Reach and Why? ISR Working Paper. Hawthorne, Institute for Social Research, 2007. http://library.bsl.org.au/jspui/bitstream/1/875/1/Whois_htr.pdf

17.	National Institute of Clinical Excellence. Tuberculosis. NICE guideline (NG33). www.nice.org.uk/guidance/ng33 Date last accessed: June 27, 2018. Date last updated: May, 2016.

18.	Gerrish K, Naisby A, Ismail M. The meaning and consequences of tuberculosis among Somali people in the United Kingdom. *J Adv Nurs* 2012; 68: 2654–2663.

19.	Kalengayi FKN, Hurtig AK, Ahlm C, *et al.* Fear of deportation may limit legal immigrants' access to HIV/AIDS-related care: a survey of Swedish language school students in Northern Sweden. *J Immigr Minor Health* 2012; 14: 39–47.

20.	Williamson J, Ramirez R, Wingfield T. Health, healthcare access, and use of traditional *versus* modern medicine in remote Peruvian Amazon communities: a descriptive study of knowledge, attitudes, and practices. *Am J Trop Med Hyg* 2015; 92: 857–864.

21.	National Institute of Clinical Excellence. HIV testing: increasing uptake among people who may have undiagnosed HIV. NICE guideline (NG60). www.nice.org.uk/guidance/ng60/chapter/Recommendations Date last accessed: August 29, 2018. Date last updated: December, 2016.

22.	Vukovic DS, Nagorni-Obradovic LM. Knowledge and awareness of tuberculosis among Roma population in Belgrade: a qualitative study. *BMC Infect Dis* 2011; 11: 284.

23.	Kauffman KS, Dosreis S, Ross M, *et al.* Engaging hard-to-reach patients in patient-centered outcomes research. *J Comp Eff Res* 2013; 2: 313–324.

24.	Department of Health. Addressing inequalities – reaching the hard-to-reach groups. National Service Frameworks. A Practical Aid to Implementation in Primary Care. London, Department of Health, 2002. http://webarchive.nationalarchives.gov.uk/20120504011517/http://www.dh.gov.uk/prod_consum_dh/groups/dh_digitalassets/@dh/@en/documents/digitalasset/dh_4065397.pdf

25.	Wingfield T, Tovar MA, Huff D, *et al.* A randomized controlled study of socioeconomic support to enhance tuberculosis prevention and treatment, Peru. *Bull World Health Organ* 2017; 95: 270–280.

26.	Wingfield T, Tovar MA, Huff D, *et al.* Socioeconomic support to improve initiation of tuberculosis preventive therapy and increase tuberculosis treatment success in Peru: a household-randomised, controlled evaluation. *Lancet* 2017; 389: S16.

https://doi.org/10.1183/2312508X.10022117

27. Dolan K, Wirtz AL, Moazen B, *et al.* Global burden of HIV, viral hepatitis, and tuberculosis in prisoners and detainees. *Lancet* 2016; 388: 1089–1102.

28. Wingfield T, Wilkins E. Opportunistic infections in HIV disease. *Br J Nurs* 2010; 19: 621–627.

29. Brewer TF, Heymann SE, Krumplitsch SM, *et al.* Strategies to decrease tuberculosis in US homeless populations: a computer simulation model. *JAMA* 2001; 286: 831–842.

30. Andrews JR, Basu S, Dowdy DW, *et al.* The epidemiological advantage of preferential targeting of tuberculosis control to the poor. *Int J Tuberc Lung Dis* 2015; 2: 147–185.

31. Walker TM, Lalor MK, Broda A, *et al.* Europe PMC Funders Group assessment of *Mycobacterium tuberculosis* transmission in Oxfordshire, UK, 2007–12, with whole pathogen genome sequences: an observational study. *Lancet Infect Dis* 2015; 2: 285–292.

32. Dodd PJ, Looker C, Plumb ID, *et al.* Original contribution age- and sex-specific social contact patterns and incidence of *Mycobacterium tuberculosis* infection. *Am J Epidemiol* 2016; 183: 156–166.

33. Johnstone-Robertson SP, Mark D, Morrow C, *et al.* Practice of epidemiology social mixing patterns within a South African township community: implications for respiratory disease transmission and control. *Am J Epidemiol* 2011; 174: 1246–1255.

34. Craig GM, Zumla A. The social context of tuberculosis treatment in urban risk groups in the United Kingdom: a qualitative interview study. *Int J Infect Dis* 2015; 32: 105–110.

35. Hens N, Jit M, Beutels P, *et al.* Social contacts and mixing patterns relevant to the spread of infectious diseases. *PLoS Med* 2008; 5: e74.

36. Jit M, Stagg HR, Aldridge RW, *et al.* Dedicated outreach service for hard to reach patients with tuberculosis in London: observational study and economic evaluation. *BMJ* 2011; 343: 1–11.

37. Guo Y, Xu X, Fu G, *et al.* Risk behaviours and prevalences of HIV and sexually transmitted infections among female sex workers in various venues in Changzhou, China. *Int J STD AIDS* 2017; 28: 1135–1142.

38. Manopaiboon C, Prybylski D, Subhachaturas W, *et al.* Unexpectedly high HIV prevalence among female sex workers in Bangkok, Thailand in a respondent-driven sampling survey. *AIDS Behav* 2013; 24: 34–38.

39. Musyoki H, Kellogg TA, Muraguri N, *et al.* Prevalence of HIV, sexually transmitted infections, and risk behaviours among female sex workers in Nairobi, Kenya: results of a respondent driven sampling survey. *AIDS Behav* 2016; 19: Suppl. 1, S46–S58.

40. Yuen WWY, Tran L, Wong CKH, *et al.* Psychological health and HIV transmission among female sex workers: a systematic review and meta-analysis. *AIDS Care* 2016; 28: 816–824.

41. Ulibarri MD, Strathdee SA, Patterson TL. Sexual and drug use behaviors associated with HIV and other sexually transmitted infections among female sex workers in the Mexico–US border region. *Curr Opin Psychiatry* 2012; 100: 215–220.

42. Mayer KH, Grinsztejn B, El-Sadr WM. Transgender people and HIV prevention: what we know and what we need to know, a call to action. *J Acquir Immune Defic Syndr* 2016; 72: 207–209.

43. Poteat T, Scheim A, Xavier J, *et al.* Global epidemiology of HIV infection and related syndemics affecting transgender people. *J Acquir Immune Defic Syndr* 2016; 72: 210–219.

44. Kosenko K, Rintamaki L, Raney S, *et al.* Transgender patient perceptions of stigma in health care contexts. *Med Care* 2013; 51: 31829.

45. White Hughto JM, Reisner SL, Pachankis JE. Transgender stigma and health: a critical review of stigma determinants, mechanisms, and interventions. *Soc Sci Med* 2016; 147: 222–231.

46. Velayutham BRV, Nair D, Chandrasekaran V, *et al.* Profile and response to anti-tuberculosis treatment among elderly tuberculosis patients treated under the TB control programme in South India. *PLoS One* 2014; 9: e88045.

47. Patra S, Lukhmana S, Tayler Smith K, *et al.* Profile and treatment outcomes of elderly patients with tuberculosis in Delhi, India: implications for their management. *Trans R Soc Trop Med Hyg* 2013; 107: 763–768.

48. Storla DG, Yimer S, Bjune GA. A systematic review of delay in the diagnosis and treatment of tuberculosis. *BMC Public Health* 2008; 8: 1–9.

49. MacPherson P, Houben RM, Glynn JR, *et al.* Pre-treatment loss to follow-up in tuberculosis patients in low- and lower-middle-income countries and high-burden countries: a systematic review and meta-analysis. *Bull World Health Organ* 2014; 92: 126–138.

50. Finnie RKC, Khoza LB, van den Borne B, *et al.* Factors associated with patient and health care system delay in diagnosis and treatment for TB in sub-Saharan African countries with high burdens of TB and HIV. *Trop Med Int Health* 2011; 16: 394–411.

51. Wingfield T, Tovar MA, Huff D, *et al.* Beyond pills and tests: addressing the social determinants of tuberculosis. *Clin Med* 2016; 16: Suppl. 6, s79–s91.

52. Rocha C, Montoya R, Zevallos K, *et al.* The Innovative Socio-economic Interventions Against Tuberculosis (ISIAT) project: an operational assessment. *Int J Tuberc Lung Dis* 2011; 15: Suppl. 2, 50–57.

53. Bonevski B, Randell M, Paul C, *et al.* Reaching the hard-to-reach: a systematic review of strategies for improving health and medical research with socially disadvantaged groups. *BMC Med Res Methodol* 2014; 14: 1–29.

54.   Woodward A, Howard N, Wolffers I. Health and access to care for undocumented migrants living in the European Union: a scoping review. *Health Policy Plan* 2014; 29: 818–830.

55.   Gil-Gonzalez D, Carrasco-Portino M, Vives-Cases C, *et al.* Is health a right for all? An umbrella review of the barriers to health care access faced by migrants. *Ethn Health* 2015; 20: 523–542.

56.   Laurence Y V, Griffiths UK, Vassall A. Costs to health services and the patient of treating tuberculosis: a systematic literature review. *Pharmacoeconomics* 2015; 33: 939–955.

57.   Kumwenda M, Desmond N, Hart G, *et al.* Treatment-seeking for tuberculosis-suggestive symptoms: a reflection on the role of human agency in the context of universal health coverage in Malawi. *PLoS One* 2016; 11: 1–12.

58.   Ukwaja KN. Alobu I, Igwenyi C, *et al.* The high cost of free tuberculosis services: patient and household costs associated with tuberculosis care in Ebonyi State, Nigeria. *PLoS One* 2013; 8: e73134.

59.   Laokri S, Weil O, Drabo KM, *et al.* Removal of user fees no guarantee of universal health coverage: observations from Burkina Faso. *Bull World Health Organ* 2013; 91: 277–282.

60.   Basnet R, Shrestha BR, Nagaraja SB, *et al.* Universal health coverage in a regional Nepali hospital: who is exempted from payment? *Public Health Action* 2013; 3: 90–92.

61.   Wei X, Zou G, Yin J, *et al.* Effective reimbursement rates of the rural health insurance among uncomplicated tuberculosis patients in China. *Trop Med Int Health* 2015; 20: 304–311.

62.   Mauch V, Woods N, Kirubi B, *et al.* Assessing access barriers to tuberculosis care with the Tool to Estimate Patients' Costs: pilot results from two districts in Kenya. *BMC Public Health* 2011; 11: 43.

63.   WHO. Global Tuberculosis Report 2017. Geneva, WHO, 2017. http://www.who.int/tb/publications/global_report/gtbr2017_main_text.pdf

64.   Tanimura T, Jaramillo E, Weil D, *et al.* Financial burden for tuberculosis patients in low- and middle-income countries: a systematic review. *Eur Respir J* 2014; 43: 1763–1775.

65.   Lönnroth K, Glaziou P, Weil D, *et al.* Beyond UHC: monitoring health and social protection coverage in the context of tuberculosis care and prevention. *PLoS Med* 2014; 11: e1001693.

66.   International Labour Organization. World Social Protection Report. Geneva, International Labour Organization, 2017. Available from: www.ilo.org/global/publications/books/WCMS_604882/lang–en/index.htm

67.   WHO. Guidelines for Treatment of Drug Susceptible Tuberculosis and Patient Care, 2017 Update. Document WHO/HTM/TB/2017.05. Geneva, WHO, 2017. www.who.int/tb/publications/2017/dstb_guidance_2017/en/

68.   Wei X, Liang X, Liu F, *et al.* Decentralising tuberculosis services from county tuberculosis dispensaries to township hospitals in China: An intervention study. *Int J Tuberc Lung Dis* 2008; 12: 538–547.

69.   Loveday M, Wallengren K, Voce A, *et al.* Comparing early treatment outcomes of MDR-TB in a decentralized setting in KwaZulu-Natal, South Africa. *Int J Tuberc Lung Dis* 2012; 16: 209–215.

70.   Cox H, Daniels J, Muller O, *et al.* Impact of decentralized care and the Xpert MTB/RIF test on rifampicin-resistant tuberculosis treatment initiation in Khayelitsha, South Africa. *Open Forum Infect Dis* 2015; 2: 1–7.

71.   Datiko DG, Lindtjørn B. Health extension workers improve tuberculosis case detection and treatment success in southern Ethiopia: a community randomized trial. *PLoS One* 2009; 4: 1–7.

72.   Ho J, Byrne AL, Linh NN, *et al.* Decentralized care for multidrug-resistant tuberculosis: a systematic review and meta-analysis. *Bull World Health Organ* 2017; 95: 584–593.

73.   WHO. Systematic Screening for Active Tuberculosis: Principles and Recommendations. Geneva, WHO, 2013. www.who.int/tb/tbscreening/en/

74.   Lönnroth K, Migliori GB, Abubakar I, *et al.* Towards tuberculosis elimination: an action framework for low incidence countries. *Eur Respir J* 2015; 45: 928–952.

75.   van Hoorn R, Jaramillo E, Collins D, *et al.* The effects of psycho-emotional and socio-economic support for tuberculosis patients on treatment adherence and treatment outcomes – a systematic review and meta-analysis. *PLoS One* 2016; 11: e0154095.

76.   Bock NN, Sales R, Rogers T, *et al.* A spoonful of sugar…: improving adherence to tuberculosis treatment using financial incentives. *Int J Tuberc Lung Dis* 2001; 5: 96–98.

77.   Munro SA, Lewin SA, Smith HJ, *et al.* Patient adherence to tuberculosis treatment: a systematic review of qualitative research. *PLoS Med* 2007; 4: e238.

78.   Müller AM, Osório CS, Silva DR, *et al.* Interventions to improve adherence to tuberculosis treatment: systematic review and meta-analysis. *Int J Tuberc Lung Dis* 2018; 22: 731–740.

79.   M'Imunya JM, Kredo T, Volmink J. Patient education and counselling for promoting adherence to treatment for tuberculosis. *Cochrane Database Syst Rev* 2012; 5: CD006591.

80.   Salleras Sanmarti L, Alcaide Megias J, Altet Gomez MN, *et al.* Evaluation of the efficacy of health education on the compliance with antituberculosis chemoprophylaxis in school children. A randomized clinical trial. *Tuber Lung Dis* 1993; 74: 28–31.

81.   White MC, Tulsky JP, Goldenson J, *et al.* Randomized controlled trial of interventions to improve follow-up for latent tuberculosis infection after release from jail. *Arch Intern Med* 2002; 162: 1044–1050.

82.   Morisky DE, Malotte CK, Ebin V, *et al.* Behavioral interventions for the control of tuberculosis among adolescents. *Public Health Rep* 2001; 116: 568–574.

https://doi.org/10.1183/2312508X.10022117

83. Tola HH, Shojaeizadeh D, Tol A, *et al.* Psychological and educational intervention to improve tuberculosis treatment adherence in Ethiopia based on health belief model: a cluster randomized control trial. *PLoS One* 2016; 11: e0155147.

84. Kaliakbarova G, Pak S, Zhaksylykova N, *et al.* Psychosocial support improves treatment adherence among MDR-TB patients: experience from East Kazakhstan. *Open Infect Dis J* 2013; 7: 60–64.

85. Lutge EE, Wiysonge CS, Knight SE, *et al.* Incentives and enablers to improve adherence in tuberculosis. *Cochrane Database Syst Rev* 2015; 9: CD007952.

86. Martins N, Morris P, Kelly PM. Food incentives to improve completion of tuberculosis treatment: randomised controlled trial in Dili, Timor-Leste. *BMJ* 2009; 339: b4248.

87. Malotte CK, Hollingshead JR, Rhodes F. Monetary *versus* nonmonetary incentives for TB skin test reading among drug users. *Am J Prev Med* 1999; 16: 182–188.

88. Malotte CK, Hollingshead JR, Larro M. Incentives *versus* outreach workers for latent tuberculosis treatment in drug users. *Am J Prev Med* 2001; 20: 103–107.

89. Pilote L, Tulsky J, Zolopa A, *et al.* Tuberculosis prophylaxis in the homeless: a trial to improve adherence to referral. *Arch Intern Med* 1996; 156: 161–165.

90. White MC, Tulsky JP, Reilly P, *et al.* A clinical trial of a financial incentive to go to the tuberculosis clinic for isoniazid after release from jail. *Int J Tuberc Lung Dis* 1998; 2: 506–512.

91. Souza MSPL, Pereira SM, Marinho JM, *et al.* Characteristics of healthcare services associated with adherence to tuberculosis treatment. [Características dos serviços de saúde associadas à adesão ao tratamento da tuberculose.] *Rev Saude Publica* 2009; 43: 997–1005.

92. Torrens AW, Rasella D, Boccia D, *et al.* Effectiveness of a conditional cash transfer programme on TB cure rate: a retrospective cohort study in Brazil. *Trans R Soc Trop Med Hyg* 2016; 110: 199–206.

93. Nery JS, Rodrigues LC, Rasella D, *et al.* Effect of Brazil's conditional cash transfer programme on tuberculosis incidence. *Int J Tuberc Lung Dis* 2017; 21: 790–796.

94. DiStefano MJ, Schmidt H. mHealth for tuberculosis treatment adherence: a framework to guide ethical planning, implementation, and evaluation. *Glob Health Sci Pract* 2016; 4: 211–221.

95. WHO. mHealth: New Horizons for Health Through Mobile Technologies. Geneva, WHO, 2011. www.who.int/goe/publications/goe_mhealth_web.pdf

96. WHO. Consolidated Guidelines on the Use of Antiretroviral Drugs for Treating and Preventing HIV Infection: Recommendations for a Public Health Approach. 2nd Edn. Geneva, WHO, 2013. Available from: www.who.int/hiv/pub/arv/arv-2016/en/

97. Finitsis DJ, Pellowski JA, Johnson BT. Text message intervention designs to promote adherence to antiretroviral therapy (ART): a meta-analysis of randomized controlled trials. *PLoS One* 2014; 9: e88166.

98. Liu X, Lewis JJ, Zhang H, *et al.* Effectiveness of electronic reminders to improve medication adherence in tuberculosis patients: a cluster-randomised trial. *PLoS Med* 2015; 12: 1–18.

99. Narasimhan P, Bakshi A, Kittusami S, *et al.* A customized m-Health system for improving tuberculosis treatment adherence and follow-up in south India. *Health Technol* 2014; 4: 1–10.

100. Saunders MJ, Wingfield T, Tovar MA, *et al.* Mobile phone interventions for tuberculosis should ensure access to mobile phones to enhance equity – a prospective, observational cohort study in Peruvian shantytowns. *Trop Med Int Health* 2018; 23: 850–859.

Disclosures: None declared.

Chapter 18

Monitoring during and after treatment

Jan-Willem C. Alffenaar[1], Onno W. Akkerman[2,3] and
Graham Bothamley[4,5,6]

TB treatment is long and often complicated by adverse reactions. Baseline assessment can reduce the likelihood of adverse reactions, especially DILI. Regular monitoring can ensure treatment efficacy and prevent serious complications. A slow response to treatment may indicate poor adherence, an inadequate treatment regimen or acquired drug resistance. Adherence can be addressed by the use of directly observed therapy in a supportive environment. To avoid under- and overdosing, plasma drug concentrations can be measured to tailor the dose to the individual needs of a patient (*i.e.* TDM). To assess treatment response, the 2-month sputum test is an important time-point for decision making during treatment. Confirmation of treatment response at the end of treatment and the absence of relapse over at least the ensuing 12 months is essential to determine cure. To conclude, monitoring at the start, during and after TB treatment is a simple but necessary task for the TB team to ensure the optimal course and outcome of TB treatment.

Cite as: Alffenaar J-WC, Akkerman OW, Bothamley G. Monitoring during and after treatment. *In:* Migliori GB, Bothamley G, Duarte R, *et al.*, eds. Tuberculosis (ERS Monograph). Sheffield, European Respiratory Society, 2018; pp. 308–325 [https://doi.org/10.1183/2312508X.10022217].

🐦 @ERSpublications
TB treatment is long and often complicated by adverse reactions. Monitoring at the start, during and after TB treatment is a simple but necessary task for the TB team to ensure the optimal course and outcome of TB treatment. http://ow.ly/cfVQ30lqCfE

Treatment for TB is long and often complicated by adverse drug reactions. Regular monitoring of the patient will ensure that adverse reactions are identified early, adherence is supported and effective treatment given. In this chapter we discuss which parameters are important to assess the condition of the patient, the efficacy and safety of anti-TB drugs, and treatment outcome.

[1]University of Groningen, University Medical Center Groningen, Dept of Clinical Pharmacy and Pharmacology, Groningen, The Netherlands. [2]University of Groningen, University Medical Center Groningen, Dept of Pulmonary Diseases and Tuberculosis, Groningen, The Netherlands. [3]University of Groningen, University Medical Center Groningen, Tuberculosis Center Beatrixoord, Haren, The Netherlands. [4]Homerton University Hospital, London, UK. [5]Blizard Institute, Barts and The London School of Medicine and Dentistry, Queen Mary University of London, London, UK. [6]London School of Hygiene and Tropical Medicine, London, UK.

Correspondence: Jan-Willem C. Alffenaar, University of Groningen, University Medical Center Groningen, Dept of Clinical Pharmacy and Pharmacology, PO Box 30.001, 9700 RB Groningen, The Netherlands. E-mail: j.w.c.alffenaar@umcg.nl

Copyright ©ERS 2018. Print ISBN: 978-1-84984-099-6. Online ISBN: 978-1-84984-100-9. Print ISSN: 2312-508X. Online ISSN: 2312-5098.

https://doi.org/10.1183/2312508X.10022217

Before the start of treatment, a baseline assessment should be made against which subsequent measurements will detect improvement or worsening of the patient's condition. During the first 2 weeks, an effective regimen must be established and the patient made aware of the importance of continuing treatment for the full course. Drug dosing has traditionally been normalised by body weight (*e.g.* mg·kg^{-1}) or by stratified weights. However, both first- and second-line drugs may deliver up to a 100-fold difference in plasma levels in different patients with standard dosing. TDM ensures that dosages are increased to provide a therapeutic effect in case of low plasma drug concentrations and to prevent drug toxicity if plasma drug concentrations are too high [1, 2].

In the continuation phase of treatment, monitoring of TB treatment is largely concerned with efficacy and cure. The 2-month appointment is the most important time-point. Where sputum conversion has not occurred, TDM is important before regimen change. TDM is especially important in DR-TB, including cases of isoniazid resistance. Confirmation of the expected treatment response is required at the end of treatment. Where culture of material is not available to define a cure, the absence of relapse over at least the ensuing 12 months is essential in meeting the patient's expectations of a cure.

This chapter aims to provide a concise overview of monitoring clinical parameters, drug concentrations and outcome. Adverse events from TB drugs are discussed in detail elsewhere in this *Monograph* [3], but mention will be made here when routine tests may be affected. Management issues for MDR-TB are discussed elsewhere in this *Monograph* [4]. This chapter has therefore been limited to the essentials of monitoring and the more specialised topic of TDM.

Initial assessment

The key indicators before the start of treatment include evidence confirming the diagnosis of TB, weight and chest radiography appearance, as discussed further elsewhere in this *Monograph* in chapters on laboratory/clinical diagnosis and imaging [5–7].

Sputum examination

Sputum examination is essential, as those with a positive sputum smear are potentially infectious and require respiratory isolation and attention to cough hygiene (as discussed elsewhere in this *Monograph* [8]). The option of molecular testing for rifampicin resistance using Xpert MTB/RIF ensures that an adequate treatment regimen is given from the start [9]. Sputum smear and time to culture act as a proxy for the bacillary load [10].

Blood tests

A full blood count is useful as a baseline. Linezolid use is associated with many haematological abnormalities [11, 12] and bone marrow failure with flu-like symptoms is associated with intermittent rifampicin use; both are reasons to discontinue the respective drugs. Urea, creatinine and electrolytes can be useful in assessing renal function [13], especially in the elderly [14], and help determine the dose of ethambutol or injectable agents. A low sodium level can be seen, as a result of the syndrome of inappropriate secretion of antidiuretic hormone due to TB, and acts like a "reverse erythrocyte sedimentation rate", with normalising levels confirming a response to treatment. Hyper- and hypokalaemia can contribute to the risk of a cardiac arrhythmia (see the later section on ECG), the former with renal impairment and the latter often found in those drinking alcohol to excess. In LFTs, alanine aminotransferase (ALT) and/or aspartate aminotransferase (AST) levels may be raised due to TB as much as to associated comorbidities such as alcohol abuse [15, 16]. A baseline bilirubin level is important if rifampicin use later causes obstructive liver damage; albumin levels can, with globulin, confirm a response to TB treatment.

TDM is routine with the first dose of SLIDs. Plasma levels of aminoglycosides are measured 90 min after the first injection to ensure that the dose used is not toxic. Subsequently (days 3–5), a pre- and post-dose measurement will guide the dose and the spacing of the doses. If there is an increase in post-dose levels, monitoring should continue at weekly intervals until the plasma levels are stable (table 1).

Chest radiography

A baseline chest radiograph should be obtained for all patients before the start of TB treatment. Current doses of radiation are low (~2 years of background radiation). In EPTB, radiological examinations are helpful in supporting the diagnosis, but repeated tests are not usually of value without a change in clinical symptoms. In MDR-TB, a computed tomography (CT) scan is often useful as a baseline test, as treatment responses can be slower and more difficult to define.

Comedication

Exploration of the use of other drugs is important before the start of anti-TB drugs due to the interactions of some of these drugs. Rifampicin is a strong cytochrome CYP3A inducer and has interactions with many other drugs. Rifampicin lowers the exposure of prednisolone and the contraceptive pill, anticoagulants (e.g. coumarin/warfarin), opiates, treatments for epilepsy, proton pump inhibitors, and some antipsychotics, as well as many antiviral agents. A urinary drug screen is often helpful in alerting the physician to the use of nonprescribed drugs.

Electrocardiography

TB itself rarely causes ECG abnormalities, although in TB pericarditis the QRS complex can be of low voltage with large effusions [18]. For MDR-TB, an ECG should be routine, as quinolones, clofazimine, bedaquiline and delamanid as well as opiates, metoclopramide and antipsychotics (table 1) can all contribute to prolonging the QT interval [19, 20] and would not be normally used in those with QT >500 ms. A urinary drug screen at the time of the ECG may also be helpful in excluding opiates, etc., as the cause of a prolonged corrected QT interval.

Assessment of nutritional status

The prevalence of malnutrition in patients with TB is an estimated 70%. The risk of death in patients with TB associated with malnutrition is twofold [21]. In addition, malnutrition is an important risk factor for reactivation of TB [22]. Malnutrition can lead to malabsorption of TB treatment, leading to a decreased bioavailability of anti-TB drugs

https://doi.org/10.1183/2312508X.10022217

Table 1. Treatment monitoring in MDR/XDR-TB after the TBNET consensus document [17]

	BL	2 weeks	Time months																		
			1	2	3	4	5	6	7	8	10	12	14	16	18	20	24	28	32	38	44
Sputum smear#	✓	✓	✓	✓	✓	✓	✓	✓	✓	✓	✓	✓	✓	✓	✓	✓	✓	✓	✓	✓	✓
TB culture¶	✓	✓	✓	✓	✓	✓	✓	✓	✓	✓	✓	✓	✓	✓	✓	✓	✓	✓	✓	✓	✓
Molecular testing for drug resistance	✓			✓+																		
Phenotypic DST from culture	✓			✓+																		
Full blood count	✓	✓	✓	✓	✓	✓	✓	✓	✓	✓	✓	✓	✓	✓	✓	✓					
Renal function tests/LFTs	✓	✓	✓	✓	✓	✓	✓	✓	✓	✓	✓	✓	✓	✓	✓	✓					
Calcium and magnesium (PTH and vitamin D)§	✓		✓§	✓§	✓§	✓§	✓§	✓§	✓§	✓§											
TSH testƒ	✓				✓			✓				✓									
Hepatitis B and C serology	✓																				
HIV test	✓																				
Pregnancy test	✓																				
Weight	✓	✓	✓	✓	✓	✓	✓	✓	✓	✓	✓	✓	✓	✓	✓	✓	✓	✓	✓	✓	✓
Height	✓																				
Audiometry	✓	✓¶¶	✓##	✓##	✓##	✓##	✓##	✓##	✓##	✓##											
Visual acuity	✓	✓¶¶	✓¶¶	✓¶¶	✓¶¶	✓¶¶	✓¶¶	✓¶¶	✓¶¶	✓¶¶	✓¶¶	✓¶¶	✓¶¶	✓¶¶	✓¶¶	✓¶¶					
Depression score++	✓											✓				✓					
Chest radiography	✓			✓				✓		✓		✓				✓					

Continued

Table 1. Continued

| | BL | 2 weeks | Time months | | | | | | | | | | | | | | | | | | |
			1	2	3	4	5	6	7	8	10	12	14	16	18	20	24	28	32	38	44
Thoracic CT[§§]	✓									✓					✓						
ECG[ff,##]	✓	✓			✓			✓				✓									
Drug levels[¶¶¶]		✓[+++]																			

BL: baseline; PTH: parathyroid hormone; TSH: thyroid-stimulating hormone; CT: computed tomography. [#]: monthly sputum samples should be sent if possible until negative culture on three separate occasions, each 1 month apart. This is especially important at the end of the initial phase of treatment (8 months) and at treatment completion to confirm cure. Regular sputum sampling throughout the course of treatment is highly recommended to identify early treatment failure. [¶]: in EPTB, the attending physician should decide on the feasibility and frequency of taking additional samples. [+]: this should be repeated if the sputum smear or culture is still positive after 2 months of adequate treatment or at any time if there is evidence of relapse. [§]: calcium and magnesium should be monitored monthly if capreomycin is used; many recommend measurements of PTH and vitamin D at baseline to improve macrophage function if vitamin D levels are low. [f]: TSH if treatment regimen includes ethionamide, prothionamide or PAS. [##]: regular audiometry should be performed while SLIDs are being used. [¶¶]: visual acuity should be checked if using ethambutol or linezolid for as long as these drugs are used. [++]: depression scores should be measured at baseline and repeated if cycloserine is being used either at regular (monthly) intervals or when symptoms arise. [§§]: CT scans can also be used when there is a concern about poor treatment response or relapse. [ff]: ECGs should be used to monitor all drugs which prolong the corrected QT interval, including those used for comorbidities or symptomatic relief. [###]: urine for nonprescribed drugs should be taken with the ECG. [¶¶¶]: first dose levels should be measured for aminoglycosides; fluoroquinolone blood levels should be routinely checked to avoid underdosing. Some physicians recommend pre-emptive nerve conduction studies for those taking linezolid at monthly intervals. [+++]: in patients failing to respond to treatment, concentrations of other drugs can be measured. Reproduced and modified from [17] with permission.

https://doi.org/10.1183/2312508X.10022217

that may result in low drug exposure [22]. Disease-related malnutrition leads to loss of fat-free mass, even in overweight or obese patients. Therefore, a normal or high body mass index can still occur in those who are severely malnourished. The assessment of nutritional status is complex as malnutrition is defined as a lack of intake or uptake of nutrition that leads to altered body composition (decreased fat-free mass) and body cell mass, leading to diminished physical and mental function and impaired clinical outcome from disease [23].

Neurological tests

Optic neuropathy is the most important adverse effect of ethambutol and the second-line drug linezolid (discussed elsewhere in this *Monograph* [3]). Vision should be screened before the start of treatment using an eye chart (*e.g.* Snellen or Jaegar charts to measure visual acuity) and the Ishihara test (to test colour vision). Testing should be monthly until ethambutol or linezolid are no longer used in the treatment regimen. Toxicity is more common with doses of ethambutol of $\geqslant 25$ mg·kg^{-1} and with prolonged use. As ethambutol is used in the standard RHZE (rifampicin, isoniazid, pyrazinamide and ethambutol) regimen to protect against drug resistance, a bacteriostatic dose of 15 mg·kg^{-1} is most commonly employed [24, 25], except in the treatment of DR-TB.

A baseline assessment of peripheral neuropathy is especially important in those with DM. Isoniazid is the drug most commonly associated with peripheral neuropathy, which can be prevented by giving pyridoxine in those likely deficient. The risk of developing peripheral neuropathy is higher for patients with HIV co-infection [26] and those with an alcohol problem, who therefore receive pyridoxine routinely so that isoniazid cannot be implicated as the cause.

Biomarkers

No set of biomarkers has yet been shown to benefit the management of TB. However, an increased C-reactive protein (CRP) level is often used, with a normal neutrophil count, to raise the suspicion of TB. If increased, CRP can be measured at a later stage to confirm a response to treatment if there are any concerns.

Comorbidities

Comorbidities are discussed in more detail elsewhere in this *Monograph* [27].

HIV

The presence of HIV co-infection and hepatitis B/C viruses is important in terms of managing TB [28, 29], recognising their greater incidence of DILI and paradoxical reactions, respectively. Comorbidities should have appropriate measurements, *e.g.* viral load and CD4 count in those with HIV co-infection. HIV and TB are linked, with 1.5 million people having both infections annually, causing 400 000 deaths per year. Some antiretroviral drugs have interactions with rifampicin, causing lower levels of the antiretroviral drugs. HIV itself can also cause absorption problems in TB patients [30].

Diabetes mellitus

DM is an increasing epidemic in affluent countries. DM has been associated with a higher risk for reactivation of TB [31–33]. Diabetes can cause gastroparesis that itself can lead to a prolonged absorption time of anti-TB drugs, resulting in lower levels of the drugs. Diabetes can cause peripheral neuropathy, which makes peripheral neuropathy caused by anti-TB drugs such as isoniazid and linezolid more difficult to exclude [11, 12, 34]. Peripheral neuropathy can be seen even more often in patients with both DM and receiving TB treatment [34]. Screening for DM can be done by testing for fasting glucose or glycated haemoglobin.

Continuous monitoring (especially during the first 2 weeks)

As with all conditions that require >1 week of treatment, the first 2 weeks are critical in establishing the treatment regimen. To this end, the treatment for TB should be acceptable to the patient, a decision made regarding whether self-administered treatment (SAT) or directly observed therapy (DOT) is to be used, all initial adverse effects managed, and a plan made for future visits by the key worker with an appointment for a physician's review to maximise adherence. The patient should be encouraged to report any new symptoms or matters of concern immediately when they occur; at each visit, the key worker should enquire whether any adverse effects have occurred.

All comorbidities should be addressed, especially any psychiatric illnesses that might affect adherence to TB treatment, alcohol and opiate addiction requiring support and harm reduction, HIV co-infection with a plan when to start ART if not already started, as well as support with the management of DM as required. Often a patient's concerns are not primarily with the treatment for TB. For example, if they are homeless, then arrangements should be made for emergency housing in order to ensure that DOT can be given effectively. A visit to the patient's address should be part of contact tracing (some homes may have frequent visitors or be part of informal child care, such that these contacts are not included in the initial list of household members) and to ensure that the address is correct (e.g. a parent's address may be given by the patient, when the patient is actually living at their partner's address).

Adherence to treatment

The DOT record should be inspected at 2 weeks and regularly at each patient visit thereafter. For those taking SAT, a pill count should be undertaken together with a spot urine test for rifampicin (the urine becomes red) at a morning visit. If <80% of the tablets have been taken, then DOT should be initiated. Patients should be questioned about their tablets to ensure that they are taken before food and in the correct quantities. The 2-week visit is especially important in making a medical assessment whether there have been any adverse effects, so that these can be addressed immediately. Questioning regarding adverse effects should be done continuously throughout treatment at each clinic or home visit.

Response to treatment

Sputum should be taken at 2 weeks for mycobacterial culture. The time to culture positivity can be taken as an estimate of bacterial load [35] and should lengthen with treatment

https://doi.org/10.1183/2312508X.10022217

duration. Some have suggested that monthly sputum samples be taken until the cultures are negative [17, 36], and this is especially important at the end of the intensive phase and towards the end of treatment. In MDR-TB, the WHO definition of a cure requires three negative sputum cultures, each >1 month apart, during the continuation phase of treatment.

Monitoring liver function

If initial LFTs were normal, then further tests are only required if the patient develops any symptoms (table 2) [37, 38]. Regular testing is recommended if: LFTs were initially abnormal (*e.g.* weekly until normal), the patient has hepatitis B or C, the patient is pregnant, or the patient is given a drug associated with liver damage, *e.g.* prothionamide or ethionamide (thionamides). As drug-induced hepatitis is especially common after the age of 55 years, some would advocate monthly testing in older patients (the TB Bureau of New York City [36] recommends this in patients >35 years of age).

DILI is relatively common (5–10%). Variations exist in the literature as to whether the treatment should be temporarily suspended if ALT or AST is >3 times the upper limit of normal (ULN) (some would not in the absence of symptoms such as nausea until the levels are 5×ULN). The only RCT of re-introduction of treatment found no difference between regimens recommended by the TB Bureau of New York City [36] or by the British Thoracic Society [39], or by simultaneous introduction of all four drugs [40]. Approximately 90% tolerated re-introduction without any problem. Drugs can be re-introduced when AST or ALT is <2×ULN and monitoring should be weekly until levels remain within the normal range.

Other monitoring is drug specific and most often associated with the use of second-line drugs (see table 1 and elsewhere in this *ERS Monograph* [4]). Renal function and hearing

Table 2. Routine monitoring in the treatment of drug-susceptible (DS)-TB					
Test	Day 0	At any time: if any new symptom	2 weeks	2 months	6 months
Sputum smear	Yes	No	No	Yes	Yes
TB culture	Yes	No[#]	No	PTB	PTB
Chest radiography	Yes	No	No	PTB	PTB
Urea and electrolytes; LFTs; CRP	Yes	Yes	No	EPTB	EPTB
Full blood count	Yes	Yes	No	No	Yes
Eye test	Yes	Visual symptoms; refer to ophthalmologist	Yes	Not required	No
Weight	Yes	Yes	Yes	Yes	Yes
TDM			Yes[¶]	Yes[¶]	

CRP: C-reactive protein. [#]: if change at site of disease [37]; [¶]: TDM is indicated in patients with DS-TB and risk factors associated with low drug exposure (see table 3) and those failing to respond after 2 months of treatment [38].

should be assessed at least monthly if an aminoglycoside or capreomycin is given. Thyroid function should be assessed monthly if PAS or a thionamide is included in the regimen. A monthly full blood count is required in patients taking linezolid.

Therapeutic drug monitoring

Pharmacokinetics and pharmacodynamics

Pharmacokinetics describes the process of drug absorption, distribution, metabolism and clearance from the body. Patient characteristics such as age, sex, body weight and kidney/liver function can have an effect on drug exposure. These characteristics have to be taken into account when prescribing anti-TB drugs, *e.g.* to adjust the dose in relation to renal function. Pharmacodynamics describes the effect of a drug. When pharmacokinetics and pharmacodynamics are combined, the concentration of the drug is combined with the effect of the drug [41]. The concentration range in which a drug is active against bacteria but not yet too toxic for patients is considered to be the therapeutic window of the drug (figure 1).

TDM is an activity focused on measuring drug concentrations in human samples in order to optimise drug exposure. In the case of high concentrations associated with toxicity, the dose can be lowered before toxicity occurs. In the case of low concentrations there is the risk of a slow response to treatment and, more worrisome, acquired drug resistance [1, 2, 42, 43]. The relation between pharmacokinetics and pharmacodynamics has to be elucidated in order to determine the target concentration of a drug (figure 2). The pharmacokinetic/pharmacodynamic relation has been investigated in *in vitro*, *in vivo* and in clinical studies. *In vitro* hollow fibre infection model studies [44] mimic human drug exposure. Animal studies and early bactericidal activity studies [45], often testing the effect of a single drug, have shown that the cumulative drug exposure during a 24-h period (area under the concentration–time curve (AUC)) in relation to the susceptibility (MIC) of *Mycobacterium tuberculosis* (AUC/MIC; figure 2) is the pharmacokinetic/pharmacodynamic parameter that best predicts the efficacy of most anti-TB drugs. For WHO SLIDs, the peak concentration (C_{max})/MIC (figure 2) is the most predictive parameter; for WHO β-lactam antimicrobial drugs, the time the concentration exceeds the MIC (T>MIC; figure 2) is the most predictive

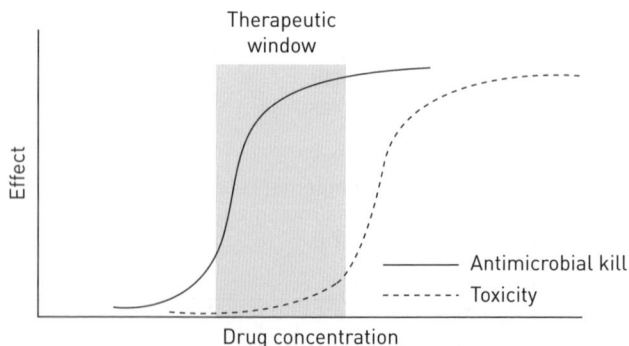

Figure 1. Therapeutic window of anti-TB drugs.

https://doi.org/10.1183/2312508X.10022217

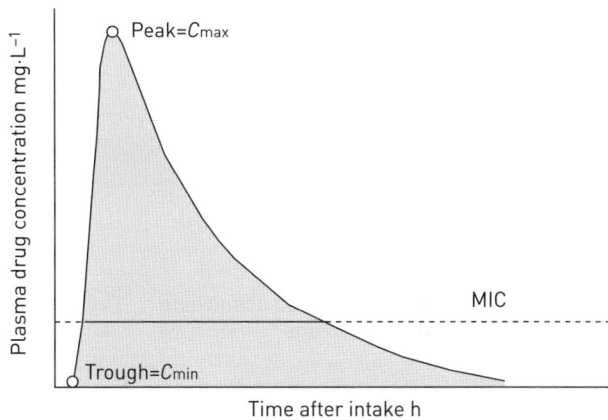

Figure 2. Pharmacokinetic/pharmacodynamic parameters of anti-TB drugs. C_{max}: maximum (peak) concentration; C_{min}: minimum (trough) concentration; AUC: area under the concentration–time curve. AUC/MIC: AUC (shaded area) over 24 h in steady-state divided by the MIC; C_{max}/MIC ratio: peak level divided by the MIC; T>MIC: cumulative percentage of a 24-h period that the drug concentration exceeds the MIC at steady-state (solid line section).

parameter. If pharmacokinetic/pharmacodynamic targets are not met, the maximum response to the drug is not reached and selection of less susceptible bacteria can occur [46].

TDM indications

Response to treatment is high in the case of drug-susceptible (DS)-TB, but urgent improvement of treatment is required in the case of drug resistance [47]. However, not all patients receiving the standard first-line four-drug RHZE regimen for DS-TB do well. In patients with problems in drug absorption, distribution, metabolism or excretion, standard dosing may not result in the desired effect [1, 2]. Although empirical dose adjustments have been applied, an informed decision based on actual drug concentrations may be a better approach [48]. An RCT on TDM is missing, but observational studies have shown that concentrations in the therapeutic window result in better outcome [49]. Recently, the American Thoracic Society, CDC and Infectious Diseases Society of America included TDM for specific indications in their guideline for TB treatment (table 3) [38].

In addition to patient characteristics that influence drug exposure, some drugs are associated with severe adverse events. Attempts have been made to reduce the toxicity of these drugs by making dose adjustments. TDM benefits patients taking linezolid, aminoglycosides and cycloserine (table 3) [12, 50–54].

Prevention of acquired drug resistance is important as it is associated with increased treatment failure and higher mortality [55, 56]. In particular, low isoniazid, rifampicin and fluoroquinolone concentrations are associated with acquired drug resistance (table 3). Large cohort studies have shown that ~10% of patients receiving a standard dose of fluoroquinolone acquire drug resistance [57]. Being the most important drug for MDR-TB treatment, fluoroquinolone dose optimisation by TDM or using a high dose seems warranted [58, 59]. Unfortunately, a high dose does not always result in adequate drug exposure. Drug absorption is likely severely compromised in these patients.

Table 3. Indications for TDM

Patient characteristics	Treatment-related factors	Drug-related factors
Severe gastrointestinal abnormalities: severe gastroparesis, short bowel syndrome, chronic diarrhoea with malabsorption[#]	Poor response to TB treatment despite adherence and fully drug-susceptible *Mycobacterium tuberculosis* strain[#]	Drug–drug interactions[#]
Impaired renal clearance: renal insufficiency, peritoneal dialysis, critically ill patients on continuous renal replacement[#]	Treatment using second-line drugs[#]	Prevention of toxicity: linezolid; aminoglycosides; cycloserine
HIV infection[#]		Prevention of acquired drug resistance: fluoroquinolones; isoniazid[¶]; rifampicin[¶]
DM[#]		Occurrence of drug concentration-related toxicity

In brief, TDM is indicated at week 2 of treatment when risk factors for low drug exposure are present, at month 2 when a patient is failing to respond and at any time during when adverse drug reactions, drug–drug interactions or other events that require TDM occur. [#]: as suggested by the American Thoracic Society/CDC/Infectious Diseases Society of America [38]; [¶]: in case of re-treatment.

Sampling procedures, sampling time and specimens

Traditionally, plasma samples for TDM are collected 2 and 6 h after drug intake [1]. This will provide information on an estimated C_{max} and potential delayed absorption. This strategy is not suitable for pharmacokinetic/pharmacodynamic-based dose optimisation for most drugs as the total drug exposure (AUC) cannot be estimated. Limited sampling strategies using two or three selected time-points based on population pharmacokinetics data enable a more precise estimation of the drug exposure. Limited sampling strategies have been developed for several anti-TB drugs that can be applied in routine care [11, 60–64]. Other types of specimens, such as dried blood spots or saliva, may replace plasma samples for reasons that include sample stability and patient-friendly sample collection [65, 66].

Assay

Several analytical techniques can be employed to measure drug concentrations. High-performance liquid chromatography coupled with an ultraviolet detector (HPLC-UV) is a relatively easy, affordable technique. A range of assays have been published to support TDM of anti-TB drugs. Liquid chromatography coupled with tandem mass spectrometry (LC-MS/MS) is nowadays the preferred method due to its higher sensitivity and specificity [67]. Multianalyte assays are easier and more cost-effective when performed using LC-MS/MS compared with HPLC-UV because extensive sample preparation and long run times can be avoided. In addition, LC-MS/MS can also be used for dried blood spot analysis because of its higher sensitivity compared with HPLC-UV. External quality control by means of participation in a laboratory proficiency programme will ensure that adequate performance can be guaranteed [68].

Setting up a therapeutic drug monitoring protocol

Setting up a TDM protocol requires background information on the local setting. It is likely that, because of budget limitations, TDM in selected patients is the most cost-effective strategy [48]. A TB referral hospital with complicated cases probably has more patients that qualify for TDM than a TB outpatient clinic mainly treating uncomplicated DS-TB. Including a TDM protocol in a local or national TB treatment programme will help to guide healthcare workers in performing TDM [69]. Indications for TDM, drugs for which TDM can be performed, plasma or DBS sampling strategies, reference values, dose adjustment strategies and where the samples can be analysed should be included in any protocol. It seems logical to follow the same strategy for TDM as for other diagnostic procedures. A strategy (figure 3) including local, regional and central facilities for TDM has been described by GHIMIRE et al. [70]. As TDM requires at least some insight into pharmacology, pharmacokinetics and pharmacodynamics, it seems logical that local expertise should be established and maintained, e.g. by attending postgraduate courses on TB pharmacology.

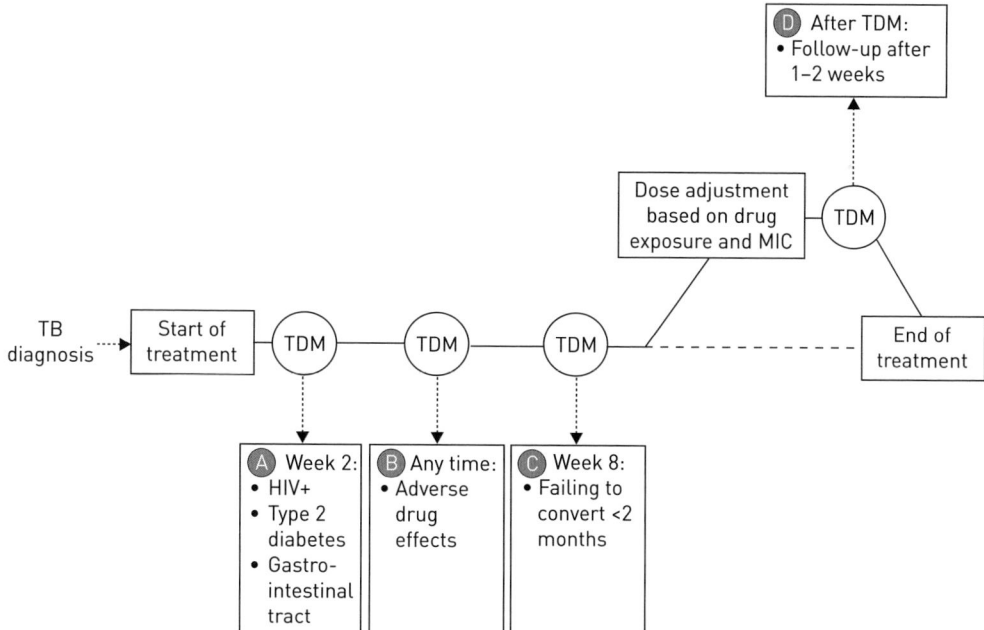

Figure 3. TDM in a programmatic setting. During treatment, TDM should be initiated by patient characteristics potentially resulting in reduced drug exposure (A), adverse drug effects that may happen at any point in time during treatment (B) or patients failing to convert their sputum (microscopy and/or culture) within 2 months (C). Dose adjustment should be followed by verification if drug exposure is adequate (D). Reproduced from [69] with permission.

Ensuring treatment has been effective

Early monitoring of TB treatment is particularly concerned with safety, whether the patient can tolerate the drugs used and whether the organism is sensitive to the chosen regimen. Drug levels may also be reduced in those who consume >40 g alcohol per week [71], take concomitant food [72] or have DM [73]. Late (≥2 months) monitoring of TB treatment is particularly concerned with treatment efficacy and cure.

The 2-month medical appointment

The attendance 2 months after the start of treatment is a turning point in the treatment of TB, whether fully sensitive or drug resistant. Close attention at this stage will prevent the development of drug resistance.

With fully sensitive TB, the decision is whether the intensive regimen can be converted to the two-drug regimen of rifampicin and isoniazid in the continuation phase. The aim is to prevent drug resistance and ensure a good outcome (table 4).

The majority will show a good response to standard treatment [74]. A poor response to treatment is indicated by persistence of symptoms, lack of weight gain, positive sputum smear or culture after 2 months of treatment and failure for either the chest radiograph in PTB or inflammatory markers in EPTB to improve. If the response to treatment is poor,

Table 4. The 2-month appointment

Area of assessment	Evidence required
Adherence	Urine test for rifampicin Patient's understanding of treatment Directly observed therapy charts inspected or tablet counts on unscheduled visits Tablets are correct and right number are taken Tablets taken 30–60 min before breakfast [72] No missed doses No missed appointments
Adverse effects	LFTs if any symptom Snellen/Jaegar charts and/or Ishihara test (for ethambutol and linezolid) Rash or itching? Nausea?
Response to treatment	Symptoms improved Weight gain (except extrathoracic lymph node TB) Chest radiograph improved or now normal Sputum smear-negative
DST	Test results viewed Regimen corresponded to resistance pattern, if any
Other considerations	HIV test result seen Alcohol excess? Other medication (legal and other) checked Pregnancy? Symptoms of pyridoxine antagonism Symptoms of vitamin D deficiency

                                        https://doi.org/10.1183/2312508X.10022217

then the evidence of adherence should be re-investigated [75]. Without a good response to treatment, if SAT had been used, then DOT should be started immediately. A sputum sample or material from the site of disease should be sent again for genetic and microbiological analysis. The marked variation of rifampicin levels after ingestion [76, 77] is a surprisingly common reason for failure to improve. In terms of drug regimen, an informed decision based on phenotypic DST and/or whole-genome sequencing is always better than an empirical regimen [78, 79]. All four drugs in the standard RHZE regimen should be continued until DST is available. A SINGLE DRUG SHOULD NEVER BE ADDED TO A FAILING REGIMEN. Some may add an injectable agent and fluoroquinolone when treatment response is poor, while awaiting the results of the DST [38].

The 2-month appointment may be the first occasion that drug resistance comes to light. The DST results should be checked against the regimen. In any patient with isoniazid resistance, rifampicin levels should be measured to ensure that MDR-TB does not arise. If moxifloxacin is used, then measurement of the levels of this drug is also important, as the 400 mg tablet does not readily produce the serum levels required (3–5 mg·L^{-1}) [1]. If there is MDR-TB, the poor bactericidal effect of pyrazinamide means that resistance to both pyrazinamide and ethambutol is likely if a standard RHZE regimen has been used [80]. A new sample from the site of disease must be sent for genetic and microbiological analysis, and the new regimen planned on the basis of these results. In patients with MDR-TB [4], in addition to the aforementioned routine monitoring, a further sample for microbiological analysis and DST is essential [17].

End of treatment

The appointment at the end of treatment is the next step in confirming efficacy. This is most commonly at 6 months for fully sensitive TB or 9–12 months for isoniazid-resistant TB. Monitoring for microbiological conversion in MDR-TB should have occurred monthly during the intensive phase and on at least three occasions during the continuation phase, together with an end-of-treatment sample.

Evidence of a response to treatment is essential. Items from table 4 can be used in addition to microbiological evidence of a cure. The latter is more difficult in those with EPTB, where inflammatory markers such as CRP can be used as a surrogate. If the chest radiograph remains abnormal, the disease was extrapulmonary or there was any drug resistance, then follow-up is required to ensure a cure. Epidemiologists use treatment completion as a marker of success for the process of treatment, but this is unacceptable to patients and clinicians, whose concerns are for a cure. This is especially important in those with MDR-TB, where relapse is much more common than with DS-TB. Relapse was included in the early Laserson criteria [81] and has a considerable impact on the outcome assessment [82].

Monitoring for relapse

In patients with fully sensitive PTB, those with a normal chest radiograph do not require any follow-up. However, for those with an abnormal chest radiograph at the end of treatment, a 2-month appointment with a further chest radiograph is reasonable. This is about the time that a positive sputum culture might be expected to develop if relapse were to occur. Clinical judgement should determine whether further follow-up, *e.g.* at 6 months and 1 year after treatment completion, is warranted. In most cases the chest radiograph shows further improvement with more linear than fluffy shadowing and further follow-up is not required. Relapse is defined as obtaining a positive culture 1–2 years after treatment completion; there should be genetic identity with the initial strain [83].

For patients with EPTB, the efficacy of the standard RHZE regimen is such that they also do not require any follow-up, although they should be asked to contact the TB team if they have further symptoms. Extrathoracic lymph node enlargement is relatively common after treatment completion, due to immune reconstitution inflammatory syndrome, and no further treatment should be given unless a positive culture is obtained (steroids can be given; most commonly the lymph node is removed as part of the diagnostic process) [84]. Some have suggested that positron emission tomography scanning can be used to indicate relapse, most notably in spinal TB, but continued inflammation towards dead bacilli, whose cell walls and some proteins are especially difficult for macrophages to digest, rather than recurrence of live TB is the more common cause of a positive scan and re-treatment should only be instigated with a positive TB culture.

For MDR-TB, concerns about relapse are especially problematic. As noted earlier, microbiological evidence of relapse is required, especially as new patterns of resistance may determine the nature of an effective regimen. In pulmonary disease, a CT scan at treatment completion is especially helpful to compare with a CT at 1 or 2 years after the end of treatment (table 1). This can direct the physician to an area for bronchoscopic examination if standard sputum culture does not confirm the clinical suspicion of relapse.

Conclusion

Before the start of TB treatment, a baseline assessment should be made against which subsequent measurements during treatment will detect improvement or worsening of the patient's condition. During the first 2 weeks, an effective regimen must be established and the patient made aware of the importance of continuing treatment for the full course.

Patients who are not doing well on standard treatment, *e.g.* lack of response or serious adverse drugs reactions, may benefit from TDM. Patients with expected problems in drug absorption, distribution, metabolism or excretion may also benefit. TDM for some drugs may be indicated for all patients because of toxicity (linezolid or aminoglycosides) or risk for acquired drug resistance (fluoroquinolones). A framework including dried blood spot analysis and limited sampling can be implemented to facilitate programmatic TDM.

To assess treatment response, the 2-month sputum test is an important time-point for decision making during treatment, *i.e.* TDM and change in regimen. Confirmation of treatment response at the end of treatment and the absence of relapse over at least the ensuing 12 months is essential to determine cure.

References

1. Alsultan A, Peloquin C. Therapeutic drug monitoring in the treatment of tuberculosis: an update. *Drugs* 2014; 74: 839–854.
2. Zuur MA, Bolhuis MS, Anthony RM, *et al.* Current status and opportunities for therapeutic drug monitoring in the treatment of tuberculosis. *Expert Opin Drug Metab Toxicol* 2016; 12: 509–521.

https://doi.org/10.1183/2312508X.10022217

3. Caminero JA, Lasserra P, Piubello A, et al. Adverse anti-tuberculosis drugs events and their management. In: Migliori GB, Bothamley G, Duarte R, et al. eds. Tuberculosis (ERS Monograph). Sheffield, European Respiratory Society, 2018; pp. 205–227.

4. Caminero JA, Scardigli A, van der Werf T, et al. Treatment of drug-susceptible and drug-resistant tuberculosis. In: Migliori GB, Bothamley G, Duarte R, et al. eds. Tuberculosis (ERS Monograph). Sheffield, European Respiratory Society, 2018; pp. 152–178.

5. Tagliani E, Nikolayevskyy V, Tortoli E, et al. Laboratory diagnosis. In: Migliori GB, Bothamley G, Duarte R, et al. eds. Tuberculosis (ERS Monograph). Sheffield, European Respiratory Society, 2018; pp. 99–115.

6. Chesov D, Botnaru V. Imaging for diagnosis and management. In: Migliori GB, Bothamley G, Duarte R, et al. eds. Tuberculosis (ERS Monograph). Sheffield, European Respiratory Society, 2018; pp. 116–136.

7. Zellweger J-P, Sousa P, Heyckendorf J. Clinical diagnosis. In: Migliori GB, Bothamley G, Duarte R, et al. eds. Tuberculosis (ERS Monograph). Sheffield, European Respiratory Society, 2018; pp. 83–98.

8. Nardell E, Volchenkov G. Transmission and control: a refocussed approach. In: Migliori GB, Bothamley G, Duarte R, et al. eds. Tuberculosis (ERS Monograph). Sheffield, European Respiratory Society, 2018; pp. 364–380.

9. Boehme CC, Nabeta P, Hillemann D, et al. Rapid molecular detection of tuberculosis and rifampin resistance. N Engl J Med 2010; 363: 1005–1015.

10. Fregonese F, Ahuja SD, Akkerman OW, et al. Comparison of different treatments for isoniazid-resistant tuberculosis: an individual patient data meta-analysis. Lancet Respir Med 2018; 6: 265–275.

11. Kamp J, Bolhuis MS, Tiberi S, et al. Simple strategy to assess linezolid exposure in patients with multi-drug-resistant and extensively-drug-resistant tuberculosis. Int J Antimicrob Agents 2017; 49: 688–694.

12. Bolhuis MS, Tiberi S, De Lorenzo S, et al. Linezolid tolerability in multidrug-resistant tuberculosis: a retrospective study. Eur Respir J 2015; 46: 1205–1207.

13. Mehta RL, Kellum JA, Shah SV, et al. Acute Kidney Injury Network: report of an initiative to improve outcomes in acute kidney injury. Crit Care 2007; 11: R31.

14. Chang C-H, Chen Y-F, Wu V-C, et al. Acute kidney injury due to anti-tuberculosis drugs: a five-year experience in an aging population. BMC Infect Dis 2014; 14: 23.

15. Saukkonen JJ, Cohn DL, Jasmer RM, et al. An official ATS statement: hepatotoxicity of antituberculosis therapy. Am J Respir Crit Care Med 2006; 174: 935–952.

16. Bénichou C. Criteria of drug-induced liver disorders. Report of an International Consensus Meeting. J Hepatol 1990; 11: 272–276.

17. Lange C, Abubakar I, Alffenaar J-WC, et al. Management of patients with multidrug-resistant/extensively drug-resistant tuberculosis in Europe: a TBNET consensus statement. Eur Respir J 2014; 44: 23–63.

18. Smedema J, Katjitae I, Reuter H, et al. Twelve-lead electrocardiography in tuberculous pericarditis. Cardiovasc J S Afr 2001; 12: 31–34.

19. Pranger AD, Van Altena R, Aarnoutse RE, et al. Evaluation of moxifloxacin for the treatment of tuberculosis: 3 years of experience. Eur Respir J 2011; 38: 888–894.

20. Nguyen TVA, Cao TBT, Akkerman OW, et al. Bedaquiline as part of combination therapy in adults with pulmonary multi-drug resistant tuberculosis. Expert Rev Clin Pharmacol 2016; 9: 1025–1037.

21. Bhargava A, Chatterjee M, Jain Y, et al. Nutritional status of adult patients with pulmonary tuberculosis in rural central India and its association with mortality. PLoS One 2013; 8: e77979.

22. Dheda K, Barry CE, Maartens G. Tuberculosis. Lancet 2016; 387: 1211–1226.

23. Cederholm T, Barazzoni R, Austin P, et al. ESPEN guidelines on definitions and terminology of clinical nutrition. Clin Nutr 2017; 36: 49–64.

24. Hasenbosch RE, Alffenaar JWC, Koopmans SA, et al. Ethambutol-induced optical neuropathy: risk of overdosing in obese subjects. Int J Tuberc Lung Dis 2008; 12: 967–971.

25. Alffenaar J-W, Van Der Werf T. Dosing ethambutol in obese patients. Antimicrob Agents Chemother 2010; 54: 4044–4045.

26. Masuka JT, Chipangura P, Nyambayo PP, et al. A comparison of adverse drug reaction profiles in patients on antiretroviral and antitubercular treatment in Zimbabwe. Clin Drug Investig 2018; 38: 9–17.

27. Magis-Escurra C, Carvalho ACC, Kritski AL, et al. Comorbidities. In: Migliori GB, Bothamley G, Duarte R, et al. eds. Tuberculosis (ERS Monograph). Sheffield, European Respiratory Society, 2018; pp. 276–290.

28. Kim WS, Lee SS, Lee CM, et al. Hepatitis C and not Hepatitis B virus is a risk factor for anti-tuberculosis drug induced liver injury. BMC Infect Dis 2016; 16: 50.

29. De Castro L, do Brasil PE, Monteiro TP, et al. Can hepatitis B virus infection predict tuberculosis treatment liver toxicity? Development of a preliminary prediction rule. Int J Tuberc Lung Dis 2010; 14: 332–340.

30. Daskapan A, De Lange WCM, Akkerman OW, et al. The role of therapeutic drug monitoring in individualised drug dosage and exposure measurement in tuberculosis and HIV co-infection. Eur Respir J 2015; 45: 569–571.

31. Lachmandas E, Thiem K, van den Heuvel C, et al. Patients with type 1 diabetes mellitus have impaired IL-1β production in response to Mycobacterium tuberculosis. Eur J Clin Microbiol Infect Dis 2018; 37: 371–380.

https://doi.org/10.1183/2312508X.10022217

32. Lachmandas E, Van Den Heuvel CNAM, Damen MSMA, *et al.* Diabetes mellitus and increased tuberculosis susceptibility: the role of short-chain fatty acids. *J Diabetes Res* 2016; 2016: 6014631.

33. van Crevel R, van de Vijver S, Moore DAJ. The global diabetes epidemic: what does it mean for infectious diseases in tropical countries? *Lancet Diabetes Endocrinol* 2017; 5: 457–468.

34. Leung CC, Yew WW, Mok TYW, *et al.* Effects of diabetes mellitus on the clinical presentation and treatment response in tuberculosis. *Respirology* 2017; 22: 1225–1232.

35. Perrin FMR, Woodward N, Phillips PPJ, *et al.* Radiological cavitation, sputum mycobacterial load and treatment response in pulmonary tuberculosis. *Int J Tuberc Lung Dis* 2010; 14: 1596–1602.

36. Munsiff S, Nilsen D, Fujiwara P. Clinical Policies and Protocols; Bureau of Tuberculosis Control. New York City Department of Health and Mental Hygiene. 4th Edn. 2008. www1.nyc.gov/assets/doh/downloads/pdf/tb/tb-protocol.pdf Date last accessed: September 12, 2018.

37. National Institute for Health Care and Excellence. Tuberculosis: NICE Guideline NG33. 2016. www.nice.org.uk/guidance/ng33/resources/tuberculosis-pdf-1837390683589 Date last accessed: September 12, 2018.

38. Nahid P, Dorman SE, Alipanah N, *et al.* Official American Thoracic Society/Centers for Disease Control and Prevention/Infectious Diseases Society of America Clinical Practice Guidelines: Treatment of Drug-Susceptible Tuberculosis. *Clin Infect Dis* 2016; 63: e147–e195.

39. Joint Tuberculosis Committee of the British Thoracic Society. Chemotherapy and management of tuberculosis in the United Kingdom: recommendations 1998. *Thorax* 1998; 53: 536–548.

40. Sharma SK, Singla R, Sarda P, *et al.* Safety of 3 different reintroduction regimens of antituberculosis drugs after development of antituberculosis treatment-induced hepatotoxicity. *Clin Infect Dis* 2010; 50: 833–839.

41. Mouton JW, Dudley MN, Cars O, *et al.* Standardization of pharmacokinetic/pharmacodynamic (PK/PD) terminology for anti-infective drugs: an update. *J Antimicrob Chemother* 2005; 55: 601–607.

42. Pasipanodya JG, Srivastava S, Gumbo T. Meta-analysis of clinical studies supports the pharmacokinetic variability hypothesis for acquired drug resistance and failure of antituberculosis therapy. *Clin Infect Dis* 2012; 55: 169–177.

43. Chideya S, Winston CA, Peloquin CA, *et al.* Isoniazid, rifampin, ethambutol, and pyrazinamide pharmacokinetics and treatment outcomes among a predominantly HIV-infected cohort of adults with tuberculosis from Botswana. *Clin Infect Dis* 2009; 48: 1685–1694.

44. Gumbo T, Angulo-Barturen I, Ferrer-Bazaga S. Pharmacokinetic-pharmacodynamic and dose-response relationships of antituberculosis drugs: recommendations and standards for industry and academia. *J Infect Dis* 2015; 211: Suppl. 3, S96–S106.

45. Diacon AH, Donald PR. The early bactericidal activity of antituberculosis drugs. *Expert Rev Anti Infect Ther* 2014; 12: 223–237.

46. Gumbo T, Louie A, Deziel MR, *et al.* Pharmacodynamic evidence that ciprofloxacin failure against tuberculosis is not due to poor microbial kill but to rapid emergence of resistance. *Antimicrob Agents Chemother* 2005; 49: 3178–3181.

47. Alffenaar J-WC, Akkerman OW, Anthony RM, *et al.* Individualizing management of extensively drug-resistant tuberculosis: diagnostics, treatment, and biomarkers. *Expert Rev Anti Infect Ther* 2017; 15: 11–21.

48. Alffenaar J, Tiberi S, Verbeeck R, *et al.* Therapeutic drug monitoring in tuberculosis: practical application for physicians. *Clin Infect Dis* 2017; 64: 104–105.

49. Pasipanodya JG, McIlleron H, Burger A, *et al.* Serum drug concentrations predictive of pulmonary tuberculosis outcomes. *J Infect Dis* 2013; 208: 1464–1473.

50. Sotgiu G, Centis R, D'Ambrosio L, *et al.* Efficacy, safety and tolerability of linezolid containing regimens in treating MDR-TB and XDR-TB: systematic review and meta-analysis. *Eur Respir J* 2012; 40: 1430–1442.

51. Alffenaar JWC, Van Altena R, Harmelink IM, *et al.* Comparison of the pharmacokinetics of two dosage regimens of linezolid in multidrug-resistant and extensively drug-resistant tuberculosis patients. *Clin Pharmacokinet* 2010; 49: 559–565.

52. Court R, Wiesner L, Stewart A, *et al.* Steady state pharmacokinetics of cycloserine in patients on terizidone for multidrug-resistant tuberculosis. *Int J Tuberc Lung Dis* 2018; 22: 30–33.

53. Alffenaar JWC, Peloquin CA, Migliori GB. Making optimal use of available anti-tuberculosis drugs: first steps to investigate terizidone. *Int J Tuberc Lung Dis* 2018; 22: 2.

54. Van Altena R, Dijkstra JA, Van Der Meer ME, *et al.* Reduced chance of hearing loss associated with therapeutic drug monitoring of aminoglycosides in the treatment of multidrug-resistant tuberculosis. *Antimicrob Agents Chemother* 2017; 61: e01400-16.

55. Cegielski JP, Kurbatova E, Van Der Walt M, *et al.* Multidrug-resistant tuberculosis treatment outcomes in relation to treatment and initial versus acquired second-line drug resistance. *Clin Infect Dis* 2015; 62: 418–430.

56. Ershova JV, Kurbatova EV, Moonan PK, *et al.* Mortality among tuberculosis patients with acquired resistance to second-line antituberculosis drugs – United States, 1993–2008. *Clin Infect Dis* 2014; 59: 465–472.

57. Cegielski J, Dalton T, Yagui M, *et al.* Extensive drug resistance acquired during treatment of multidrug-resistant tuberculosis. *Clin Infect Dis* 2014; 59: 1049–1063.

58. Alffenaar J-WC, Gumbo T, Aarnoutse RE. Acquired drug resistance: we can do more than we think! *Clin Infect Dis* 2015; 60: 969–970.

https://doi.org/10.1183/2312508X.10022217

59. Forsman LD, Bruchfeld J, Alffenaar J-WC. Therapeutic drug monitoring to prevent acquired drug resistance of fluoroquinolones in the treatment of tuberculosis. *Eur Respir J* 2017; 49: 1700317.

60. Dijkstra JA, van Altena R, Akkerman OW, *et al.* Limited sampling strategies for therapeutic drug monitoring of amikacin and kanamycin in patients with multidrug-resistant tuberculosis. *Int J Antimicrob Agents* 2015; 46: 332–337.

61. Magis-Escurra C, Later-Nijland HM, Alffenaar JW, *et al.* Population pharmacokinetics and limited sampling strategy for first-line tuberculosis drugs and moxifloxacin. *Int J Antimicrob Agents* 2014; 44: 229–234.

62. van Rijn SP, Zuur MA, van Altena R, *et al.* Pharmacokinetic modeling and limited sampling strategies based on healthy volunteers for monitoring of ertapenem in MDR-TB patients. *Antimicrob Agents Chemother* 2017; 61: e01783-16.

63. Sturkenboom MGG, Mulder LW, de Jager A, *et al.* Pharmacokinetic modeling and optimal sampling strategies for therapeutic drug monitoring of rifampin in patients with tuberculosis. *Antimicrob Agents Chemother* 2015; 59: 4907–4913.

64. Alsultan A, An G, Peloquin CA. Limited sampling strategy and target attainment analysis for levofloxacin in patients with tuberculosis. *Antimicrob Agents Chemother* 2015; 59: 3800–3807.

65. Vu DH, Alffenaar JWC, Edelbroek PM, *et al.* Dried blood spots: a new tool for tuberculosis treatment optimization. *Curr Pharm Des* 2011; 17: 2931–2939.

66. van den Elsen S, Oostenbrink L, Heysell S, *et al.* A systematic review of salivary versus blood concentrations of anti-tuberculosis drugs and their potentials for salivary therapeutic drug monitoring. *Ther Drug Monit* 2018; 40: 17–37.

67. Veringa A, Sturkenboom MGG, Dekkers BGJ, *et al.* LC-MS/MS for therapeutic drug monitoring of anti-infective drugs. *Trends Anal Chem* 2016; 84: 34–40.

68. Aarnoutse R. An interlaboratory quality control programme for the measurement of tuberculosis drugs. *Eur Respir J* 2015; 46: 268–271.

69. van der Burgt EPM, Sturkenboom MGG, Bolhuis MS, *et al.* End TB with precision treatment! *Eur Respir J* 2016; 47: 680–682.

70. Ghimire S, Bolhuis MS, Sturkenboom MGG, *et al.* Incorporating therapeutic drug monitoring into the World Health Organization hierarchy of tuberculosis diagnostics! *Eur Respir J* 2016; 47: 1867–1869.

71. Koriakin V, Sokolova G, Grinchar N, *et al.* [Pharmacokinetics of isoniazid in patients with tuberculosis and alcoholism]. *Probl Tuberk* 1986; 12: 43–46.

72. Saktiawati AMI, Sturkenboom MGG, Stienstra Y, *et al.* Impact of food on the pharmacokinetics of first-line anti-TB drugs in treatment-naive TB patients: a randomized cross-over trial. *J Antimicrob Chemother* 2016; 71: 703–710.

73. Kumar AK, Chandrasekaran V, Kannan T, *et al.* Anti-tuberculosis drug concentrations in tuberculosis patients with and without diabetes mellitus. *Eur J Clin Pharmacol* 2017; 73: 65–70.

74. Al-Moamary MS, Black W, Bessuille E, *et al.* The significance of the persistent presence of acid-fast bacilli in sputum smears in pulmonary tuberculosis. *Chest* 1999; 116: 726–731.

75. International Union against Tuberculosis and Lung Disease. Antituberculosis regimens of chemotherapy: recommendations from the committee on treatment of the International Union against Tuberculosis and Lung Disease. *Bull IUATLD* 1988; 63: 60–64.

76. Prahl JB, Johansen IS, Cohen AS, *et al.* Clinical significance of 2 h plasma concentrations of first-line anti-tuberculosis drugs: a prospective observational study. *J Antimicrob Chemother* 2014; 69: 2841–2847.

77. Boeree MJ, Diacon AH, Dawson R, *et al.* A dose-ranging trial to optimize the dose of rifampin in the treatment of tuberculosis. *Am J Respir Crit Care Med* 2015; 191: 1058–1065.

78. World Health Organization. WHO Treatment Guidelines for Drug-resistant Tuberculosis 2106 Update. Geneva, WHO, 2016.

79. Falzon D, Schünemann HJ, Harausz E, *et al.* World Health Organization treatment guidelines for drug-resistant tuberculosis, 2016 update. *Eur Respir J* 2017; 49: 1602308.

80. World Health Organization. Guidelines for the Programmatic Management of Drug-resistant Tuberculosis: 2011 Update. Geneva, WHO, 2011.

81. Laserson KF, Thorpe LE, Leimane V, *et al.* Speaking the same language: treatment outcome definitions for multidrug-resistant tuberculosis. *Int J Tuberc Lung Dis* 2005; 9: 640–645.

82. Günther G, Lange C, Alexandru S, *et al.* Treatment outcomes in multidrug-resistant tuberculosis. *N Engl J Med* 2016: 1194–1195.

83. Bryant JM, Harris SR, Parkhill J, *et al.* Whole-genome sequencing to establish relapse or re-infection with *Mycobacterium tuberculosis*: a retrospective observational study. *Lancet Respir Med* 2013; 1: 786–792.

84. Brown CS, Smith CJ, Breen RAMC, *et al.* Determinants of treatment-related paradoxical reactions during anti-tuberculosis therapy: a case control study. *BMC Infect Dis* 2016; 16: 479.

Disclosures: None declared.

Chapter 19

Sequelae assessment and rehabilitation

Marcela Muñoz-Torrico[1], Silvia Cid-Juárez[2], Susana Galicia-Amor[3], Thierry Troosters[4,5] and Antonio Spanevello[6,7]

Despite multiple WHO strategies aimed at reducing TB burden, it remains a major cause of death worldwide. However, dyspnoea and disability caused by PTB sequelae are often neglected when managing TB.

Investigating TB sequelae with pulmonary function tests is mandatory after treatment completion. Pulmonary function tests allow the clinician to evaluate the residual lung function, and determine the mechanism of lung damage involved and the severity of pulmonary impairment. The tests also allow prediction of the patients at risk of surgical complications and death.

Pulmonary rehabilitation plays a key role in the treatment of PTB sequelae. Pulmonary rehabilitation is an individualised and multidisciplinary approach (consisting of muscle training, education, behavioural change, respiratory physiotherapy and nutritional support) aimed at improving quality of life and reducing surgical complications in candidates for surgery. Due to the enormous impact this intervention has on the physical and psychological wellbeing, it is recommended in all patients with pulmonary impairment after TB treatment.

Cite as: Muñoz-Torrico M, Cid-Juárez S, Galicia-Amor S, et al. Sequelae assessment and rehabilitation. In: Migliori GB, Bothamley G, Duarte R, et al., eds. Tuberculosis (ERSMonograph). Sheffield, European Respiratory Society, 2018; pp. 326–342 [https://doi.org/10.1183/2312508X.10022317].

@ERSpublications
Pulmonary function after TB treatment should be fully evaluated with lung function tests and standardized quality of life questionnaires. Problems with symptoms, functional status and quality of life often persist and can be tackled with rehabilitation.
http://ow.ly/cfVQ30lqCfE

Since the 1980s, highly effective anti-TB treatment has been available; however, pharmacological treatment cannot prevent lung remodelling. Lung remodelling refers to

[1]Tuberculosis Clinic, Instituto Nacional de Enfermedades Respiratorias, Mexico City, Mexico. [2]Physiology Dept, Instituto Nacional de Enfermedades Respiratorias, Mexico City, Mexico. [3]Pulmonary Rehabilitation Dept, Instituto Nacional de Enfermedades Respiratorias, Mexico City, Mexico. [4]Dept of Rehabilitation Sciences, KU Leuven, Leuven, Belgium. [5]Pulmonary Rehabilitation, UZ Gasthuisberg, Leuven, Belgium. [6]Istituti Clinici Scientifici Maugeri IRCCS, Pavia, Italy. [7]Dept of Clinical and Experimental Medicine, University of Insubria, Varese, Italy.

Correspondence: Marcela Muñoz-Torrico, Tuberculosis Clinic, Instituto Nacional de Enfermedades Respiratorias Ismael Cosio Villegas, Calzada de Tlalpan 4502, Colonia Seccion XVI, Tlalpan, Mexico City, Mexico. E-mail: dra_munoz@iner.gob.mx

Copyright ©ERS 2018. Print ISBN: 978-1-84984-099-6. Online ISBN: 978-1-84984-100-9. Print ISSN: 2312-508X. Online ISSN: 2312-5098.

anatomical and structural changes (not necessarily reversible) after pharmacological treatment; it is due to the destruction of the extracellular matrix supporting the pulmonary functional units. Pulmonary remodelling after TB treatment includes the presence of residual cavitations, bronchiectasis, pulmonary fibrosis or scarring, leading to the distortion of the pulmonary architecture and, therefore, to the loss of volume [1, 2]. TB sequelae may also lead to further complications, such as the development of aspergilloma and massive haemoptysis. By far the most common complication after TB treatment is the development of bronchiectasis, particularly in developing countries [3]. Extensive TB sequelae may also lead to a completely destroyed lung, which has a poor prognosis, especially in patients with extensive lung destruction [4].

The severity of lung destruction is variable, being related to several factors including local immune response, individual patient response and infecting strain [2]. Moreover, a delay in diagnosis and specific treatment initiation may also contribute to lung damage and higher risk of chronic respiratory disease [5]. This gap between early diagnosis and treatment initiation is particularly important in DR-TB cases.

Follow-up and functional evaluation of TB patients who complete treatment has been ignored as part of clinical care; therefore, few studies have addressed this issue. The first comprehensive review of the literature on TB sequelae and rehabilitation provided clear evidence that TB is definitively responsible for lung function impairment [6].

Unfortunately, the majority of the available studies partially addressed this issue. Therefore, there is a need for more research in order to understand the physiopathology of lung damage, its impact on quality of life and the potential role of pulmonary rehabilitation on these patients [6].

The aim of this chapter is to discuss the available literature on the impact of TB on lung function after pharmacological treatment completion, its effect on quality of life and the rationale for pulmonary rehabilitation on these patients, and finally, to discuss the principles of personalising the rehabilitation programme according to the type and severity of the lung damage.

Methods

For this chapter, we carried out a nonsystematic review of the literature based on a PubMed search. Only manuscripts written in English and Spanish were selected.

We specifically searched for studies describing 1) the epidemiology of impaired lung function post-TB treatment, and 2) pulmonary lung function and rehabilitation programme in post-TB treatment patients, using specific words and combinations, including "tuberculosis", "rehabilitation programme", "chronic pulmonary disease", "obstructive lung disease" and "lung volume measurements", without time limitations.

The main areas of focus were: 1) pulmonary function in TB and evaluation of TB sequelae; 2) quality of life after TB treatment; and 3) pulmonary rehabilitation interventions.

https://doi.org/10.1183/2312508X.10022317

Pulmonary function in tuberculosis and evaluation of tuberculosis sequelae

Patients with active PTB are 5.4 (95% CI 2.98–9.68, p<0.001) times more likely to have abnormal pulmonary function test results compared to individuals with LTBI [7]. In various population-based studies, history of PTB has been associated with chronic cough, which is a predictor of chronic bronchitis and chronic airflow obstruction in nonsmokers [8–11]. Moreover, the loss of lung function was associated with the number of TB episodes; thus, the importance of early detection and prevention of relapses is of paramount importance to prevent further lung damage [12].

At present, TB sequelae are a well-recognised independent risk factor for the development of COPD, particularly in young adults (<40 years) [13]. Obviously, this risk increases if associated with cigarette smoking and air pollution (indoor and outdoor).

Unfortunately, to date, only few studies have investigated the lung function of patients with TB sequelae, usually by means of a simple spirometry. The most prevalent alteration in this population is airflow limitation without a response to a bronchodilator test [6], due to sequelae affecting the airways both at the peripheral and central level (bronchiectasis and tracheobronchial stenosis) [14–16].

The alterations of the lung parenchyma (cavities and pulmonary fibrosis) (figure 1) or at the pleural level (chronic empyema, fibrothorax, bronchopleural fistula and pneumothorax) usually produce restrictive alterations that may be of both pulmonary (with altered gas exchange) or extrapulmonary (with normal arterial gas exchange) origin. Finally, vascular complications such as pulmonary or bronchial arteritis, thrombosis, dilatation of bronchial arteries and Rasmussen aneurysm, or cor pulmonale may be present, and lead to altered gas exchange.

TB sequelae alter respiratory physiology in a variable manner (both from the mechanical and gas exchange sides), and limit daily life activities and exercise capacity, causing disability and deteriorated quality of life. Timely detection of these functional abnormalities

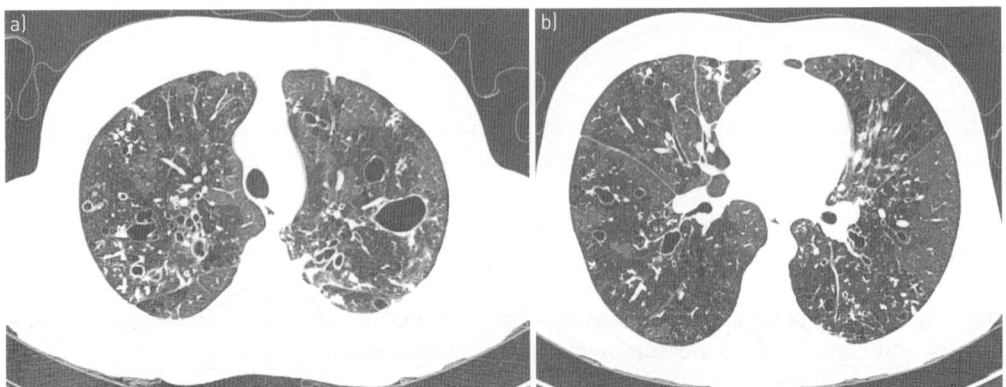

Figure 1. a and b) Chest computed tomography after 9 months of effective treatment in a 22-year-old female patient shows pulmonary sequelae as cavities; diffuse cyst bronchiectasis and mosaic attenuation pattern can be seen. This patient's lung function test results are shown in figures 2–4.

https://doi.org/10.1183/2312508X.10022317

would allow the clinician to assess the benefit of surgical treatment (*e.g.* in case of localised bronchiectasies or mycetmoma), of early initiating pharmacological treatment (bronchodilator or inhaled steroids), providing oxygen therapy and designing an adequate rehabilitation plan. The final goal of this approach is to allow the patient returning to daily life activities as soon as possible.

The proposed functional approach to TB sequelae is similar to that of any other chronic respiratory disease. Considering the necessary infection control measures to prevent transmission, respiratory functional evaluation can be performed without special precautions only once the patient is culture negative and/or TB treatment has been concluded with a positive outcome [17]. Pulmonary function tests can be performed under different conditions: 1) at rest (lung mechanics: spirometry with bronchodilator, diffusing capacity of the lung for carbon monoxide (D_{LCO}) (table 1) and arterial blood gases in all cases, and plethysmography at the initial evaluation if available) and 2) under exercise conditions (6-min walk test (6MWT) or cardiopulmonary exercise testing (CPET)), providing useful information on the physiological reserve (the results of which are associated with quality of life).

Spirometry

As previously stated, spirometry is the most widely used test to assess lung functional impairment and is the gold standard for airflow obstruction diagnosis (low forced expiratory volume in 1 s (FEV_1)/forced vital capacity (FVC) ratio) (table 1). However, when the FEV_1/FVC ratio is normal, vital capacity measurement (FVC) is useful as a lung volume measure. Low values of FEV_1 and FVC are also related to poor life expectancy [18]. The significant response to bronchodilator (increase in FEV_1 and/or FVC >12% and >200 mL) indicates the presence of air trapping [19, 20]. The majority of studies evaluating the response to a bronchodilator test (table 1) have shown that TB patients with sequelae behave as COPD patients do, without response to the bronchodilator test (figure 2); therefore, this condition has been considered a cause of COPD in nonsmokers [21, 22].

Body plethysmography

Body plethysmography is the gold standard to diagnose lung restriction (total lung capacity (TLC) is decreased); it can show the presence of air trapping (residual volume (RV) is high) and a mixed pattern (table 1) [23, 24]. However, plethysmography is not always available in all centres due to its high cost and its relatively complex management. It is not recommended as a follow-up test for restrictive pattern lung disease or air trapping since these can be assessed by spirometry when measuring FVC and bronchodilator response (figure 3). No study has used plethysmography to test TB patients so far.

Arterial blood gases

Arterial blood gas analysis is the gold standard test to diagnose hypoxaemia (arterial oxygen tension and S_{pO_2} are decreased) and hypoventilation (high arterial carbon dioxide tension (P_{aCO_2})), and to assess severity. These measurements may be altered in the presence of severe airflow obstruction, severe pulmonary restriction or pulmonary vascular disease. It is recommended to test arterial blood gases if the patient has S_{pO_2} <90% at rest or during exercise, or respiratory failure occurs (table 1) [24].

Table 1. Definitions of lung function test terms used in this chapter

Test	Definition
FEV1	Forced expiratory volume in 1 s; the total volume of air a patient is able to exhale in the first second using maximal effort.
FEV1 % pred	FEV1 expressed as a percentage of that predicted according to reference values.
FVC	Forced vital capacity; the total volume of air a patient is able to exhale for the total duration of the test using maximal effort.
FVC % pred	FVC expressed as a percentage of that predicted according to reference values.
FEV1/FVC	Percentage of the FVC expired in 1 s.
LLN	Lower limit of normal.
Bronchodilator test	The response to the bronchodilator should be evaluated 20–30 min after the administration of a short-acting β_2-agonist (salbutamol is the preferred); it is positive when there is an increase in FEV1 or FVC in adults of >12% and >200 mL.
TLC	Total lung capacity; the volume of air in the lungs at maximal inflation.
RV	Residual volume: gas volume at full expiration.
Obstructive pattern	Airflow limitation defined using spirometric tests results when the FEV1/FVC ratio is below a fixed cut-off (<70%, after GOLD) or the LLN (recommended) from reference equations that are based on values from a normal population.
Restrictive pattern	Reduced lung volumes defined as TLC <80% pred.
D_{LCO}	Diffusing capacity of the lung for carbon monoxide; measures the efficiency of the gas transfer characteristics of the lungs.
6MWD	6-min walking distance; a measure of the distance that an individual can walk as fast as possible on a hard, flat surface (usually 30-m corridor) for a period of 6 min; for interpretation, 6MWD should be compared with a mean predicted normal value and the LLN from reference equations.
CPET	Cardiopulmonary exercise testing; during CPET, the patient makes maximum effort to perform exercise. Usually, the CPET is carried out using a bicycle ergometer or treadmill. In an incremental protocol, the resistance is increased progressively and the test is limited by symptoms (the patient decides when to stop the test).
V'_{O_2max}	Maximal oxygen uptake; oxygen uptake attained during maximal exercise intensity that could not be increased despite further increases in exercise workload.
Sa_{O_2}, Sp_{O_2}	Arterial oxygen saturation; a measure of the amount of oxygen carried in the haemoglobin, measured by blood gas analysis or noninvasively by pulse oximetry.
Pa_{O_2}	Partial oxygen pressure in arterial blood.
Pa_{CO_2}	Partial carbon dioxide pressure in arterial blood.

GOLD: Global Initiative for Chronic Obstructive Lung disease.

Diffusing capacity of the lung for carbon monoxide

D_{LCO} assesses gas exchange at the pulmonary level and may be altered even when the respiratory mechanics tests (spirometry and plethysmography) are normal (figure 4). Its usefulness is variable, since it helps clinicians in the differential diagnosis of diseases with the same spirometric pattern. It is also abnormal or altered in pulmonary vascular diseases. Furthermore, D_{LCO} allows categorisation of the disease severity [25–27].

https://doi.org/10.1183/2312508X.10022317

a)

	Predicted	A1	A2	A3	A4	A5	A6	A7	A8	A9	A10	Best/predicted %
FVC L	3.81		2.29	1.98		2.45	2.58				2.58	68
FEV₁ L	3.33		1.31	1.30		1.35	1.36				1.36	41
FEV₁/FVC %			57.3	65.8		55.0	52.7				52.7	

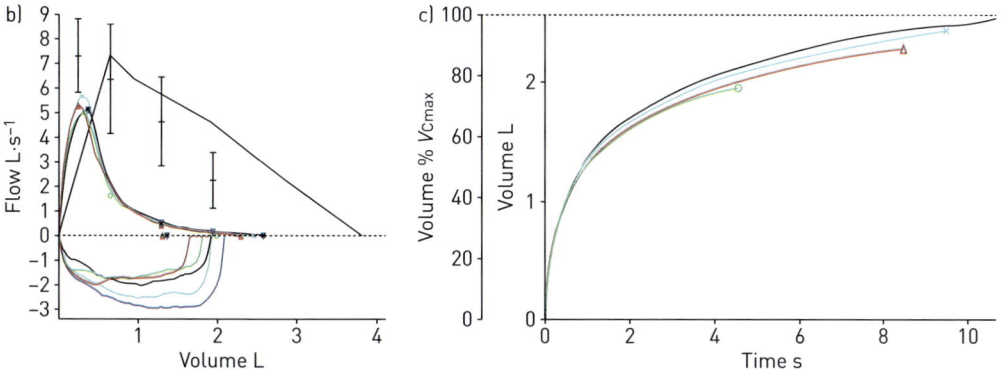

Figure 2. Forced spirometry shows severe obstruction without bronchodilation test response (forced expiratory volume in the 1 s (FEV1)/forced vital capacity (FVC) below the lower limit of normality and FEV1 <50% pred). a) Table shows measured volumes compared to predicted values; b) flow–volume curve and c) volume–time curve, both are characteristic of an obstructive pattern. VCmax: maximal vital capacity.

a)

	Predicted	Best	Best/predicted %	A1	A2	A3
ITGV L	2.74	4.59	167	4.53	4.59	4.62
RV L	1.40	4.26	303	4.37	4.28	4.28
VC L	3.86	2.36	61	2.23	2.24	2.36
IC L	2.53	2.03	80	2.08	1.93	2.03
ERV L	1.35	0.34	25	0.16	0.31	0.34
TLC L	5.17	6.62	128	6.61	6.53	6.64
RV/TLC %	27.5	64.30	234	66.2	65.6	64.4

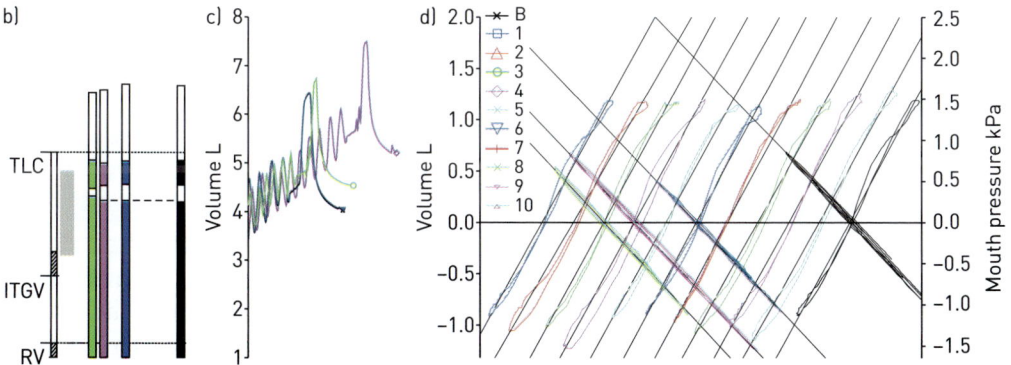

Figure 3. Body plethysmography with air trapping and hyperinflation (residual volume (RV) and total lung capacity (TLC) >120% pred). a) Table shows measured volumes compared to predicted values; b) spirogram bar graph of different lung volumes measured by body plethysmography; c) mouth pressure over shift volume during respiratory efforts for determination plethysmographic functional residual capacity and tracing of specific airway resistance loop. ITGV: intrathoracic gas volume; VC: vital capacity; IC: inspiratory capacity; ERV: expiratory reserve volume.

https://doi.org/10.1183/2312508X.10022317

a)

	Predicted	A1	A2	Best	Best/predicted %
T_{LCO} SB mL·min^{-1}·mmHg^{-1}	28.7	21.2145	21.3514	21.2745	74
V_A	5.02	3.97	4.01	3.99	79
T_{LCO}/V_A mmol·min^{-1}·kPa^{-1}·L^{-1}	1.86	1.79	1.79	1.79	96
RV/TLC-He %	27.5	32.4888	33.1437	32.8190	120
FRC/TLC-He %	49.1	42.33	45.54	43.94	89

b)

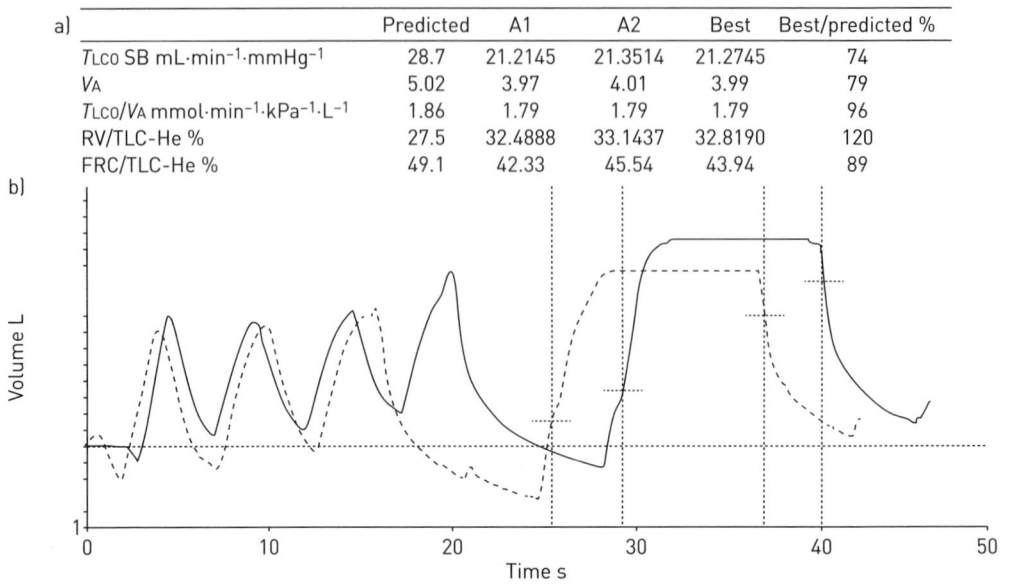

Figure 4. Mild transfer factor of the lung for carbon monoxide (T_{LCO}) decrease (<80% pred). In the same patient, on blood gas analysis, mild hypoxaemia was reported (oxygen tension 58.1 mmHg, oxygen saturation 89.8%) and 6-min walking distance was 564 m but oxygen saturation decresed to 84%. a) Table shows measured volumes compared to predicted values; b) T_{LCO} volume–time graph shows that the test accomplished quality criteria. SB: single breath; V_A: alveolar volume; RV: residual volume; TLC-He: total lung capacity by helium washout; FRC: functional residual capacity.

6-min walk test

6MWT is a simple and rapid test evaluating, in an integrated manner, the response of the respiratory, cardiovascular, metabolic, skeletal muscle and neurosensory systems to the stress imposed by the exercise (table 1). This distance in metres covered during 6 min correlates with quality of life and has prognostic value [28]. In addition, together with the measurement of the maximum oxygen consumption ($V'O_2$max), 6MWT is subject to improvement when a rehabilitation programme is carried out [29]. Few studies have used the 6MWT to study TB and TB sequelae patients, showing that the residual disability is still present at the completion of anti-TB chemotherapy, especially in MDR-TB patients [30, 31].

Cardiopulmonary exercise testing

With an incremental protocol, CPET can provide useful information on the mechanisms (respiratory: mechanical or gas exchange; cardiac and muscular) limiting the exercise capacity (table 1). Furthermore, it provides information on the cardiopulmonary reserve as well as a direct measurement of $V'O_2$max, which is a core parameter in the pre-operative assessment of surgical candidates. Based on this test, the patients whose $V'O_2$max is ≥20 mL·kg^{-1}·min^{-1} or ≥75% pred are considered at low risk of complications (7% respiratory morbidity). The patients at high risk of complications and post-operative death are those whose $V'O_2$max is ≤10 mL·kg^{-1}·min^{-1} or ≤40% of the predicted value (the respiratory morbidity being 90% and 13%, respectively) [32–34]. In patients undergoing

https://doi.org/10.1183/2312508X.10022317

pulmonary rehabilitation, $V'O_2$max can predict the exercise tolerance in the long term; it improves if the patients undergo an exercise programme [29].

CPET has been used to study patients with sequelae of TB. The test demonstrated these patients have ventilatory impairment (with a suboptimal increase in tidal volume and an increase in dead space) and gas exchange limitations (with increased haemoglobin desaturation and increased $PaCO_2$ during maximum effort). The response pattern is therefore very similar to that of COPD patients [35, 36].

Since the functional impairment after TB can be severe and disabling, it is recommended that all patients undergo a complete respiratory function evaluation regardless of the presence of respiratory symptoms.

Quality of life after tuberculosis treatment

Although there is no clear definition of the term "quality of life", the WHO defines it as the individual's perception of their position in life in the context of the culture and value systems in which they live and in relation to their goals, expectations, standards and concerns. It is a broad-ranging concept affected in a complex way by the person's physical health, psychological state, personal beliefs, social relationships and relationship to salient features of their environment.

As a result of lung destruction, PTB patients usually have persistent respiratory symptoms even after having completed treatment. Respiratory symptoms limit physical activities, which ultimately impacts on physical and psychological wellbeing, and therefore on the quality of life of those patients who are deemed to have been cured. Several studies have assessed the quality of life in patients with PTB at the beginning and end of treatment using generic questionnaires such as the 26-item Short Form health survey (SF-36). This questionnaire evaluates the physical and emotional wellbeing of the patients through eight different items; a simplified version of this questionnaire is also available (SF-12). Existing studies show that the patients' mental wellbeing is initially affected; patients experience a period of depression and anxiety (at diagnosis and when treatment starts), which usually improves during anti-TB treatment. In several studies, mental wellbeing has been associated with the patients' economic income: people with higher income have better scores compared to those with a lower one. Regarding physical wellbeing, although there is evident improvement in the patients' disease perception, the alteration in the quality of life can be seen even at the end of treatment [37–39].

The St George's Respiratory Questionnaire (SGRQ), a tool designed to measure health impairment in chronic respiratory diseases, has also been used to assess the impact of respiratory symptoms in patients with PTB sequelae. This questionnaire is composed of two parts: part 1 investigates the patients' recollection of symptoms over the preceding period (from 1 month to 1 year) while part 2 addresses the patients' current state. Using this questionnaire, it has been shown that patients with a history of active TB have significantly higher scores compared to individuals with LTBI. Furthermore, an inversely proportional relationship exists between the score in the SGRQ and the decreased lung function measured by simple spirometry [40].

The primary objective of TB control is to ensure early identification of active (infectious) cases and timely treatment to render them not infectious, thus cutting the chain of transmission. In the past, due to lack of resources, less attention was paid to individuals or forms of TB not able to transmit the disease (*e.g.* EPTB and TB in children). Similarly, little attention was given to TB patients after bacteriological cure. Unfortunately, in most cases, treatment completion may be the beginning of a new "disease". Using disability-adjusted life-years, PASIPANODYA *et al.* [41] demonstrated that pulmonary impairment after TB treatment contributes greatly (73%) to the disease burden. Therefore, it is important to assess the disease from all angles, including a complete functional evaluation, the quality of life assessment and the implementation of pharmacological and nonpharmacological measures, ideally within a pulmonary rehabilitation programme (PRP) [6].

Pulmonary rehabilitation of tuberculosis patients

PRPs for patients with chronic lung diseases are nonpharmacological strategies and have become an accepted approach in all chronic respiratory diseases including TB [6, 42].

The American Thoracic Society and the European Respiratory Society have defined pulmonary rehabilitation as "a comprehensive intervention based on a thorough patient assessment followed by patient tailored therapies that include, but are not limited to, exercise training, education, and behavior change, designed to improve the physical and psychological condition of people with chronic respiratory disease and to promote the long-term adherence to health-enhancing behaviors" [43].

The primary goal of a PRP is to improve patients' quality of life by targeting nonrespiratory consequences of chronic respiratory diseases, such as muscle disuse and deconditioning; educating patients about their disease and how to manage it (including symptom control, *e.g.* dyspnoea, fatigue and cough); and optimising functional capacity and social integration, thus improving the performance of daily life activities [44].

PRPs improve dyspnoea perception, exercise tolerance and health-related quality of life in patients suffering from COPD. Although there is less evidence [42], PRPs have also proven effective in other chronic respiratory diseases such as interstitial lung fibrosis, non-cystic fibrosis bronchiectasis and pulmonary hypertension, and also as support to the surgical approach [45, 46]. All of these can also be consequence of previous TB [6].

Most, if not all, reports in the literature are focused on rehabilitation of patients with post-TB sequelae. To the best of our knowledge, there is no reported literature on rehabilitative efforts during the acute phase of the disease [6].

During anti-TB treatment, the priority is to ensure symptom control and maintain mobility as much as possible, besides establishing high-quality pharmacological management. As long as TB is active, caution is necessary to prevent further infections; therefore, group sessions should be avoided and strict infection control measures need to be applied [16]. Active TB and its complications are not an uncommon cause of in-hospital and intensive care unit admission [47]. PRP is a useful tool in the multidisciplinary management of critically ill patients, especially those who are mechanically ventilated, as they develop muscle atrophy and loss of muscle mass [48, 49].

As pulmonary impairment and quality of life deterioration are described after TB treatment, PRP is likely to be beneficial, although few experiences and studies on this are reported in the literature [6].

https://doi.org/10.1183/2312508X.10022317

An 8-week, hospital-based PRP in eight patients assessed the impact on aerobic capacity and health-related quality of life measured by SF-36 and SGRQ. The study concluded that rehabilitation, even in a short-term programme, produced a significant improvement of both aerobic capacity and quality of life [50].

Since TB is more prevalent in economically disadvantaged settings, it should be recognised that "conventional" outpatient rehabilitation in specialised centres will often not be possible. Programmes may need to be adapted to the available logistics and community-based services. Nevertheless, the basic principle of having a multidisciplinary and individualised approach needs to be honoured. As an example, home-based PRP have been established, and evidence in COPD patients suggests that the benefit is similar to that of hospital-based PRPs [51–55]. A pilot study of a 6-week, home-based PRP including cardiovascular and low-impact exercises did not show significant improvements in exercise tolerance, symptoms or generic health status [56]. A more recent study described an experience of pulmonary rehabilitation implemented in an outpatient setting in Uganda. Significant improvements both in exercise tolerance and in health status were reported [57].

Overall only a handful of studies reported the effects of pulmonary rehabilitation in patients with post-TB sequelae [6]. These studies are summarised in table 2.

When compared to COPD patients, patients with PTB sequelae (including post-surgical patients) had no differences at baseline in their degree of disability. After a 9-week PRP (designed based on those for COPD) was offered to TB *versus* COPD patients matched by baseline 6-min walking distance (6MWD) performances, significant improvement in 6MWD, Medical Research Council dyspnoea grade, transition dyspnoea index and activities of daily living score were observed in both groups (compared to baseline); this improvement could be maintained after 6 months. There was no significant difference in the magnitude of improvement between the two groups for the different variables [59]. These results suggest that the effect of PRPs can be maintained in patients with post-TB lung disorders as well as in patients with COPD if an appropriate support programme is provided.

Table 2. Summary of the studies reporting functional exercise effects of personal rehabilitation programmes in TB sequelae patients

First author [ref.]	Year	Duration	Design	Test	Functional exercise effect
Tada [58]	2002	NR	Cohort (n=29)	6MWT	+36 m
Ando [59]	2003	9 weeks, outpatient	Cohort (n=32)	6MWT	+42 m
Yoshida [28]	2006	2 weeks, inpatient daily walks	Cohort (n=10)	6MWT	+68 m
Jones [57]	2017	6 weeks, outpatient	Cohort (n=34)	ISWT	+90 m
De Grass [56]	2014	6 weeks, home based	RCT (n=34)		+11 m (control +16 m, NS)
Betancourt-Peña [60]	2015	8 weeks, outpatient	Cohort (n=11)	6MWT	+110.2 m

NR: not reported in abstract (full article in Japanese); 6MWT: 6-min walk test; ISWT: incremental shuttle walk test; NS: nonsignificant.

Most rehabilitation interventions have been developed for COPD patients, including respiratory physiotherapy, exercise training, patient education and self-management support, and nutritional and psychosocial support [6, 43, 61], as well as promotion of physical activity. According to the available evidence, PRP in patients with TB sequelae should be carried out based on the same approach [6, 60]. Patients likely to benefit from pulmonary rehabilitation need to be identified and then individualised PRPs designed accordingly.

TB sequelae include a wide spectrum of pulmonary lesions at the bronchial, parenchymal, vascular and even mediastinal level, all able to produce functional changes (table 3). In

Table 3. TB sequelae and lung function test abnormalities

TB sequelae	Functional alteration		Main PR intervention[#]
	Respiratory mechanics	Gas exchange	
Peripheral airway	Air flow obstruction[+] Air trapping and hyperinflation[§]	Decreased D_{LCO} Hypoxaemia at rest; there may be hypoventilation	Pulmonary physiotherapy Physical conditioning
Central airway	Air flow obstruction[+] Flattened flow–volume curve	Normal D_{LCO} and ABG	Aerobic exercise
Widespread parenchymal lung damage	Reduced lung volumes[f]	Decreased D_{LCO} Exercise-induced hypoxaemia; there may be hypoxaemia at rest	Pulmonary physiotherapy If possible, aerobic exercise[##]
Localised parenchymal lung damage	Spirometry and plethysmography may be normal If >1 L difference between TLCpleth and TLCD$_{LCO}$, suggests nonventilated lung volume (cysts or cavitations)	Normal D_{LCO} and ABG	Aerobic exercise
Pleural compromise	Reduced lung volumes[f]	Normal D_{LCO} and ABG	Aerobic exercise
Vascular compromise[¶]	Normal lung volume	Decreased D_{LCO} Rest and exercise-induced hypoxaemia	Breathing exercises Daily life activity management If possible, aerobic exercise[##]

PR: pulmonary rehabilitation; D_{LCO}: diffusing capacity of the lung for carbon monoxide; ABG: arterial blood gases; TLCpleth: total lung capacity measured by plethysmography; TLCD$_{LCO}$: total lung capacity determined from D_{LCO}. [#]: all patients must be included in a complete rehabilitation programme; however, this can be individualised according to the type and severity of lung damage. [¶]: thrombosis, aneurysms, pulmonary arterial hypertension and chronic cor pulmonale. [+]: decreased forced expiratory volume in 1 s/forced vital capacity ratio. [§]: increased residual volume and TLC. [f]: decreased vital capacity and TLC. [##]: type of exercise must be individualised before including patient into a constant load exercise, neuromuscular electrical stimulation or interval exercise.

principle, all kinds of TB sequelae can benefit from a PRP. However, the conditions most likely to benefit from it are bronchiectasis, restrictive and obstructive pulmonary disease, and pre-surgery preparation (either for resection, as part of the treatment or for managing late TB complications like aspergilloma [62] or local bronchiectasis).

Non-cystic fibrosis bronchiectasis

Chronic cough, purulent sputum, recurrent infections and dyspnoea are the hallmark of non-cystic fibrosis bronchiectasis, which includes patients with TB sequelae. PRPs for these patients are similar to those with applied to patients with cystic fibrosis but modifications and special considerations are made to individualise the approach for each patient. The main goal of PRP in bronchiectasis patients is to encourage airway clearing techniques, while improving ventilatory capacity and exercise tolerance. Two systematic reviews have addressed the role of physical training and airway clearance techniques (ACTs) in non-cystic fibrosis bronchiectasis. The available evidence suggests that there is benefit on exercise capacity, quality of life and respiratory muscle function at 8 weeks if inspiratory muscle are trained [63], and ACTs are useful to reduce respiratory symptoms, facilitate sputum expectoration, lower pulmonary hyperinflation and, overall, to improve health-related quality of life [64]. As no further details are available in the two reviews, is still unclear which is the most effective technique; as of today, the recommendation is to individualise the approach based on each patient's needs. Therefore, further research investigating pros and cons of different PRP in patients with bronchiectasis will be needed.

Restrictive lung disease

Diffuse parenchymal lung damage (destroyed lung) and pleural sequelae such as fibrothorax produce restriction of lung capacity similar to that caused by pulmonary fibrosis [6]. Although there is evidence of the usefulness of PRP in these patients, the pathophysiology of the disease is different from that of COPD; therefore, the utility of PRP is limited and the benefits are not maintained over time [65–67].

There are few experiences described in the literature on patients whose TB sequelae was characterised by a severe restrictive lung damage. Intermittent noninvasive ventilation devices (nasal and mouth devices) proved to be useful by improving arterial blood gases, exercise endurance and dyspnoea perception [68, 69]. However, these are isolated experiences and their long-term benefits need to be confirmed by further research.

Lung surgery: aspergilloma and localised bronchiectasis

Due to the emergence of DR-TB, the indications for surgery in TB patients have increased during the last 20 years [70]. The rationale for operating on TB patients (resectional surgery) is not only to reduce the bacillary load (in combination with appropriate chemotherapy) but also to manage complications of TB sequelae such as aspergilloma or localised bronchiectasis [71]. In both cases, PRP should be a standard of care performed (ideally) in the pre-surgical phase in order to prevent infections and to avoid subsequent muscle disuse and deconditioning. During the post-operative period, PRP has to be aimed at avoiding inadequate management of secretions caused by pain when breathing, moving and/or coughing. In the absence of these interventions, the patient's condition will further deteriorate, with additional respiratory complications as atelectasis and/or pneumonia.

Any surgical procedure in patients with chronic respiratory diseases requires an optimal and stable clinical situation; PRP is, therefore, an essential element of the therapeutic approach to these patients which contributes to prevent further complications [72]. The benefits of pre- and post-operative PRP have been described in patients undergoing surgical resection due to lung cancer, lung volume reduction in COPD and lung transplantation [43, 45, 73, 74]. Pre-operative PRP contributes to optimising the patient's pre-operative conditions and may decrease post-surgery pulmonary complications [46]. An adequate and short pre-operative PRP can improve baseline $V'O_2max$ and exercise performance, increasing the number of patients who will be candidates for the surgical approach [75–78].

Nutritional assessment

The association between TB and malnutrition is well recognised; malnutrition may predispose to TB and TB can lead to malnutrition due to persistent catabolism. Weight loss and underweight in TB patients have been associated with increased mortality [79]. Nutritional assessment and adequate nutrition are essential components of the PRP multidisciplinary management of patients with TB sequelae.

Setting: in- *versus* outpatient pulmonary rehabilitation

There is no evidence favouring in- *versus* outpatient management to offer rehabilitation in TB. However, most reports were carried out in an outpatient setting of centres where rehabilitation facilities were available and multidisciplinary management was feasible. However, in resource-limited settings other options (*e.g.* home-based PRP) may be easier and sustainable.

Other models to deliver pulmonary rehabilitation, successfully used in COPD patients include community-based rehabilitation. In low-resource settings, less instrumented programmes were also successful; for example, elastic bands can replace resistance training equipment for performing resistance training [57]. In COPD patients, more evidence is emerging on how well-designed programmes (in terms of exercise prescription, individual tailoring and multidisciplinary input) may indeed be effective even if limited equipment is available [80]. There is no reason to believe that this would be different in patients suffering from post-TB sequelae.

Conclusion

Pulmonary impairment after TB treatment largely contributes to the burden of chronic respiratory diseases, particularly within economically productive age groups in developing countries [6]. Most TB programmes, often with the support of international partners, try to ensure adequate diagnosis and pharmacological treatment as the first priority. However, the work is not finished when bacteriological cure has been achieved; if daily life activities are limited in these patients, health-related costs increase (for the patient, the so-called "catastrophic costs" and for the society).

Although the pulmonary functional assessment performed in the available studies is not complete, there is no doubt that functional impairment exists following TB treatment. Therefore, any effort needs to be directed to prevent TB and its spread, as a way to prevent also the development of long-term sequelae.

As TB can cause functional impairment in various ways and with different degrees of severity, a complete functional evaluation (as described above) is recommended for all patients completing their anti-TB treatment.

As this topic has recently raised scientific and media attention, well designed clinical research studies are necessary to evaluate the real impact of TB on lung function and on quality of life at the end of anti-TB chemotherapy, the best way to identify the candidates for pulmonary rehabilitation and the (cost-)effectiveness of different PRP approaches.

Quality PRPs in patients with TB sequelae require a multidisciplinary approach (including functional evaluation, education, pulmonary physiotherapy, physical conditioning, nutrition and psychosocial support) delivered either at institutional level, or following home- or community-based models.

References

1. Dheda K, Booth H, Jim F, *et al.* Lung remodeling in pulmonary tuberculosis. *J Infect Dis* 2005; 192: 1201–1210.
2. Ravimohan S, Kornfeld H, Weissman D, *et al.* Tuberculosis and lung damage: from epidemiology to pathophysiology. *Eur Respir Rev* 2018; 27: 170077.
3. Chandrasekaran R, Mac Aogáin M, Chalmers JD, *et al.* Geographic variation in the aetiology, epidemiology and microbiology of bronchiectasis. *BMC Pulm Med* 2018; 18: 83.
4. Ryu YJ, Lee JH, Chun EM, *et al.* Clinical outcomes and prognostic factors in patients with tuberculous destroyed lung. *Int J Tuberc Lung Dis* 2011; 15: 246–250.
5. Lee CH, Lee MC, Lin HH, *et al.* Pulmonary tuberculosis and delay in anti-tuberculous treatment are important risk factors for chronic obstructive pulmonary disease. *PLoS One* 2012; 7: e37978.
6. Muñoz-Torrico M, Rendon A, Centis R, *et al.* Is there a rationale for pulmonary rehabilitation following successful chemotherapy for tuberculosis? *J Bras Pneumol* 2016; 42: 374–385.
7. Pasipanodya JG, Miller TL, Vecino M, *et al.* Pulmonary impairment after tuberculosis. *Chest* 2007; 131: 1817–1824.
8. Menezes AM, Hallal PC, Perez Padilla R, *et al.* Tuberculosis and airflow obstruction: evidence from the PLATINO study in Latin America. *Eur Respir J* 2007; 30: 1180–1185.
9. Buist S, Vollmer WM, McBurnie MA. Worldwide burden of COPD in high- and low-income countries. Part I. The burden of obstructive lung disease (BOLD) initiative. *Int J Tuberc Lung Dis* 2008; 12: 703–708.
10. Ehrlich RI, White N, Norman R, *et al.* Predictors of chronic bronchitis in South African adults. *Int J Tuberc Lung Dis* 2004; 8: 369–376.
11. Lee SW, Kim YS, Kim DS, *et al.* The risk of obstructive lung disease by previous pulmonary tuberculosis in a country with intermediate burden of tuberculosis. *J Korean Med Sci* 2011; 26: 268–273.
12. Hnizdo E, Singh T, Churchyard G. Chronic pulmonary function impairment caused by initial and recurrent pulmonary tuberculosis following treatment. *Thorax* 2000; 55: 32–38.
13. Byrne AL, Marais BJ, Mitnick CD, *et al.* Tuberculosis and chronic respiratory disease: a systematic review. *Int J Infect Dis* 2015; 32: 138–146.
14. Kallan BM, Kishan J. Clinicoradiological status of patients of pulmonary tuberculosis after adequate treatment. *Indian J Med Sci* 1988; 42: 4–8.
15. Poey C, Verhaegen F, Giron J, *et al.* High resolution chest CT in tuberculosis: evolutive patterns and signs of activity. *J Comput Assist Tomogr* 1997; 21: 601–607.
16. Rufino RL, Capone R, Capone D, *et al.* Pattern of chest computed tomography before and after treatment in patients with proven pulmonary tuberculosis. *Am J Respir Crit Care Med* 2015; 191.
17. World Health Organization. WHO policy on TB infection control in health-care facilities, congregate settings and households. WHO/HTM/TB/2009.419. Geneva, World Health Organization, 2009.
18. Neas LM, Schwartz J. Pulmonary function levels as predictors of mortality in a national sample of US adults. *Am J Epidemiol* 1998; 147: 1011–1018.
19. D'Urzo AD, Tamari I, Bouchard J, *et al.* New spirometry interpretation algorithm. *Can Fam Physician* 2011; 57: 1148–1152.

20. Al-Ashkar F, Mehra R, Mazzone P. Interpreeting pulmonary function test: recognize the pattern and the diagnosis will follow. *Clev Clinic J Med* 2003; 70: 866–881.

21. Baez-Saldaña R, López-Arteaga Y, Bizarrón-Muro A, *et al.* A novel scoring system to measure radiographic abnormalities and related spirometric values in cured pulmonary tuberculosis. *PLoS One* 2013; 8: e78926.

22. Lee JH, Chang JH. Lung function in patients with chronic airflow obstruction due to tuberculous destroyed lung. *Respir Med* 2003; 97: 1237–1242.

23. Criée CP, Sorichter S, Smith HJ, *et al.* Body plethysmography – its principles and clinical use. *Respir Med* 2011; 105: 959–971.

24. Puente Maestú L, García de Pedro J. Las pruebas funcionales respiratorias en las decisiones clínicas. *Arch Bronconeumol* 2012; 48: 161–169.

25. Pellegrino R, Viegi G, Brusasco V, *et al.* Interpretative strategies for lung function tests. *Eur Respir J* 2005; 26: 948–968.

26. Collard HR, King TE Jr, Bartelson BB, *et al.* Changes in clinical and physiologic variables predict survival in idiopathic pulmonary fibrosis. *Am J Respir Crit Care Med* 2003; 168: 538–542.

27. Kiakouama L, Cottin V, Glerant JC, *et al.* Conditions associated with severe carbon monoxide diffusion coefficient reduction. *Respir Med* 2011; 105: 1248–1256.

28. Meyyappan D, Chockalingam P. Evaluation of respiratory impairment and health related quality of life in pulmonary tuberculosis sequeale patients. *Inte J Adv Med* 2018; 5: 276–280.

29. Yoshida N, Toshiyama T, Asai E, *et al.* Exercise training for the improvent of exercise perfomance of patients with pulmonary tuberculosis sequelae. *Intern Med* 2006; 45: 399–403.

30. Ralph AP, Kenangalem E, Waramori G, *et al.* High morbidity during treatment and residual pulmonary disability in pulmonary tuberculosis: under-recognised phenomena. *PloS One* 2013; 8: e80302.

31. Di Naso FC, Pereira JS, Schuh SJ, *et al.* Functional evaluation in patients with pulmonary tuberculosis sequelae [Article in Portuguese]. *Rev Port Pneumol* 2011; 17: 216–221.

32. Brunelli A, Kim AW, Berger KI, *et al.* Physiologic evaluation of the patient with lung cancer being considered for resectional surgery: Diagnosis and management of lung cancer, 3rd edition: American College of Chest Physicians evidence-based clinical practice guidelines. *Chest* 2013; 143: Suppl., e166S–e190S.

33. Brunelli A, Charloux A, Bolliger CT, *et al.* The European Respiratory Society and European Society of Thoracic Surgeons clinical guidelines for evaluating fitness for radical treatment (surgery and chemoradiotherapy) in patients with lung cancer. *Eur J Cardiothoracic Surg* 2009; 36: 181–184.

34. Cid S, León P, Mejía R, *et al.* Evaluación de la función respiratoria en pacientes que van a ser sometidos a cirugía de resección pulmonary [Preoperative functional assessment for lung resection candidates]. *Neumol Cir Torax* 2018; 77: 38–46.

35. Horie J, Itou KI, Fujii H, *et al.* Exercise limitation factors of patients with chronic respiratory failure: a comparison of chronic obstructive pulmonary disease and sequelae of pulmonary tuberculosis. *J Phys Ther Sci* 2009; 21: 155–161.

36. Miki K, Maekura R, Hiraga T, *et al.* Exertional dyspnea-related acidotic and sympathetic responses in patients with sequelae of pulmonary tuberculosis. *J Physiol Sci* 2010; 60: 187–193.

37. Muhammad Atif M, Sulaiman SA, Shafie AA, *et al.* Impact of tuberculosis treatment on health-related quality of life of pulmonary tuberculosis patients: a follow-up study. *Health Qual Life Outcomes* 2014; 12: 19.

38. Kruijshaar ME, Lipman M, Essink-Bot ML, *et al.* Health status of UK patients with active tuberculosis. *Int J Tuberc Lung Dis* 2010; 14: 296–302.

39. Marra C, Marra F, Colley L, *et al.* Health-related quality of life trajectories among adults with tuberculosis: differences between latent and active infection. *Chest* 2008; 133: 396–403.

40. Pasipanodya JG, Miller TL, Vecino M. Using the St. George Respiratory Questionnaire to ascertain health quality in persons with treated pulmonary tuberculosis. *Chest* 2007; 132: 1591–1598.

41. Pasipanodya JG, McNabb SJ, Hilsenrath P, *et al.* Pulmonary impairment after tuberculosis and its contribution to TB burden. *BMC Public Health* 2010; 10: 259.

42. Holland AE, Wadell K, Spruit MA. How to adapt the pulmonary rehabilitation programme to patients with chronic respiratory disease other than COPD. *Eur Respir Rev* 2013; 22: 577–586.

43. Spruit MA, Singh SJ, Garvey C, *et al.* ATS/ERS Task Force on Pulmonary Rehabilitation. An official American Thoracic Society/European Respiratory Society statement: key concepts and advances in pulmonary rehabilitation. *Am J Respir Crit Care Med* 2013; 188: e13–e64.

44. Osadnik CR, Rodrigues FM, Camillo CA, *et al.* Principles of rehabilitation and reactivation. *Respiration* 2015; 89: 2–11.

45. Vagvolgyi A, Rozgonyi Z, Kerti M, *et al.* Effectiveness of perioperative pulmonary rehabilitation in thoracic surgery. *J Thorac Dis* 2017; 9: 1584–1591.

46. Saito H, Hatakeyama K, Konno H, *et al.* Impact of pulmonary rehabilitation on postoperative complications in patients with lung cancer and chronic obstructive pulmonary disease. *Thorac Cancer* 2017; 8: 451–460.

47. Munoz M, Tiberi S, Gomez R, *et al.* Desenlaces de casos graves de tuberculosis en América Latina y Europa. Mexico city, Mexico, ALAT, 2018.

https://doi.org/10.1183/2312508X.10022317

48. Burtin C, Clerckx B, Robbeets C, et al. Early exercise in critically ill patients enhances short-term functional recovery. Crit Care Med 2009; 37: 2499–2505.
49. Parker A, Sricharoenchai T, Needham DM. Early rehabilitation in the intensive care unit: preventing physical and mental health impairments. Curr Phys Med Rehabil Rep 2013; 1: 307–314.
50. Rivera JA, Wilches-Luna EC, Mosquera R, et al. Pulmonary rehabilitation on aerobic capacity and health- related quality of life in patients with sequelae of pulmonary TB. Physiotherapy 2015; 101: Suppl. 1, e1288.
51. Maltais F, Bourbeau J, Shapiro S, et al. Effects of home-based pulmonary rehabilitation in patients with chronic obstructive pulmonary disease: a randomized trial. Ann Intern Med 2008; 149: 869–878.
52. Wijkstra PJ, Ten Vergert EM, van Altena R, et al. Long term benefits of rehabilitation at home on quality of life and exercise tolerance in patients with chronic obstructive pulmonary disease. Thorax 1995; 50: 824–828.
53. Cambach W, Chadwick-Straver RV, Wagenaar RC, et al. The effects of a community-based pulmonary rehabilitation programme on exercise tolerance and quality of life: a randomized controlled trial. Eur Respir J 1997; 10: 104–113.
54. Strijbos JH, Postma DS, van Altena R, et al. Comparison between an outpatient hospital-based pulmonary rehabilitation program and a home-care pulmonary rehabilitation program in patients with COPD. A follow-up of 18 months. Chest 1996; 109: 366–372.
55. Hernández MT, Rubio TM, Ruiz FO, et al. Results of a home-based training program for patients with COPD. Chest 2000; 118: 106–114.
56. de Grass D, Manie S, Amosun SL. Effectiveness of a home-based pulmonary rehabilitation programme in pulmonary function and health related quality of life for patients with pulmonary tuberculosis: a pilot study. Afr Health Sci 2014; 14: 866–872.
57. Jones R, Kirenga BJ, Katagira W, et al. A pre–post intervention study of pulmonary rehabilitation for adults with post-tuberculosis lung disease in Uganda. Int J Chron Obstruct Pulmon Dis; 12: 3533–3539.
58. Tada A, Matsumoto H, Soda R, et al. Effects of pulmonary rehabilitation in patients with pulmonary tuberculosis sequelae. Nihon Kokyuki Gakkai Zasshi 2002; 40: 275–281.
59. Ando M, Mori A, Esaki H, et al. The effect of pulmonary rehabilitation in patients with post-tuberculosis lung disorder. Chest 2003; 123: 1988–1995.
60. Betancourt-Peña J, Muñoz-Erazo BE, Hurtado-Gutiérrez H. Efecto de la rehabilitación pulmonar en la calidad de vida y la capacidad funcional en pacientes con secuelas de tuberculosis [Effect of pulmonary rehabilitation in quality of life and functional capacity in patients with tuberculosis sequela]. Nova; 13: 47–54.
61. Güell Rous MR, Díaz Lobato S, Rodríguez Trigo G, et al. Pulmonary rehabilitation. Sociedad Española de Neumología y Cirugía Torácica (SEPAR). Arch Bronconeumol 2014; 50: 332–344.
62. Denning DW, Pleuvry A, Cole DC. Global burden of chronic pulmonary aspergillosis as a sequel to pulmonary tuberculosis. Bull World Health Organ 2011; 89: 864–872.
63. Bradley J, Moran F, Greenstone M. Physical training for bronchiectasis. Cochrane Database Syst Rev 2002; CD002166.
64. Lee AL, Burge AT, Holland AE. Airway clearance techniques for bronchiectasis. Cochrane Database Syst Rev 2015; CD008351.
65. Holland AE, Hill CJ, Conron M, et al. Short term improvement in exercise capacity and symptoms following exercise training in interstitial lung disease. Thorax 2008; 63: 549–554.
66. Kozu R, Senjyu H, Jenkins SC, et al. Differences in response to pulmonary rehabilitation in idiopathic pulmonary fibrosis and chronic obstructive pulmonary disease. Respiration 2011; 81: 196–205.
67. Holland A, Hill C. Physical training for interstitial lung disease. Cochrane Database Syst Rev 2008; 4: CD006322.
68. Yang GF, Alba A, Lee M. Respiratory rehabilitation in severe restrictive lung disease secondary to tuberculosis. Arch Phys Med Rehabil 1984; 65: 556–558.
69. Tsuboi T, Ohi M, Chin K, et al. Ventilatory support during exercise in patients with pulmonary tuberculosis sequelae. Chest 1997; 112: 1000–1007.
70. Moran JF. Surgical treatment of pulmonary tuberculosis. In: Sabiston DC Jr, Spencer FC, eds. Surgery of the chest. 6th Edn. Philadelphia, W.B. Saunders Company, 1995; pp. 752–772.
71. Subotic D, Yablonskiy P, Sulis G, et al. Surgery and pleuro-pulmonary tuberculosis: a scientific literature review. J Thorac Dis 2016; 8: E474–E485.
72. Celli BR. Chronic respiratory failure after lung resection: The role of pulmonary rehabilitation. Thorac Surg Clin 2004; 14: 417–428.
73. Takaoka ST, Weinacker AB. The value of preoperative pulmonary rehabilitation. Thorac Surg Clin 2005; 15: 203–211.
74. Rochester CL. Pulmonary rehabilitation for patients who undergo lung-volume-reduction surgery or lung transplantation. Respir Care 2008; 53: 1196–1202.
75. Bobbio A, Chetta A, Ampollini L, et al. Preoperative pulmonary rehabilitation in patients undergoing lung resection for non-small cell lung cancer. Eur J Cardiothorac Surg 2008; 33: 95–98.
76. Divisi D, Di Francesco C, Di Leonardo G, et al. Preoperative pulmonary rehabilitation in patients with lung cancer and chronic obstructive pulmonary disease. Eur J Cardiothorac Surg 2013; 43: 293–296.

77. Weiner P, Man A, Weiner M, *et al.* The effect of incentive spirometry and inspiratory muscle training on pulmonary function after lung resection. *J Thorac Cardiovasc Surg* 1997; 113: 552–557.

78. Wilson DJ. Pulmonary rehabilitation exercise program for high-risk thoracic surgical patients. *Chest Surg Clin N Am* 1997; 7: 697–706.

79. Miyata S, Tanaka M, Ihaku D. Usefulness of the Malnutrition Screening Tool in patients with pulmonary tuberculosis. *Nutrition* 2012; 28: 271–274.

80. Alison JA, McKeough ZJ. Pulmonary rehabilitation for COPD: are programs with minimal exercise equipment effective? *J Thorac Dis* 2014; 6: 1606–1614.

Disclosures: None declared.

Acknowledgements: The authors wish to thank G.B. Migliori (WHO Collaborating Centre for TB and Lung Diseases, Istituti Clinici Scientifici Maugeri IRCCS, Tradate, Italy), who significantly contributed to the development this chapter at various stages, and Lia D'Ambrosio (Public Health Consulting Group, Lugano, Switzerland) for her useful comments on the manuscript.

https://doi.org/10.1183/2312508X.10022317

Chapter 20

Towards a new vaccine

Morten Ruhwald[1], Peter L. Andersen[1] and Lewis Schrager[2]

Despite extensive administration of the BCG vaccine to infants throughout the world, the global TB epidemic continues, with TB representing the world's leading infectious cause of death. Developing a TB vaccine capable of preventing TB disease, primarily in adolescents and adults, the most important sources of *Mycobacterium tuberculosis* spread, represents a critical need in efforts to stem the global TB epidemic, including the spread of *M. tuberculosis* strains resistant to multiple TB drugs. 13 TB vaccine candidates are currently in clinical trials. Results from two recently completed trials have demonstrated protective efficacy, and new broader strategies to TB vaccine development, including the diversification of *M. tuberculosis* antigens, vaccine platforms and routes of vaccine administration are being pursued. In this chapter, we review the current status of the TB vaccine pipeline as well as the future directions in the critically important effort to develop new TB vaccines.

Cite as: Ruhwald M, Andersen PL, Schrager L. Towards a new vaccine. *In:* Migliori GB, Bothamley G, Duarte R, *et al.*, eds. Tuberculosis (ERS Monograph). Sheffield, European Respiratory Society, 2018; pp. 343–363 [https://doi.org/10.1183/2312508X.10022417].

@ERSpublications
It is an exciting time in the field of TB vaccines. This review provides an up to date overview of the clinical vaccine candidates, results from recent efficacy trials and future directions. http://ow.ly/cfVQ30lqCfE

In 2016 an estimated 10.4 million people became ill with TB and 1.7 million people died of the disease, despite significant advances in diagnosis and treatment [1]. Neonatal BCG vaccination is almost universally implemented in TB endemic regions but remains only partial efficacious protecting infants and young children, and this protection is not sustained in adolescents and adults, the main drivers of the epidemic [2].

Without new and better TB vaccines, it will be impossible to reach the ambitious WHO End TB Strategy targets [3]. In addition, as vaccines are expected to be equally effective against both drug-resistant and drug-sensitive strains of TB vaccine intervention is the ultimate tool to contain the accelerating spread of MDR-TB [3].

[1]Center for Vaccine Research, Statens Serum Institut, Copenhagen, Denmark. [2]Schrager BioPharma Consulting, LLC, Bethesda, MD, USA.

Correspondence: Morten Ruhwald, Human Immunology, Center for Vaccine Research, Statens Serum Institut, Artillerivej 5, 2300 S, Denmark. E-mail moru@ssi.dk

A new and improved vaccine for TB is not a low hanging fruit. TB is a complex disease that has co-evolved with humans for millennia, and we only have an incomplete understanding of the type of immune response required to control or eliminate the infection [4, 5]. The absence of valid animal models to mimic human infection and disease, reliable correlate(s) of protection, and controlled human challenge models for early triage of candidates represent major bottlenecks slowing the pace of the TB vaccine research agenda and heightening the importance of testing vaccine candidates in human efficacy trials [6].

The early stage development of TB vaccines is driven mainly by academic institutions, largely due to the perception of an unfavourable cost-to-benefit assessment of TB vaccine development, which has limited the interest of industry in this effort [7]. The TB vaccine development community, although small relative to the size of vaccine development communities for other important infectious diseases such as HIV and malaria, is characterised by a high degree of global collaboration made possible by the long-term and coordinated commitments of major donors including the European Commission, the Wellcome Trust (UK), the National Institutes of Health (USA) and the Bill and Melinda Gates Foundation (USA) [7, 8]. These investments have allowed implementation of portfolio management principles and industry-like stage gate criteria, to encourage efficient use of funds and advance only the most promising vaccine candidates in trials with comparable outcomes due to the use of standardised clinical end-points [6, 9]. More recently, WHO has developed preferred product characteristics, optimised criteria for a TB vaccine intended to "provide guidance to scientists, funding agencies and industry groups developing TB vaccine candidates intended for WHO prequalification and policy recommendations" [10].

In this chapter we will provide an overview of the TB vaccines in clinical development, including a review of the various development strategies currently being pursued, new strategic directions being explored, and the major challenges in getting a new vaccine to the market.

Strategies for protection

Mycobacterium tuberculosis infection and TB disease is a spectrum, where a complex interplay of host and bacterial factors determine the outcome [4, 11], and offer opportunities for both preventive and therapeutic vaccine strategies (figure 1) [6, 13–16]. Detailed, controlled studies in non-human primates in which *M. tuberculosis* infection was tracked using genetically "bar-coded" bacteria that permit researchers to determine the fate of single *M. tuberculosis* organisms, combined with serial positron emission tomography (PET)-computed tomography (CT) scans and detailed pathology, has led to an increased appreciation of the importance of designing vaccines to stimulate immune responses located in the pulmonary parenchyma at or near the sites of *M. tuberculosis* entry capable of responding within a few days of initial infection [4, 5, 17, 18].

There are three main strategic targets for TB vaccines: 1) preventing PTB disease (prevention of disease (POD)); 2) preventing sustained *M. tuberculosis* infection (prevention of infection (POI)), where sustained infection is defined by durable conversion of IGRAs; and 3) preventing recurrent TB disease in individuals completing successful treatment for TB

https://doi.org/10.1183/2312508X.10022417

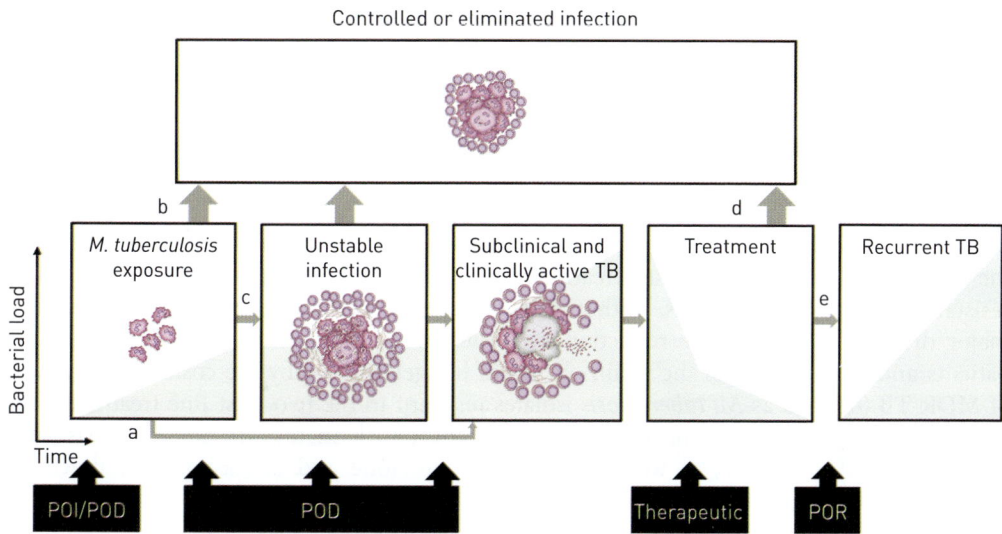

Figure 1. Schematic presentation of the spectrum of TB infection and disease. Grey shaded areas illustrate bacterial load. Following exposure and infection, a complex interaction between host and bacteria determines the outcome. A small fraction will progress directly to active disease (a); however, for the majority there seems to be a critical period where the trajectory of the infection is determined, at least in part, by predisposing host factors (nutritional status, diabetes, immune balance including impact of HIV infection, etc.). A proportion of individuals may eliminate Mycobacterium tuberculosis or exert highly effective control in the granuloma, and be at very low risk of reactivation (b); in others, M. tuberculosis control is unstable (c) with suboptimal granuloma containment and potential to progress in response to a variety of precipitating factors affecting the immune control (nutritional status, viral infections, HIV, anti-tumour necrosis factor-α treatment, pregnancy, etc.). Prior to clinical manifestation, these individuals may pass through a subclinical phase of active infection which may last months. During this phase, risk may be assessed in the transcriptomic profile, and later M. tuberculosis isolated by culture or pathology may be visible through imaging prior to symptomatic presentation. During treatment, the bacterial load declines at a rapid rate in the initial phase, with a less rapid decline during a later phase, suggesting that there are subpopulations of bacteria that differ in their drug susceptibility (rate of replication) and/or availability to drug exposure (encapsulation in a thick walled granuloma). The majority of patients will have a successful outcome of treatment (d); however, some patients, for example those with structural lung damage, drug-resistant TB or poor treatment compliance, may have persistent infection in either a controlled (d) or unstable/subclinical form with an increasing risk for progression to recurrent TB disease (e). Strategies for vaccine interventions are highlighted (black boxes). Prevention of infection (POI) and disease (POD) represent classic preventive strategies for TB infection control. In particular, if also effective in those already infected these strategies will have the largest impact on the epidemic. Therapeutic vaccination and vaccines capable of preventing recurrence (POR) will have only modest impact on the epidemic, but could play a major role in combatting drug resistance, shortening drug treatment regimens and improving patient wellbeing. Information from [4, 5, 11, 12].

(preventing recurrence (POR)). Models suggest that a POD vaccine targeting adolescents and adults will have the largest and most immediate impact on the epidemic and thus represents the highest priority target for TB vaccine developers [10, 19, 20]. Preventing PTB disease in this group is also expected to be a highly efficient means of preventing *M. tuberculosis* infection in infants and young children as adolescent and adult household contacts with TB are the primary sources for *M. tuberculosis* infection in the younger age groups. Further, a vaccine also capable of preventing progression to disease in persons already infected with *M. tuberculosis* would be the most efficient prevention strategy to reduce the incidence of TB disease in the short term [19, 21, 22].

Another important goal of TB vaccine developers is to improve upon the protective efficacy already provided by BCG. A vaccine targeting infants with superior efficacy and longer duration of protection than BCG, as well as improved safety in immunosuppressed infants including those with HIV infection, is theoretically valuable. Because such a vaccine would not be expected to have an immediate impact on the global TB epidemic, and would probably be more costly than BCG, it will need to show clear evidence of superiority over BCG to drive WHO policy change for BCG replacement [10, 19, 22].

In addition to these preventive vaccine indications, immunotherapeutic vaccines also are being developed. These strategies aim to improve the outcome of drug treatment or shorten the duration of lengthy TB drug treatment regimens for both drug-sensitive and drug-resistant *M. tuberculosis* strains. Although a therapeutic vaccine is not expected to be a major driver of TB incidence reduction, it would be of significant benefit for individual patients and relieve some of the strain on health budgets caused by the costly management of MDR-TB (defined as *M. tuberculosis* isolates resistant to the two, first-line treatments for TB: rifampicin (RIF) and isoniazid (INH)) and XDR-TB (defined as *M. tuberculosis* isolates resistant to INH and RIF, as well as any fluoroquinolone and at least one of the three SLIDs (amikacin, kanamycin or capreomycin)) [3, 10, 23].

Overview of designs of pivotal trials

When a vaccine candidate has proven safe and immunogenic in phase I and IIa trials, further evaluation of promising candidates requires direct assessments of clinical efficacy given the lack of either correlates of immune protection or a controlled human infection model (CHIM) for TB. Due to the large size, high cost and lengthy duration of POD trials, early clinical proof-of-concept trials with standardised biologically relevant end-points, such as POI and POR, are being promoted. POI and POR trials are faster, and provide lower-cost assessments of clinically relevant biological activity of the vaccine candidates intended to reduce the risk of a decision to advance promising candidates in to long and expensive POD trials (figure 1 and table 1) [6, 10, 13, 14, 24].

There are risks inherent in this strategy. One such risk is assuming that a positive POI or POR outcome will predict success of the vaccine for a POD outcome, given the possibility that different protective immune mechanisms may be needed to achieve POR, POI and POD outcomes, respectively. A second, related risk is to assume that a vaccine candidate that fails to demonstrate efficacy in preliminary POI or POR trials will fail to do so in a POD trial as well, as it may be more difficult for a vaccine to demonstrate POI or prevent disease recurrence in individuals who already manifest a susceptibility to develop TB disease, compared with improved *M. tuberculosis* containment in a POD trial. Nevertheless, as POI and POR trials require less time and resources to conduct than POD trials, and given the absence of immune correlates of protection against developing TB disease or a CHIM for TB, phase II POI and POR trial outcomes represent "go/no-go" milestones in the clinical development plans of many TB vaccine developers (table 1).

Two recent pivotal trials have generated significant optimism in the field. A landmark POD trial of the M72/AS01E vaccine demonstrated 54% vaccine efficacy in IGRA positive against placebo [25]. A POI trial comparing BCG revaccination and H4:IC31 to placebo, generated a positive signal in the BCG revaccination arm that opens the doors for possible POD trials for BCG revaccination while leaving the prospects for future development of the H4:IC31 vaccine uncertain [26]. As phase IIb and phase III efficacy data from two additional studies

https://doi.org/10.1183/2312508X.10022417

Table 1. Trial design and concepts in TB vaccine development

TB vaccine indications	Typical trial design to demonstrate efficacy	Example[#]
Prevention of disease (POD)	POD trials study the ability of TB vaccine candidates to prevent active, microbiologically confirmed TB in persons who are either *M. tuberculosis* infected (IGRA-positive) or uninfected (IGRA-negative), in a high-TB endemic setting. Smaller trials are possible in populations with higher risk (*e.g.* IGRA positive contacts or HIV-positive persons).	Identifier: NCT01755598. M72/AS01E, 3573 volunteers, HIV-negative, IGRA-positive, two-arm trial with 3 years of follow-up. Assuming a 0.55% disease rate in the controls this trial has 80% power to detect 70% efficacy when 21 cases have accrued.
Prevention of recurrence (POR)	POR trials assess vaccine efficacy for preventing the recurrence of TB in TB patients vaccinated around the time of completing drug treatment for TB. Given the high rate of TB recurrence, this type of trial can be powered to include 4–5 times fewer enrollees than for POD trials, and with follow-up limited to the first year following completion of drug treatment.	Identifier: NCT03512249. H56:IC31, 900 volunteers, HIV-negative, two-arm trial, 1 year of follow-up. Assuming a 4% recurrence rate in controls this trial has 80% power to detect 60% vaccine efficacy when 21 cases have accrued. See also NCT03152903.
Prevention of infection (POI)	POI enrol IGRA-negative adolescents and/or adults at high risk of acquiring *M. tuberculosis* infection. Subjects are followed for sustained IGRA conversion, defined by IGRA-positive tests on at least two consecutive assessments. When conducted in high endemic settings, *M. tuberculosis* infection can occur in up to 10% per year, allowing for a 10-fold reduction in sample size compared to a POD trial in the same population.	Identifier: NCT02075203. H4:IC31 and BCG revaccination, 990 volunteers (330 per arm), HIV-negative, 2 years of follow-up. Assuming 8% conversion rate in controls, this trial was powered for 80% one-sided power to detect a 60% reduction in IGRA conversion.
Therapeutic	Vaccination of TB (or MDR-TB) patients during treatment, follow-up for biological end-points like sputum conversion or TB recurrence, *e.g.* in a non-inferiority trial with shortened drug regimen.	No trials available.
BCG replacement	Vaccination of infants to prevent active PTB and/or severe, disseminated TB, *e.g.* in a non-inferiority trial against BCG.	No trials available.

M. tuberculosis: *Mycobacterium tuberculosis*. [#]: trials are registered at clinicaltrials.gov with the identifier numbers listed.

with other TB vaccine candidates are scheduled for release in the next 2–3 years, this represents a significant period for TB vaccine development. Data from these trials, along with immunological studies using banked biological specimens collected from the clinical trial participants, will provide an opportunity to identify correlates of immune protection that will probably determine the future direction of the TB vaccine development effort in the years to come.

Overview of the vaccines in clinical development

The TB vaccine candidate pipeline currently comprises 13 clinical candidates including live whole cell vaccines, killed whole mycobacterial cells or mycobacterial cell extracts, adjuvanted protein subunit vaccines, or viral-vectored vaccines (table 2).

Live, attenuated, whole mycobacterial cell vaccines

The family of live, attenuated whole cell vaccines include BCG and several novel and promising candidates. While many were developed initially as a replacement for the BCG priming vaccination in infants, they are also being assessed for use in adolescents and adults given the high priority of targeting these age groups when attempting to curtail the global TB epidemic. These vaccines offer potential advantages as they include a full genome of potential antigens and induce a wide and complex immune response. However, as these vaccines work by inducing a transient infection, they are associated with a higher risk of adverse local reactions and potentially disseminated infection, particularly in immunocompromised hosts [15].

Bacille Calmette–Guérin

BCG currently is the only globally licensed vaccine against TB. BCG is administered as a single intradermal dose to ~85% of the annual global birth cohort as a proven means to protect infants from life-threatening disseminated TB disease. Albert Calmette and Camille Guérin, working in the laboratories of the Pasteur Institute in Lille, France, developed this live attenuated bacillus by passaging *Mycobacterium bovis* 230 times from 1908 to 1921 in potato bile media, during which several genomic segments were lost, including the RD-1 segment encoding the unique ESX-1 secretion system responsible for expression of major virulence factors including ESAT-6 and CFP10 [27, 28]. A number of sub-strains have been established after BCG was distributed throughout the world during the 20th century. These regional BCG strains vary in their genomic deletions and there is little knowledge of how these sub-strains differ in terms of vaccine safety, immunogenicity and efficacy [27, 29].

The underlying immune mechanisms behind the protective efficacy of BCG remain elusive. Being a live, whole cell mycobacterial vaccine, BCG administration results in an established infection, exposing the immune system to a complex antigen repertoire including mycobacterial proteins, lipids and glycolipids, and allows for interaction with innate immune cells and induction of both conventional and unconventional T-cell responses as well as antibody responses [28]. In addition, BCG seems capable of inducing "trained immunity" in the form of epigenetic changes in monocytes, which specifically enhance their capacity to control not only mycobacteria, but also other pathogens, which at least in high endemic regions has been associated with a reduction in morbidity and improved all-cause mortality [30, 31].

Meta-analyses of studies assessing BCG efficacy have demonstrated a high degree of protection in infants and toddlers against lethal meningeal and miliary TB, and it is estimated to prevent 120 000 childhood deaths a year [32–34]. The ability of BCG to

https://doi.org/10.1183/2312508X.10022417

Table 2. Overview, strategy and status of TB vaccine candidates in clinical development

Candidate; developers	Description	Target population	Clinical trial status
Live vaccines			
MTBVAC; Biofabri (Spain), University of Zaragoza (Spain), TBVI (Netherlands), Aeras/IAVI (USA)	Attenuated *M. tuberculosis*, by deletions of the PhoP and fadD26 genes required for trascription of virulence genes and synthesis of cell surface lipids.	BCG replacement in infants, single dose. Potential for revaccination in adolescents/adults is (also) being pursued as secondary target.	A phase IIb trial in infants and a phase Ib trial in adolescents, both to be conducted in South Africa, will start in 2018.
VPM1002; Serum Institute of India (India), Vakzine Project Management (Germany)	Recombinant BCG, with a listeriolysin knock-in and a urease gene knock-out permitting bacterial escape from the lysosome, inducing autophagy and augmenting stimulation of innate immunity.	BCG replacement in infants, single dose; POR infection in adolescents and adults.	Several large trials planned and ongoing, including a phase III comparison of safety and non-inferior efficacy to BCG in 10 000 infants (expected to close in 2021), and a phase IIb–III trial assessing POR in adolescents and adults in India (initiated in 2018).
BCG and BCG revaccination; several manufacturers	Attenuated *Mycobacterium bovis* developed 1907–1921, through serial passage of BCG in potato bile broth.	Adolescents, as a BCG boost.	BCG revaccination recently demonstrated 45% efficacy for POI in South Africa, further trials are expected.
Adjuvanted protein subunit vaccines			
H4:IC31; Sanofi Pasteur (France), Statens Serum Institut (Denmark), Valneva (Austria), Aeras/IAVI (USA)	Fusion protein of Ag85B and TB10.4, in adjuvant IC31 (anti-bacterial peptide (KLK) and non-CpG immunostimulatory oligonucleotide (ODN1a)), signals through TLR9, resulting in a T-cell bias and sustained CD4 responses.	Prevention of TB disease in BCG vaccinated adolescents and adults, administered as two intramuscular doses.	Two trials assessing H4:IC31 immunogenicity aligned with the EPI schedule and a trial exploring potential correlates for POI trials are ongoing. Plans for future development of H4:IC31 are unclear following the demonstration of only modest protection against infection in a phase II POI trial.

Continued

Table 2. Continued

Candidate; developers	Description	Target population	Clinical trial status
H56:IC31; Statens Serum Institut (Denmark), Valneva (Austria), Aeras/IAVI (USA)	Fusion protein of Ag85B and ESAT-6 and Rv2660c, in adjuvant IC31, designed as a multistage vaccine inducing a sustained T-cell memory response against early, constitutive and latency-associated antigens.	Prevention of TB disease in BCG vaccinated adolescents and adults; also designed to provide post-exposure protection and as a therapeutic vaccine. Administered in two doses.	A trial exploring potential correlates for POI trials is ongoing. An open label trial assessing safety when vaccinating at month 3 for potential therapeutic potential is ongoing. A POR trial is planned to start in South Africa and Tanzania in 2018.
M72/AS01E; GSK, Aeras/IAVI (USA)	Fusion protein of Mtb39A and Mtb32A in adjuvant AS01E.	Prevention of TB disease in BCG vaccinated adolescents and adults. Administered in two doses.	Phase IIb trial demonstrated 54% protection against TB disease in HIV negative, IGRA positive individuals. Further studies are expected.
ID93+GLA-SE; IDRI (USA)	Fusion protein of Rv1813, Rv2608, Rv3619 and Rv3620 in adjuvant GLA-SE. Designed as a multistage vaccine, with a synthetic TLR-4 agonist in a squalene oil in a water nano-emulsion, to induce a T-cell response.	Primarily designed to supplement drug treatment as an immunotherapeutic agent.	Phase IIa completed, a phase IIb POR trial is being planned.
Viral vectored vaccines			
Ad5Ag85A; McMaster University (Canada), CanSino (China)	Adenovirus-based vaccine that employs serotype 5 (Ad5) as a vector to deliver *M. tuberculosis* antigen 85A.	Adolescents, as a BCG boost.	Assessing safety and immunogenicity of aerosol delivery in phase I, results expected mid-2020.
ChAdOx185A/MVA85A; Oxford University (UK)	Several approaches being explored, including heterologous prime boost with chimp adenovirus and MVA-vectored vaccines expressing antigen 85A.	Prevention of TB disease in BCG primed persons.	Phase I, experimental medicine studies.

Continued

https://doi.org/10.1183/2312508X.10022417

Table 2. Continued

Candidate; developers	Description	Target population	Clinical trial status
Killed whole cell or extract vaccines			
RUTI; University of Badalona (Spain), Archival Pharma (Spain)	Cell wall fragments of *M. tuberculosis* formulated in a liposome suspension.	Prevention of recurrent TB after treatment for TB and MDR-TB; shorting or supplementing drug treatment.	A phase IIa trial, assessing safety and immunogenicity in MDR-TB patients favourably responding to standard MDR-TB treatment, is being planned.
DAR-901; Geisel School of Medicine, Dartmouth (USA)	Broth-grown, whole cell, heat-inactivated *Mycobacterium obuense*, a NTM closely related to *M. tuberculosis.*	Prevention of TB disease in BCG vaccinated adolescents and adults, administered in three intradermal doses.	A phase II POI trial is ongoing, results expected late 2018. A POD trial is planned for 2020.
Vaccae; Anhui Zhifei Longcom Biologic Pharmacy (China)	Heat-killed preparation of *Mycobacterium vaccae*, a NTM closely related to *M. obuense*, administered ×6 (licensed for use in China as adjunctive immnotherapy to drug treatment of active TB).	Adjunctive immunotherapy for drug treatment of active TB.	A phase III trial assessing POD in TST positive adults is completed but not reported.

M. tuberculosis: *Mycobacterium tuberculosis*; POR: prevention of recurrence; TLR: Toll-like receptor 9; EPI: Expanded Program on Immunization; POI: prevention of infection; MVA: modified vaccinia Ankara; POD: prevention of disease.

protect against PTB in adults, however, is more variable. BCG efficacy is negatively impacted by past exposure to environmental mycobacteria, thus supporting the recommendation that infants receive BCG vaccination as soon as possible after birth [2]. The duration of protection also may be impacted by geographical latitude [35], with only limited evidence for sustained protection beyond the first decade in tropical climates [2] and more prolonged protection further from the equator [31]. A recently completed trial demonstrated that BCG-revaccination of adolescents protected against infection (vaccine efficacy (VE) 45.4%, 95% CI 6.4–68.1%), defined as sustained IGRA conversion, among IGRA-negative adolescents at high risk for acquiring *M. tuberculosis* infection in a high transmission setting in the Western Cape in South Africa [26]. This unexpected degree of efficacy resulting from BCG revaccination contrasts with other trials from Brazil and India, which did not demonstrate a beneficial effect on TB incidence from revaccinating persons previously vaccinated with BCG [36–38], but illustrates that there is still much to learn about the ability of BCG to prevent TB.

In addition to its protective effects on TB, BCG is also partially efficacious against *Mycobacterium leprae* and may have nonspecific, protective effects against other infectious diseases, factors that will have to be considered when making policy decisions concerning the potential replacement of BCG with new TB vaccines [39]. BCG also is used as an adjunctive, immunotherapeutic agent in treating noninvasive bladder cancer [40].

VPM1002

BCG *ΔureC::hly* (VPM1002) is a recombinant BCG developed as a TB vaccine to replace BCG in infants, and as a booster vaccine in adults to prevent TB recurrence. In addition, the vaccine is being developed for noninvasive bladder cancer [41].

In VPM1002, a listeriolysin gene has been added and a urease gene deleted in BCG Prague, which permits it to escape the macrophage lysosome allowing antigens to be processed in the cytosol, as occurs for *M. tuberculosis* but not BCG. This promotes autophagy and apoptosis, and the generation of a broader immune response than the already broad immune profile of BCG [42, 43].

VPM1002 was recently licensed by Vakzine Projekt Management (VPM; Hannover, Germany) to the Serum Institute of India PVT LTD (Pune, India), which has initiated an ambitious clinical development plan for VPM1002. The vaccine has passed phase 1 clinical trials in Germany and South Africa, demonstrating its safety and immunogenicity in young adults. It was also successfully tested in a phase IIa RCT in healthy South African newborns and is currently undergoing a phase IIb study in HIV exposed and unexposed newborns powered for non-inferiority to BCG. A phase IIb/phase III POR trial was initiated in India in 2017 [41].

An additional benefit that would result from VPM1002 licensing is the potential to relieve the chronic global shortages that commonly develop in the BCG supply chain. VPM1002 can be manufactured using modern, highly effective fermentation processes at a plant capable of delivering 100 million annual doses [34].

MTBVAC

The MTBVAC vaccine, being developed by the University of Zaragoza (Spain) and their industry partner Biofabri, in close collaboration with the TB Vaccine Initiative (TBVI) and Aeras/IAVI, is a recombinant *M. tuberculosis* developed primarily for BCG replacement in

https://doi.org/10.1183/2312508X.10022417

newborns. Exploring its potential to prevent TB disease in adolescents and adults represents an additional, important development target. MTBVAC is unique in that it represents the first live, attenuated vaccine derived from *M. tuberculosis* to be tested in clinical trials. The vaccine was rationally constructed by making two independent and stable deletions in a clinical isolate of *M. tuberculosis*: 1) deletion of the phoP gene, which controls the transcription of key *M. tuberculosis* virulence genes permitting its survival in host cells; and 2) deletion of the fadD26 gene, required for the synthesis of cell surface lipids that play a critical role in *M. tuberculosis* pathogenicity [44]. As MTBVAC is derived directly from *M. tuberculosis* it possesses an estimated 48% more epitopes than those retained in BCG after the attenuation by passage of *M. bovis* [45]. Importantly, MTBVAC retains the major *M. tuberculosis* immunodominant antigens ESAT-6 and CFP10, both of which are missing from BCG as a result of the loss of the RD-1 region [45].

Preclinical studies have demonstrated that MTBVAC is as safe as BCG and protects better than BCG in different animal models [46]. In addition, MTBVAC-induced immunity to ESAT-6 and CFP10 correlated with improved efficacy relative to BCG in these animal challenge studies, increasing the optimism for potential clinical efficacy [47]. A phase I trial conducted in Swiss adults with no history of BCG vaccination showed that MTBVAC is safe and immunogenic [48], and preliminary results of a phase Ib trial in 36 South African babies demonstrated that MTBVAC is safe and immunogenic in newborns (C. Martin, University of Zaragoza, Zaragoza, Spain; personal communication). In 2018, a phase IIb trial in 99 newborns and another phase Ib/IIa trial in 120 healthy adults, with and without LTBI, started in South Africa to define the dose for future efficacy studies of MTBVAC. One as yet unresolved challenge with MTBVAC is that vaccination can drive false-positive IGRA test responses due to ESAT-6 and CFP10 expressed by the vaccine, but nevertheless it seems a promising candidate for improved protection against childhood TB.

Killed whole mycobacterial cell vaccines and mycobacterial cell extracts

Because BCG vaccination and, to some extent, LTBI protects against the development of TB disease [49], several groups are pursuing vaccines based on killed whole mycobacterial cells, or mycobacterial cell extracts, to safely induce complex immune patterns against multiple *M. tuberculosis* antigens [15].

Vaccae
Vaccae is a whole cell, heat-killed *Mycobacterium vaccae* preparation manufactured by Anhui Zhifei Longcom Biologic Pharmacy in China. It is currently licensed in China for use as an adjunctive therapy to shorten TB treatment, but has not been licensed elsewhere for this purpose. The licensed regimen calls for six intramuscular administrations of the vaccine, making the regimen a challenging one to adhere to. A recent meta-analysis suggested that Vaccae may have some efficacy in preventing smear and culture conversion at month 1–2 following vaccine administration and for sputum smear negativity at the end of treatment, but no evidence of protective efficacy for culture negativity at the end of treatment or a reduction in mortality were demonstrated. The risk for recurrent TB was not assessed [50]. A large phase III trial assessing POD in 10 000 TST-positive adults using the same 6 *i.m.* administration regimen licensed for immunotherapeutic use was completed in 2016. Results from this study, however, have not been made available to the public.

DAR-901

DAR-901 is a preparation of whole-cell, heat inactivated *Mycobacterium obuense*, a NTM closely related to *M. vaccae*. The vaccine is being developed by Geisel School of Medicine at Dartmouth (USA) to prevent TB disease in adolescents and adults previously vaccinated with BCG, when administered as three intradermal injections 2 months apart. DAR-901 was derived from the Master Cell Bank of SRL172, a vaccine in development from 1994–2008, which advanced through phase II trials in Finland and Zambia [51, 52]. A phase III trial of SRL172 administered five times among 2013 HIV-infected subjects in Tanzania concluded in 2008 and demonstrated 39% efficacy for prevention of culture-confirmed TB disease [53]. SRL172, however, required growth on agar and therefore was not scalable. DAR-901 was derived from the SRL172 Master Cell Bank *via* a selection process seeking to identify organisms adapted for growth in liquid media, thereby enhancing scalability. A Phase I trial in BCG-primed adults demonstrated the safety and immunogenicity of DAR-901 [54]. A phase IIb RCT for POI was initiated in 2016 among 650 BCG-primed, healthy Tanzanian adolescents at high risk of acquiring *M. tuberculosis* infection. The three-dose series of immunisations has been completed in all subjects and has confirmed the safety and tolerability of the vaccine. Results of POI efficacy end-points are expected in quarter 4 2019 and a POD trial is planned for 2020.

RUTI

The RUTI, an *M. tuberculosis* extract, is being developed by University of Badalona (Spain) and Archivel Farma as a therapeutic vaccine administered as a single subcutaneous dose to supplement drug therapy for TB. The vaccine is comprised of cell wall fragments of *M. tuberculosis* grown under stress conditions. RUTI has successfully completed phase I and IIa trials, demonstrating an acceptable safety and immunogenicity profile in both HIV-uninfected and HIV-infected individuals, as well as in people with pre-existing *M. tuberculosis* infection [55]. The RUTI vaccine is supported by preclinical data in several animal models, demonstrating both therapeutic and prophylactic potential. RUTI will next be evaluated in a phase IIa trial in MDR-TB patients who have successfully completed the intensive phase, multidrug induction TB therapy. If the results are promising, further trials exploring the therapeutic efficacy in MDR-TB patients are being planned.

Adjuvanted protein subunit vaccines

Adjuvanted protein subunit vaccines are comprised of one or more protein antigens, often covalently linked as a fusion protein, which are administered with adjuvants capable of directing the adaptive immunological responses to the protein subunits towards a desired quality. Adjuvanted protein subunit vaccines represent a significant advance in vaccine technology as they are better defined, easier to produce and safer than other types of vaccines, particularly those derived from whole cells. As the understanding of protective immunity to *M. tuberculosis* increases, particularly our understanding of correlates of immune protection from TB, allowing critical antigens to be selected for inclusion in vaccine candidates, adjuvanted protein subunit vaccines should allow vaccine developers to target the critical protein components of the bacillus with the right type of immune response required for protection.

M72/AS01E

M72/AS01E is a subunit vaccine developed by GSK and Aeras/IAVI to prevent TB disease in adolescents and adults. The M72 construct is comprised of two proteins: Mtb39A, a membrane-associated protein, expressed early in the *M. tuberculosis* life cycle, which

https://doi.org/10.1183/2312508X.10022417

putatively has been identified as an immune evasion factor; and Mtb32A, a constitutively expressed secreted protein, identified as a putative serine protease. Both proteins are found in BCG and *M. tuberculosis*. The AS01E adjuvant consist of liposomes, monophosphoryl lipid A and *Quillaja saponaria* fraction (QS-21), driving a strong and sustained polyfunctional $CD4^+$ T-cell and $CD8^+$ T-cell response as well as induction of vaccine-specific antibodies [56–58].

M72/AS01E has completed 11 phase I and II trials, assessing safety and immunogenicity in a variety of relevant cohorts, including HIV-infected adults and adults with active TB disease (reviewed in [25]). Very recently, a preliminary analysis in a large phase IIb, POD trial in 3573 IGRA positive, HIV-negative adults in Zambia, Kenya and South Africa demonstrated 54.0% (95% CI 2.9–78.2; p=0.04) protection against active pulmonary disease, without evident safety concerns. Of note, protection was highest in participants 25 years of age or younger. These promising results suggest further evaluation of M72/AS01E as a possible vaccination strategy against tuberculosis [25].

H4:IC31

The H4:IC31 subunit vaccine is being developed by Sanofi Pasteur, in collaboration with Aeras/IAVI, Statens Serum Institut (Denmark) and Valneva Austria GmbH (Vienna, Austria). The H4 construct comprises two *M. tuberculosis* antigens: TB10.4, a member of the ESAT-6 family of proteins; and Ag85B, a protein secreted by replicating bacteria in the early stage of infection. The adjuvant, IC31, is manufactured by Valneva and consists of an anti-bacterial peptide (KLK) that results in a depot effect, increasing antigen and adjuvant uptake by antigen-presenting cells, and a non-CpG immunostimulatory oligonucleotide, ODN1a, which stimulates antigen-presenting cells *via* toll-like receptor (TLR)-9 signalling [59], driving mainly a polyfunctional $CD4^+$ T-cell response towards both TB10.4 and Ag85B [60, 61].

H4:IC31 has completed four clinical phase I/IIa trials, determining dose, safety and immunogenicity in adults in both Europe and South Africa. A safety, immunogenicity and dose-ranging study in 229 healthy, BCG-vaccinated, IGRA- and HIV-negative infants, aligned with the Expanded Program on Immunization (EPI) schedule, is ongoing in South Africa with results expected in 2019. One trial assessing potential immune correlates relevant for POI trials is comparing H4:IC31, H56:IC31 and BCG revaccination. Data from this study is expected in early 2019.

Recently a Phase IIb POI trial including 990 healthy, BCG unvaccinated, IGRA- and HIV-negative adolescents, designed to compare H4:IC31 and BCG revaccination against placebo, was completed. Although H4:IC31 failed to demonstrate protective efficacy against the primary end-point, "any IGRA conversion", it demonstrated a VE of 30.5% (95% CI −15.8–58.3%) reduction in new, sustained *M. tuberculosis* infection as compared with placebo recipients for the secondary end-point, "sustained IGRA conversion" [26].

H56:IC31

H56:IC31 is an adjuvanted protein subunit vaccine, developed by Statens Serum Institut, in collaboration with Aeras/IAVI and with support from the European and Developing Countries Clinical Trial Partnership (EDCTP) and other funders. This vaccine is being assessed for POD and POR in adolescents and adults, as well as its potential for use as immunotherapy in persons with active TB disease. The H56:IC31 protein construct is comprised of three antigens: Ag85B; ESAT-6, a premiere virulence-associated antigen constitutively expressed throughout all stages of infection; and Rv2660c, a stress-induced antigen strongly upregulated during latency. As with the H4 vaccine, IC31 (Valneva) serves as the adjuvant. By targeting antigens expressed during the entire infectious cycle, H56:IC31 is designed as a multistage vaccine, and its development is supported by a large preclinical dataset demonstrating protective efficacy for prevention, post-exposure and immunotherapeutic use [62–65].

H56:IC31 builds on the H1:IC31 vaccine, which contained both Ag85B and ESAT-6 but was lacking the Rv2660 antigen. H1:IC31 has completed five phase I/IIa trials demonstrating a positive safety and immunogenicity profile, including safety in HIV-infected individuals, which has allowed for an accelerated development of H56:IC31 [66–68]. H56:IC31 has proven to be safe and immunogenic in completed clinical trials in healthy persons, IGRA-positive individuals, and patients who had completed treatment for active TB [69, 70]. One ongoing, open label phase IIa trial in Norway is assessing the safety and immunogenicity of H56:IC31 given 3 months into active TB treatment as adjunctive immunotherapy. The trial is nearing completion and no safety signal has been reported (A.M. Dyrhol-Riise, Oslo University hospital, Oslo, Norway; personal communication). The immune profile is dominated by polyfunctional CD4$^+$ T-cells with a central memory profile, and strong boosting of ESAT-6 responses when administered post-exposure [69].

In 2018, a POR trial will be initiated in Tanzania and South Africa co-sponsored by Statens Serum Institut and Aeras South Africa, with support from EDCTP. The trial will randomise 900 TB patients at completion of TB treatment and follow-up for 1 year for recurrence or reinfection. Parallel to the efficacy assessment, specimens will be collected to establish a biobank which will be used to advance the understanding of vaccine immunogenicity and to further the efforts to identify immune correlates of protection.

ID93/GLA-SE

ID93 is the lead TB vaccine antigen candidate developed by the Infectious Disease Research Institute (IDRI, USA) for the prevention of PTB and as an immunotherapeutic agent to improve the outcome of drug treatment for active TB. ID93 is a fusion protein comprised of four highly immunodominant antigens: Rv1813, a protein up-regulated under hypoxic conditions; Rv2608, a PE/PPE protein associated with the *M. tuberculosis* outer-membrane; and the ESAT-6 family members Rv3619 and Rv3620 [71]. ID93 is adjuvanted with GLA-SE, which contains a synthetic TLR4 agonist, glucopyranosyl lipid adjuvant (GLA), formulated in a stable nano-emulsion of squalene oil-in-water (SE). The vaccine induces a polyfunctional CD4$^+$ T-cell response as well as a humoral response [72, 73].

Three phase I/IIa trials have been completed in the USA and South Africa, including IGRA-negative and IGRA-positive individuals as well as TB patients at completion of drug treatment. ID93/GLA-SE has proven both safe and immunogenic and has been demonstrated to boost a pre-existing immune response to *M. tuberculosis*. A phase IIa trial is expected to report findings in 2018 and a POR trial is being planned.

Viral vectored tuberculosis vaccines

Another strategy used to generate an immune response to specific antigenic proteins of *M. tuberculosis* relies on live, attenuated, non-replicating viruses engineered to deliver antigen-encoding genes into host cells. Such vaccines trigger intracellular production of the

https://doi.org/10.1183/2312508X.10022417

antigen *in vivo* and can induce both CD4$^+$ and CD8$^+$ T-cell-mediated immunity. In addition, the vector has the potential to activate innate immunity, therefore obviating the need for adjuvants. One viral vectored candidate, MVA85A, developed by the University of Oxford (UK), used a modified vaccinia Ankara (MVA) virus to deliver the Ag85A antigen as a BCG booster vaccine. In a phase IIb efficacy trial in 2795 South African infants randomised to receive MVA85A or placebo, the vaccine failed to demonstrate clinical efficacy for POD, or for exploratory end-points like POI [74]. Although the efficacy outcomes of this trial were disappointing to the TB vaccine community, the results of this and another MVA85A phase IIb trial, which also did not demonstrate efficacy [75], has led to significant advances in the understanding of vaccine immunogenicity and development of biomarkers [76]. New viral-vectored vaccine candidates are being designed with a broader, multistage antigen-specific immunity that can be administered as a heterologous prime boost or through routes other than injection, for example *via* the intranasal route in an effort to induce mucosal antigen-specific cellular immunity in the lung tissue [77].

ChAdOx185a/MVA85A

A TB vaccine strategy currently being advanced by researchers at the University of Oxford is to develop a recombinant viral vector regime using a recombinant simian adenoviral vector prime and an MVA boost, with both vectors expressing four or five antigens which have been demonstrated to be protective in mouse challenge studies [78]. The immunogenicity of an adenoviral vector prime-MVA boost vaccine regimen for TB has previously been demonstrated [79]. In parallel with the antigen identification and optimisation of a prime-boost regimen, the safety and immunogenicity of these vectors delivered directly to the respiratory mucosa is also being evaluated [77]. The aim of this strategy is to maximise mucosal and systemic cellular and humoral immunity using these vectors in small, highly focused clinical studies (experimental medicine studies) to identify the optimum delivery regimen to use when developing these multi-antigenic constructs.

Ad5Ag85A

Ad5Ag85A is another adenovirus-vectored vaccine delivering the Ag85A antigen. This vaccine was developed by McMaster University (Canada) and has been in commercial development by CanSino (China), in collaboration with Aeras, since 2011. The Ad5Ag85A vaccine has completed phase I testing in BCG naïve and BCG vaccinated adults and has been shown to be safe and immunogenic [80, 81]. Ad5Ag85A delivered to the respiratory tract is currently undergoing further evaluation in a phase IIa trial.

Future directions in tuberculosis vaccine research and development

After the disappointing efficacy results of the MVA85A trial [74], the TB vaccine field has sought to diversify the clinical and preclinical pipeline of TB vaccines. One diversification effort centres on attempts to develop vaccines that generate immune responses beyond human leukocyte antigen (HLA)-1-restricted CD4$^+$ T-cell immunity directed at *M. tuberculosis* antigens used as immunogenicity selection criteria for advancing the current vaccine candidates into clinical trials. Interest has focused on the potential utility of donor unrestricted T-cell responses, as well as HLA-E restricted CD8$^+$ T-cell immunity [82]. The potential value of developing TB vaccines generating stronger antibody responses, either alone or in conjunction with T-cells, is being considered [83], as are strategies to stimulate T-helper (Th)17 cells and tissue-resident T-cell effector responses in the pulmonary parenchyma [18, 84, 85].

One novel strategy to diversifying the vaccine platform has shown promise in late stage preclinical studies. This approach uses live cytomegalovirus (CMV) as a vector to deliver a permanent expression of TB antigens for lifelong immune priming (Oregon Health Science University, Portland, OR, USA and Vir Biotechnologies, San Francisco, CA, USA). CMV vectored vaccines induce massive and boostable, antigen-specific CD4$^+$ and CD8$^+$ T-cell vaccine responses that occupy ~10% of the total peripheral T-cell repertoire even 10 months after the second CMV-vectored TB vaccine immunisation [86]. Because CMV represents a persistent viral infection, regulatory concerns regarding safety will have to be addressed before licensing is possible [87]. This approach, however, has shown a degree of protective efficacy unmatched by candidates currently in clinical trials as it cleared *M. tuberculosis* infection in a third of infected rhesus macaques. These results raise hope for generating substantial protective efficacy in humans as well as providing an opportunity to identify immune correlates of protection that could prove greatly beneficial to the field as new TB vaccines are being developed [86].

Diversification strategies have also been applied to methods of vaccine administration. Although BCG initially was administered as an oral vaccine to infants, it and the vast majority of vaccine candidates being assessed in clinical trials are administered *via* either *i.m.* or intradermal injection. As *M. tuberculosis* is an inhaled infectious agent, with the lung as the primary site of initial infection, interest has grown in assessing aerosol delivery of vaccines, with the intent of stimulating an immune response against *M. tuberculosis* in the respiratory mucosa and, possibly, improving the nature of the immune response generated in the pulmonary parenchyma as compared to vaccines administered *via* injection. In addition to administering a single vaccine candidate *via* aerosol, heterologous prime-boost strategies, in which one vaccine is administered *via* injection and the other *via* aerosol administration, are being evaluated in phase I studies. Recently, investigators have been assessing the potential for administering TB vaccines *via* an intravenous route. *i.v.* BCG administration was compared with the standard intradermal route and inhaled aerosolised BCG in an *M. tuberculosis* challenge model in rhesus macaques [88]. The *i.v.* route was proven highly immunogenic and protective even after high-dose *M. tuberculosis* challenge, supporting studies performed half a century ago [89]. While an *i.v.* administration strategy for live, attenuated vaccines such as BCG may not be feasible due to safety concerns, the impressive degree of protection conveyed after *i.v.* administration provides a unique opportunity to understand the types and location of immune responses induced by this route, and the potential for generating such responses by other, safer means.

Future directions in TB vaccine research and development also include increased use of experimental medicine studies, in which vaccine concepts not projected as candidates for full-blown clinical development, or varied vaccine administration strategies, including aerosol and/or *i.v.* administration, are tested in a small number of individuals, permitting extensive studies of the immune response engendered by the vaccine concepts. Another important future direction is to develop a CHIM for TB vaccines. Key issues in developing a TB CHIM are 1) to make the challenge strain safe; and 2) to make the challenge strain detectable, an effort highly dependent on the planned route of challenge. Efforts to make *M. tuberculosis* sufficiently safe for administration to volunteers in a CHIM include building in "kill switches" in *M. tuberculosis* through a timed expression of toxins or development of auxotroph organisms with dependence on non-natural amino acids.

https://doi.org/10.1183/2312508X.10022417

One possible route of administration of the *M. tuberculosis* challenge in a TB CHIM is *via* the intradermal route [90]. A detection system using mycobacteria genetically engineered to produce fluorescence is being assessed as a possible reporter system for this strategy. For CHIMs in which pulmonary challenge *via* inhalation is planned, a leading detection strategy is the engineering of *M. tuberculosis* strains to produce volatile reporter molecules for simple breath monitoring. Advances in preclinical assessment techniques, including the use of PET-CT scans, to assess the efficacy of TB vaccine candidates soon after challenge, offer the potential to reduce the time and cost of important TB vaccine assessment steps, thereby accelerating vaccine development [24, 91, 92].

Conclusion

With 13 TB vaccine candidates in clinical trials, promising results from two new efficacy evaluations [25, 26], and two phase IIb/III efficacy trials scheduled to be unblinded in the next few years, these are exciting times for the TB vaccine research and development community. In particular the very recent results demonstrating efficacy of the M72/AE01E subunit vaccine, are a cause for optimism and supports prioritised pursuit with this class of vaccines. M72/AS01E is based on only two antigens, and it would be tempting to speculate if the observed 54% efficacy could be increased by the inclusion of additional antigens [93]. Additional results from this and the ongoing efficacy trials will be essential in pointing the way to new and better TB vaccine development strategies. Completed phase II efficacy trials of MVA85A, H4:IC31 and BCG revaccination have stimulated the field to seek greater diversification of vaccine strategies. These include an expansion of immunological targets to stimulate a wider variety of immunological responses including different categories of donor-unrestricted T-cells and possibly antibodies; diversification in vaccine platforms, including a persistent CMV-vectored vaccine that has shown great promise in rhesus macaque challenge studies; and diversification in administration approaches, with greater focus on aerosol vaccine delivery. Efforts to identify correlates of immune protection and to develop a TB CHIM are ongoing and offer the potential for greatly increasing the efficiency of TB vaccine development efforts in the future. It will be important to learn from both successful and disappointing outcomes of advanced clinical efficacy trials as we move forward with efforts to develop this critically important tool that is essential to controlling the global TB epidemic, including the spread of MDR- and XDR-TB, in future years.

References

1. World Health Organization. Global tuberculosis report 2017. Geneva, World Health Organization, 2017. Available from: http://www.who.int/tb/publications/global_report/gtbr2017_main_text.pdf
2. World Health Organization. BCG vaccine: WHO position paper, February 2018 – Recommendations. *Vaccine* 2018; 36: 3408–3410.
3. Fletcher HA, Schrager L. TB vaccine development and the End TB Strategy: importance and current status. *Trans R Soc Trop Med Hyg* 2016; 110: 212–218.
4. Esmail H, Barry CE, Young DB, *et al.* The ongoing challenge of latent tuberculosis. *Philos Trans R Soc Lond B Biol Sci* 2014; 369: 20130437.
5. Cadena AM, Fortune SM, Flynn JL. Heterogeneity in tuberculosis. *Nat Rev Immunol* 2017; 17: 691–702.
6. Voss G, Casimiro D, Neyrolles O, *et al.* Progress and challenges in TB vaccine development. *F1000Research* 2018; 7: 199.
7. Frick M. Funding for tuberculosis research—an urgent crisis of political will, human rights, and global solidarity. *Int J Infect Dis* 2017; 56: 21–24.
8. Kaufmann SHE, Dockrell HM, Drager N, *et al.* TBVAC2020: advancing tuberculosis vaccines from discovery to clinical development. *Front Immunol* 2017; 8: 1203.

9. Barker L, Hessel L, Walker B. Rational approach to selection and clinical development of TB vaccine candidates. *Tuberculosis (Edinb)* 2012; 92: Suppl. 1, S25–S29.

10. World Health Organization. Tuberculosis vaccine development. www.who.int/immunization/research/development/tuberculosis/en/ Date last updated: June 14, 2018. Date last accessed: May 7, 2018.

11. Barry CE, Boshoff HI, Dartois V, *et al.* The spectrum of latent tuberculosis: rethinking the biology and intervention strategies. *Nat Rev Microbiol* 2009; 7: 845–855.

12. Horsburgh CR, Barry CE, Lange C. Treatment of tuberculosis. *N Engl J Med* 2015; 373: 2149–2160.

13. Ellis RD, Hatherill M, Tait D, *et al.* Innovative clinical trial designs to rationalize TB vaccine development. *Tuberculosis (Edinb)* 2015; 95: 352–357.

14. Hawn TR, Day TA, Scriba TJ, *et al.* Tuberculosis vaccines and prevention of infection. *Microbiol Mol Biol Rev* 2014; 78: 650–671.

15. Kaufmann SHE, Weiner J, von Reyn CF. Novel approaches to tuberculosis vaccine development. *Int J Infect Dis* 2017; 56: 263–267.

16. Evans TG, Churchyard GJ, Penn-Nicholson A, *et al.* Epidemiologic studies and novel clinical research approaches that impact TB vaccine development. *Tuberculosis (Edinb)* 2016; 99: S21–S25.

17. Lin PL, Maiello P, Gideon HP, *et al.* PET CT identifies reactivation risk in Cynomolgus Macaques with latent *M. tuberculosis. PLoS Pathog* 2016; 12: e1005739.

18. Griffiths KL, Ahmed M, Das S, *et al.* Targeting dendritic cells to accelerate T-cell activation overcomes a bottleneck in tuberculosis vaccine efficacy. *Nat Commun* 2016; 7: 13894.

19. Knight GM, Griffiths UK, Sumner T, *et al.* Impact and cost-effectiveness of new tuberculosis vaccines in low- and middle-income countries. *Proc Natl Acad Sci USA* 2014; 111: 15520–15525.

20. Abu-Raddad LJ, Sabatelli L, Achterberg JT, *et al.* Epidemiological benefits of more-effective tuberculosis vaccines, drugs, and diagnostics. *Proc Natl Acad Sci USA* 2009; 106: 13980–13985.

21. Shah NS, Auld SC, Brust JCM, *et al.* Transmission of extensively drug-resistant tuberculosis in South Africa. *N Engl J Med* 2017; 376: 243–253.

22. Harris RC, Sumner T, Knight GM, *et al.* Systematic review of mathematical models exploring the epidemiological impact of future TB vaccines. *Hum Vaccines Immunother* 2016; 12: 2813–2832.

23. Gröschel MI, Prabowo SA, Cardona P-J, *et al.* Therapeutic vaccines for tuberculosis—A systematic review. *Vaccine* 2014; 32: 3162–3168.

24. O'Shea MK, McShane H. A review of clinical models for the evaluation of human TB vaccines. *Hum Vaccines Immunother* 2016; 12: 1177–1187.

25. Van Der Meeren O, Hatherill M, Nduba V, *et al.* Phase 2b controlled trial of M72/AS01E vaccine to prevent tuberculosis. *N Engl J Med* 2018; in press [https://doi.org/10.1056/NEJMoa1803484].

26. Nemes E, Geldenhuys H, Rozot V, *et al.* Prevention of *M. tuberculosis* infection with H4:IC31 vaccine or BCG revaccination. *N Engl J Med* 2018; 379: 138–149.

27. Brosch R, Gordon SV, Garnier T, *et al.* Genome plasticity of BCG and impact on vaccine efficacy. *Proc Natl Acad Sci USA* 2007; 104: 5596–5601.

28. Dockrell HM, Smith SG. What have we learnt about BCG vaccination in the last 20 years? *Front Immunol* 2017; 8: 1134.

29. Cernuschi T, Malvolti S, Nickels E, *et al.* Bacillus Calmette-Guérin (BCG) vaccine: A global assessment of demand and supply balance. *Vaccine* 2018; 36: 498–506.

30. Netea MG, Joosten LAB, Latz E, *et al.* Trained immunity: a program of innate immune memory in health and disease. *Science* 2016; 352: aaf1098.

31. Verma D, Parasa VR, Raffetseder J, *et al.* Anti-mycobacterial activity correlates with altered DNA methylation pattern in immune cells from BCG-vaccinated subjects. *Sci Rep* 2017; 7: 12305.

32. Mangtani P, Abubakar I, Ariti C, *et al.* Protection by BCG vaccine against tuberculosis: a systematic review of randomized controlled trials. *Clin Infect Dis* 2014; 58: 470–480.

33. Roy A, Eisenhut M, Harris RJ, *et al.* Effect of BCG vaccination against *Mycobacterium tuberculosis* infection in children: systematic review and meta-analysis. *BMJ* 2014; 349: g4643.

34. Harris RC, Dodd PJ, White RG. The potential impact of BCG vaccine supply shortages on global paediatric tuberculosis mortality. *BMC Med* 2016; 14: 138.

35. Wilson ME, Fineberg HV, Colditz GA. Geographic latitude and the efficacy of bacillus Calmette-Guérin vaccine. *Clin Infect Dis* 1995; 20: 982–991.

36. Barreto ML, Pereira SM, Pilger D, *et al.* Evidence of an effect of BCG revaccination on incidence of tuberculosis in school-aged children in Brazil: second report of the BCG-REVAC cluster-randomised trial. *Vaccine* 2011; 29: 4875–4877.

37. Rodrigues LC, Pereira SM, Cunha SS, *et al.* Effect of BCG revaccination on incidence of tuberculosis in school-aged children in Brazil: the BCG-REVAC cluster-randomised trial. *Lancet* 2005; 366: 1290–1295.

38. Karonga Prevention Trial Group. Randomised controlled trial of single BCG, repeated BCG, or combined BCG and killed *Mycobacterium leprae* vaccine for prevention of leprosy and tuberculosis in Malawi. *Lancet* 1996; 348: 17–24.

https://doi.org/10.1183/2312508X.10022417

39. Kandasamy R, Voysey M, McQuaid F, *et al.* Non-specific immunological effects of selected routine childhood immunisations: systematic review. *BMJ* 2016; 355: i5225.

40. Morales A. BCG: A throwback from the stone age of vaccines opened the path for bladder cancer immunotherapy. *Can J Urol* 2017; 24: 8788–8793.

41. Nieuwenhuizen NE, Kulkarni PS, Shaligram U, *et al.* The recombinant bacille Calmette–Guérin vaccine VPM1002: ready for clinical efficacy testing. *Front Immunol* 2017; 8: 1147.

42. Grode L, Ganoza CA, Brohm C, *et al.* Safety and immunogenicity of the recombinant BCG vaccine VPM1002 in a phase 1 open-label randomized clinical trial. *Vaccine* 2013; 31: 1340–1348.

43. Loxton AG, Knaul JK, Grode L, *et al.* Safety and Immunogenicity of the recombinant *Mycobacterium bovis* BCG vaccine VPM1002 in HIV-unexposed newborn infants in South Africa. *Clin Vaccine Immunol* 2017; 24: e00439-16.

44. Arbues A, Aguilo JI, Gonzalo-Asensio J, *et al.* Construction, characterization and preclinical evaluation of MTBVAC, the first live-attenuated *M. tuberculosis*-based vaccine to enter clinical trials. *Vaccine* 2013; 31: 4867–4873.

45. Gonzalo-Asensio J, Marinova D, Martin C, *et al.* MTBVAC: Attenuating the human pathogen of tuberculosis (TB) toward a promising vaccine against the TB epidemic. *Front Immunol* 2017; 8: 1803.

46. Marinova D, Gonzalo-Asensio J, Aguilo N, *et al.* MTBVAC from discovery to clinical trials in tuberculosis-endemic countries. *Expert Rev Vaccines* 2017; 16: 565–576.

47. Aguilo N, Gonzalo-Asensio J, Alvarez-Arguedas S, *et al.* Reactogenicity to major tuberculosis antigens absent in BCG is linked to improved protection against *Mycobacterium tuberculosis*. *Nat Commun* 2017; 8: 16085.

48. Spertini F, Audran R, Chakour R, *et al.* Safety of human immunisation with a live-attenuated *Mycobacterium tuberculosis* vaccine: a randomised, double-blind, controlled phase I trial. *Lancet Respir Med* 2015; 3: 953–962.

49. Andrews JR, Noubary F, Walensky RP, *et al.* Risk of progression to active tuberculosis following reinfection with *Mycobacterium tuberculosis*. *Clin Infect Dis* 2012; 54: 784–791.

50. Huang C-Y, Hsieh W-Y. Efficacy of *Mycobacterium vaccae* immunotherapy for patients with tuberculosis: a systematic review and meta-analysis. *Hum Vaccines Immunother* 2017; 13: 1960–1971.

51. Waddell RD, Chintu C, Lein AD, *et al.* Safety and immunogenicity of a five-dose series of inactivated *Mycobacterium vaccae* vaccination for the prevention of HIV-associated tuberculosis. *Clin Infect Dis* 2000; 30: Suppl. 3, S309–S315.

52. Vuola JM, Ristola MA, Cole B, *et al.* Immunogenicity of an inactivated mycobacterial vaccine for the prevention of HIV-associated tuberculosis: a randomized, controlled trial. *AIDS*; 17: 2351–2355.

53. von Reyn CF, Mtei L, Arbeit RD, *et al.* Prevention of tuberculosis in bacille Calmette-Guérin-primed, HIV-infected adults boosted with an inactivated whole-cell mycobacterial vaccine. *AIDS* 2010; 24: 675–685.

54. von Reyn CF, Lahey T, Arbeit RD, *et al.* Safety and immunogenicity of an inactivated whole cell tuberculosis vaccine booster in adults primed with BCG: a randomized, controlled trial of DAR-901. *PLoS One* 2017; 12: e0175215.

55. Nell AS, D'lom E, Bouic P, *et al.* Safety, tolerability, and immunogenicity of the novel antituberculous vaccine RUTI: randomized, placebo-controlled Phase II clinical trial in patients with latent tuberculosis infection. *PLoS One* 2014; 9: e89612.

56. Gillard P, Yang P-C, Danilovits M, *et al.* Safety and immunogenicity of the M72/AS01E candidate tuberculosis vaccine in adults with tuberculosis: a phase II randomised study. *Tuberculosis (Edinb)* 2016; 100: 118–127.

57. Penn-Nicholson A, Geldenhuys H, Burny W, *et al.* Safety and immunogenicity of candidate vaccine M72/AS01E in adolescents in a TB endemic setting. *Vaccine* 2015; 33: 4025–4034.

58. Leroux-Roels I, Forgus S, De Boever F, *et al.* Improved CD4+ T cell responses to *Mycobacterium tuberculosis* in PPD-negative adults by M72/AS01 as compared to the M72/AS02 and Mtb72F/AS02 tuberculosis candidate vaccine formulations: a randomized trial. *Vaccine* 2013; 31: 2196–2206.

59. Szabo A, Gogolak P, Pazmandi K, *et al.* The two-component adjuvant IC31° boosts type I interferon production of human monocyte-derived dendritic cells *via* ligation of endosomal TLRs. *PLoS One* 2013; 8: e55264.

60. Norrby M, Vesikari T, Lindqvist L, *et al.* Safety and immunogenicity of the novel H4:IC31 tuberculosis vaccine candidate in BCG-vaccinated adults: two phase I dose escalation trials. *Vaccine* 2017; 35: 1652–1661.

61. Geldenhuys H, Mearns H, Miles DJC, *et al.* The tuberculosis vaccine H4:IC31 is safe and induces a persistent polyfunctional CD4 T cell response in South African adults: a randomized controlled trial. *Vaccine* 2015; 33: 3592–3599.

62. Lin PL, Dietrich J, Tan E, *et al.* The multistage vaccine H56 boosts the effects of BCG to protect cynomolgus macaques against active tuberculosis and reactivation of latent *Mycobacterium tuberculosis* infection. *J Clin Invest* 2012; 122: 303–314.

63. Aagaard C, Hoang T, Dietrich J, *et al.* A multistage tuberculosis vaccine that confers efficient protection before and after exposure. *Nat Med* 2011; 17: 189–194.

64. Billeskov R, Tan EV, Cang M, *et al.* Testing the H56 vaccine delivered in 4 different adjuvants as a BCG-booster in a non-human primate model of tuberculosis. *PLoS One* 2016; 11: e0161217.

65. Hoang T, Aagaard C, Dietrich J, *et al.* ESAT-6 (EsxA) and TB10.4 (EsxH) based vaccines for pre- and post-exposure tuberculosis vaccination. *PLoS One* 2013; 8: e80579.

66. Mearns H, Geldenhuys HD, Kagina BM, *et al.* H1:IC31 vaccination is safe and induces long-lived TNF-α$^+$IL-2$^+$CD4 T cell responses in *M. tuberculosis* infected and uninfected adolescents: a randomized trial. *Vaccine* 2017; 35: 132–141.

67. Hussein J, Zewdie M, Yamuah L, *et al.* A phase I, open-label trial on the safety and immunogenicity of the adjuvanted tuberculosis subunit vaccine H1/IC31® in people living in a TB-endemic area. *Trials* 2018; 19: 24.

68. Reither K, Katsoulis L, Beattie T, *et al.* Safety and Immunogenicity of H1/IC31®, an adjuvanted TB subunit vaccine, in HIV-infected adults with CD4$^+$ lymphocyte counts greater than 350 cells/mm^3: a phase II, multi-centre, double-blind, randomized, placebo-controlled trial. *PLoS One* 2014; 9: e114602.

69. Luabeya AKK, Kagina BMN, Tameris MD, *et al.* First-in-human trial of the post-exposure tuberculosis vaccine H56:IC31 in *Mycobacterium tuberculosis* infected and non-infected healthy adults. *Vaccine* 2015; 33: 4130–4140.

70. Suliman S, Luabeya AKK, Geldenhuys H, *et al.* Dose optimization of H56:IC31 vaccine for TB endemic populations: a double-blind, placebo-controlled, dose-selection trial. *Am J Respir Crit Care Med* 2018; in press [https://doi.org/10.1164/rccm.201802-0366OC].

71. Baldwin SL, Ching LK, Pine SO, *et al.* Protection against tuberculosis with homologous or heterologous protein/vector vaccine approaches is not dependent on CD8$^+$ T cells. *J Immunol* 2013; 191: 2514–2525.

72. Coler RN, Bertholet S, Pine SO, *et al.* Therapeutic immunization against *Mycobacterium tuberculosis* is an effective adjunct to antibiotic treatment. *J Infect Dis* 2013; 207: 1242–1252.

73. Penn-Nicholson A, Tameris M, Smit E, *et al.* Safety and immunogenicity of the novel tuberculosis vaccine ID93 + GLA-SE in BCG-vaccinated healthy adults in South Africa: a randomised, double-blind, placebo-controlled phase 1 trial. *Lancet Respir Med* 2018; 6: 287–298.

74. Tameris MD, Hatherill M, Landry BS, *et al.* Safety and efficacy of MVA85A, a new tuberculosis vaccine, in infants previously vaccinated with BCG: a randomised, placebo-controlled phase 2b trial. *Lancet* 2013; 381: 1021–1028.

75. Ndiaye BP, Thienemann F, Ota M, *et al.* Safety, immunogenicity, and efficacy of the candidate tuberculosis vaccine MVA85A in healthy adults infected with HIV-1: a randomised, placebo-controlled, phase 2 trial. *Lancet Respir Med* 2015; 3: 190–200.

76. Fletcher HA, Snowden MA, Landry B, *et al.* T-cell activation is an immune correlate of risk in BCG vaccinated infants. *Nat Commun* 2016; 7: 11290.

77. Satti I, Meyer J, Harris SA, *et al.* Safety and immunogenicity of a candidate tuberculosis vaccine MVA85A delivered by aerosol in BCG-vaccinated healthy adults: a phase 1, double-blind, randomised controlled trial. *Lancet Infect Dis* 2014; 14: 939–946.

78. Stylianou E, Harrington-Kandt R, Beglov J, *et al.* Identification and evaluation of novel protective antigens for the development of a candidate TB subunit vaccine. *Infect Immun* 2018; 86: e00014-18.

79. Sheehan S, Harris SA, Satti I, *et al.* A phase I, open-label trial, evaluating the safety and immunogenicity of candidate tuberculosis vaccines AERAS-402 and MVA85A, administered by prime-boost regime in BCG-vaccinated healthy adults. *PLoS One* 2015; 10: e0141687.

80. Jeyanathan M, Damjanovic D, Yao Y, *et al.* Induction of an immune-protective T-Cell repertoire with diverse genetic coverage by a novel viral-vectored tuberculosis vaccine in humans. *J Infect Dis* 2016; 214: 1996–2005.

81. Smaill F, Jeyanathan M, Smieja M, *et al.* A human type 5 adenovirus-based tuberculosis vaccine induces robust T cell responses in humans despite preexisting anti-adenovirus immunity. *Sci Transl Med* 2013; 5: 205ra134.

82. Joosten SA, Sullivan LC, Ottenhoff TH. Characteristics of HLA-E restricted T-cell responses and their role in infectious diseases. *J Immunol Res* 2016; 2016: 2695396.

83. Achkar JM, Casadevall A. Antibody-mediated immunity against tuberculosis: implications for vaccine development. *Cell Host Microbe* 2013; 13: 250–262.

84. Woodworth JS, Cohen SB, Moguche AO, *et al.* Subunit vaccine H56/CAF01 induces a population of circulating CD4 T cells that traffic into the *Mycobacterium tuberculosis*-infected lung. *Mucosal Immunol* 2016; 10: 555–564.

85. Andersen P, Woodworth JS. Tuberculosis vaccines – rethinking the current paradigm. *Trends Immunol* 2014; 35: 387–395.

86. Hansen SG, Zak DE, Xu G, *et al.* Prevention of tuberculosis in rhesus macaques by a cytomegalovirus-based vaccine. *Nat Med* 2018; 24: 130–143.

87. Aiello AE, Chiu Y-L, Frasca D. How does cytomegalovirus factor into diseases of aging and vaccine responses, and by what mechanisms? *GeroScience* 2017; 39: 261–271.

88. Sharpe S, White A, Sarfas C, *et al.* Alternative BCG delivery strategies improve protection against *Mycobacterium tuberculosis* in non-human primates: protection associated with mycobacterial antigen-specific CD4 effector memory T-cell populations. *Tuberculosis (Edinb)* 2016; 101: 174–190.

89. Barclay WR, Anacker RL, Brehmer W, *et al.* Aerosol-induced tuberculosis in subhuman primates and the course of the disease after intravenous BCG vaccination. *Infect Immun* 1970; 2: 574–582.

90. Blazevic A, Xia M, Turan A, *et al.* Pilot studies of a human BCG challenge model. *Tuberculosis (Edinb)* 2017; 105: 108–112.

91. Herzmann C, Ernst M, Lange C, *et al.* Pulmonary immune responses to *Mycobacterium tuberculosis* in exposed individuals. *PLoS One* 2017; 12: e0187882.

https://doi.org/10.1183/2312508X.10022417

92. Esmail H, Lai RP, Lesosky M, *et al.* Characterization of progressive HIV-associated tuberculosis using 2-deoxy-2-[18F]fluoro-D-glucose positron emission and computed tomography. *Nat Med* 2016; 22: 1090–1093.

93. Bloom BR. New promise for vaccines against tuberculosis. *N Engl J Med* 2018; in press [https://doi.org/10.1056/NEJMe1812483].

Disclosures: M. Ruhwald is employed by SSI, who develop vaccines for TB, including the H4:IC31 and the H56:IC31 vaccines which are described in the paper. He has no financial relationship to said vaccines. P.L. Andersen is employed by SSI, who develop vaccines for TB, including the H4:IC31 and the H56:IC31 vaccines, which are described in the paper. P.L. Andersen is recognised as an inventor on patents (numbers WO2006136162 for H56 vaccine and WO0011214 for Rv 2660c); all rights have been assigned to SSI.

Support statement: Morten Ruhwald and Peter L. Andersen receive funding from European Commission H2020 program [grant number TBVAC2020 643381] and Research Council Norway [GLOBVAC 248042/H10].

Acknowledgements: Thanks for excellent input from colleges in the TB vaccine field, in particular Rhea Coler Infectious Disease Research Institute (IDRI, USA); Carlos Martin, University of Zaragoza (Spain); Helen McShane, University of Oxford (UK); Leander Grode, Vakzine Projekt Management GmbH (Germany) and Ford von Reyn, Geisel School of Medicine at Dartmouth (USA).

Chapter 21

Transmission control: a refocused approach

Edward Nardell[1] and Grigory Volchenkov[2]

Ongoing transmission, infection and reinfection, in both community and congregate settings, is fuelling the global TB epidemic. This is despite longstanding comprehensive WHO TB transmission control policies and training, suggesting generally ineffective implementation strategies. Traditional transmission control efforts in institutions tend to focus on known TB patients; many already on effective therapy and not the source of most transmission. Longstanding evidence suggests that TB patients on effective therapy become rapidly noninfectious, and that unsuspected, untreated cases (and unsuspected drug resistance) account for most transmission. In this chapter we argue for a refocused TB transmission control strategy based on active case finding (community and institutional), rapid molecular diagnosis and DST, followed by prompt, fully supervised effective treatment, in the community rather than the hospital or clinic. In Eastern Europe and Central Asia, prolonged hospitalisation combined with delayed diagnosis of drug resistance and poor ventilation in cold climates has resulted in hyper-transmission, resulting in rates of MDR-TB of ⩾25% among new cases, compared with <7% in most other countries. Despite screening, some infectious cases will be missed, especially in crowded ambulatory settings. We discuss the pros and cons of natural ventilation, mechanical ventilation systems, upper room germicidal ultraviolet air disinfection, fit-tested respirators on healthcare workers, and short-term use of masks on coughing patients before effective treatment is initiated. We discourage the use of portable room air cleaners.

Cite as: Nardell E, Volchenkov G. Transmission control: a refocused approach. *In:* Migliori GB, Bothamley G, Duarte R, *et al.*, eds. Tuberculosis (ERS Monograph). Sheffield, European Respiratory Society, 2018; pp. 364–380 [https://doi.org/10.1183/2312508X.10022517].

@ERSpublications
Diagnosing and effectively treating unsuspected TB patients is the most effective means of transmission control. Upper room germicidal ultraviolet air disinfection is an underused complement to natural ventilation. http://ow.ly/cfVQ30lqCfE

While global rates of drug-susceptible cases are declining incrementally, drug-resistant cases are not declining but are increasing in many areas [1]. Although transmission control is essential for both drug-susceptible and drug-resistant disease, we focus on drug

[1]Division of Global Health Equity, Brigham and Women's Hospital, Boston, MA, USA. [2]Vladimir Regional TB Control Center, Vladimir, Russian Federation.

Correspondence: Edward Nardell, Division of Global Health Equity, Brigham and Women's Hospital, 75 Francis Street, Boston, MA, 02115, USA. E-mail: enardell@gmail.com

resistance because of the greater threat it poses to individuals and to global TB control. Moreover, interventions that reduce MDR-TB transmission will reduce all TB transmission, as most transmission arises from those with unsuspected TB or unsuspected drug resistance [2].

In many high-burden countries, MDR-TB cases result from transmission in congregate settings (for example, hospitals, clinics, prisons and various crowded-living situations) more quickly than slowly emerging treatment programmes are able to cure them [3]. In 2016, an estimated 22% of the incident MDR cases worldwide were started on treatment, and the rest continue to transmit throughout the natural history of their disease [1]. It is not surprising, therefore, that the vast majority of new and previously treated cases of MDR-TB are a result of transmission and not poor treatment as was once suspected [4]. Transmission from unrecognised or inadequately treated MDR-TB and XDR-TB cases is a critically important factor that is fuelling the global DR-TB epidemic; this is particularly the case in parts of the world where patients are hospitalised for prolonged periods, and in places where HIV infection is also prevalent [5, 6].

Our focus on transmission does not dispute the widely understood importance of erratic treatment and poor treatment supervision in selecting for drug-resistant *Mycobacterium tuberculosis* strains. We believe that community-based treatment supervision can greatly reduce drug resistance by preventing the selection of resistant strains, by halting transmission through effective treatment, and by avoiding or minimising hospitalisation [7–10]. However, when mutant organisms are selected by poor chemotherapy, we emphasise the urgency of controlling their highly efficient airborne spread in congregate settings [11].

By far the most important way to control transmission of MDR TB in institutions as well as in the community is through prompt diagnosis and effective treatment [12]. However, we do acknowledge that not every case of TB will be diagnosed promptly, especially in crowded ambulatory settings; with this in mind, we review the environmental controls designed to reduce transmission from unsuspected cases in situations where unsuspected TB or unsuspected drug resistance is common [13–16]. We discuss respiratory protection for healthcare workers and surgical masks on infectious patients; these are important in certain high-risk circumstances but are secondary in terms of stopping transmission generally [17].

We follow the conventional TB transmission control hierarchy of administrative, environmental and respiratory protection; however, this chapter emphasises the use of FAST (Find cases Actively by cough surveillance and rapid molecular testing, Separate temporarily, and Treat effectively based on molecular DST results), a refocused combination of administrative controls [12, 18].

As not every case of unsuspected TB or unsuspected drug resistance will be identified, we also emphasise the use of upper room germicidal ultraviolet (GUV) as a safe and highly effective supplement or alternative to natural ventilation; this is especially important in very cold and very hot climates [14].

How *Mycobacterium tuberculosis* is transmitted

There are few infectious diseases, other than TB, whose transmission from person to person is almost exclusively airborne [19]. *M. tuberculosis* is initially an infection of the alveolar macrophages, requiring inhalation of particles fine enough (1–5 μm) to transit to the upper respiratory tract and reach the distal lung where alveolar macrophages reside [20]. Such fine particles remain airborne, diluted in moving room air, unless they are inhaled by occupants or exhausted outdoors [21]. Inhaled particles containing viable, virulent *M. tuberculosis* may be engulfed by alveolar macrophages and destroyed, or they may replicate in the macrophages, initiating specific microbial mechanisms to avoid intracellular lysosomal killing, eventually triggering autophagy with the release of organisms into the lung tissue, with progressive infection [22]. Little is known about how often inhaled organisms fail to initiate or sustain infection, although early artificial aerosol studies suggested that there was a relatively good correlation between colony forming units and guinea pig infections when droplets were of a respirable size [21]. Allowing for considerable variation due to chance and other factors, the percentage of transient (aborted), sustained and progressive infection is likely to be determined by the virulence of *M. tuberculosis* and the effectiveness of host innate and early adaptive immunity. The effective dose of *M. tuberculosis* is believed to be as little as one viable, virulent organism, or one droplet nucleus containing several organisms. Multiple foci on radiographs are uncommon in primary TB infection in children, consistent with rapid dilution in room air to relatively low concentrations [23]. Another manifestation of dose, however, is repeated inhalation of *M. tuberculosis* over time in high-risk settings, increasing the probability that at least one will successfully establish sustained infection and progress [24]. The average number of inhaled organisms (rarely known) that is statistically likely to establish sustained infection of most exposed hosts in a population is called a "quantum of infection", which is estimated to be as low as one organism for susceptible hosts, but much higher in hosts with established (innate or adaptive) immunity or with low-virulence *M. tuberculosis* strains [21].

Infectious droplet nuclei (dried residua of larger respiratory droplets) are generated by those with PTB who cough, but also by quiet breathing as alveoli pop open with inhalation [25]. Caseous necrosis is a hallmark of TB pathogenesis and results in lung cavitation, containing up to 10^8 organisms. When cavities erode into the airways, large numbers of organisms suddenly have access to the environment and are aerosolised through cough and other respiratory manoeuvres. Cough frequency, cavities on chest radiographs and strongly positive sputum smears for *M. tuberculosis* have traditionally been correlated with infectiousness, but recently cough aerosol sampling (a research tool) has been shown to correlate better with household transmission because the patient's ability to generate aerosol is also quantified [26]. *M. tuberculosis* aerosol generation rate varies greatly from patient to patient but so does *M. tuberculosis* virulence, host resistance and environmental conditions, making TB transmission very difficult to predict with any one factor [27]. TB is occasionally spread from extrapulmonary sites, such as a tissue abscesses, during surgery and at the autopsy table [28].

Later in this chapter, we review the interventions used to reduce transmission (figure 1): 1) by decreasing source strength (*M. tuberculosis* aerosol-generation rate); 2) through air disinfection and; 3) through respiratory protection. No intervention is more effective than identifying infectious TB patients and quickly starting DST-based effective treatment [29]. Combined with active case finding and rapid molecular diagnosis, the core administrative intervention package, FAST, discussed later, should be the highest priority in institutional TB transmission control [12].

How common is unsuspected tuberculosis?

When institutional TB transmission control is implemented, it generally focuses on known TB cases that are already receiving therapy and are pending microbial confirmation.

https://doi.org/10.1183/2312508X.10022517

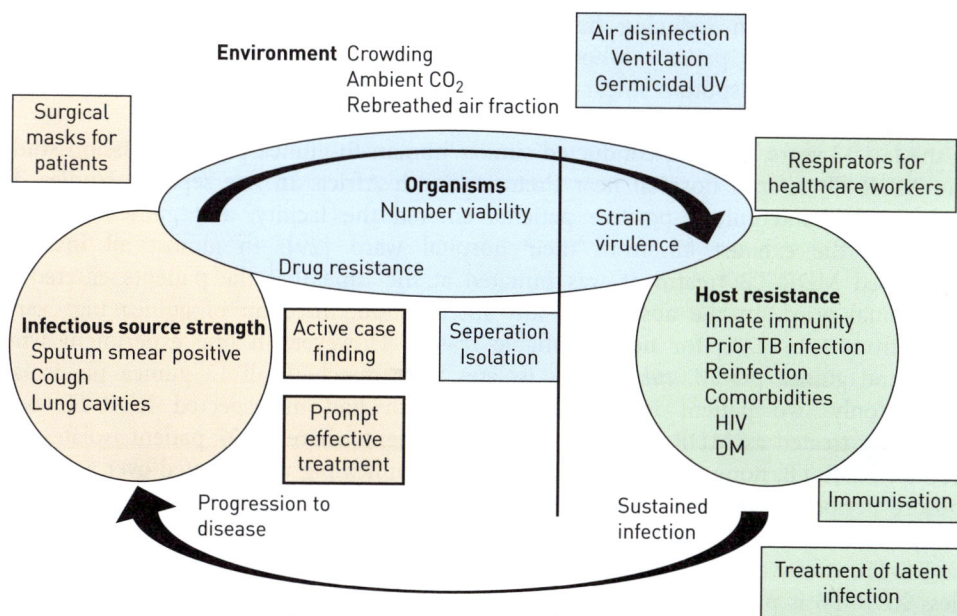

Figure 1. The four major factors in the transmission of *Mycobacterium tuberculosis*: environment; infectious source strength; organisms; and host resistance. The boxes describe interventions at each step in the TB propagation. Active case finding and prompt effective treatment are the single most important interventions to reduce transmission.

However, it has long been known that the greater risk in hospitals is posed by unsuspected and untreated cases. The number of unsuspected TB patients, including drug-resistant cases, is rarely documented. Over the course of a year, WILLINGHAM *et al.* [30] screened 250 patients admitted to a large female ward for TB in a busy general hospital in Lima (Peru). They found 40 patients who were TB-culture positive, including 26 (65%) who were smear positive and 13 (33%) who were unsuspected for TB. Of the 40 culture-positive cases, eight had MDR-TB (six unsuspected, three of whom were smear-positive cases). Without prompt identification of TB and drug resistance, followed by effective treatment, transmission from such patients continues. Other screening efforts, in Zambia for example, have had similar results [2].

The rapid impact of treatment on transmission

A study conducted in Madras, India, in the 1960s showed that, compared to treatment in hospital, treatment at home did not increase the risk to close contacts of infection or disease or over the following 5 years [31]. Other epidemiological studies that were performed slightly later, confirmed the safety of treating TB in the community, and the disassociation between smear and culture positivity and infectiousness in treated patients [32–35]. However, the most direct evidence of the impact of treatment on the reduction of TB transmission can be found in an animal experiment, in which a large number of sentinel guinea pigs (a well-established animal model used to quantify TB transmission) breathed the air exhausted from experimental TB wards [36]. In R.L. Riley's first study, performed over 60 years ago, all transmission to guinea pigs stopped when sputum smear-positive patients who had just started receiving effective therapy for drug-susceptible (DS)-TB were admitted to the ward, and resumed when sputum smear-positive drug-resistant patients receiving ineffective treatment were admitted [37]. In Riley's second, 2–year study, the rapid effect of treatment on reducing transmission was prospectively demonstrated: sputum smear-positive DS-TB patients who had started receiving treatment were only 2% as infectious as untreated sputum smear-positive patients [36].

For the last 13 years, we have conducted similar human-to-guinea pig transmission studies at an MDR-TB referral hospital near Pretoria, South Africa. In five separate studies, 109 mostly smear- and culture-positive patients entered the facility, and guinea pigs were exposed to the exhaust air from their hospital ward [29]. In almost all instances, standardised MDR-TB treatment was initiated at the time that the patients entered the experimental ward. In the absence of any intervention, infection of guinea pigs varied greatly, from 1 to 77%, for no identifiable reason. However, in one experiment where patient and guinea pig *M. tuberculosis* isolates were matched, all 13 guinea pig isolates matched only two patient isolates, both of which had unsuspected XDR-TB being ineffectively treated as MDR-TB. In another experiment where all 27 patient isolates were tested for XDR-TB, none were found, and only one guinea pig was infected over a 4-month exposure period. In the other three experiments, in which 10, 53 and 77% guinea pigs became infected, patients had unsuspected XDR-TB that was being treated as MDR-TB. Like DS-TB, effective MDR treatment appears to rapidly and profoundly stop transmission, unless XDR-TB is present. Not all treatment promptly stops transmission. A recent, as yet unpublished study of the early effect of adding bedaquiline and linezolid to patients with XDR-TB failed to show any reduction in human-to-guinea pig transmission in the first 11 days of treatment (A. Stoltz, University of Pretoria, Hatfield, South Africa; personal communication). This is consistent with the pharmokinetics of the drugs, which require weeks to reach therapeutic levels [38, 39].

Hyper-transmission and reinfection

KENDALL *et al.* [40] recently published a model that estimated the percentage of MDR-TB transmitted and acquired as a result of poor treatment, both globally and in selected countries at high and low risk of MDR-TB. Overall, their model showed that WHO's global estimate of 3.5% MDR-TB among new cases and 20.5% among retreated cases translated to a median of 96% transmitted among all incident cases and 61% among retreated cases. Table 1 presents the country-specific estimates found in the study.

With the exception of the low MDR rate in Bangladesh presented in table 1, most MDR-TB results from transmission, not from poor treatment. In the 2016 WHO report, the rate of MDR-TB amongst new cases was 38% in Belarus, 26% in Kazakhstan, 27% in

Table 1. Estimation of transmitted MDR-TB cases in selected countries with varying rates of MDR-TB among new cases [40]

	MDR among new cases %	Transmitted %
Bangladesh	1.2	48
Ethiopia	1.5	92
Malawi	0.3	82
Peru	3.9	95
Philippines	2.0	76
Uzbekistan	27	99

https://doi.org/10.1183/2312508X.10022517

Kyrgyzstan, 26% in Moldova, 27% in Russia, 22% in Tajikistan and 27% in Ukraine [1]. Clearly, these distinctly high MDR-TB rates represent hyper-transmission, resulting, we propose, from a combination of prolonged hospitalisation, delayed DR-TB diagnosis and poor ventilation in generally cold climates in Eastern Europe and Central Asia [41–43]. With the introduction of universal rapid molecular DST on admission, however, this could change dramatically, as will be discussed further later [44]. The following scenario from Tomsk, Russia, provides insight into why hyper-transmission has been happening in Eastern Europe and Central Asia.

A retrospective study of risk factors for MDR-TB in Tomsk unexpectedly found that hospitalisation among adherent patients during an initial course of treatment for DS-TB was the major risk factor (odds ratio >6) for MDR-TB development compared with adherent patients treated in an ambulatory setting [45]. As they had previously been treated, these cases would have been routinely classified as acquired drug resistance rather than primary MDR-TB, but that is clearly not the case. In many Former Soviet Union countries, patients are admitted to hospital and treated for DS-TB based on smear test or chest radiography with culture pending. Only after months of failing treatment clinically, are DSTs ordered, and MDR-TB diagnosed and effectively treated. In the meantime, other patients are admitted to the same poorly ventilated congregate rooms, and many with DS-TB become re-infected with DR-TB. Prompt diagnosis and effective treatment based on rapid molecular testing can stop hyper-transmission and re-infection, as demonstrated below.

In Voronezh and Petrozavodsk, Russia, investigators implemented universal Xpert MTB/ RIF (Cepheid, Sunnyvale, CA, USA) testing on patient admission to 800-bed and 120-bed facilities, respectively, followed by prompt treatment of DS-TB and RR-TB [44]. Patients were in hospital an average of 20.7 weeks before implementation of rapid molecular testing, and 20.0 weeks after implementation. Before implementation of universal Xpert MTB/RIF testing, it took an average of 76.5 days before MDR-TB was diagnosed and patients began effective treatment. Out of a total of 450 patients who were HR sensitive on admission before implementation, 12.2% were diagnosed with MDR-TB within 12 months of finishing treatment. Out of 259 patients who were isoniazid and rifampin sensitive after implementation of universal molecular testing and prompt treatment, only 3.1% were subsequently diagnosed with MDR-TB within 12 months of finishing treatment. This is a 78% odds reduction in MDR acquisition through the interruption of transmission by effective treatment of an MDR-TB case in hospital.

Transmission and re-infection are driving the epidemic in warm as well as cold climates. Without comparing the molecular fingerprints of original and relapse isolates (which are infrequently available), there are no specific tests for re-infection and it is rarely discussed. Re-infection is an important distinction in TB pathogenesis because it usually implies recent transmission, whereas reactivation does not [46]. The widely publicised report of rapidly fatal XDR-TB cases in South Africa called the world's attention to the potential for rapid spread from one or more unsuspected XDR-TB case to HIV-infected patients in the multi-bed wards that are common to resource-limited regions [5]. Of the 53 cases initially reported, 55% had not been treated previously but two-thirds had been hospitalised, and 85% had isolates with the same genotypes. This strongly suggested transmission and largely re-infection among previously infected adults. Moreover, due to the soaring temperatures and humidity caused by climate change, ductless air conditioning is being introduced widely, in India for example [47]; the use of air conditioning results in windows being closed and, therefore, an increased risk of transmission. Although rapid diagnosis and effective treatment is essential to prevent the spread of DS-TB and MDR-TB, stopping XDR transmission may depend more on isolation and air disinfection, as there is no evidence of a rapid treatment effect from current drug regimens, even with the addition of bedaquiline and lenazolid. However, in our South African human-to-guinea pig transmission facility, recent unpublished studies indicate that a delamamid-like drug containing regimen promptly stopped XDR transmission [44].

FAST: a refocused administrative approach to transmission control

Recognition of the importance of transmission from those with unsuspected TB or with unsuspected drug resistance, who not on therapy or on ineffective therapy, combined with the availability of rapid molecular diagnostics, and a renewed understanding of the rapid impact of effective treatment, has led to a refocused administrative approach to institutional transmission control called FAST [12, 18]. The FAST acronym is intended to help prioritise active case finding, rapid diagnosis and effective treatment, the most important activities required to stop transmission in institutions and in the community. FAST is being widely adopted around the world with preliminary results published from Bangladesh and Russia, as previously noted [18, 44]. Vietnam is implementing FAST nationwide, and preliminary results have been submitted for publication (D. Tierney, Brigham & Women's Hospital, Division of Global Health Equity, Boston, MA, USA; personal communication).

The case for community-based treatment

Some hospitalisation is certainly required for socially and medically complicated cases, especially in rural areas; however, in locations as diverse as Peru, Lesotho, Cambodia and Karachi (Pakistan), there is growing evidence of enhanced treatment adherence with favourable clinical and presumably transmission control consequences, as well as a much-reduced programme cost [8, 9, 48, 49]. The National Tuberculosis Program decision regarding where DR-TB patients should be treated is often complex (it is influenced by national, regional and local community policies as well as customary practise) and is sometimes compromised by a perverse financial incentive to fill beds [43]. Programmes also require a viable alternative of established and effective community-based care. The choice can often be influenced by outmoded perceptions of the relative risk of transmission in each environment. And yet these choices are frequently made without full consideration of the impact of institutional transmission on the propagation of the disease, particularly in areas with a high prevalence of HIV [16]. There are not enough hospital beds in the world for the initial 6 months of treatment for the estimated 1.3 million DR-TB cases requiring treatment. Because effective outpatient follow-up is needed after discharge in order to complete 18–24 months of conventional treatment (or a 9-month short treatment) of those patients started in hospital, the incremental programmatic investment necessary to develop a fully community-based treatment programme should be cost-effective, assuming that it would not only improve treatment outcomes, but greatly reduce hospitalisation and hospital-related transmission [50].

Interventions in institutions

The widely accepted standard approach to TB transmission control includes administrative interventions, engineering or environmental measures, and respiratory protection [51]. This approach is detailed in both the published WHO TB infection control policy (under revision,

https://doi.org/10.1183/2312508X.10022517

expected first quarter of 2019) and the companion facility-level implementation document (soon to be updated) [51, 52]. If more detail on conventional approaches is required, these sources should be consulted, as well as the current CDC guidelines, although the latter are written primarily for low-prevalence, resource-rich settings [53].

The process of TB transmission control in institutions begins with the creation of an administratively empowered and funded multidisciplinary TB infection control team. This team is responsible for: institutional transmission risk assessment; policy development; plan implementation; and monitoring of the process and its outcomes. In high-risk settings, one of the most relevant and readily available metrics of risk and risk reduction is the annual rate of active TB among institutional workers (*e.g.* nurses, doctors, laboratory workers or prison staff) [51]. It can be assumed that if institutional workers are protected, transmission amongst patients, prisoners and other institutional residents will reduce.

Administrative controls are often the least expensive and most effective interventions. FAST, which includes active case finding, rapid molecular diagnosis and effective community-based treatment, involves both administrative and environmental policy components [12]. FAST is likely to be successful and cost-effective both in terms of treatment outcome and transmission prevention.

Conventional institutional TB transmission control also involves environmental control and the targeted use of respiratory protection [51]. Depending on existing conditions, new building construction or renovation may be required to ensure natural ventilation in a favourable setting [54, 55]. Where natural ventilation is inadequate or unreliable, a greater understanding and selective application of sustainable upper room germicidal air disinfection with air mixing is essential (thought currently underused) [14, 15, 56–64].

Hospital and clinic design for multidrug-resistant tuberculosis transmission control

Overcrowded hospital wards increase the risk of TB transmission for two reasons: more patients on the ward means that there is a higher chance that some will be infectious and overcrowding increases the number of other patients exposed. In an unpublished study of medical student skin test conversion in Lima (Peru) Accinelli and colleagues reported a 25.5% conversion risk among students who underwent clinical training in a hospital with a room volume of 16.2 m^3 per bed, compared with 12.7% for students training in a hospital with 41.4 m^3 per bed (R. Accinelli, Cayetano Heredia University, Lima, Peru; personal communication). Both hospitals served poor populations in urban areas at high risk of TB. The hospital with large room volumes also had very high ceilings; this accommodated tall windows, which allowed for copious natural ventilation. The hospital with the smaller room volumes had lower ceilings, fewer and smaller windows, and a generally ineffective mechanical ventilation system.

The need for architects and engineers who are trained in airborne infection control is growing. An example of a recent renovation/new construction that capture the state of the art in resource-limited settings can be seen in Karachi (Pakistan). Here, a new clinic- and community-based MDR-TB programme based on the Peru model required the design and construction of a new ambulatory treatment centre and laboratory. The design included covered outdoor waiting areas, a novel patient flow scheme, and a building which fully

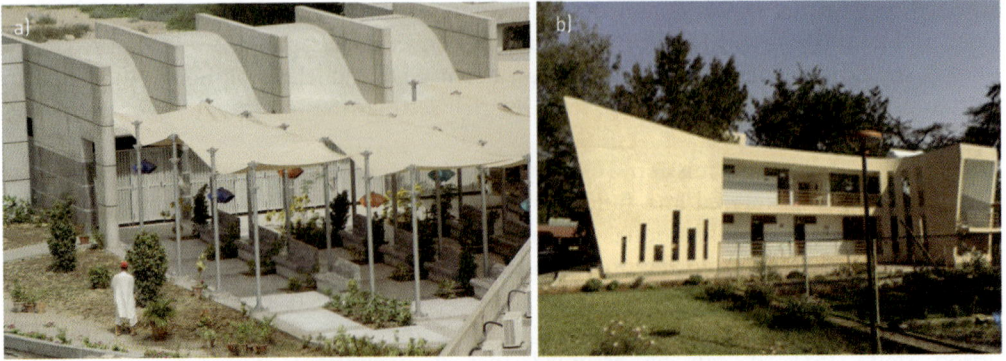

Figure 2. Two examples of MDR-TB clinics designed for natural ventilation. a) The Indus Hospital MDR-TB Clinic in Karachi (Pakistan), designed by T. Quasir with "wind scoops" for maximum interior ventilation, and a covered outdoor waiting area. b) The Alert Hospital MDR-TB clinic in Addis Ababa (Ethiopia), designed by M. Girma, with exterior corridors to prevent room-to-room flow of contaminated air through central corridors. Both architects received special training on building design and engineering for airborne transmission control. As noted, highly effective natural ventilation requires compatible climates and specific designs. In existing buildings in cold climates, mechanical ventilation and/or upper room germicidal air disinfection are recommended.

takes advantage of natural ventilation, including metal stacks that heat up in the sun to generate additional airflow through the building (figure 2). This design, however, is climate-specific and would not work for much of the year in cold Eastern European and Central Asian countries. Figure 2b is another example of an MDR-TB clinic in Ethiopia where the architect avoids interior corridors that can be conduits for cross-contamination.

Ambient carbon dioxide levels as a surrogate for environmental risk

RUDNICK and MILTON [65] have suggested that ambient carbon dioxide (CO_2) levels can serve as a good surrogate for "rebreathed air fraction", as humans routinely exhale CO_2 at 40 000 ppm, which is immediately diluted by room volume and ventilation to levels between those found outdoors (now 350–400 ppm) and those commonly found indoors (400–1000 ppm). Ambient indoor CO_2 represents the combined effect of occupancy and ventilation and as such is a good surrogate for the risk of airborne infection. However, as important are source strength (the generation rate of infectious droplet nuclei) and exposure duration, which is influenced by many factors including active case finding and prompt, effective treatment of otherwise unsuspected TB cases or drug resistance. Monitoring of ambient CO_2 in an individual's environment has been used to understand when and where (in combination with a geographic positioning system) in the course of a day airborne risks are highest [66]. Finally, portable, personal CO_2 monitoring is being used to assess building design (and use) by cohorts of hospital workers to assess the effectiveness of buildings and their use (J. Nice, South African Council for Scientific and Industrial Research, Pretoria, South Africa; personal communication).

The pros and cons of natural ventilation and mechanical ventilation

Facilities in warm climates can take advantage of outdoor waiting areas, covered open walkways and open windows much of the year. In studies where CO_2 has been used as a

https://doi.org/10.1183/2312508X.10022517

tracer gas, very high indoor exchange rates have been found in some settings when windows are open compared with when they are closed [55]. While facilities planners are encouraged to take full advantage of natural ventilation, there are limitations that must be fully understood. Effective natural ventilation is rarely as simple as opening a window. It is essential that the volume and direction of airflow in various climate conditions and at different times of day should be studied. Wind direction often changes. The effects of opening and closing interior doors (*e.g.* examination room doors) should also be considered. WHO recently issued comprehensive, evidence-based guidelines on natural ventilation to control airborne infections in the healthcare setting [67]. The guidelines propose a number of minimal hourly average ventilation rates, taking into account fluctuations in conditions: 160 $L \cdot s^{-1} \cdot patient^{-1}$ for new airborne infection isolation rooms or major renovations; 60 $L \cdot s^{-1} \cdot patient^{-1}$ for general wards and outpatient departments; and 2.5 $L \cdot s^{-1} \cdot m^{-3}$ for corridors and other transient spaces without a fixed number of patients. Ideally, the direction of airflow should be from the source patient to the outside. Despite guidelines, however, existing structures and climate conditions often mean interior conditions are less than optimal. As previously noted, global warming is resulting in wider use of ductless air conditioning, which requires that windows are closed. When ventilation rates and airflow direction cannot be reliably achieved with natural ventilation alone, mechanical ventilation or mixed-mode systems are recommended [53].

Upper room germicidal air disinfection is more affordable and sustainable than mechanical ventilation, and can be used as a complementary system to natural ventilation at night or during cold/hot seasons when windows may be closed, for example [13]. "Room air cleaners" rarely provide "clean air delivery rates" sufficient to produce the equivalent of six to 12 room air changes per hour [16, 68]. More commonly, room air cleaners add the equivalent of one or two air changes per hour, which is not effective air disinfection and is falsely reassuring.

The pros and cons of upper room germicidal ultraviolet air disinfection

With the exception of natural ventilation, no other engineering intervention offers as much potential benefit for as little cost as properly designed and installed upper room GUV air disinfection [13–16, 56–58, 69–73]. This is particularly true in cold climates where natural ventilation or high-volume mechanical ventilation systems are not appropriate. However, upper room GUV is poorly understood and frequently poorly applied [72].

Germicidal lamps are used in three different ways: 1) for direct, unshielded room disinfection; 2) for disinfection of ventilation ducts or room air cleaners; and 3) for upper room air disinfection. In Eastern Europe, unshielded GUV (UV-C, 254 nm UV) is commonly used to disinfect entire unoccupied room surfaces. However, this application of ultraviolet germicidal irradiation (UVGI) is not effective for TB transmission control because: 1) there is little evidence that once it has settled on surfaces, *M. tuberculosis* can be resuspended as particles small enough to reach the alveoli of the lung where infection must begin; 2) although widely used, UV is not an ideal surface decontaminant because it misses shadowed surfaces; and 3) air disinfection is most useful for protecting room occupants at the same time that the infectious source is present, not empty rooms [13].

UVGI in ventilation ductwork can reduce recirculated contagion but is of little benefit in reducing transmission within a room or hospital ward, which is the main goal. Similarly,

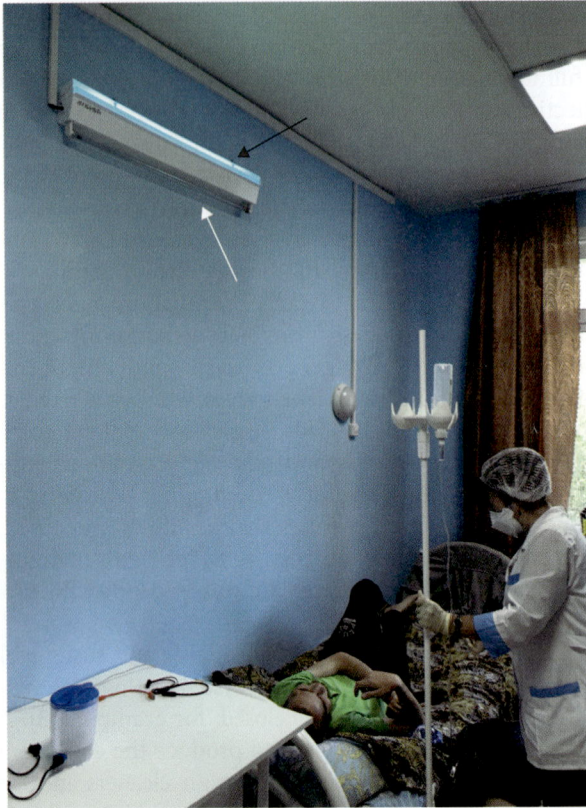

Figure 3. Upper room germicidal ultraviolet (GUV) fixture in use in Vladimir, Russia. Note that this locally favoured fixture has two GUV lamps. The visible blue light (black arrow) reflects a shielded lamp designed for upper room air disinfection as discussed. The lower bare UV lamp (white arrow) is favoured locally but is not recommended for TB transmission control. It is intended to be used periodically on sterilise surfaces in unoccupied rooms, but is not effective for preventing person-to-person TB transmission. Such lamps are being widely used to reduce contact pathogens such as drug-resistant *Staphylococcus* or *Clostridium difficile*, common sources of nosocomial infections.

GUV in a properly designed room air cleaner will effectively disinfect the air going through it, but the overall effect is limited to the number of germ-free equivalent room air changes (clean air delivery rate) added per hour, as previously noted [68]. Small air cleaning units with very low clean air delivery rates are often mounted to the walls of corridors or placed in patient rooms, but unless the room is very small, these are of little or no benefit. These units are often sold as a quick and easy solution for TB transmission control, but they simply create a false sense of security and provide no meaningful risk reduction. The same limitations apply to room air cleaners that use filters, with or without germicidal lamps.

In contrast, upper room UVGI fixtures can disinfect a large volume of room air at once [14]. Vertical air mixing (optimally aided by low velocity paddle fans) efficiently disinfects air in the lower room at high rates (20–30 equivalent air changes) that are difficult to achieve with mechanical ventilation alone (figure 3).

Recent controlled studies in hospitals in South America and South Africa have demonstrated air disinfection efficacy of 70–80%, inactivating patient-generated TB aerosols

https://doi.org/10.1183/2312508X.10022517

at rates equivalent to an added ⩾10–20 room air changes per hour [14, 59]. These results are highly dependent on the technical details of the installation: specifically, the total GUV wattage delivered (exiting the fixture) per m^3 room volume or the average upper room UV fluence rate (irradiation dose from multiple sources) and the amount of vertical room air mixing [14, 61, 74]. Fortunately, with well-designed fixtures, commonly available low-velocity ceiling fans and simple installation guidelines, highly effective and safe upper room GUV systems can be applied in most indoor settings where they are needed.

There are currently two major technical barriers to the wider use of upper room GUV. First, GUV technology does not belong to any one professional discipline. Engineers are not taught about its use, partly because the field is not fully developed. Architects and lighting designers are equally unfamiliar with its applications. An international team of engineers and architects fully trained in applying this intervention is needed. With this goal in mind, GUV experts are developing international standards based on the best available evidence [14]. The free website, Global Health Delivery Online (www.ghdonline.org) is also a good source of TB infection control advice, including identifying knowledgeable international consultants on all air disinfection modalities.

A second barrier is the lack of good-quality, low-cost GUV fixtures available for use in resource-limited settings. Once performance specifications are available, local manufacturers should be encouraged to produce compliant fixtures for standardised testing by universities or health and safety agencies. Fixtures that meet standards should be recommended for local or regional use. The two critical parameters are: how much total GUV wattage exits the fixture (0.5 W is a reasonable goal); how well it is confined to the upper room so that room occupants are not overexposed. Special laboratory measurements are required to measure total GUV output from the fixture, not just a simple meter measurement of UV intensity.

Finally, there is the barrier of UV safety [60, 72, 75]. Modern germicidal lamps predominantly generate 254 nm UV irradiation (UV-C) and produce very little ozone. While unprotected airborne microbes are readily inactivated at even low-exposure levels to 254 nm UV, most human exposure is absorbed by the outer dead layer of skin, with very little irradiation penetrating to reach the viable skin layers or the lens of the eye [76]. Therefore, skin cancer and cataracts, two major complications of the longer, more penetrating wavelength UV found in sunlight, are highly unlikely to be caused by GUV. Two recent publications demonstrate the low risk of properly applied upper room GUV to room occupants [60, 75]. Data on GUV maintenance have also been published [57]. Maintenance requirements are limited to keeping lamps clean of dust with a periodic alcohol wipe and changing lamps on a regular basis. As with ventilation, contracting with a knowledgeable company to regularly service a GUV system will assure its continued effectiveness.

Healthcare worker surveillance and protection

Like patients, healthcare workers and staff are at increased risk of TB infection and re-infection [77–79]. TB infection and disease among nursing and medical students has long been used to estimate the risk of transmission in hospitals, and is currently a recommended outcome measure of TB transmission control efficacy [51]. Moreover, healthcare workers disabled by TB directly reduce the critical workforce needed to effectively treat TB, MDR-TB and HIV patients, and fear of nosocomial infection indirectly undermines the staffing of inpatient, ambulatory and community-based treatment programmes. Although effective TB transmission measures in hospitals will protect healthcare workers as well as patients, extra protective measures are warranted where risk has been demonstrated. Respiratory protection has a role for healthcare workers, less so for visitors and other patients, as discussed later. Of course, nosocomially acquired TB disease must be promptly and effectively treated with due concern for confidentiality. More controversial and challenging is monitoring and treating healthcare workers for LTBI with periodic TST or IGRA [79–82]. High background rates of BCG and prior TB infection present difficulties, as does the absence of a test for recent re-infection. Some healthcare workers believe that they might lose the considerable protection associated with latent infection if they agree to treatment, although there is no scientific basis for that fear. Rates of isoniazid (INH) resistance of 10–20% render INH the less than optimal drug; where MDR is being widely transmitted, there is as yet no proven preventive regimen. The newer MDR drugs as well as prevention of infection and re-infection with novel vaccines or host-directed therapies are potential protective strategies [83].

Targeted respiratory protection

The personal respiratory protection intervention that is recommended for TB infection control is a respirator not a surgical mask (figure 4). Surgical masks are not designed to protect the wearer but are commonly used in the short-term by contagious TB patients or coughing patients with presumptive TB in the hours or days before treatment becomes effective [84–87]. A surgical mask acts as a simple physical barrier, like a hand or a tissue,

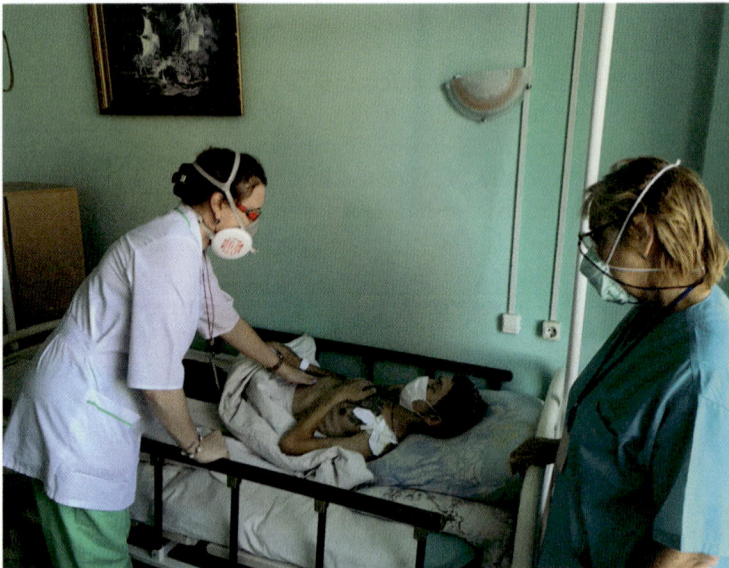

Figure 4. Respiratory protection being used in Vladimir, Russia. The healthcare worker on the left is wearing a fitted elastomeric respirator with replaceable N-95 filtration cartridges. More commonly used in industry, elastomeric respirators provide a better fit, can be cleaned and are more cost-effective than typical disposable N-95 or FFP2 respirators (as worm by the healthcare worker on the right). The patient is wearing a surgical mask, not a respirator, designed to reduce the generation of infectious particles by impaction near the source. Surgical masks do not protect the wearer and are not recommended for healthcare worker use.

https://doi.org/10.1183/2312508X.10022517

impacting large particles in exhaled air and reducing the number that can evaporate into droplet nuclei. The use of surgical masks has been estimated to reduce TB transmission risk by half under study conditions [87].

Certified disposable (or elastomeric face piece) respirators are recommended for use by healthcare workers and other room occupants in high TB transmission-risk areas [88]. Respirators, if fitted and donned properly, remove aerosol particles from the wearer's inhaled air *via* fine filtration. To act as an effective air filter there should be minimal detectable leakage of unfiltered air into the wearer's breathing zone. This can be achieved by wearing a respirator of the appropriate model and size, by correct donning, and by being sure that the respirator is not damaged or deformed. For healthcare workers in high TB-transmission areas, certified respirators N95 (US 42CFR84 standard) or FFP2 (European EN149 standard) are recommended [89]. As the use of a respirator can create some level of discomfort and can complicate communication, the healthcare worker's respirator use time should be limited by administrative measures (such as creating low-risk isolated areas for staff, implementing warning signage in high-risk areas, limiting aerosol-generating procedures, safe working practises, *etc.*) and by air disinfection. All personnel working in high-risk areas should be trained how to correctly and safely put on, store and dispose of respirators [89]. Disposable respirators can be reused by the same worker if they are not damaged, remain dry and clean, are not grossly contaminated and still provide a good fit. A simple procedure of qualitative respirator fit testing should be conducted for all at-risk healthcare workers in order to choose the appropriate model and size and to learn correct donning and fit checking. Respirator procurement for healthcare workers should be based on fit testing results, requiring the availability of several models and sizes to fit different shape faces. Disposal of used respirators and surgical masks should be organised in compliance with national regulations for contaminated medical waste. Since generation of fine aerosols from used respirators is extremely unlikely, there is no measurable TB transmission risk from used respirators [86].

Conclusion

In conclusion, it is our contention that long-term control and eradication of DR-TB and DS-TB will require: 1) an unprecedented massive scale up of more effective regimens and treatment delivery systems: 2) a shift away from the hospital and clinic to community-based treatment; 3) a focus on active case finding and prompt, DST-based effective treatment(*i.e.* FAST); 4) more effective air disinfection, especially in extreme (cold or hot) climates; and 5) effective but targeted use of respiratory protection.

References

1. World Health Organization. Global Tuberculosis Report. Geneva, WHO, 2016. http://apps.who.int/medicinedocs/documents/s23098en/s23098en.pdf
2. Bates M, O'Grady J, Mwaba P, *et al.* Evaluation of the burden of unsuspected pulmonary tuberculosis and co-morbidity with non-communicable diseases in sputum producing adult inpatients. *PLoS One* 2012; 7: e40774.
3. Sharma A, Hill A, Kurbatova E, *et al.* Estimating the future burden of multidrug-resistant and extensively drug-resistant tuberculosis in India, the Philippines, Russia, and South Africa: a mathematical modelling study. *Lancet Infect Dis* 2017; 17: 707–715.
4. Kendall EA, Azman AS, Cobelens FG, *et al.* MDR-TB treatment as prevention: the projected population-level impact of expanded treatment for multidrug-resistant tuberculosis. *PLoS One* 2017; 12: e0172748.

5. Gandhi NR, Moll A, Sturm AW, *et al.* Extensively drug-resistant tuberculosis as a cause of death in patients co-infected with tuberculosis and HIV in a rural area of South Africa. *Lancet.* 2006; 368: 1575–1580.

6. Moodley P, Shah NS, Tayob N, *et al.* Spread of extensively drug-resistant tuberculosis in KwaZulu-Natal province, South Africa. *PLoS One* 2011; 6: e17513.

7. Shenoi SV, Moll AP, Brooks RP, *et al.* Integrated tuberculosis/human immunodeficiency virus community-based case finding in rural South Africa: implications for tuberculosis control efforts. *Open Forum Infect Dis* 2017; 4: ofx092.

8. Loveday M, Wallengren K, Brust J, *et al.* Community-based care *versus* centralised hospitalisation for MDR-TB patients, KwaZulu-Natal, South Africa. *Int J Tuberc Lung Dis* 2015; 19: 163–171.

9. Shin S, Furin J, Bayona J, *et al.* Community-based treatment of multidrug-resistant tuberculosis in Lima, Peru: 7 years of experience. *Soc Sci Med* 2004; 59: 1529–1539.

10. Wandwalo E, Kapalata N, Egwaga S, *et al.* Effectiveness of community-based directly observed treatment for tuberculosis in an urban setting in Tanzania: a randomised controlled trial. *Int J Tuberc Lung Dis* 2004; 8: 1248–1254.

11. Basu S, Friedland GH, Medlock J, *et al.* Averting epidemics of extensively drug-resistant tuberculosis. *Proc Natl Acad Sci USA* 2009; 106: 7672–7677.

12. Barrera E, Livchits V, Nardell E. F-A-S-T: a refocused, intensified, administrative tuberculosis transmission control strategy. *Int J Tuberc Lung Dis* 2015; 19: 381–384.

13. Nardell EA. Indoor environmental control of tuberculosis and other airborne infections. *Indoor Air* 2016; 26: 79–87.

14. Mphaphlele M, Dharmadhikari AS, Jensen PA, *et al.* Institutional tuberculosis transmission. controlled trial of upper room ultraviolet air disinfection: a basis for new dosing guidelines. *Am J Respir Crit Care Med* 2015; 192: 477–484.

15. Miller SL. Upper room germicidal ultraviolet systems for air disinfection are ready for wide implementation. *Am J Respir Crit Care Med* 2015; 192: 407–409.

16. Nardell EA. Transmission and institutional infection control of tuberculosis. *Cold Spring Harb Perspect Med* 2015; 6: a018192.

17. Fennelly KP. Personal respiratory protection and prevention of occupational tuberculosis. *Int J Tuberc Lung Dis* 2005; 9: 476.

18. Nathavitharana RR, Daru P, Barrera AE, *et al.* FAST implementation in Bangladesh: high frequency of unsuspected tuberculosis justifies challenges of scale-up. *Int J Tuberc Lung Dis* 2017; 21: 1020–1025.

19. Riley RL, O'Grady F. Airborne Infection: Transmission and Control. New York, The Macmillan Company, 1961.

20. Queval CJ, Brosch R, Simeone R. The macrophage: a disputed fortress in the battle against *Mycobacterium tuberculosis. Front Microbiol.* 2017; 8: 2284.

21. Wells W. Airborne Contagion and Air Hygiene. Cambridge, Harvard University Press, 1955.

22. Khan N, Vidyarthi A, Javed S, *et al.* Innate immunity holding the flanks until reinforced by adaptive immunity against *Mycobacterium tuberculosis* infection. *Front Microbiol* 2016; 7: 328.

23. Cruz AT, Starke JR. Pediatric tuberculosis. *Pediatr Rev* 2010; 31: 13–25.

24. Smith D, Wiengeshaus E. What animal models can teach us about the pathogenesis of tuberculosis in humans. *Rev Infect Dis* 1989; 11: S385–S393.

25. Edwards DA, Man JC, Brand P, *et al.* Inhaling to mitigate exhaled bioaerosols. *Proc Natl Acad Sci USA* 2004; 101: 17383–17388.

26. Jones-Lopez EC, Acuna-Villaorduna C, Ssebidandi M, *et al.* Cough aerosols of *Mycobacterium tuberculosis* in the prediction of incident tuberculosis disease in household contacts. *Clin Infect Dis* 2016; 63: 10–20.

27. Sultan L, Nyka C, Mills C, *et al.* Tuberculosis disseminators - a study of variability of aerial infectivity of tuberculosis patients. *Am Rev Respir Dis* 1960; 82: 358–369.

28. Hutton MD, Stead WW, Cauthen GM, *et al.* Nosocomial transmission of tuberculosis associated with a draining abscess. *J Infect Dis* 1990; 161: 286–295.

29. Dharmadhikari AS, Mphahlele M, Venter K, *et al.* Rapid impact of effective treatment on transmission of multidrug-resistant tuberculosis. *Int J Tuberc Lung Dis* 2014; 18: 1019–1025.

30. Willingham FF, Schmitz TL, Contreras M, *et al.* Hospital control and multidrug-resistant pulmonary tuberculosis in female patients, Lima, Peru. *Emerg Infect Dis* 2001; 7: 123–127.

31. Ramakrishnan CV, Andrews RH, Devadatta S, *et al.* Prevalence and early attack rate of tuberculosis among close family contacts of tuberculous patients in South India under domiciliary treatment with isoniazid plus PAS or isoniazid alone. *Bull World Health Organ* 1961; 26: 361–407.

32. Riley RL, Moodie AS. Infectivity of patients with pulmonary tuberculosis in inner city homes. *Am Rev Respir Dis* 1974; 110: 810–812.

33. Brooks SM, Lassiter N, Young E. A pilot study concerning the infection risk of sputum positive with tuberculosis patients on chemotherapy. *Am Rev Respir Dis* 1973; 108: 799–804.

34. Gunnels J, Bates J, Swindoll H. Infectivity of sputum positive tuberculosis patients on chemotherapy. *Am Rev Resp Dis* 1974; 109: 323.

35. Rouillon A, Perdrizet S, Parrot R. Transmission of tubercle bacilli: the effects of chemotherapy. *Tubercle* 1976; 57: 275–299.

https://doi.org/10.1183/2312508X.10022517

36. Riley RL, Mills CC, O'Grady F, et al. Infectiousness of air from a tuberculosis ward. Ultraviolet irradiation of infected air: comparative infectiousness of different patients. *Am Rev Respir Dis* 1962; 85: 511–525.

37. Riley RL. Mills C, Nyka W, et al. Aerial dissemination of pulmonary tuberculosis: a two-year study of contagion in a tuberculosis ward: 1959. *Am J Epidemiol* 1995; 142: 3–14.

38. Cholo MC, Mothiba MT, Fourie B, et al. Mechanisms of action and therapeutic efficacies of the lipophilic antimycobacterial agents clofazimine and bedaquiline. *J Antimicrob Chemother* 2017; 72: 338–353.

39. Svensson EM, Dosne AG, Karlsson MO. Population pharmacokinetics of bedaquiline and metabolite M2 in patients with drug-resistant tuberculosis: the effect of time-varying weight and albumin. *CPT Pharmacometrics Syst Pharmacol* 2016; 5: 682–691.

40. Kendall EA, Fofana MO, Dowdy DW. Burden of transmitted multidrug resistance in epidemics of tuberculosis: a transmission modelling analysis. *Lancet Respir Med* 2015; 3: 963–972.

41. Atun RA, Samyshkin Y, Drobniewski F, et al. Costs and outcomes of tuberculosis control in the Russian Federation: retrospective cohort analysis. *Health Policy Plan* 2006; 21: 353–364.

42. Floyd K, Hutubessy R, Samyshkin Y, et al. Health-systems efficiency in the Russian Federation: tuberculosis control. *Bull World Health Organ* 2006; 84: 43–51.

43. Atun RA, Samyshkin YA, Drobniewski F, et al. Barriers to sustainable tuberculosis control in the Russian Federation health system. *Bull World Health Organ* 2005; 83: 217–223.

44. Miller AC, Livchits V, Ahmad Khan F, et al. Turning off the tap: using the FAST approach to stop the spread of drug-resistant tuberculosis in Russian Federation. *J Infect Dis* 2018; 218: 654–658.

45. Gelmanova IY, Keshavjee S, Golubchikova VT, et al. Non-adherence, default, and the acquisition of multidrug resistance in a tuberculosis treatment program in Tomsk, Siberia. *Bulletin of the World Health Organization* 2007; 85: 703–711.

46. Andrews JR, Gandhi NR, Moodley P, et al. Exogenous reinfection as a cause of multidrug-resistant and extensively drug-resistant tuberculosis in rural South Africa. *J Infect Dis* 2008; 198: 1582–1589.

47. Greenstone M. India's air-conditioning and climate change quandary. *New York Times* 26 October 2016. https://www.nytimes.com/2016/10/27/upshot/indias-air-conditioning-and-climate-change-quandary.html

48. Mitnick C, Bayona J, Palacios E, et al. Community-based therapy for multidrug-resistant tuberculosis in Lima, Peru. *N Engl J Med* 2003; 348: 119–128.

49. Farmer P, Kim J. Community based approaches to the control of multidrug resistant tuberculosis: introducing "DOTS-plus". *BMJ* 1998; 317: 671–674.

50. Fitzpatrick C, Floyd K. A systematic review of the cost and cost effectiveness of treatment for multidrug-resistant tuberculosis. *Pharmacoeconomics* 2012; 30: 63–80.

51. WHO. WHO Policy on TB Infection Control in Health-Care Facilities, Congregate Settings and Households. Geneva, WHO, 2009. http://www.who.int/tb/publications/2009/infection_control/en/

52. WHO. Implementing the WHO policy on TB infection control:[150 p.].

53. CDC. Guideline for preventing the transmission of *Mycobacterium tuberculosis* in health-care facilities, 1994. Centers for Disease Control and Prevention. *MMWR Morb Mortal Wkly Rep* 1994; 43: 1–132.

54. Nardell EA, Keegan J, Cheney SA, et al. Airborne infection. Theoretical limits of protection achievable by building ventilation. *Am Rev Respir Dis* 1991; 144: 302–306.

55. Escombe AR, Oeser CC, Gilman RH, et al. Natural ventilation for the prevention of airborne contagion. *PLoS Med* 2007; 4: e68.

56. Milonova S, Rudnick S, McDevitt J, et al. Occupant UV exposure measurements for upper-room ultraviolet germicidal irradiation. *J Photochem Photobiol B* 2016; 159: 88–92.

57. Nardell E, Vincent R, Sliney DH. Upper-room ultraviolet germicidal irradiation (UVGI) for air disinfection: a symposium in print. *Photochem Photobiol* 2013; 89: 764–769.

58. Miller SL, Linnes J, Luongo J. Ultraviolet germicidal irradiation: future directions for air disinfection and building applications. *Photochem Photobiol* 2013; 89: 777–781.

59. Escombe AR, Moore DA, Gilman RH, et al. Upper-room ultraviolet light and negative air ionization to prevent tuberculosis transmission. *PLoS Med* 2009; 6: e43.

60. Nardell EA, Bucher SJ, Brickner PW, et al. Safety of upper-room ultraviolet germicidal air disinfection for room occupants: results from the Tuberculosis Ultraviolet Shelter Study. *Public Health Rep* 2008; 123: 52–60.

61. Rudnick SN, First MW. Fundamental factors affecting upper-room ultraviolet germicidal irradiation - part II. Predicting effectiveness. *J Occup Environ Hyg* 2007; 4: 352–362.

62. Nardell EA. Environmental infection control of tuberculosis. *Semin Respir Infect* 2003; 18: 307–319.

63. First M, Nardell E, Chaisson W, et al. Guidelines for the application of upper-room ultraviolet germicidal irradiation for preventing transmission of airborne contagion - Part II: Design and operations guidance. *ASHRAE Transactions* 1999; 105: 877–887.

64. First M, Nardell E, Chaisson W, et al. Guidelines for the application of upper-room ultraviolet germicidal irradiation for preventing transmission of airborne contagion - Part I: Basic principles. *ASHRAE Transactions* 1999; 105: 869–876.

65. Rudnick SN, Milton DK. Risk of indoor airborne infection transmission estimated from carbon dioxide concentration. *Indoor Air* 2003; 13: 237–245.

66. Andrews JR, Morrow C, Walensky RP, *et al.* Integrating social contact and environmental data in evaluating tuberculosis transmission in a South African township. *J Infect Dis* 2014; 210: 597–603.

67. Atkinson J, Chartier Y, Pessoa-Silva CL, *et al.* Natural ventilation for infection control in health care settings. Geneva, WHO, 2009. http://www.who.int/water_sanitation_health/publications/natural_ventilation/en/

68. Shaughnessy RJ, Sextro RG. What is an effective portable air cleaning device? A review. *J Occup Environ Hyg* 2006; 3: 169–181.

69. Reed NG. The history of ultraviolet germicidal irradiation for air disinfection. *Pub Health Reports* 2010; 125: 15–24.

70. Nardell E, Dharmadhikari A. Turning off the spigot: reducing drug-resistant tuberculosis transmission in resource-limited settings. *Int J Tuberc Lung Dis* 2010; 14: 1233–1243.

71. Radonovich LJ, Martinello RA, Hodgson M, *et al.* Influenza and ultraviolet germicidal irradiation. *Virol J* 2008; 5: 149.

72. Nardell EA. Use and misuse of germicidal UV air disinfection for TB in high-prevalence settings. *Int J Tuberc Lung Dis* 2002; 6: 647–648.

73. Ko G, First MW, Burge HA. The characterization of upper-room ultraviolet germicidal irradiation in inactivating airborne microorganisms. *Environ Health Perspect* 2002; 110: 95–101.

74. First M, Rudnick SN, Banahan KF, *et al.* Fundamental factors affecting upper-room ultraviolet germicidal irradiation - part I. Experimental. *J Occup Environ Hyg* 2007; 4: 321–331.

75. First MW, Weker RA, Yasui S, *et al.* Monitoring human exposures to upper-room germicidal ultraviolet irradiation. *J Occup Environ Hyg* 2005; 2: 285–292.

76. Bruls W. Transmission of human epidermis and stratum corneum as a function of thickness in the ultravilolet and visible wavelengths. *Photochem Photobiol* 1984; 40: 485–494.

77. Seaworth BJ, Armitige LY, Aronson NE, *et al.* Recommendations for reducing risk during travel for healthcare and humanitarian work. *Ann Am Thorac Soc* 2014; 11: 286–295.

78. Szep Z, Kim R, Ratcliffe SJ, *et al.* Tuberculin skin test conversion rate among short-term health care workers returning from Gaborone, Botswana. *Travel Med Infect Dis* 2014; 12: 396–400.

79. Joshi R, Reingold AL, Menzies D, *et al.* Tuberculosis among health-care workers in low- and middle-income countries: a systematic review. *PLoS Med* 2006; 3: e494.

80. Nathavitharana RR, Bond P, Dramowski A, *et al.* Agents of change: the role of healthcare workers in the prevention of nosocomial and occupational tuberculosis. *Presse Med* 2017; 46: e53–e62.

81. Pai M, Dendukuri N, Wang L, *et al.* Improving the estimation of tuberculosis infection prevalence using T-cell-based assay and mixture models. *Int J Tuberc Lung Dis* 2008; 12: 895–902.

82. Menzies D, Joshi R, Pai M. Risk of tuberculosis infection and disease associated with work in health care settings. *Int J Tuberc Lung Dis* 2007; 11: 593–605.

83. Vaccine Prevention of Sustained Mycobacterium tuberculosis Infection Summary G. Developing vaccines to prevent sustained infection with *Mycobacterium tuberculosis*: Conference proceedings: National Institute of Allergy and Infectious Diseases, Rockville, Maryland USA, November 7, 2014. *Vaccine* 2015; 33: 3056–3064.

84. Lee K, Slavcev A, Nicas M. Respiratory protection against *Mycobacterium tuberculosis*: quantitative fit test outcomes for five type N95 filtering-facepiece respirators. *J Occup Environ Hyg* 2004; 1: 22–28.

85. Fennelly KP, Nardell EA. The relative efficacy of respirators and room ventilation in preventing occupational tuberculosis. *Infect Control Hosp Epidemiol* 1998; 19: 754–759.

86. Fennelly KP. Personal respiratory protection against Mycobacterium tuberculosis. *Clin Chest Med* 1997; 18: 1–17.

87. Dharmadhikari AS, Mphahlele M, Stoltz A, *et al.* Surgical face masks worn by patients with multidrug-resistant tuberculosis: impact on infectivity of air on a hospital ward. *Am J Respir Crit Care Med* 2012; 185: 1104–1109.

88. Nicas M, Neuhaus J. Variability in respiratory protection and the assigned protection factor. *J Occup Environ Hyg* 2004; 1: 99–109.

89. Campbell DL, Coffey CC, Jensen PA, *et al.* Reducing respirator fit test errors: a multi-donning approach. *J Occup Environ Hyg* 2005; 2: 391–399.

Disclosures: None declared.

https://doi.org/10.1183/2312508X.10022517

Chapter 22

Diagnosis and treatment of latent tuberculosis infection

Adrian Rendon[1], Delia Goletti[2] and Alberto Matteelli[3,4]

Current concepts of diagnosis and treatment of LTBI will be reviewed in detail and the rationality to use IGRA for diagnosis will be explained. The new regimens that include rifampicin or rifapentine and the main groups to be considered for treatment are fully described.

Cite as: Rendon A, Goletti D, Matteelli A. Diagnosis and treatment of latent tuberculosis infection. *In:* Migliori GB, Bothamley G, Duarte R, *et al.*, eds. Tuberculosis (ERS Monograph). Sheffield, European Respiratory Society, 2018; pp. 381–398 [https://doi.org/10.1183/2312508X.10022617].

@ERSpublications
Treatment of LTBI is an important strategy to eliminate TB. New diagnostic tests and new shorter treatment regimens are now available. Treatment of LTBI is not for everybody and should be targeted for those risk groups who will get the greatest benefit. http://ow.ly/cfVQ30lqCfE

TB is caused by *Mycobacterium tuberculosis* and represents a major public health problem. In 2017, 9.0 to 11.1 million new active TB cases and 1.2 to 1.4 million deaths have been estimated [1]. Almost a quarter of the world population, 1.7 billion subjects, is estimated to have LTBI [2], and 5–10% of them may progress to active TB in their lifetime [3, 4]. LTBI treatment has been scarcely used in the past in many countries around the world. The WHO is now recommending the reinstatement of this approach if we want to reach TB eradication goals. New data related to the diagnosis and treatment of LTBI is already available and even more will surface over the coming years. In this chapter, we will review how LTBI is currently defined and diagnosed and to whom testing should be systematically directed. An analysis of the current role of TST and IGRA in the LTBI diagnosis will be made. We will discuss why treatment of LTBI is indispensable in the WHO End TB Strategy and which risk groups should be tested and treated. Regimens currently recommended by the WHO will be described and recommendations for specific risk groups will be presented. We now have better diagnostic tests, such as IGRA, and several effective regimens to choose from. Safe shorter regimens to treat LTBI are necessary to increase treatment completion rates and to make the TB elimination dream a reality.

[1]TB Dept, University Hospital of Monterrey, Monterrey, Mexico. [2]Translational Research Unit, National Institute for Infectious Diseases L Spallanzani, Rome, Italy. [3]WHO Collaborating Centre for TB/HIV and TB elimination. [4]Dept of Infectious and Tropical Diseases, University of Brescia, Brescia, Italy.

Correspondence: Adrian Rendon, Pulmonary services, Hospital Universitario de Nuevo Leon, CIPTIR AV. Madero y Gonzalitos Mitras Centro, Monterrey, Nuevo Leon, 64460 Mexico. E-mail: adrianrendon@hotmail.com

In the following sections these arguments will be expanded. It is expected that, when new data is released, our current approach will have to be readjusted.

Latent tuberculosis infection: definition and diagnosis

According to the WHO, LTBI is defined as a status characterised by the presence of immune responses to *M. tuberculosis* but without clinical evidence of active TB [3, 4]. The TST or IGRA may be used to measure the immune response, which are based on the specific recognition of mycobacterial antigens [5, 6]. It has become clear that LTBI has to be considered as a broad spectrum of infection states which differ by the degree of pathogen replication, host resistance and inflammation [6–9]. We will use the current WHO definition throughout.

By measuring the transverse diameter of induration resulting from intradermal injection of purified protein derivative (PPD), TST response can be evaluated. PPD is a crude mixture of antigens, many of which are shared by *M. tuberculosis* and other mycobacteria, in particular BCG. The cause of the suboptimal specificity of the test for *M. tuberculosis* infection is due to the absence of the specificity of the antigens used in this assay [5, 6, 10]. This is particularly relevant in people coming from high TB endemic countries where BCG vaccination is commonly performed very early in life [11]. An induration $\geqslant$10 mm is considered a positive reaction but $\geqslant$5 mm is the cut-off in individuals living with HIV or other immunosuppressive conditions. In some countries, such as the UK and USA, the 5 mm cut-off is also used while screening contacts. However, different cut-off sizes that allow an estimation of the risk to develop TB, based on factors such as age, BCG vaccination and immune suppression diseases, are also considered [12]. Definitions for conversion and boosting have also been established; conversion is defined as an induration >10 mm with an increase of at least 6 mm over the previous result [13]. Although broadly used, TST has limitations. Sensitivity may be reduced by malnutrition, severe active TB disease and immunodeficiency status, as for HIV infection or therapy with biological drugs inhibiting tumour necrosis factor (TNF). A reduced specificity is associated with exposure to NTM and, as reported above, is associated with BCG vaccination, although after 10 years or more the effect of the BCG vaccination on TST reactions is limited if the vaccination was given in infancy [14]. Moreover, subjective variability in performing the test or in reading it is possible. From a logistical point of view, TST involves two healthcare visits, one for the PPD injection and the other to measure the induration, leading to a loss of reading in 10% of cases [15]. However, a positive TST, especially if large, red and itchy, may encourage the patient to attend the clinic and subsequently adhere to treatment.

In contrast to TST, IGRA are blood laboratory tests and include QuantiFERON Plus (QFT-P; Qiagen, Hilden, Germany) and T-SPOT.TB (Oxford Immunotec, Abingdon, UK). The assays involve a negative control, a positive control (mitogen stimulus) and a specific *M. tuberculosis* stimulation. IFN-γ production is measured after 16–20 h in whole blood or peripheral blood mononuclear cells (PBMCs), using ELISA or enzyme-linked immunospot (ELISPOT) assay, respectively [5–7]. The stimulation is performed using *M. tuberculosis*-specific peptides spanning the *M. tuberculosis* antigens ESAT-6 and CFP-10, and are restricted to a region of the *M. tuberculosis* genome deleted from *Mycobacterium bovis* BCG and which is not present in most environmental mycobacteria [16, 17]. QFT-P is the updated version of the QFT Gold-In Tube [10, 18, 19], and, includes an additional antigen tube containing peptides designed to induce a CD8 T-cell response in addition to the CD4

https://doi.org/10.1183/2312508X.10022617

T-cell response [10, 18–21]. The peptides stimulating CD8 T-cells are included to increase the sensitivity for active TB detection as this specific response is associated with active TB more than LTBI, in both HIV-uninfected and -infected subjects [22–24]. IGRA are more specific than TST for the diagnosis of TB due to the higher specificity of the antigens used. An additional important advantage of *in vitro* testing is that the laboratory test takes into account background signals or general T-cell responsiveness, having stimulation reactions with negative and positive controls (carried out in parallel). These assays' characteristics are then very important in the setting of immunodeficiency where an impaired mitogen response may additionally be interpreted as a meaningful measure for assessing the overall extent of immunosuppression. Therefore, unlike TST, *in vitro* tests may be able to discriminate true-negative responses from anergy. It is important to note that ESAT-6 and CFP-10 are also present in *M. kansasii*, *M. marinum* and *M. szulgai*. Having more diagnostic tools available, NTM infections are more commonly diagnosed today, this fact needs to be acknowledged since it could be a cause of false-positive results [25, 26].

However, immune suppressive regimens such as those based on glucocorticoids or anti-TNF may negatively impact on the score of both TST and IGRA, leading to false-negative results [27]. *In vitro* studies have shown that the addition of dexamethasone on QFT-Gold-In Tube causes a reversion of the results from positive to negative in 30% of the LTBI subjects tested [28]. Table 1 shows a comparison of the available diagnostic tests.

Finally, a new skin test for LTBI detection, named C-Tb, has been described [29]. It uses recombinant ESAT-6 and CFP-10 as antigens and is applied as the TST. This assay has the advantages of both TST (low cost and ease of use) and IGRA (high specificity analogous) technologies. TST and IGRA are acceptable for LTBI screening based on the WHO recommendations [30]. If possible, clinicians may consider starting with IGRA in those with a history of BCG vaccination to increase the specificity of LTBI detection. If the index of suspicion for LTBI is high, independently of BCG vaccination, both IGRA and TST may be performed in immune compromised subjects, especially in HIV-infected subjects and prior to initiating TNF-α inhibitor therapy. Corticosteroids at doses >20 mg for >2 weeks have an impact in reducing TST sensitivity for detecting LTBI [31, 32]

Table 1. Characteristics of the routinely used immune-based tests for LTBI diagnosis

	TST	QFT-IT/QFT-P	T-SPOT TB
Laboratory test with internal controls	No	Yes	Yes
Mycobacterium tuberculosis specific antigen	No	Yes	Yes
T-cell anergy diagnosed	No	Yes	Yes
Time required for results	48–72 h	16–20 h	16–20 h
Impact of cortisone on the lower reliability of the result	High	Medium	Medium
Impact of immune suppression on the reliability of the result	High	Medium	Medium
Cut-off established depending on age, immune suppression and BCG	Yes	No	No
Accuracy for active TB from LTBI discrimination	No	No	No
Accuracy to detect those at high risk of developing active TB	Low	Low	Low

QFT-IT: QuantiFERON-In-Tube; QFT-P: QuantiFERON Plus. Data from [27, 28].

The inability to distinguish between active TB and LTBI is an important limitation of both TST and IGRA [33]. Thus, several approaches have previously been performed to increase the accuracy of these tests, as assays based on the response to antigens associated with latency (*e.g.* heparin-binding hemagglutinin [34–36] or those regulated by the Dos-Regulon [37–39]), or tests based on the detection of memory response [40, 41]. The predictive value for TB development of TST and IGRA has been reported as low [42, 43]. The PREDICT study recently reported some of these findings [44]. The aim of PREDICT was to estimate the predictive values of three TST scores (5 mm, 10 mm and 15 mm) and two IGRAs (QFT Gold-In Tube and T-SPOT.TB) in high-risk groups (*i.e.* people in recent contact with active TB cases and from high-burden countries) for the development of active TB. In those who tested negatively the annual incidence of TB was very low in all tests (1.2 per 1000 person-years for TST 5 mm to 1·9 per 1000 person-years for QFT-Gold In-Tube). This is an important characteristic because the negative result could be used to reassure the patients on the low probability of progression to disease. In participants who tested positively, the annual incidence was highest for T-SPOT.TB (13.2 per 1000 person-years), TST 15 mm (11.1 per 1000 person-years) and QFT-Gold In-Tube (10.1 per 1000 person-years). The PREDICT study confirms that the predictive value for active TB progression is not that high, therefore, several attempts to generate new tests have been developed. In a study conducted in South Africa and later validated in Gambia, a new mRNA signature was described. It consists of 16 transcripts associated with active TB with a discrete accuracy for TB development 6 months earlier of the disease [10, 45, 46]. Recent studies identified smaller (n=3 or 4) gene signatures associated with active TB [47, 48]. Some signatures have been also described in HIV-infected subjects [49]. These signatures have the potential to enter routine clinical use if validated in larger studies.

Who needs to be screened and treated for latent tuberculosis infection?

The risk of progressing from LTBI to active TB is greater in some populations, including: recent contacts [50], children aged <5 years [51–53], immigrants from high TB-burden countries [54–58], people living with HIV [59, 60] subjects exposed to biological therapy [3, 4, 6, 61–66] and healthcare workers [67–70]. These groups are considered a high priority to be screened and treated for LTBI. Specific consideration for them and for other particular risk populations will be reviewed later.

Role of latent tuberculosis infection treatment in tuberculosis elimination

The goal of the WHO is to eliminate TB by 2050, reducing the annual incidence of TB to less than one case per million people. Among the several approaches to undertake, this goal can be achieved identifying and eliminating LTBI by preventive treatment whose purpose is killing of replicating mycobacteria. This leads to a reduction in the development of the disease in single individuals and the community, thus limiting the transmission of infection from individuals who are at a higher risk of progression to active TB [41, 65]. The expected reduction varies according to the risk factor that is present. The group with the highest reduction derived from any preventive treatment is people living with HIV (RR 0.68, 95% CI 0.54–0.85) and the benefit is even higher among those with a positive TST (RR 0.38, 95% CI 0.25–0.57) [71].

https://doi.org/10.1183/2312508X.10022617

The RR of developing active TB in non-HIV infected persons is 0.40 (95% CI 0.31–0.52) when they receive preventive therapy with isoniazid (INH) for 6 or 12 months [72].

Treatment of LTBI is an important component of the WHO model for the decline of TB from 2015 to 2035. The current global trend, in which treatment of LTBI is almost not performed, is a 1.5% decline per year. Implementing diagnosis and treatment of LTBI may improve the decline to -17%. Without pursuing the diagnosis and treatment of LTBI, it would not be possible to reach the TB elimination goals [73].

Treatment regimens for latent tuberculosis infection

The WHO has recently turned its attention to an old approach that had been neglected for years: treatment of LTBI, also called preventive chemotherapy of TB or chemoprophylaxis [74].

The USA is possibly the most experienced country in the world on this matter, given that they have been performing studies with INH since 1957 [75]. Based on the results of several early studies of the United States Public Health Service, joint recommendations by the Center of Disease Control and American Thoracic Society were issued in 1965 [76]. The first review of the large-scale United States Public Health Service trials was performed in 1970 [77], with results showing that INH preventive therapy led to 60% overall protection against active TB. Guidelines for the treatment of LTBI have evolved in response to the surge of new data, new challenges and new drugs. Originally, INH (300 mg a day) was the only drug used and it was recommended for periods as short as 6 months or as long as 12 months. The range of INH reduction of TB has been reported as 54–90% in several studies [30, 78]. Presently, INH is not the only recommended drug: rifampicin and rifapentine are also part of the armamentarium. The use of these last two drugs, alone or in combination with INH, has allowed shortened treatment regimens, which in turn increases their completion rates without losing effectiveness or increasing toxicity. In addition, fluoroquinolones are now recommended for particular situations such as exposure to MDR-TB cases. In 2015, the WHO launched its guidelines on the management of LTBI [74], followed by an updated and consolidated version of that document in 2018 [50].

Those guidelines include several different, but effective, regimens for the treatment of LTBI plus two other regimens for special circumstances (i.e. HIV infection in high-prevalence and frequent exposure communities and MDR-TB exposure). Herein, we will describe these regimens and others still not recommended by the WHO. Table 2 presents the doses of the most commonly used drugs.

Regimens containing only isoniazid

The duration of the regimens using only INH ranges from 6 to 12 months [79, 80]. It has been proven that the longer the duration, the higher the efficacy. 9 months are better than 6 months and 12 months are better than 9 months, but the increment in efficacy after 9 months is small [80]. In the USA, the most commonly used INH preventive therapy regimen is 9 months [81], but many countries use the 6-month regimen. The WHO recommends either the 6 or the 9-month regimens, which are prescribed daily by self-administered therapy [50]. There is a 36-month INH regimen recommended by the WHO for use mainly in people with HIV infection who live in high TB-prevalence settings

Table 2. Common drugs used to treat LTBI*

	Daily dose		Maximum dose[#]	Weekly dose		Maximum dose[#]	Toxicity[¶]	Interactions with ART[+]
	Children	Adults		Children	Adults			
INH	10 mg·kg^{-1}	5 mg·kg^{-1}	300 mg	25 mg·kg^{-1}	15 mg·kg^{-1}	900 mg	Hepatitis, peripheral neuritis	Can be used with ART
Rifampicin	15 mg·kg^{-1}	10 mg·kg^{-1}	600 mg				Hepatitis, rash, thrombocytopenia	Not recommended with protease inhibitors or nevirapine
Rifapentine				300–750[§] mg	900[§] mg	900 mg	Hepatitis, rash, thrombocytopenia, flu-like illness	Not recommended with protease inhibitors, nevirapine or dolutegravir

*: regimens and their duration are addressed below. #: children and adults. ¶: anti-TB drugs toxicity and its management is discussed in another chapter. +: because of their interactions, regimens containing rifampicin or rifapentine should be used with caution in patients receiving other drugs (common finding for patients living with HIV). §: doses recommended by the WHO: 0.0–14.0 kg=300 mg, 14.1–25.0 kg=450 mg, 25.1–32.0 kg=600 mg, 32.1–50.0 kg=750 mg, >50 kg=900 mg [50].

https://doi.org/10.1183/2312508X.10022617

and have frequent exposure. Such strategies can further decrease the risk of active TB not only by treating current LTBI but also by preventing a new infection or a re-infection [82].

Regimens containing only rifampicin

The main advantages of regimens using only rifampicin are to shorten the length of the regimen to 3–4 months, to protect contacts of INH resistant cases, and as an alternative when INH hepatitis develops. A 2014 meta-analysis [83], recently updated in 2017 [84], showed that rifampicin protection was similar to that offered by a 6-month INH regimen, but with a lower toxicity rate. The most recent RCT, published in 2018 [85], compared 4-month rifampicin against 9-month INH. The results showed that both regimens were similar, but more patients completed the rifampicin regimen and toxicity was also lower in that group. Rifampicin regimens are administered daily under observation but can also be self-administered.

Regimens containing isoniazid and rifampicin

A 3- or 4-month regimen of daily INH plus rifampicin is recommended by the WHO [50] and the Public Health Agency of Canada [86]. The two meta-analyses mentioned earlier [71, 72] showed that a 6-month regimen of INH was similar to a regimen of 3–4 months of INH plus rifampicin in terms of efficacy and toxicity. The same findings were observed in two other studies involving children [87, 88]. Again, shorter regimens had a better completion rates. Regimens with daily INH plus rifampicin can be administered under observation or can be self-administered.

Regimen containing isoniazid and rifapentine

This is the newest regimen recommended by the WHO [50] and it is currently the most commonly prescribed regimen in the USA [81]. It is administered once a week for 12 weeks under DOT: INH and rifapentine are given in a high dose with a maximum of 900 mg each [89]. Original studies applying this regimen compared it against 6–9 months of INH and included groups at high risk for developing active TB such as close contacts, HIV-infected patients and those with fibrotic changes on the chest radiograph. Results showed a similar efficacy but a higher rate of completion and fewer side-effects for the weekly regimen in all the studied groups [89, 90]. Later studies also showed the same efficacy and safety in children and pregnant women [91, 92].

Regimen recommended to prevent multidrug-resistant tuberculosis

There is no well-designed effective regimen that could be recommended for preventing TB in people exposed to MDR-TB cases. Available data is scanty but offers some hope that regimens containing either moxifloxacin or levofloxacin (alone or combined with other drugs) could give some protection if the source case is sensitive to those drugs [93, 94]. Concordance of resistance patterns among source cases and secondary cases is >50% [95]. Prevention of MDR-TB will be reviewed further at the end of the chapter.

Future regimens

A new regimen lasting only 1 month with daily INH plus rifapentine in HIV patients has been recently presented at several international meetings. When compared against the

9-month INH regimen, both regimens had similar effectiveness and safety. However, the INH plus rifapentine regimen showed a higher completion rate [96].

Several ongoing trials are studying regimens for preventing MDR-TB: VQUIN and TB-CHAMP are comparing levofloxacin against placebo and PHOENIx is evaluating delamanid compared to INH. Results are not expected any time soon [97].

The decision to treat latent TB should be based on the presence of risk factors for developing active TB. The regimen to be used should be chosen based on available drugs and resistance patterns in the source case (if known). Current shorter regimens that include rifampicin or rifapentine are effective, safe and have a greater completion rate.

General recommendations and comments for specific groups

In countries in which the incidence of TB is low, reactivation of LTBI accounts for the majority of new TB cases [98]. It is not surprising that prevention of active TB disease by treatment of LTBI is a critical component of the WHO End TB Strategy [99]. For implementation of LTBI programmes, the first step is to weigh up the risk and benefit of diagnosing and treating LTBI, which should be performed at individual rather than a population level. The potential benefit of treatment should be carefully balanced against the risk for drug-related adverse events. Population-wide mass screening and treatment of LTBI are unfeasible due to weak tests, high costs, poor sustainability, uncertain cost-effectiveness, and risk of serious and fatal side-effects. A recent study of untargeted community-wide provision of INH preventive therapy among 79 000 gold miners in South Africa, with 3–4% TB prevalence, concluded that no population-level effect in decreasing TB incidence and prevalence was achieved [100].

The lifetime risk of reactivation TB for a person with a positive TST is usually estimated to be 5–10%; this estimate is based on a large body of data collected before treatment for latent TB was routinely recommended. However, that estimate is a mean value that underestimates the risk for some patients and overestimates the risk for others, because the risk is strongly influenced by several factors, mainly the immunological status of the host [30] and early age [102]; the chance of developing active TB in a young child with a positive TST is close to 10% while a teenager may have a lifetime risk of 1–3% [101]. Therefore, the definition of the risk of reactivation TB in population groups is essential to balance the potential benefits of LTBI treatment.

According to the WHO (unpublished 2015 guidelines), the ideal methodology to identify at risk populations for LTBI is to measure the incidence rate ratio of TB in cohorts of individuals with LTBI carrying the condition with the relevant incidence rate ratio in individuals with LTBI in the general population. However, such studies are very difficult to conduct and very rarely published. A systematic review [74] conducted among 24 pre-defined at-risk population groups as part of the guidelines development process only identified eight individual studies providing evidence of increased risk of progression in the following: people with HIV, adult contacts of TB cases, patients undergoing dialysis, people who are underweight, people with fibrotic radiologic lesions, and recent converters to the TST. For the majority of other populations this type of evidence is not available. Therefore, additional composite methodology was used to identify populations who might benefit from preventive treatment or for whom TST or IGRA testing would be indicated, using evidence on increased risk of LTBI or increased risk of incident TB. The prevalence of

 https://doi.org/10.1183/2312508X.10022617

LTBI, as measured either by TST or IGRA, was assessed using a systematic review as meta-analyses could not be performed due to the high degree of heterogeneity. Using LTBI prevalence estimates derived from modelling, a comparison between LTBI prevalence among risk groups and prevalence among the general population was made and pooled risk ratios were calculated for the risk groups. In at least 65% of the studies for the following risk groups Increased prevalence of LTBI was reported for both TST and IGRA: prisoners, the homeless and elderly, immigrants from high TB-burden countries, adult and child TB contacts and illicit drug users.

In order to compare the pooled incidence rate ratio of active TB in the pre-defined risk groups compared with the general population, a second systematic review was conducted [102]. Data of increased risk of active TB were reported in the following: people with HIV, adult and child contacts of a TB case, patients with silicosis, healthcare workers (including students), immigrants from high TB-burden countries, prisoners, homeless people, patients receiving dialysis, patients receiving anti-TNF drugs, patients with cancer, people with DM, people with harmful alcohol use, tobacco smokers and underweight people.

Based on this approach, the WHO identified six at risk population for whom systematic screening and treatment of LTBI is universally recommended, five at risk populations for whom the recommendation to screen and treat should be taken at a country level, and four populations for whom current evidence recommends against systematic screening and treatment [102]. Table 3 summarise these findings.

Populations that should be universally screened

People living with HIV

Even in the era of wide access to ART, TB remains the most frequent cause of AIDS-related deaths worldwide [103]. In 2017, it caused more than 300000 deaths among people living with HIV, which represents one-third of all HIV deaths. Global data indicated that in 2017 people living with HIV were 21 times (95% CI 16–27) more likely to develop active TB than those without HIV infection [1].

Almost 20 years ago the biological proof of an increased risk of progression to active disease was obtained in a prospective cohort of intravenous drug users with HIV infection [104], and in a prospective cohort study in HIV-infected homeless persons stratified by LTBI status, using HIV-negative homeless persons as a control (proxy of the general population) [105]. The benefit of INH preventive therapy in reducing active TB among persons living with HIV has been systematically demonstrated in a number of clinical trials and confirmed by meta-analyses. A systematic review of 12 RCTs of 8578 people living with HIV found that preventive treatment reduced the overall risk of TB by 33% (RR 0.67, 95% CI 0.51–0.87) [71]. The benefit of INH is demonstrated in persons living with HIV with high CD4 and who take antiretroviral medicines. A 6-month course of INH in persons living with HIV enrolling in care has been shown to reduce mortality by 37% after 5 years in a major study from West Africa [59]. INH preventive therapy for 36 months or longer is conditionally recommended by the WHO in settings with high TB transmission (as defined by local authorities), due to the high risk of re-infection that reduces the duration of protection [50]. Clinical trials of repeated courses of preventive treatment are ongoing and will probably shed more light on this complex issue.

Table 3. Summary of recommendations on target risk population groups according to the WHO[#]

Risk population groups	Strength of recommendation
People living with HIV Adult and child PTB contacts Patients initiating anti-tumour necrosis factor treatment Patients receiving dialysis Patients preparing for transplantation Patients with silicosis	Strong: systematic testing and treatment should be performed (low to very low quality of evidence)
Prisoners Healthcare workers Immigrants from high-burden countries Homeless persons Illicit drug user	Conditional: systematic testing and treatment should be considered (low to very low quality of evidence)
Patients with diabetes People with harmful alcohol use Tobacco smokers Underweight people	Conditional: systematic testing and treatment is not recommended unless they belong in the upper two groups (very low quality of evidence)

[#]: recommendations for low TB-burden countries. Data from [102].

The evidence of protective efficacy of INH for 6 months among children living with HIV is less clear, with two RCTs showing both significant reduction in mortality and protection against TB [106], and no benefit in infants with no known exposure to a TB case [107]. In another trial, the incidence of TB was lower in those given preventive treatment than in those who were not amongst 167 children receiving ART, but the difference was not statistically significant (incidence rate ratio 0.51, 95% CI 0.15–1.75) [108]. A cohort study suggested an additive protective effect of preventive treatment in children receiving ART [109].

Overall, in light of the evidence in adults and the increased risk of TB in children compared to adults, children living with HIV should be prioritised among candidate populations for treatment of LTBI. Although most evidence on the additive effect of INH preventive therapy over ART comes from high TB-incidence countries, the recommendation about INH preventive therapy for persons living with HIV extends to low-incidence countries as well. Despite overwhelming evidence of efficacy and safety, and more than 20 years after the WHO issued a clear policy to support it, the roll out of INH preventive therapy on a global scale remains very limited, mainly due to programmatic issues.

Close contacts
Investigation of people exposed to cases of infectious TB (contact investigation) to identify and treat persons with LTBI is a key component of TB control programmes in countries with low TB incidence. In a retrospective, population-based cohort study of close contact with a person with infectious TB using casual contacts as a control (proxy of the general population), the TB incidence rate ratio ranged from 5.2 to 10.6 depending on the level of the TST induration at baseline. In a systematic review and meta-analysis of LTBI in close contacts, the prevalence of infection was 51.4% (95% CI 50.6–52.2, I^2=99.4%) with substantial heterogeneity in all analyses [110].

    https://doi.org/10.1183/2312508X.10022617

In high-incidence countries, contact tracing for LTBI management is commonly only performed in children under the age of 5 years. In recent years the debate about the opportunity to extend the recommendation for screening and treatment of LTBI to adult household contacts in high-incidence countries has increased. In 2017 the WHO performed an updated systematic review with the aim of determining the prevalence of LTBI, the progression to active TB disease and the cumulative prevalence of active TB among household contacts stratified by age (WHO unpublished data). The prevalence of LTBI was higher among children and adolescents aged >15 years and adults than in children aged <5 years. The pooled risk ratios for progression to active TB were lower in children aged 5–15 years (0.28, 95% CI 0.12–0.65; four studies) and >15 years (0.22, 95% CI 0.08–0.60; three studies) in comparison to children aged <5 years. Regardless of their age or LTBI status, all household contacts were at a substantially higher risk for progression to active TB than the general population. Based on this evidence, the WHO currently conditionally recommends testing and treatment for LTBI in adult contacts in high-incidence countries [50].

Immunocompromising conditions

A large number of conditions characterised by reduced levels of immune competency have been associated with an increased risk of progression from latent infection to overt disease. However, sound evidence for such an effect is currently available for a very limited number of population groups. In a prospective cohort study of patients undergoing dialysis, the relative risk of progression was determined using an age-matched control group in the general population and supported by the national TB registry: the adjusted risk ratio varied from 8 to 41, depending on the TST induration at baseline [111].

Because studies providing direct evidence of increased risk of disease progression were not available in other risk populations, a series of systematic reviews were conducted to determine the incidence rate ratio for active TB in a number of candidate populations in comparison with year-adjusted national estimates derived from the 2013 WHO Global TB report. In these analyses, recipients of anti-TNF drugs had particularly high relative risks for incident TB (16.2; 95% CI 14.6–18; unpublished data). These results were in line with previous individual cohort analyses in recipients of TNF inhibitors [112].

The number of subjects exposed to biological therapy is increasing. The therapeutic armamentarium for inflammatory rheumatic disorders is impressive. Around 20 years ago, anti- -TNFs infliximab and etanercept were licensed and, over the following years, other anti-TNFs such as adalimumab, golimumab and certolizumab pegol have been approved [61, 62]. Although they are effective, an increased risk of developing active TB has been described in those with LTBI. Indeed, the block of TNF negatively affects granuloma formation and maintenance, favouring *M. tuberculosis* replication. Screening procedures and preventive treatment has decreased TB incidence in this population group; however, an increased risk of TB reactivation in anti-TNF exposed patients is still currently observed [3, 4, 62–66]. In this category of patients, there is a risk of false-negative diagnostic tests for LTBI due to either the diseases themselves or the treatments used. Because of that, the decision to treat LTBI should consider not only the test results but also the risk stratification.

During the past 10 years, new inflammatory pathways sustained by CD20 and CD28 lymphocytes and cytokines other than TNF, including interleukin (IL)-6, IL-12, IL-23 and IL-17, have been discovered with the research and development of new biologics. They have showed a safer profile in rheumatological patients with LTBI. Indeed, only sporadic cases of active TB, whose frequency is not higher than that recorded in the general population, were reported in tocilizumab- (inhibiting IL-6), rituximab- (inhibiting CD20) and abatacept-exposed patients (inhibiting CD28) with rheumatoid arthritis, and no cases were associated with ustekinumab (targeting IL12/IL-23) and secukinumab (targeting IL-17) in patients with ankylosing spondylitis [62]. Nivolumab, a novel programmed death receptor (PD)-1, that acts as a check point inhibitor, has also recently been associated with active TB [113]. Patients receiving these new treatments should be routinely screened and treated for LTBI.

Exposure to silica dust is also associated with increased risk of TB [114]. Recently, the combination of HIV and silicosis in South African miners has contributed to an explosive epidemic of TB in this population [115].

People who are candidates for solid organ or haematological transplantation were added to the list of priority populations based mainly on good clinical practise [116].

Healthcare workers

Healthcare workers are at risk of acquiring TB even in countries with low TB incidence. It has been estimated that the average annual risk for developing TB disease is up to three-fold higher for healthcare workers compared to the general population. Moreover, healthcare workers are at a higher risk of contracting MDR-TB, being up to six times more likely to be hospitalised for MDR-TB than the population they care [67–70]. This is due to delayed diagnosis, less effective treatment and longer contact periods with infectious patients that altogether may increase the risk of transmission. Therefore, the screening procedures of the healthcare workers are crucial for TB control in the work place [102].

Populations with national indication for screening

For other populations there is evidence of benefits in the systematic testing and treatment of LTBI, but the extent of such benefits may vary significantly in different epidemiological settings, or be perceived differently in different socio-political contexts, resulting in a conditional recommendation from the WHO. For example, a large number of studies demonstrate a higher incidence of TB among prisoners [117] and illicit drug users [118]. However, the decision to implement TB control activities in the prison sector or among illicit drug users is often influenced by the national legal framework and the political context. Other populations, for which there is consistent evidence of a greater risk of TB, may be highly relevant in low-incidence settings, but perceived as a lower priority in high-burden countries. That would not be the case of recent immigrants from countries that have a high TB burden [119].

Populations that should not be screened

For a few populations, the WHO has issued a recommendation against systematic testing and treatment of LTBI; namely diabetic patients, people with harmful alcohol use, tobacco smokers and people who are underweight [102]. The case of diabetic patients is paradigmatic. There is evidence from the literature of an increased risk of TB in diabetic patients, both from meta-analysis of observational studies (relative risk 3.11, 95% CI 2.27–4.26) and prospective cohorts (adjusted hazard ratio 2.09; 95% C 1.10–3.95) [120, 121].

https://doi.org/10.1183/2312508X.10022617

Although the number of diabetes-associated TB cases globally is large, the expected benefits for the individual with diabetes from LTBI treatment are relatively marginal. Weighing such benefits against the potential harms of currently available treatment regimens results in a trade-off that is probably not favourable to treatment of the individual. That could not be the case in countries with high prevalence of both conditions, such as Mexico, where around 25% of TB cases and 50% of MDR-TB cases coexist with diabetes [1, 122].

In addition, there are a number of possible risk populations for whom no evidence is in fact available; this is the case, for example, of persons receiving glucocorticoids [123]. In this case, the large variability in glucocorticoids regimen (type of drug, dose and duration), patients and underlying diseases prevent any informative analysis from the extensive data available from the literature. This question can only be addressed by carefully planned prospective studies that, however, are extremely complex to perform.

Exposure to multidrug-resistant tuberculosis

An unpublished systematic review of the effectiveness of preventive treatment for contacts of people with MDR-TB was conducted by the WHO for the preparation of the 2018 LTBI guidelines [50]. 10 studies were identified, but only four enrolled more than 20 participants and two of those did not report TB cases in either the intervention or the control arm [124, 125]. In one of the two remaining studies [93], 119 exposed individuals were enrolled, 104 contacts with LTBI initiated fluoroquinolone-based preventive treatment, of whom 93 (89%) completed treatment, and none developed active TB; while three (20%) out of 15 contacts who refused treatment developed MDR-TB (OR 0.02, 95% CI 0.00–0.39). Confirmed or probable TB developed in two (4.9%) out of 41 children receiving tailored preventive treatment and in 13 (20.3%) out of 64 children who did not receive proper preventive treatment (OR 0.2, 95% CI 0.04–0.949) in the other study [94]. Fluoroquinolones (*e.g.* moxifloxacin and levofloxacin) with or without other agents (*e.g.* ethambutol and ethionamide) were the drugs mainly used in these studies. Although one study reported that no serious adverse events could be attributed to fluoroquinolone-based preventive treatment, no study included a comparison of the risk for adverse events [93, 94]. The median proportion of participants who discontinued treatment because of adverse events in all the studies was 5.1% (interquartile range 1.9–30.2%). As stated above, the drug resistance pattern of the MDR-TB source case can help to predict the resistance pattern in the secondary cases in >50% of the cases [95].

Three cluster-randomised superiority clinical trials have been initiated and their results will be pivotal for policy development. In the TB-CHAMP trial, children aged 0–5 years in South Africa exposed to fluoroquinolone-sensitive MDR-TB strains will receive levofloxacin paediatric dispersible tablets or placebo, with incident MDR-TB being the primary outcome [126]. In the V-Quin clinical trial, an exposed individual of any age in Vietnam will receive either levofloxacin or placebo and incident MDR-TB will be measured [127]. Finally, in the multicenter, multinational PHOENIx clinical trial exposed children aged 0–5 years and with HIV co-infection will be randomly allocated to receive delamanid or INH and incident MDR-TB will be comparatively measured [128].

While awaiting the results of the above trials, we have very weak evidence of a potential benefit of quinolone-based preventive therapy (for both adults and children) in contacts of MDR-TB cases. It is important to note that in some cases, even though the identified contact was an MDR-TB patient, the LTBI could be caused by an INH sensitive strain. Therefore, some physicians add INH to the fluoroquinolone.

A regimen of preventive treatment of MDR-TB contacts should be based on reliable information on the drug resistance profile of the source case, according to the WHO recommendations [50]. Unless the strain of the source case is resistant to later generation fluoroquinolones (*e.g.* levofloxacin and moxifloxacin), they are important components of a preventive treatment regimen. Because retardation of cartilage development has been shown in animals, there has been concern about the use of fluoroquinolones in children [129]; however, similar effects have not been demonstrated in humans [130]. There is very weak evidence for the duration of treatment, and this should be based on clinical judgement. In the studies conducted to date, the regimens were given for 6, 9 and 12 months.

Diagnosis and treatment of LTBI is evolving. Implementation of strategies to fight LTBI in the national TB programmes is challenging. More resources and political commitment are needed to support pillar three of the End TB strategy, which includes the issue of preventing active TB by tackling LTBI.

References

1.   World Health Organization. Global tuberculosis report 2018. Geneva, World Health Organization, 2018.
2.   Houben RM, Dodd PJ. The global burden of latent tuberculosis infection: a re-estimation using mathematical modelling. *PLoS Med* 2016; 13: e1002152.
3.   Flynn JL, Goldstein MM, Chan J, *et al.* Tumor necrosis factor-alpha is required in the protective immune response against *Mycobacterium tuberculosis* in mice. *Immunity* 1995; 2: 561–572.
4.   Pai M, Behr MA, Dowdy D, *et al.* Tuberculosis. *Nat Rev Dis Primers* 2016; 2: 16076.
5.   Goletti D, Sanduzzi A, Delogu G. Performance of the tuberculin skin test and interferon-gamma release assays: an update on the accuracy, cut-off stratification, and new potential immune-based approaches. *J Rheumatol Suppl* 2014; 91: 24–31.
6.   Delogu G, Goletti D. The spectrum of tuberculosis infection: new perspectives in the era of biologics. *J Rheumatol Suppl* 2014; 91: 11–16.
7.   Barry CE 3rd, Boshoff HI, Dartois V, *et al.* The spectrum of latent tuberculosis: rethinking the biology and intervention strategies. *Nat Rev Microbiol* 2009; 7: 845–855.
8.   Esmail H, Barry CE 3rd, Young DB, *et al.* The ongoing challenge of latent tuberculosis. *Philos Trans R Soc Lond B Biol Sci* 2014; 369: 20130437.
9.   Dorhoi A, Kaufmann SH. Pathology and immune reactivity: understanding multidimensionality in pulmonary tuberculosis. *Semin Immunopathol* 2016; 38: 153–166.
10.   Petruccioli E, Scriba TJ, Petrone L, *et al.* Correlates of tuberculosis risk: predictive biomarkers for progression to active tuberculosis. *Eur Respir J* 2016; 48: 1751–1763.
11.   Zwerling A, Pai M. The BCG world atlas: a new, open-access resource for clinicians and researchers. *Expert Rev Anti Infect Ther* 2011; 9: 559–561.
12.   Bucher HC, Griffith LE, Guyatt GH, *et al.* Isoniazid prophylaxis for tuberculosis in HIV infection: a meta-analysis of randomized controlled trials. *AIDS* 1999; 13: 501–507.
13.   Trajman A, Steffen RE, Menzies D. Interferon-gamma release assays *versus* tuberculin skin testing for the diagnosis of latent tuberculosis infection: an overview of the evidence. *Pulm Med* 2013; 2013: 601737.
14.   Farhat M, Greenaway C, Pai M, *et al.* False-positive tuberculin skin tests: what is the absolute effect of BCG and non-tuberculous mycobacteria? *Int J Tuberc Lung Dis* 2006; 10: 1192–1204.
15.   Diel R, Ernst M, Doscher G, *et al.* Avoiding the effect of BCG vaccination in detecting *Mycobacterium tuberculosis* infection with a blood test. *Eur Respir J* 2006; 28: 16–23.
16.   Mahairas GG, Sabo PJ, Hickey MJ, *et al.* Molecular analysis of genetic differences between *Mycobacterium bovis* BCG and virulent *M. bovis*. *J Bacteriol* 1996; 178: 1274–1282.
17.   Andersen P, Munk ME, Pollock JM, *et al.* Specific immune-based diagnosis of tuberculosis. *Lancet* 2000; 356: 1099–1104.
18.   Barcellini L, Borroni E, Brown J, *et al.* First evaluation of QuantiFERON-TB Gold Plus performance in contact screening. *Eur Respir J* 2016; 48: 1411–1419.

https://doi.org/10.1183/2312508X.10022617

19. Petruccioli E, Chiacchio T, Pepponi I, *et al.* First characterization of the CD4 and CD8 T-cell responses to QuantiFERON-TB Plus. *J Infect* 2016; 73: 588–597.

20. Petruccioli E, Vanini V, Chiacchio T, *et al.* Analytical evaluation of QuantiFERON-Plus and QuantiFERON-Gold In-tube assays in subjects with or without tuberculosis. *Tuberculosis (Edinb)* 2017; 106: 38–43.

21. Mori T, Sakatani M, Yamagishi F, *et al.* Specific detection of tuberculosis infection: an interferon-gamma-based assay using new antigens. *Am J Respir Crit Care Med* 2004; 170: 59–64.

22. Chiacchio T, Petruccioli E, Vanini V, *et al.* Polyfunctional T-cells and effector memory phenotype are associated with active TB in HIV-infected patients. *J Infect* 2014; 69: 533–545.

23. Day CL, Abrahams DA, Lerumo L, *et al.* Functional capacity of *Mycobacterium tuberculosis*-specific T cell responses in humans is associated with mycobacterial load. *J Immunol* 2011; 187: 2222–2232.

24. Rozot V, Patrizia A, Vigano S, *et al.* Combined use of *Mycobacterium tuberculosis*-specific CD4 and CD8 T-cell responses is a powerful diagnostic tool of active tuberculosis. *Clin Infect Dis* 2015; 60: 432–437.

25. Vordermeier HM, Brown J, Cockle PJ, *et al.* Assessment of cross-reactivity between *Mycobacterium bovis* and *M. kansasii* ESAT-6 and CFP-10 at the T-cell epitope level. *Clin Vaccine Immunol* 2007; 14: 1203–1209.

26. Bosserman RE, Thompson CR, Nicholson KR, *et al.* Esx paralogs are functionally equivalent to ESX-1 proteins but are dispensable for virulence in *Mycobacterium marinum. J Bacteriol* 2018; 200: e00726-17.

27. Wong SH, Gao Q, Tsoi KK, *et al.* Effect of immunosuppressive therapy on interferon-γ release assay for latent tuberculosis screening in patients with autoimmune diseases: a systematic review and meta-analysis. *Thorax* 2016; 71: 64–72.

28. Edwards A, Gao Y, Allan RN, *et al.* Corticosteroids and infliximab impair the performance of interferon-gamma release assays used for diagnosis of latent tuberculosis. *Thorax* 2017; 72: 946–949.

29. Ruhwald M, Aggerbeck H, Gallardo RV, *et al.* Safety and efficacy of the C-Tb skin test to diagnose *Mycobacterium tuberculosis* infection, compared with an interferon gamma release assay and the tuberculin skin test: a phase 3, double-blind, randomised, controlled trial. *Lancet Respir Med* 2017; 5: 259–268.

30. Getahun H, Chaisson RE, Raviglione M. Latent *Mycobacterium tuberculosis* infection. *N Engl J Med* 2015; 373: 1179–1180.

31. Carmona L, Gomez-Reino JJ, Rodriguez-Valverde V, *et al.* Effectiveness of recommendations to prevent reactivation of latent tuberculosis infection in patients treated with tumor necrosis factor antagonists. *Arthritis Rheum* 2005; 52: 1766–1772.

32. Goletti D, Petrone L, Ippolito G, *et al.* Preventive therapy for tuberculosis in rheumatological patients undergoing therapy with biological drugs. *Expert Rev Anti Infect Ther* 2018; 16: 501–512.

33. Goletti D, Vincenti D, Carrara S, *et al.* Selected RD1 peptides for active tuberculosis diagnosis: comparison of a gamma interferon whole-blood enzyme-linked immunosorbent assay and an enzyme-linked immunospot assay. *Clin Diagn Lab Immunol* 2005; 12: 1311–1316.

34. Chiacchio T, Delogu G, Vanini V, *et al.* Immune characterization of the HBHA-specific response in *Mycobacterium tuberculosis*-infected patients with or without HIV infection. *PLoS One* 2017; 12: e0183846.

35. Delogu G, Chiacchio T, Vanini V, *et al.* Methylated HBHA produced in *M. smegmatis* discriminates between active and non-active tuberculosis disease among RD1-responders. *PLoS One* 2011; 6: e18315.

36. Delogu G, Vanini V, Cuzzi G, *et al.* Lack of response to HBHA in HIV-infected patients with latent tuberculosis infection. *Scand J Immunol* 2016; 84: 344–352.

37. Goletti D, Butera O, Vanini V, *et al.* Response to Rv2628 latency antigen associates with cured tuberculosis and remote infection. *Eur Respir J* 2010; 36: 135–142.

38. Leyten EM, Arend SM, Prins C, *et al.* Discrepancy between *Mycobacterium tuberculosis*-specific gamma interferon release assays using short and prolonged *in vitro* incubation. *Clin Vaccine Immunol* 2007; 14: 880–885.

39. Black GF, Thiel BA, Ota MO, *et al.* Immunogenicity of novel DosR regulon-encoded candidate antigens of *Mycobacterium tuberculosis* in three high-burden populations in Africa. *Clin Vaccine Immunol* 2009; 16: 1203–1212.

40. Butera O, Chiacchio T, Carrara S, *et al.* New tools for detecting latent tuberculosis infection: evaluation of RD1-specific long-term response. *BMC Infect Dis* 2009; 9: 182.

41. de Paus RA, van Meijgaarden KE, Prins C, *et al.* Immunological characterization of latent tuberculosis infection in a low endemic country. *Tuberculosis (Edinb)* 2017; 106: 62–72.

42. Rangaka MX, Wilkinson KA, Glynn JR, *et al.* Predictive value of interferon-gamma release assays for incident active tuberculosis: a systematic review and meta-analysis. *Lancet Infect Dis* 2012; 12: 45–55.

43. Zellweger JP, Sotgiu G, Block M, *et al.* Risk assessment of tuberculosis in contacts by IFN-gamma release assays. A Tuberculosis Network European Trials Group Study. *Am J Respir Crit Care Med* 2015; 191: 1176–1184.

44. Abubakar I, Drobniewski F, Southern J, *et al.* Prognostic value of interferon-γ release assays and tuberculin skin test in predicting the development of active tuberculosis (UK PREDICT TB): a prospective cohort study. *Lancet Infect Dis* 2018; 18: 1077–1088.

45. Zak DE, Penn-Nicholson A, Scriba TJ, *et al.* A blood RNA signature for tuberculosis disease risk: a prospective cohort study. *Lancet* 2016; 4: 387–388.

46. Kik SV, Cobelens F, Moore D. Predicting tuberculosis risk. *Lancet* 2016; 16: 227–238.

47. Maertzdorf J, Repsilber D, Parida SK, *et al.* Human gene expression profiles of susceptibility and resistance in tuberculosis. *Genes Immun* 2011; 12: 15–22.

48. Sweeney TE, Braviak L, Tato CM, *et al.* Genome-wide expression for diagnosis of pulmonary tuberculosis: a multicohort analysis. *Lancet Respir Med* 2016; 4: 213–224.

49. Esmail H, Lai RP, Lesosky M, *et al.* Complement pathway gene activation and rising circulating immune complexes characterize early disease in HIV-associated tuberculosis. *Proc Natl Acad Sci USA* 2018; 115: E964–E973.

50. World Health Organization. Latent tuberculosis infection: updated and consolidated guidelines for programmatic management. Geneva, World Health Organization, 2018.

51. Marais BJ, Gie RP, Hesseling AH, *et al.* Adult-type pulmonary tuberculosis in children 10–14 years of age. *Pediatr Infect Dis J* 2005; 24: 743–744.

52. Marais BJ, Gie RP, Schaaf HS, *et al.* The spectrum of disease in children treated for tuberculosis in a highly endemic area. *Int J Tuberc Lung Dis* 2006; 10: 732–738.

53. Marais BJ, Gie RP, Schaaf HS, *et al.* The clinical epidemiology of childhood pulmonary tuberculosis: a critical review of literature from the pre-chemotherapy era. *Int J Tuberc Lung Dis* 2004; 8: 278–285.

54. International Organization for Migration. World migration report 2018. Geneva, International Organization for Migration, 2018.

55. Dara M, Solovic I, Goletti D, *et al.* Preventing and controlling tuberculosis among refugees in Europe: more is needed. *Eur Respir J* 2016; 48: 272–274.

56. Dara M, Solovic I, Sotgiu G, *et al.* Call for urgent actions to ensure access to early diagnosis and care of tuberculosis among refugees: Statement of the European Respiratory Society and the European Region of the International Union Against Tuberculosis and Lung Disease. *Eur Respir J* 2016; 47: 1345–1347.

57. Dara M, Solovic I, Sotgiu G, *et al.* Tuberculosis care among refugees arriving in Europe: a ERS/WHO Europe region survey of current practices. *Eur Respir J* 2016; 48: 808–817.

58. Kunst H, Burman M, Arnesen TM, *et al.* Tuberculosis and latent tuberculous infection screening of migrants in Europe: comparative analysis of policies, surveillance systems and results. *Int J Tuberc Lung Dis* 2017; 21: 840–851.

59. Danel C, Moh R, Gabillard D, *et al.* A trial of early antiretrovirals and isoniazid preventive therapy in Africa. *N Engl J Med* 2015; 373: 808–822.

60. Lawn SD, Myer L, Edwards D, *et al.* Short-term and long-term risk of tuberculosis associated with CD4 cell recovery during antiretroviral therapy in South Africa. *AIDS* 2009; 23: 1717–1725.

61. Ramiro S, Sepriano A, Chatzidionysiou K, *et al.* Safety of synthetic and biological DMARDs: a systematic literature review informing the 2016 update of the EULAR recommendations for management of rheumatoid arthritis. *Ann Rheum Dis* 2017; 76: 1101–1136.

62. Cantini F, Nannini C, Niccoli L, *et al.* Risk of tuberculosis reactivation in patients with rheumatoid arthritis, ankylosing spondylitis, and psoriatic arthritis receiving non-anti-TNF-targeted Biologics. *Mediators Inflamm* 2017; 2017: 8909834.

63. Cantini F, Goletti D. Biologics and tuberculosis risk: the rise and fall of an old disease and its new resurgence. *J Rheumatol Suppl* 2014; 91: 1–3.

64. Cantini F, Nannini C, Niccoli L, *et al.* Guidance for the management of patients with latent tuberculosis infection requiring biologic therapy in rheumatology and dermatology clinical practice. *Autoimmun Rev* 2015; 14: 503–509.

65. Minozzi S, Bonovas S, Lytras T, *et al.* Risk of infections using anti-TNF agents in rheumatoid arthritis, psoriatic arthritis, and ankylosing spondylitis: a systematic review and meta-analysis. *Expert Opin Drug Saf* 2016; 15: 11–34.

66. Souto A, Maneiro JR, Salgado E, *et al.* Risk of tuberculosis in patients with chronic immune-mediated inflammatory diseases treated with biologics and tofacitinib: a systematic review and meta-analysis of randomized controlled trials and long-term extension studies. *Rheumatology (Oxford)* 2014; 53: 1872–1885.

67. Fennelly KP, Iseman MD. Health care workers and tuberculosis: the battle of a century. *Int J Tuberc Lung Dis* 1999; 3: 363–364.

68. Baussano I, Nunn P, Williams B, *et al.* Tuberculosis among health care workers. *Emerging Infect Dis* 2011; 17: 488–494.

69. Napoli C, Ferretti F, Di Ninno F, *et al.* Screening for tuberculosis in health care workers: experience in an Italian teaching hospital. *Biomed Res Int* 2017; 2017: 7538037.

70. O'Donnell MR, Jarand J, Loveday M, *et al.* High incidence of hospital admissions with multidrug-resistant and extensively drug-resistant tuberculosis among South African health care workers. *Ann Inter Med* 2010; 153: 516–522.

71. Akolo C, Adetifa I, Shepperd S, *et al.* Treatment of latent tuberculosis infection in HIV infected persons. *Cochrane Database Syst Rev* 2010; 20: CD000171.

72. Smieja MJ, Marchetti CA, Cook DJ, *et al.* Isoniazid for preventing tuberculosis in non-HIV infected persons. *Cochrane Database Syst Rev* 2000: CD001363.

73. World Health Organization. The End TB Strategy. 2015, Geneva, World Health Organization,

74. World Health Organization. Guidelines for the management of latent tuberculosis infection. Geneva, World Health Organization, 2015.

https://doi.org/10.1183/2312508X.10022617

75. United States Public Health Service. United States Public Health Service tuberculosis prophylaxis trial. Prophylactic effects of isoniazid on primary tuberculosis in children: preliminary report. *Am Rev Tuberc* 1957; 76: 942–963.

76. American Thoracic Society. Preventive treatment in tuberculosis. A Statement by the Committee on Therapy. *Am Rev Respir Dis* 1965; 91: 297–298.

77. Ferebee SH. Controlled chemoprophylaxis trials in tuberculosis. A general review. *Adv Tuberc Res* 1970; 17: 28–106.

78. Comstock GW, Woolpert SF. Preventive therapy. *In*: Kubica GP, Wayne LG, eds. The Mycobacteria: A Sourcebook. New York, Dekker, 1984; pp. 1071–1082.

79. Comstock GW, Fereber SH, Hammes LM. A controlled trial of community-wide isoniazid prophylaxis in Alaska. *Am Rev Respir Dis* 1969; 95: 935–943.

80. Comstock GW. How much isoniazid is needed for prevention of tuberculosis among immunocompetent adults? *Int J Tuberc Lung Dis* 1999; 3: 847–850.

81. Centers for Disease Control and Prevention. Treatment Regimens for Latent TB Infection (LTBI). www.cdc.gov/tb/topic/treatment/ltbi.htm Date last updated June 29 2017. Date last accessed October 11, 2018.

82. Den Boon S, Matteelli A, Ford N, *et al.* Continuous isoniazid for the treatment of latent tuberculosis infection in people living with HIV. *AIDS* 2016; 30: 797–801.

83. Zenner D, Beer N, Harris RJ, *et al.* Treatment of latent tuberculosis infection: an updated network meta-analysis. *Ann Inter Med* 2017; 167: 248–255.

84. Stagg HR, Zenner D, Harris RJ, *et al.* Treatment of latent tuberculosis infection: a network meta-analysis. *Ann Intern Med* 2014; 161: 419–428.

85. Menzies D, Adjobimey M, Ruslami R, *et al.* Four months of rifampin or nine months of isoniazid for latent tuberculosis in adults. *N Engl J Med* 2018; 379: 440–453.

86. Menzies D, Alvarez G, Khan K. Treatment of latent tuberculosis infection. *In*: Canadian Tuberculosis Standards. 7th Edn. Ottawa, Public Health Agency of Canada, 2014.

87. Spyridis NP, Spyridis PG, Gelesme A, *et al.* The effectiveness of a 9-month regimen of isoniazid alone *versus* 3- and 4-month regimens of isoniazid plus rifampin for treatment of latent tuberculosis infection in children: results of an 11-year randomized study. *Clin Infect Dis* 2007; 45: 715–722.

88. Van Zyl S, Marais BJ, Hesseling AC, *et al.* Adherence to anti-tuberculosis chemoprophylaxis and treatment in children. *Int J Tuberc Lung Dis* 2006; 10: 13–18.

89. Sterling TR, Villarino ME, Borisov AS, *et al.* Three months of rifapentine and isoniazid for latent tuberculosis infection. *N Engl J Med* 2011; 365: 2155–2166.

90. Martinson NA, Barnes GL, Moulton LH, *et al.* New regimens to prevent tuberculosis in adults with HIV infection. *N Engl J Med* 2011; 365: 11–20.

91. Villarino ME, Scott NA, Weis SE, *et al.* Treatment for preventing tuberculosis in children and adolescents: a randomized clinical trial of a 3-month, 12-dose regimen of a combination of rifapentine and isoniazid. *JAMA Pediatr* 2015; 169: 247–255.

92. Moro R, Scott N, Vernon A, *et al.* Pregnancy safety assessment of 3 months of once-weekly rifapentine and isoniazid and 9 months of daily isoniazid: a post-hoc analysis of the PREVENT TB and the iAdhere trials. *Am J Respir Crit Care Med* 2016; 193: A7859.

93. Bamrah S, Brostrom R, Dorina F, *et al.* Treatment for LTBI in contacts of MDR-TB patients, Federated States of Micronesia, 2009–2012. *Int J Tuberc Lung Dis* 2014; 18: 912–918.

94. Schaaf HS, Gie RP, Kennedy M, *et al.* Evaluation of young children in contact with adult multidrug-resistant pulmonary tuberculosis: a 30-month follow-up. *Pediatrics* 2002; 109: 765–771.

95. Shah NS, Yuen CM, Heo M, *et al.* Yield of contact investigations in households of patients with drug-resistant tuberculosis: systematic review and meta-analysis. *Clin Infect Dis* 2014; 58: 381–391.

96. Swindells S, Ramchandani R, Gupta A, *et al.* One month of rifapentin/isoniazid to prevent TB in people with HIV: BRIEF-TB/A5279. www.croiconference.org/sessions/one-month-rifapentineisoniazid-prevent-tb-people-hiv-brief-tba5279 Date last updated: March 2018. Date last accessed: October 11 2018.

97. Tang P, Johnston J. Treatment of latent tuberculosis infection. *Curr Treat Options Infect Dis* 2017; 9: 371–379.

98. Shea KM, Kammerer JS, Winston CA, *et al.* Estimated rate of reactivation of latent tuberculosis infection in the United States, overall and by population subgroup. *Am J Epidemiol* 2014; 179: 216–225.

99. Uplekar M, Weil D, Lonnroth K, *et al.* WHO's new end TB strategy. *Lancet* 2015; 385: 1799–1801.

100. Churchyard GJ, Fielding KL, Lewis JJ, *et al.* A trial of mass isoniazid preventive therapy for tuberculosis control. *N Engl J Med* 2014; 370: 301–310.

101. Comstock GW, Livesay VT, Woolpert SF. The prognosis of a positive tuberculin reaction in childhood and adolescence. *Am J Epidemiol* 1974; 99: 131–138.

102. Getahun H, Matteelli A, Abubakar I, *et al.* Management of latent *Mycobacterium tuberculosis* infection: WHO guidelines for low tuberculosis burden countries. *Eur Respir J* 2015; 46: 1563–1576.

103. Ford N, Matteelli A, Shubber Z, *et al.* TB as a cause of hospitalization and in-hospital mortality among people living with HIV worldwide: a systematic review and meta-analysis. *J Int AIDS Soc* 2016; 19: 20714.

104. Selwyn PA, Hartel D, Lewis VA, *et al.* A prospective study of the risk of tuberculosis among intravenous drug users with human immunodeficiency virus infection. *N Engl J Med* 1989; 320: 545–550.

105. Moss AR, Hahn JA, Tulsky JP, *et al.* Tuberculosis in the homeless. A prospective study. *Am J Respir Crit Care Med* 2000; 162: 460–464.

106. Zar HJ, Cotton MF, Strauss S, *et al.* Effect of isoniazid prophylaxis on mortality and incidence of tuberculosis in children with HIV: randomised controlled trial. *BMJ* 2007; 334: 136.

107. Madhi SA, Nachman S, Violari A, *et al.* Primary isoniazid prophylaxis against tuberculosis in HIV-exposed children. *N Engl J Med* 2011; 365: 21–31.

108. Gray DM, Workman LJ, Lombard CJ, *et al.* Isoniazid preventive therapy in HIV-infected children on antiretroviral therapy: a pilot study. *Int J Tuberc Lung Dis* 2014; 18: 322–327.

109. Frigati LJ, Kranzer K, Cotton MF, *et al.* The impact of isoniazid preventive therapy and antiretroviral therapy on tuberculosis in children infected with HIV in a high tuberculosis incidence setting. *Thorax* 2011; 66: 496–501.

110. Morrison J, Pai M, Hopewell PC. Tuberculosis and latent tuberculosis infection in close contacts of people with pulmonary tuberculosis in low-income and middle-income countries: a systematic review and meta-analysis. *Lancet Infect Dis* 2008; 8: 359–368.

111. Christopoulos AI, Diamantopoulos AA, Dimopoulos PA, *et al.* Risk factors for tuberculosis in dialysis patients: a prospective multi-center clinical trial. *BMC Nephrol* 2009; 10: 36.

112. Keane J, Bresnihan B. Tuberculosis reactivation during immunosuppressive therapy in rheumatic diseases: diagnostic and therapeutic strategies. *Curr Opin Rheumatol* 2008; 20: 443–449.

113. Fujita K, Terashima T, Mio T. Anti-PD1 antibody treatment and the development of acute pulmonary tuberculosis. *J Thorac Oncol* 2016; 11: 2238–2240.

114. Ringshausen FC, Nienhaus A, Schablon A, *et al.* Frequent detection of latent tuberculosis infection among aged underground hard coal miners in the absence of recent tuberculosis exposure. *PLoS One* 2013; 8: e82005.

115. Corbett EL, Churchyard GJ, Clayton TC, *et al.* HIV infection and silicosis: the impact of two potent risk factors on the incidence of mycobacterial disease in South African miners. *AIDS* 2000; 14: 2759–2768.

116. Al-Anazi KA, Al-Jasser AM, Alsaleh K. Infections caused by *Mycobacterium tuberculosis* in recipients of hematopoietic stem cell transplantation. *Front Oncol* 2014; 4: 231.

117. Baussano I, Williams BG, Nunn P, *et al.* Tuberculosis incidence in prisons: a systematic review. *PLoS Med* 2010; 7: e1000381.

118. Getahun H, Baddeley A, Raviglione M. Managing tuberculosis in people who use and inject illicit drugs. *Bull World Health Organ* 2013; 91: 154–156.

119. European Centre for Disease Prevention and Control (ECDC). Tuberculosis surveillance and monitoring in Europe. Stockholm, ECDC, 2017.

120. Jeon CY, Murray MB. Diabetes mellitus increases the risk of active tuberculosis: a systematic review of 13 observational studies. *PLoS Med* 2008; 5: e152.

121. Baker MA, Lin HH, Chang HY, *et al.* The risk of tuberculosis disease among persons with diabetes mellitus: a prospective cohort study. *Clin Infect Dis* 2012; 54: 818–825.

122. CENAPRECE. www.cenaprece.salud.gob.mx/programas/interior/portada_tuberculosis.html Date last updated: March 2018. Date last accessed: October 11 2018.

123. Jick SS, Lieberman ES, Rahman MU, *et al.* Glucocorticoid use, other associated factors, and the risk of tuberculosis. *Arthritis Rheum* 2006; 55: 19–26.

124. Garcia-Prats AJ, Zimri K, Mramba Z, *et al.* Children exposed to multi drug resistant tuberculosis at a home-based day care centre: a contact investigation. *Int J Tuberc Lung Dis* 2014; 18: 1292–1298.

125. Trieu L, Proops DC, Ahuja SD. Moxifloxacin prophylaxis against MDR TB, New York, New York, USA. *Emerging Infect Dis* 2015; 21: 500–503.

126. ISRCTN register. Tuberculosis child multidrug-resistant preventive therapy: TB CHAMP trial. ISRCTN92634082. https://doi.org/10.1186/ISRCTN92634082 Date last updated: April 1 2017. Date last accessed: October 11 2018.

127. ANZCTN register. The V-QUIN MDR TRIAL: a randomized controlled trial of six months of daily levofloxacin for the prevention of tuberculosis among household contacts of patients with multi-drug resistant tuberculosis. https://anzctr.org.au/Trial/Registration/TrialReview.aspx?id=369817 Date last updated: May 23 2017. Date last accessed: October 11 2018.

128. AID Clinical TrialsGroup. PHOENIx is rising! https://actgnetwork.org/PHOENIX-rising Date last updated: April 2018. Date last accessed: October 11 2018.

129. Takizawa T, Hashimoto K, Minami T, *et al.* The comparative arthropathy of fluoroquinolones in dogs. *Hum Exp Toxicol* 1999; 18: 392–399.

130. Hampel B, Hullmann R, Schmidt H. Ciprofloxacin in pediatrics: worldwide clinical experience based on compassionate use – safety report. *Pediatr Infect Dis J* 1997; 16: 127–129.

Disclosures: None declared.

https://doi.org/10.1183/2312508X.10022617

Chapter 23

Nontuberculous mycobacteria

Sanne Zweijpfenning[1], Wouter Hoefsloot[1] and Jakko van Ingen ⓘ[2]

NTM can cause chronic severe infections, particularly of the lungs. The incidence and prevalence of these infections is increasing in most settings, particularly those where TB incidence is in decline. Owing to their ubiquity in nature, the diagnosis of NTM pulmonary disease is based on symptoms, radiology and repeated isolation of the same NTM species. NTM are intrinsically resistant to most classes of antibiotics. Treatment is multidrug, long, species specific and cumbersome. DST can help streamline these treatment regimens. In the past two decades, a lot of new knowledge on epidemiology, risk factors, microbiology, and treatment and outcome has been gathered. This chapter provides a review of the new insights in these fields, to support clinicians in the diagnosis and treatment of these severe infections.

Cite as: Zweijpfenning S, Hoefsloot W, van Ingen J. Nontuberculous mycobacteria. *In:* Migliori GB, Bothamley G, Duarte R, *et al.*, eds. Tuberculosis (ERS Monograph). Sheffield, European Respiratory Society, 2018; pp. 399–413 [https://doi.org/10.1183/2312508X.10022717].

🐦 @ERSpublications
The complex diagnosis and treatment of nontuberculous mycobacterial disease: a comprehensive review http://ow.ly/cfVQ30lqCfE

In the early 1950s, TB sanatoria in several countries were faced with patients whose supposed PTB was, in fact, caused by NTM [1, 2]. The first NTM associated with TB-like pulmonary disease was *Mycobacterium kansasii* (then dubbed "the yellow bacillus", for its pigmented colonies in culture) [1], but within the course of 5 years several cases of *Mycobacterium avium* and *Mycobacterium intracellulare* (or the "Battey bacillus", after Battey State Hospital, Rome, GA, USA) pulmonary disease were also reported [3]. All these reported patients had been TB suspects, with fibro-cavitary pulmonary disease. It took until 1992 to realise that NTM cause another important pulmonary disease, *i.e.* nodular/bronchiectatic NTM pulmonary disease (NTM-PD). Due to the peculiar phenotype of some of these patients and the hypothesis that it resulted from habitual voluntary suppression of cough, the disease was dubbed "Lady Windermere syndrome" [4], although this name is no longer used.

Nearly 70 years after their initial discovery as pulmonary pathogens, NTM are now increasingly studied and increasingly recognised as important opportunistic pathogens of

[1]Dept of Pulmonary Diseases, Radboud University Medical Center, Nijmegen, The Netherlands. [2]Dept of Medical Microbiology, Radboud University Medical Center, Nijmegen, The Netherlands.

Correspondence: Jakko van Ingen, Dept of Medical Microbiology, Radboud University Medical Center, PO Box 9101, 6500 HB Nijmegen, The Netherlands. E-mail: jakko.vaningen@radboudumc.nl

humans; NTM-PD is their most frequent clinical manifestation. The more than 150 published species differ widely in their virulence, associated diseases, drug susceptibility, and isolation frequency and geographical distribution [5]. Owing to similarities to conventional PTB in terms of clinical presentation and the overlap in diagnostic tools and treatment modalities, NTM-PD is mostly diagnosed by physicians who also treat TB patients. Hence, this *ERS Monograph* on TB [6] would not be complete if it did not include an update on NTM-PD. Within this chapter, we review the laboratory aspects, epidemiology, clinical presentation and treatment of NTM-PD.

Laboratory features of nontuberculous mycobacteria

Microscopy and culture

The diagnostic routine to visualise and culture NTM from respiratory specimens is not very different from TB diagnostics. Auramine and Ziehl–Neelsen staining techniques are equally efficient for NTM and *Mycobacterium tuberculosis* [7]. The NTM species that cause NTM-PD typically grow well at 37°C; species that prefer lower temperatures tend to cause localised or disseminated skin diseases rather than NTM-PD (*e.g. Mycobacterium marinum, Mycobacterium haemophilum* and *Mycobacterium chelonae*) [8]. Most NTM species grow well in routinely used "TB media" such as Middlebrook 7H9 broth or solid Middlebrook 7H10/7H11 agar and Löwenstein–Jensen medium. Relevant exceptions to this rule include *Mycobacterium xenopi, Mycobacterium malmoense* and *Mycobacterium genavense*; the very slow and fastidious growth of these organisms may be overcome by lowering the pH of the medium (for *M. malmoense* [9]), prolonged incubation at 42°C (for *M. xenopi* [8]) or adding charcoal and blood as well as acidifying the medium (for *M. genavense* [10]). These three NTM species may be missed by conventional culture approaches in routine diagnostics. The use of molecular detection assays is helpful for these species [8].

To optimise the sensitivity of culture-based diagnosis of NTM-PD, it is recommended to use both liquid and solid media for primary culture. Adding Löwenstein–Jensen medium to automated liquid media systems increases the sensitivity of NTM detection by 15% [8].

Identification

Molecular tools, *i.e.* specific probes, line probe assays or PCR amplification and sequencing techniques, are the most commonly used tools for identification of NTM. The probe assays are adequate to identify species to the "complex" level, *i.e. M. avium* complex (MAC) or *Mycobacterium fortuitum* complex. Identification to the species level in some of these complexes, or identification to the subspecies level of *M. abscessus*, requires gene sequencing approaches, often using multiple targets [8]. Such complicated sequencing approaches are typically restricted to reference laboratories. A new addition to the laboratory armamentarium is matrix assisted laser desorption/ionisation time-of-flight (MALDI-TOF) mass spectrometry. After breaking open the cell wall, this technique ionises the mostly ribosomal proteins and analyses their content by TOF mass spectrometry and comparison to mass spectra of NTM species in its database [11]. This technique has the potential to spread accurate NTM identification to laboratories that previously did not have good access to molecular tools, although the methodology and databases for comparisons are still in development [11].

https://doi.org/10.1183/2312508X.10022717

Drug susceptibility testing

DST of NTM started off as the main means to distinguish them from MTBC bacteria [12]. The observation that an often complete lack of susceptibility to first-line anti-TB drugs could not predict which patient would respond to treatment with combinations of these drugs fed the myth that *in vitro* susceptibility of NTM had no relation to *in vivo* outcomes of treatment [13]. Recent studies have proven that for macrolides and aminoglycoside antibiotics (primarily amikacin) there is a clear correlation between *in vitro* activity and *in vivo* outcomes of treatment, at least for MAC and *M. abscessus* disease [12].

When the macrolides were introduced into treatment regimens for MAC pulmonary disease (MAC-PD), it was observed that macrolide resistance was clearly associated with failure of macrolide-based treatment regimens for MAC-PD. In the landmark single-arm trial performed by TANAKA *et al.* [14], the culture conversion rate after 6 months of treatment with rifampicin, ethambutol, clarithromycin and initial kanamycin was 77% (24 out of 31) among patients with clarithromycin-susceptible isolates *versus* only 17% (one out of six) for those whose baseline isolates were already clarithromycin resistant after prior exposure. The clinical utility of amikacin susceptibility testing in MAC-PD was proven recently, first in a small retrospective study [15] and later in a clinical trial of amikacin liposomal inhalation solution (ALIS), in which no patient with an amikacin-resistant baseline isolate (MIC >64 mg·L^{-1}) attained culture conversion on treatment with ALIS-containing regimens [16].

Fewer data are available for *M. abscessus*, but again susceptibility to amikacin and macrolides seems to correlate with treatment outcomes with these agents as part of multidrug therapies [12]. Most strikingly, treatment outcomes of standardised macrolide-based regimens are poorer for patients with disease caused by *M. abscessus* subsp. *abscessus* or subsp. *bolletii*, with their erythromycin resistance methylase (*erm(41)*) gene-mediated inducible macrolide resistance, than for patients with disease caused by *M. abscessus* subsp. *massiliense*, in which the *erm(41)* gene is typically nonfunctional because of a large deletion. In Japan, prolonged culture conversion rates of macrolide-based regimens were 50% (11 out of 22) for patients with *M. abscessus* subsp. *massiliense* disease *versus* only 24% (17 out of 72) for those with disease caused by *M. abscessus* subsp. *abscessus* [17]. A similar study in South Korea showed culture conversion rates of 88% (*M. abscessus* subsp. *massiliense*) and 25% (*M. abscessus* subsp. *abscessus*) [18].

For *M. kansasii*, the rare occurrence of therapy failure has been linked to nonadherence and the emergence of rifampicin resistance conferred by mutations in the β subunit of RNA polymerase (*rpoB*) gene identical to those seen in rifampicin-resistant *M. tuberculosis* [12].

The *in vitro–in vivo* correlations are clear for macrolides and amikacin for MAC and *M. abscessus*, and for rifampicin for *M. kansasii*. DST to these drugs for these NTM species is thus helpful for regimen design. For other drugs and other NTM species, such correlations are less obvious or have not been studied.

Epidemiology of nontuberculous mycobacteria pulmonary disease

In the last two decades, a rise in incidence and prevalence of NTM-PD has been recorded in many settings, particularly where there is a medium to low incidence of TB [19]. The incidence and prevalence of NTM-PD in Europe appear to be lower than those measured in studies in North America, East Asia and Australia, although methodological differences hamper direct comparisons. In Oregon, USA, the incidence of NTM-PD increased from 4.8 per 100 000 per year in 2007 to 5.6 per 100 000 per year in 2012 [20]. In Japan, in 2008, an incidence of 5.7 per 100 000 per year was recorded [21], where later studies reported incidences up to 11.0 per 100 000 per year [22]. In Queensland, Australia, where NTM-PD is a notifiable disease, the incidence was 3.2 per 100 000 per year in 2005 [23]. In contrast, older studies in the Netherlands, Denmark and Croatia reported incidences of 1.8, 1.08 and 0.61 per 100 000 per year, respectively [24–26]. More recently, in Germany, an incidence rate of 2.6 per 100 000 insured persons was measured over 2010 and 2011 [27]. The reasons for the lower incidences in Europe are not completely understood; host factors, differences in health systems and diagnostic practices as well as environmental exposure likely play a role [19].

Even within countries or otherwise defined geographical areas, large differences in NTM-PD incidence can exist. In the USA, geospatial analyses revealed hotspots of NTM-PD, characterised by high population densities, large bodies of surface water and high evapotranspiration rates [28]. Focusing on hotspot areas can teach us more about modes of NTM exposure and transmission. Two interesting recent examples come from the state of Colorado in the USA and Croatia. In Colorado, a geospatial epidemiological analysis showed that cases of NTM-PD tended to cluster in two watershed areas, one rural and one urban, where the relative risk of developing NTM-PD was, respectively, ~12- and ~4-fold higher than the average risk in the whole area. The water from those two watershed areas may be an important source of NTM exposure [29]. In Croatia, too, a link between water systems and the incidence of NTM-PD was noted. In a national surveillance study in 2006–2010, the estimated annual incidence of NTM-PD was 0.23 per 100 000 population, but differed between the rural, less populated and often well-water-reliant continental region (0.17 per 100 000) and the more populous, urbanised and water-systems-reliant coastal region (0.35 per 100 000); in the latter, MAC and *M. xenopi* isolation rates were higher, driving the higher disease incidence [30].

Who gets nontuberculous mycobacteria pulmonary disease?

Risk factors

The reason why individual patients get NTM-PD often remains elusive. Environmental sources are often quoted, but rarely proven, to be the source of NTM causing NTM-PD. A case–control study in Japan revealed that MAC-PD patients had significantly more soil exposure than noninfected controls [31]. Occupational exposure to soil had previously also been linked to *M. avium* infection measured by skin test sensitisation [32]. A later case–control study in the USA did not find any associations between NTM-PD and aerosol exposures from either soil or water [33]. While soil may be a source according to case–control studies, a few cases of MAC-PD have actually been linked to home water sources by environmental sampling and bacterial genotyping. One study in the USA was able to link MAC isolates of seven out of a cohort of 37 patients to MAC isolated from their home plumbing [34]; one study in Japan found the causative MAC bacteria of two out of a cohort of 49 patients in their home bath tubs [35].

Host factors associated with NTM-PD include older age (>65 years old), female sex and chronic lung diseases, including COPD and bronchiectasis [36, 37]. The risk of NTM-PD

https://doi.org/10.1183/2312508X.10022717

in COPD patients is greatly increased if these patients use inhaled steroids [37]. Rheumatoid arthritis has also been shown to increase the risk of NTM-PD, but this is likely due to immunosuppressive mediation [38].

Immunology

Genetic mutations associated with increased host susceptibility to NTM-PD have been identified, and include mutations in the α_1-antitrypsin (*AAT*), cystic fibrosis transmembrane conductance regulator (*CFTR*) and natural resistance-associated macrophage protein 1 (*NRAMP1*) genes, as well as a mutation in the major histocompatibility complex class I chain-related A (*MICA*) gene [36, 39–44]. No associations have been found between mutations in the genes encoding IFN-γ or interleukin (IL)-12 receptors or human leukocyte antigen molecules and NTM-PD in adult patients [40–43]. The roles of Toll-like receptor 2 and vitamin D remain controversial [45–50]. Recently, PFEFFER *et al.* [51] found that patients with NTM-PD had higher levels of eosinophilia and total IgE than TB patients, and HALSTROM *et al.* [52] observed a high frequency of mutations in the *IL10* gene and increased IL-10 production by blood leukocytes of NTM-PD patients. While disseminated NTM disease is strongly linked to HIV/AIDS, that association is less strong for NTM-PD. In a large cohort study, NTM-PD as a prominent NTM manifestation was present in 2.5% of 200 AIDS patients with disseminated MAC infection [53].

Host immunity to mycobacteria may also be impaired by iatrogenic factors, *i.e.* immunosuppressive treatments. This pertains to steroids as well as to the so-called "biologicals", in particular tumour necrosis factor (TNF)-α antagonists [54]. NTM disease is more frequent than TB as a complication of TNF-α antagonist therapy [55], in part because there is no latent infection and no screening tool for subclinical infection. Other classes of "biologicals" have now become available, including human IL-1 receptor antagonists (anakinra), CD20+ B-cell antibodies (rituximab), IL-12 and IL-23 antagonists (ustekinumab), and CD4+ T-cell costimulation modulators (abatacept). Of these, only CD20+ B-cell antibody use has been associated with NTM disease [54, 55].

Taking all this into consideration, NTM-PD is now thought of as a sign of a multigene, multisystem disorder that can combine genetic traits related to subtle immunodeficiencies related to the IFN-γ/IL-12 axis, *CFTR* gene variants, airway cilia dysfunction and connective tissue diseases [56, 57]. These genetic traits, alone or in combination, may increase the susceptibility to NTM-PD, after environmental NTM exposure. If the exact contributions of these susceptibility traits become better established, this may open up important new inroads for host-directed therapies.

Clinical manifestations of nontuberculous mycobacteria pulmonary disease

Fibro-cavitary disease

Fibro-cavitary NTM-PD is a severe, slowly progressive disease that primarily affects patients with underlying pulmonary diseases, particularly COPD. As a result, patients are often males and the disease manifests in those 55–75 years old. Cavities can be thin or thick walled and typically form in the upper lobes (figure 1a). Aside from the upper lobe cavities, there are often nodular lesions and signs of bronchiolitis in other lobes; bronchiectasis may

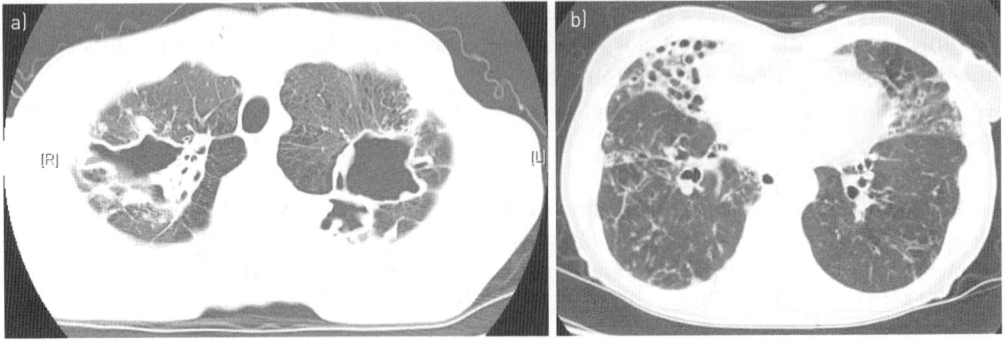

Figure 1. Computed tomography images of NTM pulmonary disease due to *Mycobacterium intracellulare*: a) fibro-cavitary disease and b) nodular/bronchiectatic disease.

be present but also be related to underlying lung disease [58]. The bacterial load is mostly high, so the sensitivity of smear and culture to diagnose this manifestation is high [8]. Untreated, this disease manifestation is progressive; its complications include haemoptysis or pulmonary haemorrhage, pneumothorax and empyema [5].

Nodular/bronchiectatic disease

Nodular/bronchiectatic NTM-PD is a milder but also progressive disease that affects patients whose pulmonary history can be otherwise unremarkable. The classic "Lady Windermere syndrome" is a nodular/bronchiectatic disease primarily affecting the lingula and middle lobe in older (>60 years old) females and, less frequently, males [4]. The dominant radiological features are nodular lesions, bronchiectasis and so-called "tree-in-bud" lesions of bronchiolitis (figure 1b). Some patients have a distinct habitus, being tall and slender with chest wall deformities and sometimes other signs compatible with connective tissue disorders, including mitral valve prolapse [4, 36, 57]. Untreated, this NTM-PD manifestation is slowly progressive; its complications include the formation of cavitary lesions which may be cystic bronchiectasis or nodules with a necrotic core [5].

Hypersensitivity pneumonitis

NTM hypersensitivity pneumonitis is mostly caused by MAC bacteria or, specifically in metalworkers, by *Mycobacterium immunogenum*. It is a subacute disease that develops in immediate response to exposure to aerosols with the causative bacteria. Hot tubs and Jacuzzis are the best known sources of exposure, particularly when used indoors. The hypersensitivity pneumonitis caused by *M. immunogenum* in metalworkers results from exposure to aerosols of metalworking fluid containing the NTM. Dyspnoea and fever are the most prominent symptoms. Radiologically, small nodules and ground-glass opacities can be seen in all lobes. Treatment is primarily by blocking exposure; in severe cases, steroids or antimycobacterial treatment may be indicated [5].

Other manifestations

In addition to fibro-cavitary and nodular/bronchiectatic disease (or mixed forms with features of both), two more rare NTM-PD manifestations exist: indolent single-lesion disease

https://doi.org/10.1183/2312508X.10022717

and aggressive infiltrative disease. Single-lesion NTM-PD consists of a single nodular lesion, mimicking pulmonary malignancy. This disease is often diagnosed by biopsies or after surgical resection. Its course is very slow and indolent; its diagnosis is often accidental [5]. It is not known whether antimycobacterial treatment after surgical resection is necessary.

The infiltrate form of NTM-PD was described by ANDRÉJAK *et al.* [59] as a rapidly progressive and very-hard-to-treat manifestation of *M. xenopi* disease. Radiologically, it is characterised by dense airspace opacities ("infiltrates") in all lobes. Its prognosis was very poor. No further reports of this manifestation exist.

Clinical relevance and diagnostic criteria

As NTM are environmental organisms, humans are likely exposed to NTM on a daily basis. The human airways are thus occasionally contaminated with NTM and this aspect implies that a single positive culture from a sample of a nonsterile body such as the human airways is insufficient to diagnose NTM disease.

The American Thoracic Society (ATS) and Infectious Diseases Society of America (IDSA) have issued statements including a set of criteria to differentiate chance NTM isolation from true NTM-PD, summarised in table 1 [5]. To diagnose NTM-PD, clinical, radiological and microbiological evidence of disease should be gathered. Symptoms are generally nonspecific, in part owing to frequent underlying pulmonary diseases. Radiological abnormalities are more specific, but the most compelling criterion to diagnose NTM-PD is

Table 1. Summary of the American Thoracic Society (ATS)/Infectious Diseases Society of America (IDSA) diagnostic criteria for NTM pulmonary disease

Clinical (all three criteria need to be fulfilled)
1   Pulmonary symptoms
2   Nodular or cavitary opacities on chest radiograph, or a high-resolution computed tomography scan that shows multifocal bronchiectasis with multiple small nodules
3   Appropriate exclusion of other diagnoses
Microbiological
1   Positive culture results from at least two separate expectorated sputum samples (if the results from the initial sputum samples are nondiagnostic, consider repeat sputum AFB smears and cultures)
    or
2   Positive culture results from at least one bronchial wash or lavage
    or
3   Transbronchial or other lung biopsy with mycobacterial histopathological features (granulomatous inflammation or AFB) and positive culture for NTM or biopsy showing mycobacterial histopathological features (granulomatous inflammation or AFB) and one or more sputum or bronchial washings that are culture positive for NTM

AFB: acid-fast bacilli. At least three consecutive respiratory samples are needed to apply these criteria. Expert consultation should be obtained when NTM are recovered that are either infrequently encountered or that usually represent environmental contamination. Patients who are suspected of having NTM lung disease but who do not meet the diagnostic criteria should be followed until the diagnosis is firmly established or excluded. Making the diagnosis of NTM lung disease does not *per se* necessitate the institution of therapy, which is a decision based on potential risks and benefits of therapy for individual patients. Information from [5].

the microbiological criterion of multiple positive cultures with the same species. This last criterion was based on the finding by TSUKAMURA [60] in Japan that pulmonary disease (infiltrates or cavitary lesions) progressed in 98% of the patients who had two or more positive sputum cultures for MAC *versus* just 2% in those with a single positive culture during 12 months of observation. For 97% of patients, the first two positive cultures grew from the initial three sputum specimens. Those latter findings are less applicable to the nodular/bronchiectatic type of NTM-PB, because these patients can have less or no sputum production. Bronchoalveolar lavage (BAL) is likely to be more sensitive than sputum culture to diagnose nodular/bronchiectatic NTM-PD [61]. In a small study of 26 patients with suspected nodular/bronchiectatic MAC-PD, BAL yielded positive cultures in 13 *versus* only six by sputum cultures [62]. In nodular/bronchiectatic NTM-PD patients who do not produce sputum, a single positive culture from BAL, preferably with histological evidence of mycobacterial disease, may be used to diagnose NTM-PD. This is incorporated in the most recent statement by the ATS/IDSA (table 1) [5]. It needs to be stressed that a diagnosis of NTM-PD from a single positive BAL culture is only appropriate in patients who cannot produce additional respiratory samples. Isolation of rare species, or species generally considered nonpathogenic (*e.g. Mycobacterium gordonae, Mycobacterium terrae* and *Mycobacterium phlei*) in this setting, may warrant a conservative approach and repeat bronchoscopy where possible.

Of all NTM cultured from pulmonary samples, *M. kansasii, Mycobacterium szulgai* and *M. malmoense* (in northwestern Europe) have been most strongly associated with true NTM-PD (figure 2) [24, 26, 30, 63, 64]. Solitary isolates of these species from pulmonary samples in patients with no additional evidence of NTM-PD are very rare [5, 24, 26, 30, 63, 64]. On the contrary, isolation of *M. gordonae*, or to a lesser extent *M. chelonae* and *Mycobacterium simiae*, is rarely associated with clinical disease [5, 24, 26, 30, 63, 64]. For these species, solitary isolates from pulmonary samples without additional evidence of NTM-PD are the rule rather than the exception. MAC and *M. xenopi* seem to form an intermediate category, as 40–70% of all isolates are considered clinically relevant in different studies [5, 24, 26, 30, 63, 64]. To prevent unwarranted diagnoses and treatment of NTM disease as well as unnecessary diagnostic delay, it would be helpful to use separate, more stringent criteria for species of low clinical relevance and less stringent criteria for species of high clinical relevance [24, 26]. Clinical relevance of NTM species may differ strongly between regions or countries (figure 2); local studies are thus required to assign species to low/high clinical relevance groups.

Treatment of nontuberculous mycobacteria pulmonary disease

Antibiotic treatment

The multidrug antibiotic treatment of NTM-PD is long, cumbersome and poorly tolerated. The goal of therapy is 12 months of sputum culture negativity while on therapy. Recommended treatment regimens for the most extensively studied NTM respiratory pathogens are listed in table 2.

There are major knowledge gaps regarding these multidrug regimens. The regimen now recommended for MAC-PD applies rifampicin and ethambutol, which are both inactive *in vitro* against MAC. In a clinical trial, a regimen of just these two drugs yielded a long-term culture conversion rate of only 27% [13]. Once the *in vitro* active macrolides were added to

https://doi.org/10.1183/2312508X.10022717

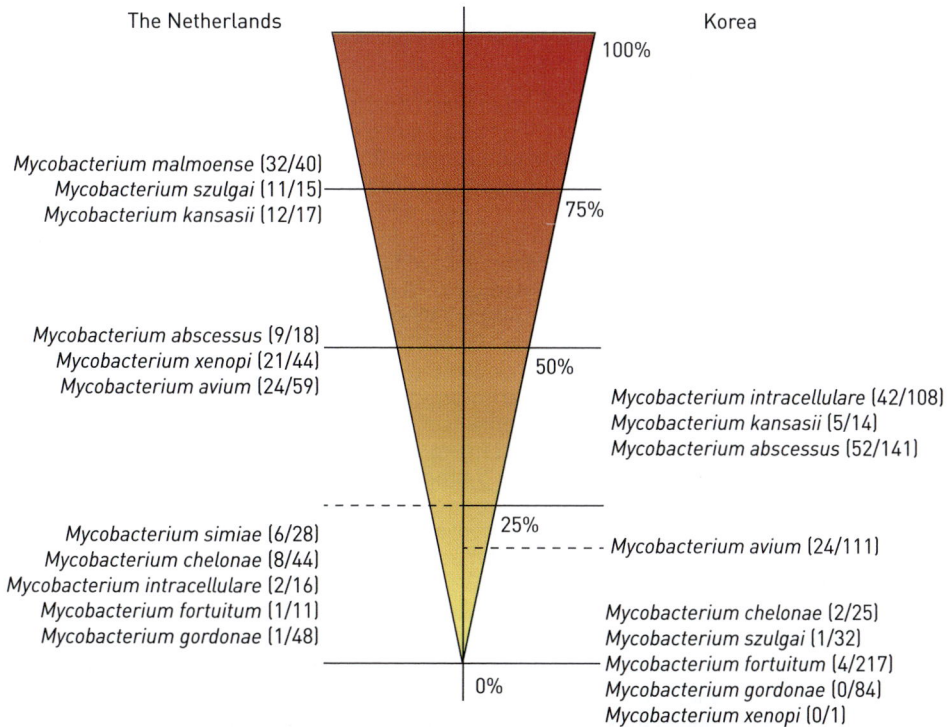

Figure 2. Clinical relevance of NTM species isolated from pulmonary specimens in two countries: the Netherlands and Korea. Clinical relevance is calculated as the percentage of patients with a pulmonary isolate of the respective species that meets American Thoracic Society (ATS)/Infectious Diseases Society of America (IDSA) diagnostic criteria for NTM pulmonary disease (table 1). Dotted lines represent the mean of all species. Data from [63, 64].

rifampicin and ethambutol, this three-drug regimen proved moderately effective, yielding culture conversion rates from 50% (for fibro-cavitary disease) to 85% (for nodular/bronchiectatic disease) [58, 66]. The *in vitro* inactive rifampicin and ethambutol are both needed, however, to prevent the emergence of macrolide resistance [67]. In severe disease, intravenous amikacin is added to the regimen in the first 3 months [5]; this is based on an RCT in which the addition of streptomycin to the rifampicin–ethambutol–clarithromycin regimen led to faster culture conversion but not to improved long-term clinical outcomes [68]. In mild nodular/bronchiectatic disease, the rifampicin–ethambutol–clarithromycin regimen can be given 3 times weekly [66].

Very few alternative regimens for MAC-PD have been studied. A large retrospective study in Canada showed that regimens featuring clofazimine instead of rifampicin yielded outcomes comparable to the rifampicin–ethambutol–macrolide regimen, at least in patients with nodular/bronchiectatic disease [69]. A regimen of clofazimine–minocycline–clarithromycin has also been tried in a small study in France and showed a culture conversion rate of 63% (14 out of 22 patients) [70]. Very recently, clinical trials have shown that adding ALIS to MAC-PD regimens in patients who had experienced treatment failure increased the rate of culture conversion [16]. Its role in primary treatment remains to be investigated.

The regimen for MAC-PD is also commonly used for NTM-PD caused by rarer, slow-growing species such as *M. malmoense*, *M. szulgai* and *Mycobacterium celatum* [71],

Table 2. Recommended treatment regimens for the most common NTM species

***Mycobacterium avium* complex**	Daily therapy[#]: rifampicin 10 mg·kg^{-1} or rifabutin 150–300 mg, with ethambutol 15 mg·kg^{-1} once daily and clarithromycin 500 mg 2 times daily/azithromycin 250–500 mg once daily Intermittent therapy[¶]: 3 times weekly rifampicin 10 mg·kg^{-1}, with ethambutol 25 mg·kg^{-1} and clarithromycin 1000 mg or azithromycin 500 mg Treatment is continued for 12 months after culture conversion
Mycobacterium kansasii	Daily therapy: rifampicin 10 mg·kg^{-1}, with ethambutol 15 mg·kg^{-1} and either isoniazid 300 mg or clarithromycin 500 mg 2 times daily or azithromycin 500 mg once daily Treatment is continued for 12 months after culture conversion
Mycobacterium abscessus	Daily therapy: clarithromycin 500 mg 2 times daily/azithromycin 250 mg[+], with amikacin 15 mg·kg^{-1} (daily to 3 times weekly) and cefoxitin (up to 12 g·kg^{-1} in multiple doses) or imipenem (500–1000 mg 2–3 times daily) and/or tigecycline (50 mg 2 times daily) Prolonged culture conversion may not be attainable; oral holding regimens (sometimes with inhaled amikacin) or periodic treatment may be warranted

[#]: amikacin should be considered for patients with cavitary disease and/or macrolide resistance; [¶]: intermittent therapy may be used for noncavitary disease; [+]: the role of macrolides for *M. abscessus* isolates with functional erythromycin resistance methylase *erm(41)* genes is controversial; they can be added to regimens but not counted as active drugs. Information from [5, 65].

but has also been successfully used in *M. kansasii* disease [72]. This regimen is also used for *M. xenopi*, although moxifloxacin is often added to this regimen or used instead of a macrolide. The outcome of antibiotic treatment of *M. xenopi* is often very poor, with very high on-treatment mortality rates; this lack of response is not completely understood [59, 71]. For some NTM species, notoriously for the extensively drug-resistant *M. simiae*, no antibiotic regimen has proven effective [5, 71].

Treatment of *M. abscessus* disease is extremely complicated and yields very poor outcomes, with culture conversion rates ranging from 30% to 50% [5, 16–18, 71, 73]. The drugs typically used in the initial phase, *i.e.* amikacin, cefoxitin or imipenem and tigecycline, all have *in vitro* activity. Their use is limited by toxicity and practical burdens of long-term *i.v.* treatments [71, 73, 74]. The oral continuation-phase treatment, according to guidelines, employs three to five drugs, including macrolides, tetracyclines, fluoroquinolones, linezolid, clofazimine and inhaled amikacin [5, 73–75]. The role of the fluoroquinolones, tetracyclines and linezolid is questionable as they are inactive *in vitro* against *M. abscessus* even in combination [65, 76]. The contributions of inhaled amikacin and oral clofazimine have never been tested in clinical trials; both are active alone and may be synergistic in combination [77]. New oral drugs for this continuation phase of *M. abscessus* treatment are urgently needed.

The role of the macrolides in *M. abscessus* treatment has become the subject of debate [74, 75]. We now know that *M. abscessus* has three distinct subspecies: *M. abscessus* subsp. *abscessus*, subsp. *bolletii* and subsp. *massiliense*. The latter is susceptible to macrolides, because of a deletion in the *erm(41)* gene [12]. Macrolide-based treatment regimens achieve higher culture conversion rates in patients with NTM-PD caused by *M. abscessus* subsp.

https://doi.org/10.1183/2312508X.10022717

massiliense (50–80%) than in those whose disease is caused by *M. abscessus* subsp. *abscessus* or subsp. *bolletii* (25%) [17, 18].

Even with the use of guideline-recommended treatment regimens, treatment outcomes are suboptimal. Outcomes differ widely between species and between disease manifestations. In general, microbiological outcomes (*i.e.* prolonged culture conversion) are better for nodular/bronchiectatic disease than for fibro-cavitary disease [58, 71]. Microbiological outcomes are better for disease caused by MAC bacteria (60–70% culture conversion) than for *M. abscessus* (40–50% culture conversion) or *M. xenopi* (20–50% culture conversion) [58, 59, 66, 71–73]. However, these outcomes are all reported by reference centres and mostly on the basis of guideline-compliant therapies. Recent studies in the USA, Europe and Japan have shown that very few patients with NTM-PD actually receive guideline-compliant therapies [78, 79], and their outcomes might be even worse.

Surgery

Surgical resection of NTM-infected segments or lobes is an important and probably underused treatment modality. Various cases series, including series of the difficult-to-treat *M. abscessus*, have shown that patients who are treated with antibiotics and surgery typically have better outcomes than those treated with antibiotics alone [66, 73]. Of course, surgery is only feasible in patients whose pulmonary function and health status allows for surgical resection of the affected areas of the lungs. To minimise the chance of surgical complications, surgery should be performed in expert centres by experienced surgeons and only if adequate post-surgical treatment can be offered [80].

Supportive treatments

A number of supportive treatments exist for patients with NTM-PD. Most of them are aimed at improving airway clearance, and include flutter devices, oscillating vests and the inhalation of hypertonic saline. While these treatments may be beneficial, they have not been properly investigated in NTM-PD patients [5, 75].

A special case: nontuberculous mycobacteria pulmonary disease in patients with cystic fibrosis

Patients with CF have long been known to have a high NTM isolation prevalence. In CF patients, MAC and *M. abscessus* are the two most frequently isolated organisms, and both are strongly associated with NTM-PD [81]. In most studies in the USA, MAC is the predominant NTM isolated from CF patients, whereas in most European studies, *M. abscessus* predominates [81]. Also, where MAC isolation in European CF patients is a late event, occurring in the second and third decades of life, *M. abscessus* isolation can occur at all ages [82]. Isolation of *M. abscessus* seems to be associated with a more severe clinical course of CF, particularly of lung involvement [82].

Risk factors for NTM isolation and disease in CF patients have been studied, but these studies have yielded conflicting results [83]. Importantly, whether macrolide maintenance therapy is a risk factor for, or protects against, NTM-PD in CF patients remains controversial [84].

The most striking feature of *M. abscessus* disease in CF patients, apart from its severity and very poor response to treatment, is the observation of disease transmission between CF patients [85, 86]. The transmission route is most likely indirect, *e.g. via* fomites, but it is clear that in select settings *M. abscessus* disease can be transmitted between CF patients by aerosol [85, 86]. Moreover, transmissible strains of *M. abscessus* also show increased resistance to antimycobacterial drugs and an increase in virulence [86]. This realisation that *M. abscessus* disease is transmissible between CF patients, although still under debate [87], has caused a stir in the CF community. Infection control policies are now under evaluation.

Conclusion

NTM-PD is now finally positioned as a chronic, difficult-to-treat pulmonary infection that all pulmonologists are likely to encounter in their clinical practice. Its many challenges, ranging from its unknown sources of infection, poor response to treatment and high recurrence rates, make this disease (or better, these diseases) very difficult to manage for all involved. Nearly 70 years after their initial description as pulmonary pathogens, the outlook for affected patients has certainly improved, but is nowhere near where it should be. Improved antibiotic treatment regimens, better identification of patients at risk and increased compliance with published guidelines are crucial next steps.

References

1. Buhler VB, Pollak A. Human infection with atypical acid-fast organisms; report of two cases with pathologic findings. *Am J Clin Pathol* 1953; 23: 363–374.
2. Manten A. Antimicrobial susceptibility and some other properties of photochromogenic mycobacteria associated with pulmonary disease. *Antonie van Leeuwenhoek* 1957; 23: 357–363.
3. Wolinsky E. Nontuberculous mycobacteria and associated diseases. *Am Rev Respir Dis* 1979; 119: 107–159.
4. Reich JM, Johnson RE. *Mycobacterium avium* complex pulmonary disease presenting as an isolated lingular or middle lobe pattern. The Lady Windermere syndrome. *Chest* 1992; 101: 1605–1609.
5. Griffith DE, Aksamit T, Brown-Elliot BA, *et al.* An official ATS/IDSA statement: diagnosis, treatment, and prevention of nontuberculous mycobacterial diseases. *Am J Respir Crit Care Med* 2007; 175: 367–416.
6. Migliori GB, Bothamley G, Duarte R, Rendon A, eds. Tuberculosis. Sheffield, European Respiratory Society, 2018.
7. Wright PW, Wallace RJ Jr, Wright NW, *et al.* Sensitivity of fluorochrome microscopy for detection of *Mycobacterium tuberculosis* versus nontuberculous mycobacteria. *J Clin Microbiol* 1998; 36: 1046–1049.
8. van Ingen J. Microbiological diagnosis of pulmonary disease caused by nontuberculous mycobacteria. *Clin Chest Med* 2015; 36: 43–54.
9. Katila ML, Mattila J, Brander E. Enhancement of growth of *Mycobacterium malmoense* by acidic pH and pyruvate. *Eur J Clin Microbiol Infect Dis* 1989; 8: 998–1000.
10. Realini L, de Ridder K, Hirschel B, *et al.* Blood and charcoal added to acidified agar media promote the growth of *Mycobacterium genavense*. *Diagn Microbiol Infect Dis* 1999; 34: 45–50.
11. Alcaide F, Amlerová J, Bou G, *et al.* How-to: identify non-tuberculous *Mycobacterium* species by using MALDI-TOF mass spectrometry. *Clin Microbiol Infect* 2018; 24: 599–603.
12. van Ingen J, Kuijper EJ. Drug susceptibility testing of nontuberculous mycobacteria. *Future Microbiol* 2014; 9: 1095–1110.
13. Research Committee of the British Thoracic Society. First randomised trial of treatments for pulmonary disease caused by *M. avium intracellulare*, *M. malmoense*, and *M. xenopi* in HIV negative patients: rifampicin, ethambutol and isoniazid versus rifampicin and ethambutol. *Thorax* 2001; 56: 167–172.
14. Tanaka E, Kimoto T, Tsuyuguchi K, *et al.* Effect of clarithromycin regimen for *Mycobacterium avium* complex pulmonary disease. *Am J Respir Crit Care Med* 1999; 160: 866–872.
15. Brown-Elliott BA, Iakhiaeva E, Griffith DE, *et al.* In vitro activity of amikacin against isolates of *Mycobacterium avium* complex with proposed MIC breakpoints and finding of a 16S rRNA gene mutation in treated isolates. *J Clin Microbiol* 2013; 51: 3389–3394.
16. Olivier KN, Griffith DE, Eagle G, *et al.* Randomized trial of liposomal amikacin for inhalation in nontuberculous mycobacterial lung disease. *Am J Respir Crit Care Med* 2017; 195: 814–823.
17. Harada T, Akiyama Y, Kurashima A, *et al.* Clinical and microbiological differences between *Mycobacterium abscessus* and *Mycobacterium massiliense* lung diseases. *J Clin Microbiol* 2012; 50: 3556–3561.

 https://doi.org/10.1183/2312508X.10022717

18. Koh WJ, Jeon K, Lee NY, *et al*. Clinical significance of differentiation of *Mycobacterium massiliense* from *Mycobacterium abscessus*. *Am J Respir Crit Care Med* 2011; 183: 405–410.

19. Prevots DR, Marras TK. Epidemiology of human pulmonary infection with non-tuberculous mycobacteria: a review. *Clin Chest Med* 2015; 36: 13–34.

20. Henkle E, Hedberg K, Schafer S, *et al*. Population-based incidence of pulmonary nontuberculous mycobacterial disease in Oregon 2007 to 2012. *Ann Am Thorac Soc* 2015; 12: 642–647.

21. Morimoto K, Iwai K, Uchimura K, *et al*. A steady increase in nontuberculous mycobacteriosis mortality and estimated prevalence in Japan. *Ann Am Thorac Soc* 2014; 11: 1–8.

22. Ide S, Nakamura S, Yamamoto Y, *et al*. Epidemiology and clinical features of pulmonary nontuberculous mycobacteriosis in Nagasaki, Japan. *PLoS One* 2015; 10: e0128304.

23. Thomson RM. Changing epidemiology of pulmonary nontuberculous mycobacteria infections. *Emerg Infect Dis* 2010; 10: 1576–1583.

24. van Ingen J, Bendien SA, de Lange WCM, *et al*. Clinical relevance of nontuberculous mycobacteria isolated in the Nijmegen-Arnhem region, the Netherlands. *Thorax* 2009; 64: 502–506.

25. Andréjak C, Thomsen VØ, Johansen IS, *et al*. Nontuberculous pulmonary mycobacteriosis in Denmark: incidence and prognostic factors. *Am J Respir Crit Care Med* 2010; 181: 514–521.

26. Jankovic M, Sabol I, Zmak L, *et al*. Microbiologic criteria in nontuberculous mycobacterial pulmonary disease, a tool for diagnosis and epidemiology. *Int J Tuberc Lung Dis* 2016; 20: 934–940.

27. Diel R, Jacob J, Lampenius N, *et al*. Burden of non-tuberculous mycobacterial pulmonary disease in Germany. *Eur Respir J* 2017; 49: 1602109.

28. Adjemian J, Olivier KN, Seitz AE, *et al*. Spatial clusters of nontuberculous mycobacterial lung disease in the United States. *Am J Respir Crit Care Med* 2012; 186: 553–558.

29. Lipner EM, Knox D, French J, *et al*. A geospatial epidemiologic analysis of nontuberculous mycobacterial infection: an ecological study in Colorado. *Ann Am Thor Soc* 2017; 14: 1523–1532.

30. Jankovic M, Samarzija M, Sabol I, *et al*. Geographical distribution and clinical relevance of non-tuberculous mycobacteria in Croatia. *Int J Tuberc Lung Dis* 2013; 17: 836–841.

31. Maekawa K, Ito Y, Hirai T, *et al*. Environmental risk factors for pulmonary *Mycobacterium avium-intracellulare* complex disease. *Chest* 2011; 140: 723–729.

32. Reed C, von Reyn CF, Chamblee S, *et al*. Environmental risk factors for infection with *Mycobacterium avium* complex. *Am J Epidemiol* 2006; 164: 32–40.

33. Dirac MA, Horan KL, Doody DR, *et al*. Environment or host? A case–control study of risk factors for *Mycobacterium avium* complex lung disease. *Am J Respir Crit Care Med* 2012; 186: 684–691.

34. Falkinham JO 3rd. Nontuberculous mycobacteria from household plumbing of patients with nontuberculous mycobacteria disease. *Emerg Infect Dis* 2011; 17: 419–424.

35. Nishiuchi Y, Maekura R, Kitada S, *et al*. The recovery of *Mycobacterium avium–intracellulare* complex (MAC) from the residential bathrooms of patients with pulmonary MAC. *Clin Infect Dis* 2007; 45: 347–351.

36. Kim RD, Greenberg DE, Ehrmantraut ME, *et al*. Pulmonary nontuberculous mycobacterial disease: prospective study of a distinct preexisting syndrome. *Am J Respir Crit Care Med* 2008; 178: 1066–1074.

37. Andréjak C, Nielsen R, Thomsen VØ, *et al*. Chronic respiratory disease, inhaled corticosteroids and risk of non-tuberculous mycobacteriosis. *Thorax* 2013; 68: 256–262.

38. Brode SK, Jamieson FB, Ng R, *et al*. Increased risk of mycobacterial infections associated with anti-rheumatic medications. *Thorax* 2015; 70: 677–682.

39. Chan ED, Kaminska AM, Gill W, *et al*. Alpha-1-antitrypsin (AAT) anomalies are associated with lung disease due to rapidly growing mycobacteria and AAT inhibits *Mycobacterium abscessus* infection of macrophages. *Scand J Infect Dis* 2007; 39: 690–696.

40. Hwang JH, Kim EJ, Koh WJ, *et al*. Polymorphisms of interferon-gamma and interferon-gamma receptor 1 genes and non-tuberculous mycobacterial lung diseases. *Tuberculosis* 2007; 87: 166–171.

41. Park HY, Kwon YS, Ki CS, *et al*. Interleukin-12 receptor β1 polymorphisms and nontuberculous mycobacterial lung diseases. *Lung* 2008; 186: 241–245.

42. Um SW, Ki CS, Kwon OJ, *et al*. HLA antigens and nontuberculous mycobacterial lung disease in Korean patients. *Lung* 2009; 187: 136–140.

43. Koh WJ, Kwon OJ, Kim EJ, *et al*. *NRAMP1* gene polymorphism and susceptibility to nontuberculous mycobacterial lung diseases. *Chest* 2005; 128: 94–101.

44. Shojima J, Tanaka G, Keicho N, *et al*. Identification of *MICA* as a susceptibility gene for pulmonary *Mycobacterium avium* complex infection. *J Infect Dis* 2009; 199: 1707–1715.

45. Ryu YJ, Kim EJ, Koh WJ, *et al*. Toll-like receptor 2 polymorphisms and nontuberculous mycobacterial lung diseases. *Clin Vaccine Immunol* 2006; 13: 818–819.

46. Yim JJ, Kim HJ, Kwon OJ, *et al*. Association between microsatellite polymorphisms in intron II of the human Toll-like receptor 2 gene and nontuberculous mycobacterial lung disease in a Korean population. *Hum Immunol* 2008; 69: 572–576.

47. Ryu YJ, Kim EJ, Lee SH, *et al.* Impaired expression of Toll-like receptor 2 in nontuberculous mycobacterial lung disease. *Eur Respir J* 2007; 30: 736–742.

48. Gelder CM, Hart KW, Williams OM, *et al.* Vitamin D receptor gene polymorphisms and susceptibility to *Mycobacterium malmoense* pulmonary disease. *J Infect Dis* 2000; 181: 2099–2102.

49. Park S, Kim EJ, Lee SH, *et al.* Vitamin D-receptor polymorphisms and non-tuberculous mycobacterial lung disease in Korean patients. *Int J Tuberc Lung Dis* 2008; 12: 698–700.

50. Jeon K, Kim SY, Jeong BH, *et al.* Severe vitamin D deficiency is associated with nontuberculous mycobacterial lung disease: a case-control study. *Respirology* 2013; 18: 983–988.

51. Pfeffer PE, Hopkins S, Cropley I, *et al.* An association between pulmonary *Mycobacterium avium-intracellulare* complex infections and biomarkers of Th2-type inflammation. *Respir Res* 2017; 18: 93.

52. Halstrom S, Thomson R, Goullee H, *et al.* Susceptibility to non-tuberculous mycobacterial disease is influenced by rs1518111 in *IL10*. *Hum Immunol* 2017; 78: 391–393.

53. Kalayjian RC, Toossi Z, Tomashefski JF Jr, *et al.* Pulmonary disease due to infection by *Mycobacterium avium* complex in patients with AIDS. *Clin Infect Dis* 1995; 20: 1186–1194.

54. van Ingen J, Boeree MJ, Dekhuijzen PNR, *et al.* Mycobacterial disease in patients with rheumatic disease. *Nat Clin Pract Rheumatol* 2008; 4: 649–656.

55. Winthrop KL, Yamashita S, Beekmann SE, *et al.* Mycobacterial and other serious infections in patients receiving anti-tumor necrosis factor and other newly approved biologic therapies: case finding through the Emerging Infections Network. *Clin Infect Dis* 2008; 46: 1738–1740.

56. Becker K, Arts P, Jaeger M, *et al.* *MST1R* mutation as a genetic cause of Lady Windermere syndrome. *Eur Respir J* 2017; 49: 1601478.

57. Szymanski EP, Leung JM, Fowler CJ, *et al.* Pulmonary nontuberculous mycobacterial infection. A multisystem, multigenic disease. *Am J Respir Crit Care Med* 2015; 192: 618–628.

58. Zweijpfenning S, Kops S, Magis-Escurra C, *et al.* Treatment and outcome of non-tuberculous mycobacterial pulmonary disease in a predominantly fibro-cavitary disease cohort. *Respir Med* 2017; 131: 220–224.

59. Andréjak C, Lescure FX, Pukenyte E, *et al.* *Mycobacterium xenopi* pulmonary infections: a multicentric retrospective study of 136 cases in north-east France. *Thorax* 2009; 64: 291–296.

60. Tsukamura M. Diagnosis of disease caused by *Mycobacterium avium* complex. *Chest* 1991; 99: 667–669.

61. Sugihara E, Hirota N, Niizeki T, *et al.* Usefulness of bronchial lavage for the diagnosis of pulmonary disease caused by *Mycobacterium avium–intracellulare* complex (MAC) infection. *J Infect Chemother* 2003; 9: 328–332.

62. Tanaka E, Amitani R, Niimi A, *et al.* Yield of computed tomography and bronchoscopy for the diagnosis of *Mycobacterium avium* complex pulmonary disease. *Am J Respir Crit Care Med* 1997; 155: 2041–2046.

63. van Ingen J, Boeree MJ, van Soolingen D, *et al.* Are phylogenetic position, virulence, drug susceptibility and in vivo response to treatment in mycobacteria interrelated? *Infect Gen Evol* 2012; 12: 832–837.

64. Koh WJ, Kwon OJ, Jeon K, *et al.* Clinical significance of nontuberculous mycobacteria isolated from respiratory specimens in Korea. *Chest* 2006; 129: 341–348.

65. Ferro BE, Srivastava S, Deshpande D, *et al.* Moxifloxacin's limited efficacy in the hollow-fiber model of *Mycobacterium abscessus* disease. *Antimicrob Agents Chemother* 2016; 60: 3779–3785.

66. Wallace RJ Jr, Brown-Elliott BA, McNulty S, *et al.* Macrolide/azalide therapy for nodular/bronchiectatic *Mycobacterium avium* complex lung disease. *Chest* 2014; 146: 276–282.

67. Griffith DE, Brown-Elliott BA, Langsjoen B, *et al.* Clinical and molecular analysis of macrolide resistance in *Mycobacterium avium* complex lung disease. *Am J Respir Crit Care Med* 2006; 174: 928–934.

68. Kobashi Y, Matsushima T, Oka M. A double-blind randomized study of aminoglycoside infusion with combined therapy for pulmonary *Mycobacterium avium* complex disease. *Respir Med* 2007; 101: 130–138.

69. Jarand J, Davis JP, Cowie RL, *et al.* Long-term follow-up of *Mycobacterium avium* complex lung disease in patients treated with regimens including clofazimine and/or rifampin. *Chest* 2016; 149: 1285–1293.

70. Roussel G, Igual J. Clarithromycin with minocycline and clofazimine for *Mycobacterium avium intracellulare* complex lung disease in patients without the acquired immune deficiency syndrome. *Int J Tuberc Lung Dis* 1998; 2: 462–470.

71. van Ingen J, Ferro BE, Hoefsloot W, *et al.* Drug treatment of pulmonary nontuberculous mycobacterial disease in HIV-negative patients: the evidence. *Expert Rev Anti Infect Ther* 2013; 11: 1065–1077.

72. Shitrit D, Baum GL, Priess R, *et al.* Pulmonary *Mycobacterium kansasii* infection in Israel, 1999–2004: clinical features, drug susceptibility, and outcome. *Chest* 2006; 129: 771–776.

73. Jarand J, Levin A, Zhang L, *et al.* Clinical and microbiologic outcomes in patients receiving treatment for *Mycobacterium abscessus* pulmonary disease. *Clin Infect Dis* 2011; 52: 565–571.

74. Ruth MM, van Ingen J. New insights in the treatment of nontuberculous mycobacterial pulmonary disease. *Future Microbiol* 2017; 12: 1109–1112.

75. Haworth CS, Banks J, Capstick T, *et al.* British Thoracic Society guidelines for the management of non-tuberculous mycobacterial pulmonary disease (NTM-PD). *Thorax* 2017; 72: ii1–ii64.

76. Ruth MM, Sangen JJN, Pennings LJ, *et al.* Minocycline has no clear role in the treatment of *Mycobacterium abscessus* disease. *Antimicrob Agents Chemother* 2018; 62: e01208.

https://doi.org/10.1183/2312508X.10022717

77. Ferro BE, Meletiadis J, Wattenberg M, *et al.* Clofazimine prevents the regrowth of *Mycobacterium abscessus* and *Mycobacterium avium* type strains exposed to amikacin and clarithromycin. *Antimicrob Agents Chemother* 2016; 60: 1097–1105.

78. Adjemian J, Prevots DR, Gallagher J, *et al.* Lack of adherence to evidence-based treatment guidelines for nontuberculous mycobacterial lung disease. *Ann Am Thorac Soc* 2014; 11: 9–16.

79. van Ingen J, Wagner D, Gallagher J, *et al.* Poor adherence to management guidelines in nontuberculous mycobacterial pulmonary diseases. *Eur Respir J* 2017; 49: 1601855.

80. Mitchell JD. Surgical management of pulmonary mycobacterial disease. *Semin Respir Crit Care Med* 2018; 39: 392–398.

81. Martiniano SL, Davidson RM, Nick JA. Nontuberculous mycobacteria in cystic fibrosis: updates and the path forward. *Pediatr Pulmonol* 2017; 52: S29–S36.

82. Catherinot E, Roux AL, Vibet MA, *et al. Mycobacterium avium* and *Mycobacterium abscessus* complex target distinct cystic fibrosis patient subpopulations. *J Cyst Fibros* 2013; 12: 74–80.

83. Coolen N, Morand P, Martin C, *et al.* Reduced risk of nontuberculous mycobacteria in cystic fibrosis adults receiving long-term azithromycin. *J Cyst Fibros* 2015; 14: 594–599.

84. Floto RA, Olivier KN, Saiman L, *et al.* US Cystic Fibrosis Foundation and European Cystic Fibrosis Society consensus recommendations for the management of non-tuberculous mycobacteria in individuals with cystic fibrosis. *Thorax* 2016; 71: 1–22.

85. Bryant JM, Grogono DM, Greaves D, *et al.* Whole-genome sequencing to identify transmission of *Mycobacterium abscessus* between patients with cystic fibrosis: a retrospective cohort study. *Lancet* 2013; 381: 1551–1560.

86. Bryant JM, Grogono DM, Rodriguez-Rincon D, *et al.* Emergence and spread of a human-transmissible multidrug-resistant nontuberculous mycobacterium. *Science* 2016; 354: 751–757.

87. Tortoli E, Kohl TA, Trovato A, *et al. Mycobacterium abscessus* in patients with cystic fibrosis: low impact of inter-human transmission in Italy. *Eur Respir J* 2017; 50: 1602525.

Disclosures: S. Zweijpfenning reports receiving personal fees (for unrelated research) from Insmed and Novartis, outside the submitted work. W. Hoefsloot reports receiving the following, outside the submitted work: an unrestricted study grant from Insmed for an investigator initiated trial on NTM; and nonfinancial support (free delivery of clofazimin) from Novartis for an investigator initiated trial on NTM. J. van Ingen reports receiving the following, outside the submitted work: a grant from Pfizer for an investigator initiatied research proposal on tigecycline. J. van Ingen has also received support from Insmed and Spero Therapeutics for advisory board membership.

Chapter 24

What next? Basic research, new treatments and a patient-centred approach

Graham Bothamley [1,2,3]

The End TB Strategy presents an ambitious target to reduce TB by 90% compared to 2015 levels over a 20-year period, ending in 2035. Already, there are developments that will revolutionise the diagnosis of TB and of drug resistance. Entirely new treatments for TB are on the horizon. Patient involvement, not only in near-patient tests but also in active case finding, data input for research and adherence, and TB support clubs will be crucial. For the longer term future, there are exciting developments in understanding the host and pathogen responses to each other, which will lead to important advances, provided clinical aspects of TB are not forgotten.

Cite as: Bothamley G. What next? Basic research, new treatments and a patient-centred approach. *In:* Migliori GB, Bothamley G, Duarte R, *et al.*, eds. Tuberculosis (ERS Monograph). Sheffield, European Respiratory Society, 2018; pp. 414–429 [https://doi.org/10.1183/2312508X.10026118].

@ERSpublications
The future of TB management lies in the interaction between basic research and clinical medicine. Molecular microbiology is redefining *Mycobacterium tuberculosis* while genes, RNA and proteomics are redefining the immune response in TB. The human element remains paramount in defeating TB. http://ow.ly/cfVQ30lqCfE

This chapter is designed to introduce the non-TB specialist to current TB research, provide starting points for TB specialists to contribute to clinically relevant studies and, as discussed elsewhere in this *Monograph* [1], to highlight some of the patient-related research that will improve the delivery of whatever treatments prove to be most effective. The End TB Strategy is aiming for a 90% reduction by 2035 in the incidence of TB compared to 2015, *i.e.* to $\leqslant$10 per 100 000 or less [2]. This chapter addresses areas where our understanding of TB will need to improve to begin to address this goal.

The scientific literature has shown an increase in articles related to TB from 1634 papers in 1981 to 7684 papers in 2016 (PubMed). Progress towards significant benefits for those with

[1]Homerton University Hospital, London, UK. [2]Blizard Institute, Barts and The London School of Medicine and Dentistry, Queen Mary University of London, London, UK. [3]London School of Hygiene and Tropical Medicine, London, UK.

Correspondence: Graham Bothamley, Dept of Respiratory Medicine, Homerton University Hospital, London E9 6SR, UK. E-mail: g.bothamley@nhs.net

TB has largely been due to operational changes in treatment delivery options, the IGRAs, molecular tests for *Mycobacterium tuberculosis* and drug resistance, and new drugs. However, the literature is swamped by repetitive case series and observational studies. A lack of meaningful interactions between scientists and clinicians means that the answers we need may be hiding in plain sight, either because the literature refers to basic science outside the TB physician's view or that the important papers are not universally accessible.

There are many interesting research topics relevant to TB. In order to try and give a clinical perspective, table 1 gives four main questions that, if answered, would lead to the transformation of the clinical management of TB.

Basic research

The tubercle bacillus has been a very successful organism in colonising the human population [4]. Rather than reiterate the detail elsewhere in this *Monograph* [5] on the pathogenesis of TB, this section will introduce some developing concepts that might be useful in answering the four questions posed in table 1.

Table 1. Four important questions in TB

Question	Why it matters	What we know	Next steps
1) Why is TB treatment so long?	Infection control and adherence are difficult	Isoniazid kills 99% of tubercle bacilli in 5 days; rifampicin kills 99% in 14 days; pyrazinamide shortens therapy	Investigate effect of drugs on *M. tuberculosis* Understand entry to and exit from latency and dormancy for *M. tuberculosis*
2) Why do only a fraction of those infected with *Mycobacterium tuberculosis* develop a form of TB disease that can be passed on?	If we prevented infectious sputum smear-positive PTB, no further transmission need occur	Primary TB is not infectious; lymph node TB is also not infectious	Understand the clinical TB spectrum Investigate more virulent strains Understand why some individuals transmit better than others
3) Why is TB a human disease?	If *M. tuberculosis* were eradicated, another mycobacterial (zoonotic) disease might take its place	3 billion people live with LTBI As TB falls, NTM species are more common	Investigate any indirect benefits of long-lasting TB immunity (BCG vaccination) [3]
4) How can we be sure that a contact does not have/will not develop TB?	Potential for drug resistance and unnecessary treatment	Immunological tests don't help Gene expression signatures may identify subclinical or incipient disease Innate immunity might be important	Cohort studies of LTBI

Microbiology

Since the publication of the genome of *M. tuberculosis* (the standard strain H37Rv) in 1998 [6], whole-genome sequencing (WGS) has become a routine laboratory practise [7]. The clinical purpose of WGS includes the early recognition of drug resistance and the definition of outbreaks. WGS has also indicated the evolution of *M. tuberculosis* into different lineages, usually associated with a racial or ethnic group [4, 8]. However, human T-cell epitopes (the small parts of an antigen that bind to the human leukocyte antigen molecules for presentation to T-cells) from *M. tuberculosis* are remarkably conserved [9]. This suggests that *M. tuberculosis* is using the immunological response in order to survive and transmit itself from one host to another.

Comparison of the genome of *M. tuberculosis*, *Mycobacterium bovis* and BCG indicated various regions of difference (RDs) [10, 11]. The first, RD1 (which contains the genes for the 6-kDa early secretory antigenic target (ESAT-6) and 10-kDa culture filtrate protein (CFP-10) as used in IGRAs), can restore virulence when added back into BCG, but not to as great an extent as virulent *M. tuberculosis* [12]. Deletion of RD1 alone from a virulent strain of *M. tuberculosis* (H37Rv:ΔRD1) resulted in a loss of virulence and toxin-related cytolysis [13]. The important genes of RD1-encoded proteins were redefined as part of a molecular secretion system (ESX-1) [14] that lyses cell membranes both at the cell surface and the phagolysosome [15, 16], and impacts on proteins that depend on ESX-1 for secretion (suggested by the effect of *M. tuberculosis* on CX3CL1 [17]). Moreover, regulation of ESX-1 by EspR (Rv3849), itself regulated by WhiB6 (which also regulates the dormancy regulon; see later) controls the amount of disease as measured by size and number of granulomas [18]. The ESX-1 secretion system also has an indirect effect by permitting the secretion of other antigens, such as EspR (Rv3849), EspA (Rv3616c), EspB (Rv3881c) and EspC (Rv3615c) in the context of Rv3870, Rv3871, Rv3877, ESAT-6 and CFP-10 [19]. However, *M. tuberculosis* H37Rv:ΔRD1 still gave rise to extensive lung inflammation in mice after more than a year [20], indicating that RD1 is important in early infection but may not explain the later phases of TB pathology.

The dormancy regulon is induced by hypoxia, nitrous oxide, acidic environments and other metabolic stresses, and in a primate model, is essential for *M. tuberculosis* persistence [21]. To date, various mechanistic and immunological correlates of this collection of genes have accumulated but as yet, there is no clear picture as to how this might change the treatment of LTBI or reduce the duration of the continuous phase of treatment. Dormancy gene-related changes include a noncoding RNA (ncRv12659) located within the Rv2660c [22] and indicates a level of regulation (the "RNA world" with regulatory elements and enzymes as well as mRNA) that has been more frequently found in human cells. The converse of the *dosR* regulon is a collection of resuscitation promoting factors (Rpf) thought to be important in reactivation [23]. An IFN-γ response to DosR and Rpf antigens appears to be higher in those with LTBI [24], suggesting the potential for clinical application.

The first *M. tuberculosis* genome sequence indicated that a very large proportion of the DNA was devoted to genes involved in lipid metabolism [6]. *M. tuberculosis* that has entered a dormant or persister state accumulates lipid droplets [25] and a lipid environment prevents the action of many anti-TB drugs [26]. In clinical terms, polyketides are associated with the form of disease, notably TB meningitis [27]. In terms of pathogenesis, phenolic glycolipid is important in escaping the first attack by

https://doi.org/10.1183/2312508X.10026118

tissue-resident macrophages [28]. Phthiocerol dimycocerosate lipids mask pathogen-associated molecular pattern recognition [29] and then epithelial CD1d (a receptor that presents lipids to immune cells) elicits an anti-inflammatory response *via* interleukin (IL)-10 [30]. Interestingly, one of the RNA transcripts used to predict who with LTBI might develop active disease [31] is that for CD1c, another molecule that presents lipids to the immune system [32].

Immunology

The general history of clinical TB has some important lessons relevant to the immune response of the human host.

- There is a clinical spectrum ranging from latent through pauci- to multibacillary TB.
- Tuberculin injection in TB patients gives a necrotic response, both locally and at more distant sites, and was associated with death (the Koch phenomenon) [33].
- Tuberculin sensitivity does not correlate with protection (in those with a BCG scar, those without a tuberculin response are as well protected against TB as those with a positive response [34]; in those where TB infection is thought responsible for the tuberculin response, the larger the response, the greater the likelihood of TB disease [35]).
- BCG was first successfully used as an oral vaccine [36] (the current intradermal injection was later used as the scar was helpful in showing whether a large tuberculin response was due to vaccination or disease).
- Effective BCG vaccination requires live bacilli [37].
- BCG affords protection against miliary TB and TB meningitis but not sputum smear-positive pulmonary disease [38] (except in tuberculin-negative adolescents, although the proportion with a positive culture and with cavitation did not differ among the nonvaccinated and two vaccinated groups) [39, 40].
- HIV infection has shown the importance of CD4$^+$ T-cells in protection: low CD4$^+$ counts result in disseminated disease but higher cell counts do not protect against TB disease [41].
- A positive IGRA is found in both healthy contacts and patients with TB. Basic research that is applicable to human TB must create hypotheses and draw conclusions that are compatible with these observations.

The earliest experiments showed that protection from BCG was transferred by cells but not serum in a mouse model [42]. This coloured the subsequent view of the immunology of TB (although antibody to the *M. tuberculosis* lipopolysaccharide coat was shown to be linked with protection against disseminated TB in children [43]). Antibodies were thought to be a defective response and indicate a failure to contain TB. This developed into the Th1/Th2 dichotomy of cellular and humoral immunity, related to different subclasses of CD4$^+$ T-cells. This distinction is now considered to be broader (and some would argue, redundant) as it has been modified to one with a genetic and cytokine-secreting definition, and also includes cells without antigen specificity, such as innate lymphoid cells [44] (table 2).

From the above table, although many of the terms may be unfamiliar and the interested reader can explore these further, it can be seen that the immune response moves between the different types of immunity, depending on the stage of infection and the number of bacilli. There are also links with the microbiome through Th17 cells and Tuft cells, which

Table 2. A simplified, modern view of the type 1/type 2 dichotomy as relevant to TB [45, 46]

	Type 1/Th1/local	Type 2/Th2/systemic with tissue repair
Definition: genetic	Th1 cells: T-bet$^+$ (and STAT-4)	Th2 cells: GATA3$^+$ (and STAT-6)
Target	Small, invasive/intracellular and rapidly multiplying microbial pathogens	Macroscopic parasites; nonmicrobial stimuli (toxins)
Aim	Destroy pathogens and infected cells	Engages whole tissue, using antibody and complement
Triggers	Pattern recognition receptors: TLRs DC-SIGN, binds to mannose (CD206) NOD-like receptor PAMPs	Hypoxia, acidification, metabolic stress IL-33, an "alarmin" (necrotic cell death, stretched cells, release of cell contents, proteolysis)
Mechanism	CD4$^+$ T-cells go to lymph nodes, proliferate and then migrate to sites of inflammation	Resident memory T-cells[#] proliferate locally and in inducible BALT
Action	Cell-mediated cytotoxicity Macrophage activation	Antibody-dependent cytotoxicity
Main cytokines	IFN-γ, TNF to stimulate IL-15 to IL-32 [47] IL-12 (positive feedback)	IL-5, IL-9 and IL-13 Later IL-4 (positive feedback)
Partner cells	Macrophages, CD8$^+$ T-cells	B-cells; eosinophils, mast cells
Inhibitors **Th17 cell (type 3[¶])** **RORγt+ (STAT3) and IL-17 family [48–51]**	IL-10 and IL-26 (TGF-β) Pro-inflammatory Recruit macrophages and Th1 cells Accelerate Th1 memory Secrete IL-17, disseminated TB results if levels are low Possible role for lipids [52]	Pro-inflammatory Induced by tissue damage (IL-6, IL-23) IL-22 (IL-10 family) promotes Th2 IL-25 (IL-17E) from Tuft cells [53] Trigger CD5L–CD36 axis [54]
Treg (type 3) **Foxp3$^+$** **(limits inflammation and supports tissue repair [55])**	Anti-inflammatory TGF-β limits Th1 suppression [56] Hypoxia limits Th1 as Treg promoted [57]	Anti-inflammatory IgG stimulates Treg cells Th2 specificity usually different to Treg specificity [58]
Macrophages [59]	M1 (Jak–STAT1) Classically activated by IFN-γ Bacteriostatic/bactericidal	M2 (MAF, PU.1 and C/EBP) Alternative pathway Homeostatic and reparative
NK cells [60]	CD56^{bright} and CD56^{dim}CD57$^-$NKG2C$^{-/+}$ Produce IFN-γ Nonspecific memory	CD56^{dim}CD57$^-$ Cytotoxic
Metabolism **Importance of the tricarboxylic acid cycle in determining immune responses [61–63]**	Glycolysis Citrate (and acetyl Co-A) accumulates Aspartate-argino-succinate shunt Nitrous oxide produced Favours Th17	Anaerobic respiration Oxidative phosphorylation Fatty acids undergo β-oxidation α-ketoglutarate and glutamine

Continued

https://doi.org/10.1183/2312508X.10026118

Table 2. Continued

	Type 1/Th1/local	Type 2/Th2/systemic with tissue repair
Metabolism **Importance of the** **tricarboxylic acid cycle** **in determining immune** **responses [61–63]** **(cont.)**		Favours Treg cells (Metformin lowers citrate, α-ketoglutarate, succinate, fumarate and malate)

Th: T-helper; T-bet: T-box expressed in T-cells; STAT: signal transducer and activator of transcription; TLR: Toll-like receptor; DC-SIGN: dendritic cell-specific intercellular adhesion molecule-3-grabbing nonintegrin; NOD: nucleotide-binding oligomerisation domain; PAMP: pathogen-associated molecular pattern; IL: interleukin; BALT: bronchial-associated lymphoid tissue; TNF: tumour necrosis factor; TGF: transforming growth factor; Treg: regulatory T-cell; Jak: Janus kinase; MAF: macrophage-activating factor; C/EBP: CCAAT enhancer-binding protein; NK: natural killer; Co-A: coenzyme A. [#]: cells that transfer protection differ from those that cause delayed-type hypersensitivity [64]. [¶]: others have divided the immune response into three types, whereby a type 3 response is more rapid and acute but also fades more quickly, and is initiated by Th17 cells and limited by Treg cells; this response then leads to a type 1 or 2 response if the infection is not controlled, as in the table.

produce IL-25 (IL-17E, systemic response in table 2) [65]. The influence of changes in the tricarboxylic acid cycle on immune responses is an area of intense current interest, especially noting that metformin improves treatment outcomes in TB [66].

Interest in type I IFNs was aroused by looking at mRNA transcripts that differ in TB disease, LTBI and health controls [67]. Type I IFNs (IFN-α and -β) are found in a variety of tissues as a response to intracellular oligonucleotides. Unexpectedly, expression of type I IFN genes was increased in TB disease compared to LTBI or controls. When looking at mRNA transcripts that were associated with the later development of TB disease in those with LTBI, 15 of the 16 genes identified in a prospective study were associated with chronic IFN activation [68]. Type I IFNs appear to cause more severe TB disease by inducing IL-10 and IL-1 receptor antagonist, and blocking tumour necrosis factor, IL-12 and IL-1β [69], *via* the cytosolic GMP–AMP synthase DNA sensor activating IFN production by the STING/TBK1/IRF3 (stimulator of IFN genes/serine–threonine protein kinase/IFN regulatory transcription factor-3) pathway [70] (mentioned only for the interested reader). Knockout mice for the IFN-αβ receptor showed lower bacillary counts when infected with *Mycobacterium africanum* [71]. Some have suggested that type I IFNs may exert their effect by altering the ratio of classically activated macrophages (M1) to a regulatory/anti-inflammatory phenotype (M2) [72, 73]. Thus, the main clinical role for measuring IFNs or their RNA is diagnostic and prognostic rather than interventional. However, their role in promoting chronic inflammation and immunosuppression means that some of the proposed tools for cancer treatments that counteract type I IFNs may have a bearing on TB [74].

The signal that determines the clinical spectrum may come at an early stage after infection. Following movement of infected alveolar macrophages into the interstitial space, different signals may determine whether haematogenous or lymphatic spread occurs [75]. High serum levels of vascular endothelial growth factor (VEGF) have been found in patients with

PTB [76]. Whether the difference between the various VEGFs determine whether TB will be infectious or merely result in enlarged extrathoracic lymph nodes is as yet unclear. Monoclonal antibodies against VEGF are used in lung cancer and serous/wet macular degeneration, and therefore these agents may have a future bearing on the management of TB.

Vaccine development in TB has been undergoing a renaissance. There is now evidence that natural killer (NK) cells can develop a nonspecific memory and "train" monocytes to respond better to nonspecific stimuli such that re-challenge with TB results in greater production of IFN-γ [77] and other cytokines [51, 78]; the duration of this effect is as yet unknown (the half-life of human NK cells is 1–2 weeks [79]). A vaccine that had a more prolonged effect might be able to prevent TB without stimulating *M. tuberculosis*-specific immunity, mimicking the effect of TB contact without a positive IGRA. The effect of both BCG re-vaccination and the antigen85/TB10.7 vaccine H4:IC31 seems to prevent sustained QuantiFERON Gold-In-Tube (Qiagen, Hilden, Germany) conversion in those previously negative living in a TB-endemic area [80]. A vaccine to prevent infectious smear-positive PTB in those who have LTBI has been suggested by the controlled trial of M72/AS01$_E$ with an efficacy of 54%, although with 95% confidence intervals ranging from 2.9 to 78.2, especially in males under the age of 26 years [81] . The problem lies in the fact that we do not yet know what causes the granulomas in the high-oxygen regions of the lung to grow and cavitate, although the Koch phenomenon suggests that it is primarily an unregulated immune response derived from circulating immune cells. Secondly, if this cavitation were initiated by an action of immune cells, does this lie along the continuum of the usual immune response or does another key immune cell act? The former would require a vaccine that restores the "homeostasis" of LTBI, the latter an immune cell-specific vaccine.

Treatment

The subject of new and repurposed drugs in the treatment of TB has been addressed elsewhere in this *Monograph* [82].

High-dose rifampicin

Therapeutic drug monitoring [83] during treatment has shown that a high proportion of patients have rifampicin levels below the therapeutic threshold [84]. This may simply be because doctors or patients do not heed the advice to take treatment on an empty stomach. However, with rifampicin, the initial expense (similar to that of bedaquiline today in real terms) meant that doses were tailored to the MIC rather than that to achieve maximal bactericidal effect. High-dose rifampicin studies have suggested that treatment for TB might be shortened, as using rifampicin at doses of 35 mg·kg^{-1} was associated with earlier sputum conversion [85, 86]. Although high doses of rifampicin might shorten treatment, only low isoniazid levels have been associated with previous TB and perhaps a poorer outcome [87].

Treatment of multidrug-resistant/extensively drug-resistant tuberculosis

As noted in elsewhere in this *Monograph* [88], drug resistance has the potential to negate the End TB Strategy. The main problem has been how to evaluate new treatments. RCTs provide the highest quality of evidence but are expensive and, for TB, require considerable periods of time both for treatment and for later follow-up. Various alternatives have been proposed but each has its weaknesses [89]. For instance, the current treatment of MDR-TB

https://doi.org/10.1183/2312508X.10026118

has been based on meta-analyses of treated patients [90, 91]. Problems with these cohort analyses, even with propensity scoring to adjust for confounding related to demographic and comorbid factors that might skew comparisons, are: 1) the definition of a regimen is at a single time-point, whereas regimen change is common [92]; 2) doses of moxifloxacin and ethambutol may have been inadequate to achieve bactericidal levels (600 mg daily and 25 mg·kg^{-1} respectively); and 3) the outcome definition included both "cured" and "completed treatment", a definition of success that produces an apparently better cure rate for XDR-TB than for MDR-TB [93]. Other, less readily addressed problems include confounding by indication (*e.g.* capreomycin may perform poorly if it is always used in subjects whose regimen was suboptimal whereas the carbapenems may appear better as their relative absence of adverse effects may permit treatment completion), variation in individual or clinical group application of WHO definitions of failure, and the difficulty in handling data for those who interrupt treatment or die during treatment. There is a move away from the use of injectable drugs, due to their many adverse effects, to entirely oral treatments with a greater emphasis on the use of bedaquiline [94]. Cohort studies have suggested that the duration of treatment with bedaquiline might be >6 months in those with a positive sputum smear and social risks associated with hepatitis C infection [95]; attempts to disentangle these two risk factors will be important. Comparison of the randomised addition of an approved drug to an optimised background regimen should be feasible for any patient being treated, if data collection can be patient centred and protocols simple enough not to attract excessive regulatory hurdles.

However, completely new regimens, comparable with the introduction of pyrazinamide to shorten TB treatment from 18 to 6 months, require an RCT. Several important RCTs of treatment are expected to report later this year to document the benefits of linezolid, pretominid and bedaquiline, especially in XDR-TB.

Operational research

Pre-diagnosis

TB is usually diagnosed as a result of patients presenting to healthcare systems. Most TB transmission occurs before diagnosis, and it should be noted that an estimated 30–40% of all TB remains undiagnosed [96]. Active case finding is a feature of contact tracing and WHO now recommends giving preventive treatment to all children of families living in a high TB incidence country where an adult has culture-positive TB [97]. Screening of those with a high risk of infection, such as people living with HIV (PLHIV) is the first priority. Other groups have been identified based on TB contact, immunosuppression and those living in settings where *M. tuberculosis* survives more readily (overcrowding, poor ventilation, high humidity and lack of ultraviolet light) who also have a high risk of TB [79]. An effective innovation has been to train patients who have successfully been treated for TB to identify and screen high-risk groups themselves [98].

A test to rule out TB that could be made available in the community (as with HIV testing on saliva) remains an important target. A negative IGRA has value in screening, as few develop TB [99]. However, in TB disease, as many as 20% may have a negative IGRA [100]. A better triage test to identify those with a high risk of TB who require further investigation would be useful. It is likely that a combination of a *M. tuberculosis*-specific test with a more general marker of inflammation in a near-patient format will be required [101].

There is as yet no equivalent marker of viral load in HIV for TB. A descriptive summary of more than 4137 proteins found in the blood in relation to genetic risk factors for disease suggests that a marker of disease activity in TB is possible [102]. Re-analysis of RNA transcriptome studies combined with new evidence in TB suggests that monitoring of NK cells, amongst many other biomarkers, might be a valuable marker of response during treatment [103]. However, these remain distant from the tubercle bacillus. Actively dividing *M. tuberculosis* secretes a number of proteins that might be detectable [104] but in cases where the dormancy regulon is active, the quantities of such dormancy-associated proteins may currently be beyond the limit of detection [105].

Diagnosis of tuberculosis

WHO introduced the use of Xpert MTB/RIF (Cepheid, Sunnyvale, CA, USA) to improve the detection of smear-negative culture-positive PTB above that attainable with a sputum smear and a chest radiograph [106]. However, a gap between those diagnosed with TB and those starting treatment soon became evident [107]. A cluster-randomised trial showed that placing the testing equipment in a primary care clinic treating PLHIV or those with a high risk of DR-TB resulted in a shorter time to starting treatment than if the equipment were placed in the laboratory of a district general hospital (1 compared to 7 days) [108]. Even in a low TB prevalence country, the routine testing of sputum samples sent for TB examination appeared to be cost-effective [109]. Cost-effectiveness was reached when ⩾6% of submitted samples proved to have TB [110]. Further roll-out of these and similar near-patient tests will continue to be an important target for the near future.

Drug-susceptibility testing and whole-genome sequencing

The UK is the first country to implement WGS for all cultures of *M. tuberculosis* as the first step in replacing routine phenotypic DST [111]; phenotypic testing will still be performed for all those with genetic mutations in order to establish important parameters such as the MIC. As resistance tends to occur in patterns (*e.g.* rifampicin resistance tends to occur after isoniazid resistance, making rifampicin-monoresistant strains rare), the greater detail afforded by WGS has permitted the development of algorithms to improve the sensitivity and specificity of genetic predictions of drug resistance [112]. The development of a potential point-of-care test for samples positive for rifampicin resistance suggested that a similar test might be valuable in deciding upon the initial regimen for those with DR-TB [113]. WGS from sputum samples is now possible [114]. Already, WGS will be cost-effective if it replaces phenotypic sensitivity testing for those with no mutations in the genes associated with drug resistance. The costs of WGS continue to fall and WGS will become the standard of the future for microbiological investigation of TB. The most important barriers to the use of genetic tests for TB appear to lie with physicians [115].

New ideas in treatment adherence

Adherence has been covered elsewhere in this *Monograph* [83, 116–118]. When the DOTS strategy was first introduced, this was an acknowledgement that patient-centred factors in the process of care were as important as, if not more so than, the drug regimen. To summarise these data, patient education and incentives in addition to directly observed treatment were more effective than staff education, psychological support and the use of mobile telephones to remind patients and monitor their adherence to medication [119].

https://doi.org/10.1183/2312508X.10026118

The cost to patients to adhere to treatment for TB can represent a significant proportion of their annual income or even put them into debt [120]. Such "catastrophic" costs, defined as >20% of annual income, or taking a loan, or selling property or livestock to deal with TB-related costs [121], have been targeted by various cash transfer schemes to defray the costs of treatment [122] and have been shown to improve outcomes [123]. However, in studies of social support as well as economic support, TB clubs with peer-led mutual support were most effective in supporting adherence to treatment and valued more highly than economic support [124]. More general approaches to improving health and food security and reducing poverty (*e.g.* Mexico's Oportunidades/Prospera and Seguro Popular programmes and Brazil's Bolsa Familia programme) might be even more effective in reducing TB [125–127]. Such social interventions will need to become part of the routine management of TB.

A world without tuberculosis

The End TB Strategy has been covered elsewhere in this *Monograph* [116]. The purpose of this section is to highlight some general principles of host–pathogen relationships and to add a cautionary note that, unlike the eradication of smallpox or polio, there may be broader consequences of TB elimination due to the complexities of the host–microbiome interactions.

In general, the virulence of a pathogen (the rate at which it kills the host) is often coupled with its transmissibility and the time taken for the host to recover [128]. The evolution of *M. tuberculosis* has shown a trend towards less pathogenic forms [4, 129] punctuated by outbreaks of more virulent forms, such as the recent rise of the Beijing lineage [130]. Indeed, commensalism might be considered a desirable state for *M. tuberculosis* survival within a vast human population in which to reside, if the problem of transmission and therefore of efforts to control TB disease might be avoided [131]. Studies of the lung and gut microbiome have suggested that interrelationships among bacteria may be much more complex [132]. Having overcome the common problems of repeatability with adequate controls [133], there are now studies that indicate that interactions with the microbiome *via* small chain fatty acids, such as propionate and butyrate, might be at least important in regulating the immune response to *M. tuberculosis* [134].

Elsewhere in this *Monograph*, RAVIGLIONE [116] indicates the enormous benefits of reducing the burden of TB, noting its prevalence in economically active young adults and effect on family life. Does infection with the *M. tuberculosis* complex provide any advantages to its human host? Using *M. bovis* BCF, as an example, neonatal BCG vaccination improves the general ability to control infections *via* NK cell and monocyte nonspecific memory (see Immunology section earlier). The International Study of Asthma and Allergies in Childhood even suggested that TB itself might be inversely related to asthma [135]. A large study in Japan also showed an inverse association between tuberculin reactivity and atopy [136]. BCG vaccination may be able to provide the same benefits in preventing atopy [137]. This is again consistent with an effect of BCG vaccination to downregulate the allergic type 2 response. However, it is to be hoped that a search for a cure rather than palliative treatment for asthma and the atopic diseases will be more directly beneficial.

Countries in which the incidence has fallen have shown both a trend towards a greater proportion of sputum smear-positive PTB in the native population and an increase in NTM infection [138]. Fortunately, most NTM infections have not been associated with person-to-person transmission. However, *Mycobacterium abscessus* is one of the few mycobacterial species that has been associated with transmission by aerosol in the context of a cystic fibrosis clinic [139] and outbreaks in a hospital environment [140]. This fast-growing mycobacterium has the potential to occupy the same ecological niche as *M. tuberculosis* but with significantly greater problems in terms of treatment options [141].

Conclusion

Progress in the control of TB must accelerate if we are to reach the targets of the End TB Strategy. There are encouraging indications that significant advances can be implemented now in terms of laboratory diagnosis, new treatments and patient involvement. The host response to TB has turned out to be much more complicated than previously thought but a greater scientific understanding of both host and pathogen is beginning to show the way forward.

References

1.   Spita G, Clegg H, Dumitru M, *et al.* The patients' perspective. *In:* Migliori GB, Bothamley G, Duarte R, *et al.*, eds. Tuberculosis (ERS Monograph). Sheffield, European Respiratory Society, 2018; pp. 1–7.

2.   World Health Organization. The End TB Strategy. www.who.int/tb/strategy/End_TB_Strategy.pdf?ua=1. Date last updated: May 2014.

3.   Colonna M. Innate lymphoid cells: diversity, plasticity and unique functions in immunity. *Immunity* 2018; 48: 1104–1117.

4.   Loddenkemper R, Murray JF, Gradmann C, *et al.* History of tuberculosis. *In:* Migliori GB, Bothamley G, Duarte R, *et al.*, eds. Tuberculosis (ERS Monograph). Sheffield, European Respiratory Society, 2018; pp. 8–27.

5.   Barreira-Silva P, Torrado E, Nebenzahl-Guimaraes H, *et al.* Aetiopathogenesis, immunology and microbiology. *In:* Migliori GB, Bothamley G, Duarte R, *et al.*, eds. Tuberculosis (ERS Monograph). Sheffield, European Respiratory Society, 2018; pp. 62–82.

6.   Cole ST, Brosch R, Parkhill J, *et al.* Deciphering the biology of *Mycobacterium tuberculosis* from the complete genome sequence. *Nature* 1998; 393: 537–544.

7.   Cabibbe AM, Trovato A, De Filippo MR, *et al.* Countrywide implementation of whole genome sequencing: an opportunity to improve tuberculosis management, surveillance and contact tracing in low incidence countries. *Eur Respir J* 2018; 51: 1800387.

8.   Comas I, Coscolla M, Luo T, *et al.* Out-of-Africa migration and Neolithic co-expansion of *Mycobacterium tuberculosis* with modern humans. *Nat Genet* 2013; 45: 1176–1182.

9.   Comas I, Chakravatti J, Small PM, *et al.* Human T cell epitopes of *Mycobacterium tuberculosis* are evolutionarily hyper-conserved. *Nat Genet* 2010; 42: 498–503.

10.   Mahairas GG, Sabo PJ, Hivkey MJ, *et al.* Molecular analysis of genetic differences between *Mycobacterium bovis*-BCG and virulent *M. bovis. J Bacteriol* 1996; 178: 1274–1282.

11.   Brosch R, Gordon SV, Marmiesse M, *et al.* A new evolutionary scenario for the *Mycobacterium tuberculosis*-complex. *Proc Natl Acad Sci USA* 2002; 99: 3684–3689.

12.   Pym AS, Brodin P, Brosch R, *et al.* Loss of RD1 contributed to the attenuation of live tuberculosis vaccines *Mycobacterium bovis*-BCG and *Mycobacterium microti. Mol Microbiol* 2002; 46: 709–717.

13.   Hsu T, Hingley-Wilson SM, Chen B, *et al.* The primary mechanism of attenuation of bacilli-Calmette Guérin is a loss of secreted lytic function required for invasion of lung interstitial tissue. *Proc Natl Acad Sci USA* 2003; 100: 12420–12425.

14.   Brodin P, Majlessi L, Marsollier L, *et al.* Dissection of ESAT-6 system 1 of *Mycobacterium tuberculosis* and impact on immunogenicity and virulence. *Infect Immun* 2006; 74: 88–98.

15.   Conrad WH, Osman MM, Shanahan JK, *et al.* Mycobacterial ESX-1 secretion system mediates host cell lysis through bacterium-contact-dependent gross membrane disruptions. *Proc Natl Acad Sci USA* 2017; 114: 1371–1376.

16.   Augenstreich J, Arbues A, Simeone R, *et al.* ESX-1 and phthiocerol dimycocerosates of *Mycobacterium tuberculosis* act in concert to cause phagosomal rupture and host cell apoptosis. *Cell Microbiol* 2017; 19: https://doi.org/10.1111/cml.12726.

17.   Hingley-Wilson SM, Connell D, Pollock K, *et al.* ESX1-dependent fractalkine mediates chemotaxis and *Mycobacterium tuberculosis* infection in humans. *Tuberculosis* 2014; 94: 262–270.

https://doi.org/10.1183/2312508X.10026118

18. Chen Z, Hu Y, Cumming BM, *et al.* Mycobacterial WhiB6 differentially regulates ESX-1 and the Dos regulon to modulate granuloma formation and virulence in zebrafish. *Cell Rep* 2016; 16: 2512–2524.

19. DiGiuseppe Champion PA, Champion MM, Manzanillo P, *et al.* ESX-1 secreted virulence factors are recognized by multiple cytosolic AAA ATPases in pathogenic mycobacteria. *Mol Microbiol* 2009; 73: 950–962.

20. Sherman DR, Guinn KM, Hickey MJ, *et al. Mycobacterium tuberculosis* H37Rv:DRD1 is more virulent than *M. bovis* Bacille Calmette-Guérin in long-term murine infection. *J Infect Dis* 2004; 190: 123–126.

21. Mehra S, Foreman TW, Didier PJ, *et al.* The DosR regulon modulates adaptive immunity and is essential for *Mycobacterium tuberculosis* persistence. *Am J Respir Crit Care Med* 2015; 191: 1185–1196.

22. Houghton J, Cortes T, Schubert O, *et al.* A small RNA encoded in the Rv2660c locus of *Mycobacterium tuberculosis* is induced during starvation and infection. *PLoS One* 2013; 8: e80047.

23. Kana BD, Gordhan BG, Downing KJ, *et al.* The resuscitation-promoting factors of *Mycobacterium tuberculosis* are required for virulence and resuscitation from dormancy but are collectively dispensable for growth *in vitro. Mol Microbiol* 2008; 67: 672–684.

24. Arroyo L, Marin D, Franken KLMC, *et al.* Potential of DosR and Rpf antigens from *Mycobacterium tuberculosis* to discriminate between latent and active tuberculosis in a tuberculosis endemic population of Medelin, Colombia. *BMC Infect Dis* 2018; 18: 26.

25. Garton NJ, Waddell SJ, Sherratt AL, *et al.* Cytological and transcript analyses reveal fat and lazy persister-like bacilli in tuberculous sputum. *PLoS Med* 2008; 5: e75.

26. Aguilar-Ayala DA, Cnockaert M, Vandamme P, *et al.* Antimicrobial activity against *Mycobacterium tuberculosis* under *in vitro* dormancy conditions. *J Med Microbiol* 2018; 67: 282–285.

27. Faksri K, Ong RT, Tan JH, *et al.* Comparative whole-genome sequence analysis of *Mycobacterium tuberculosis* isolated from tuberculous meningitis and pulmonary tuberculosis patients. *Sci Rep* 2018; 8: 4910.

28. Cambier CJ, O'Leary SM, O'Sullivan MP, *et al.* Phenolic glycolipid facilitates mycobacterial escape from microbicidal tissue-resident macrophages. *Immunity* 2017; 47: 552–565.

29. Cambier CJ, Takaki KK, Larson RP, *et al.* Mycobacteria manipulate macrophage recruitment through coordinated use of membrane lipid. *Nature* 2014; 505: 218–222.

30. Olszak T, Neves JF, Dowds CM, *et al.* Protective mucosal immunity mediated by epithelial CD1d and IL-10. *Nature* 2014; 509: 497–502.

31. Suliman S, Thompson EG, Sutherland J, *et al.* Four-gene pan-African blood signature predicts progression to tuberculosis. *Am J Respir Crit Care Med* 2018; 197: 1198–1208.

32. Adams EJ. Diverse antigen presentation by the Group 1 CD1 molecule CD1c. *Mol Immunol* 2013; 55: 182–185.

33. Danenberg AMJ. Delayed-type hypersensitivity and cell-mediated immunity in the pathogenesis of tuberculosis. *Immunol Today* 1991; 12: 228–233.

34. Hart P, Sutherland I, Thomas J. The immunity conferred by effective BCG and vole bacillus vaccines, in relation to individual variations in tuberculin sensitivity and to technical variations in the vaccines. *Tubercle* 1967; 48: 201–210.

35. Abubakar I, Drobniewski F, Southern J, *et al.* Prognostic value of interferon-γ release assays and tuberculin skin test in predicting the development of active tuberculosis (UK PREDICT TB): a prospective cohort study. *Lancet Infect Dis* 2018; 18: 1077–1087.

36. Bleiker MA, Meijer J, Stýblo K, *et al.* The persistence of tuberculin sensitivity following oral BCG vaccination in the Netherlands. *Tubercle* 1983; 64: 255–263.

37. Weiss DW. Vaccination against tuberculosis with non-living vaccines. *Am Rev Respir Dis* 1959; 80: 495–509.

38. Colditz GA, Brewer TF, Berkey CS, *et al.* Efficacy of BCG vaccine in the prevention of tuberculosis. Meta-analysis of the published literature. *JAMA* 1994; 271: 698–702.

39. Medical Research Council. BCG and vole bacillus vaccines in the prevention of tuberculosis in adolescents. *BMJ* 1956; 1: 413–427.

40. D'Arcy Hart P, Sutherland I. BCG and vole bacillus vaccines in the prevention of tuberculosis in adolescence and early adult life. *BMJ* 1977; 2: 293–295.

41. Jones BE, Young SMM, Antoniskis D, *et al.* Relationship of the manifestations of tuberculosis to CD4 counts in patients with human immunodeficiency virus infection. *Am Rev Respir Dis* 1993; 148: 1292–1297.

42. Mackanness GB. The immunology of anti-tuberculosis immunity. *Am Rev Respir Dis* 1968; 97: 337–344.

43. De L Costello AM, Kumar A, Narayan V, *et al.* Does antibody to mycobacterial antigens, including lipoarabinomannan, limit dissemination in childhood tuberculosis. *Trans R Soc Trop Med Hyg* 1992; 86: 686–692.

44. Kotas ME, Locksley RM. Why innate lymphoid cells? *Immunity* 2018; 48: 1081–1090.

45. Von Moltke J, Pepper M. Sentinels of the type 2 immune response. *Trends Immunol* 2018; 39: 99–111.

46. Colonna M. Innate lymphoid cells: diversity, plasticity, and unique functions in immunity. *Immunity* 2018; 48: 1104–1117.

47. Montoya D, Inkeles MS, Liu PT, *et al.* IL-32 is a molecular marker of a host defense network in human tuberculosis. *Sci Transl Med* 2014; 6: 250ra114.

48. Li Y, Wei C, Xu H, *et al*. The immunoregulation of Th17 in host against intracellular bacterial infection. *Mediators Inflamm* 2018; 2018: 6587296.

49. Matsuzaki G, Umemura M. Interleukin-17 family cytokines in protective immunity against infections: role of haematopoietic cell-derived and non-haematopoietic cell-derived interleukin 17s. *Microbiol Immunol* 2018; 62: 1–13.

50. Le Rouzic O, Pichavant M, Frealle E, *et al*. Th17 cytokines: novel potential therapeutic targets for COPD pathogenesis and exacerbations. *Eur Respir J* 2017; 50: 1602434.

51. Eyerich K, Dimartino V, Cavani A. IL-17 and IL-22 in immunity: driving protection and pathology. *Eur J Immunol* 2017; 47: 607–614.

52. Davis FP, Kanno Y, O'Shea JJ. A metabolic switch for Th17 pathogenicity. *Cell* 2015; 163: 1308–1310.

53. Montoro DT, Haber AL, Biton M, *et al*. A revised airway epithelial hierarchy includes CFTR-expressing ionocytes. *Nature* 2018; 560: 319–324.

54. Martinez VG, Escoda-Ferran C, Simões IT, *et al*. The macrophage soluble receptor AIM/Api6/CD5L displays a broad pathogen recognition spectrum and is involved in early response to microbial aggression. *Cell Mol Immunol* 2014; 11: 343–354.

55. Vasanthakumar A, Kallies A. The regulatory T cell: jack-of-all-trades. *Trends in Immunol* 2015; 36: 756–758.

56. Konkel JE, Zhang D, Zanvit P, *et al*. Transforming growth factor-β signalling in regulatory T cell controls T helper-17 cells and tissue-specific immune responses. *Immunity* 2017; 46: 660–674.

57. Clever D, Roychaudhuri R, Constantinides MG, *et al*. Oxygen sensing by T cells establishes an immunologically tolerant metastatic niche. *Cell* 2016; 166: 11117–11131.

58. Bacher P, Heinrich F, Stervbo U, *et al*. Regulatory T cell specificity direct tolerance *versus* allergy against aeroantigens in humans. *Cell* 2016; 167: 1067–1078.

59. Kang K, Park SH, Chen J, *et al*. Interferon-γ represses M2 gene expression in human macrophages by disassembling enhancers bound by the transcription factor MAF. *Immunity* 2017; 47: 235–250.

60. Wagstaffe HR, Mooney JP, Riley EM, *et al*. Vaccinating for natural killer effector functions. *Clin Translat Immunol* 2018: e1010.

61. Phan AT, Goldrath AW, Glass CK. Metabolic and epigenetic coordination of T cell and macrophage immunity. *Immunity* 2017; 46: 714–729.

62. Angajala A, Lim S, Phillips JB, *et al*. Diverse roles of mitochondria in immune responses: novel insights into immune-metabolism. *Front Immunol* 2018; 9: 1605.

63. Kornberg MD, Bhargava P, Kim PM, *et al*. Dimethyl fumarate targets GAPDH and aerobic glycolysis to modulate immunity. *Science* 2018; 360: 449–453.

64. Orme IM, Collins FM. Adoptive protection of the *Mycobacterium tuberculosis*-infected lung: dissociation between cells that transfer protective immunity and those that transfer delayed-type hypersensitivity to tuberculin. *Cell Immunol* 1984; 84: 113–120.

65. Ivanov II. Microbe hunting hits home. *Cell Host Microbe* 2017; 21: 282–285.

66. Singhal A, Jie L, Kumar P, *et al*. Metformin as adjunct antituberculosis therapy. *Sci Transl Med* 2014; 6: 263ra159.

67. Berry MPR, Graham CM, McNab FW, *et al*. An interferon-inducible neutrophil driven blood transcriptional signature in human tuberculosis. *Nature* 2010; 466: 973–977.

68. Zak DE, Penn-Nicholson A, Scriba TJ, *et al*. A blood RNA signature for tuberculosis disease risk: a prospective cohort study. *Lancet* 2016; 387: 2312–2322.

69. McNab FW, Ewbank J, Howes A, *et al*. Type I IFN induces IL-10 production in an IL-27-independent manner and blocks responsiveness to IFN-γ for production of IL-12 and bacterial killing in *Mycobacterium tuberculosis*-infected macrophages. *J Immunol* 2014; 193: 3600–3612.

70. Watson RO, Bell SL, MacDuff DA, *et al*. The cytosolic sensor cGAS detects *Mycobacterium tuberculosis* DNA to induce type I interferons and activate autophagy. *Cell Host Microbe* 2015; 17: 811–819.

71. Wiens KE, Ernst JD. The mechanism for type I interferon induction by *Mycobacterium tuberculosis* is bacterial strain-dependent. *PLoS Pathog* 2016; 12: e1005809.

72. Moreira-Teixeira L, Sousa J, McNab FW, *et al*. Type I IFN inhibits alternative macrophage activation during *Mycobacterium tuberculosis* infection and leads to enhanced protection in the absence of IFN-γ signalling. *J Immunol* 2016; 197: 4714–4725.

73. Bénard A, Sakwa I, Schierloh P, *et al*. B cells producing type I interferon modulate macrophage polarization in tuberculosis. *Am J Respir Crit Care Med* 2018; 197: 801–813.

74. Zevini A, Olagnier D, Hiscott J. Crosstalk between cytoplasmic RIG-1 and STING sensing pathways. *Trends Immunol* 2017; 38: 194–205.

75. Kim PM, Lee J-J, Choi D, *et al*. Endothelial lineage-specific interaction of *Mycobacterium tuberculosis* with the blood and lymphatic systems. *Tuberculosis* 2018; 111: 1–7.

76. Matsuyama W, Hashiguchi T, Matsumuro K, *et al*. Increased serum level of vascular endothelial growth factor in pulmonary tuberculosis. *Am J Respir Crit Care Med* 2000; 162: 1120–1122.

77. Zufferey C, Germano S, Dutta B, *et al*. The contribution of non-conventional T cells and NK cells in the mycobacterial-specific IFNγ response in Bacille Calmette-Guérin (BCG)-immunized infants. *PLoS One*; 8: e77334.

https://doi.org/10.1183/2312508X.10026118

78. Smith SG, Kleinnijenhuis J, Netea MG, *et al.* Whole blood profiling of Bacillus Calmette-Guérin-induced trained innate immunity in infants identifies epidermal growth factor, IL-6, platelet-derived growth factor-AB/BB and natural killer activation. *Front Immunol* 2017; 8: 644.

79. Zhang Y, Wallace DL, de Lara CM, *et al. In vivo* kinetics of human natural killer cells: the effect of ageing and acute and chronic viral infection. *Immunology* 2007; 121: 258–265.

80. Nemes E, Geldenhuys H, Rozot V, *et al.* Prevention of *M. tuberculosis* infection with H4:IC31 vaccine or BCG revaccination. *N Engl J Med* 2018; 379: 138–149.

81. Van der Meeren O, Hatherill M, Nduba V, *et al.* Phase 2b controlled trial of M72/AS01E vaccine to prevent tuberculosis. *N Engl J Med* 2018; 379: 1621–1634.

82. Krutikov M, Bruchfeld J, Migliori GB, *et al.* New and repurposed drugs. *In:* Migliori GB, Bothamley G, Duarte R, *et al.*, eds. Tuberculosis (ERS Monograph). Sheffield, European Respiratory Society, 2018; pp. 179–204.

83. Alffenaar J-WC, Akkerman OW, Bothamley G. Monitoring during and after treatment. *In:* Migliori GB, Bothamley G, Duarte R, *et al.*, eds. Tuberculosis (ERS Monograph). Sheffield, European Respiratory Society, 2018; pp. 308–325.

84. Mota L, Al-Efraij K, Campbell JR, *et al.* Therapeutic drug monitoring in anti-tuberculosis treatment: a systematic review and meta-analysis. *Int J Tuberc Lung Dis* 2016; 20: 819–826.

85. Boeree MJ, Diacon AH, Dawson R, *et al.* A dose-ranging trial to optimize the dose of rifampin in the treatment of tuberculosis. *Am J Respir Crit Care Med* 2015; 191: 1058–1065.

86. Svensson EM, Svensson RJ, Te Brake LHM, *et al.* The potential for treatment shortening with higher rifampicin doses: relating drug exposure to treatment response in patients with pulmonary tuberculosis. *Clin Infect Dis* 2018; 67: 34–41.

87. Park JS, Lee JY, Lee YJ, *et al.* Serum levels of antituberculosis drugs and their effect on tuberculosis treatment outcome. *Antimicrob Agents Chemother* 2015; 60: 92–98.

88. Duarte R, Santos JV, Santos Silva A, *et al.* Epidemiological and socioeconomic determinants. *In:* Migliori GB, Bothamley G, Duarte R, *et al.*, eds. Tuberculosis (ERS Monograph). Sheffield, European Respiratory Society, 2018; pp. 28–35.

89. Frieden TR. Evidence for health decision making – beyond randomized, controlled trials. *N Engl J Med* 2017; 377: 465–475.

90. Ahuja SD, Ashkin D, Avendano M, *et al.* Multidrug resistant pulmonary tuberculosis treatment regimens and patient outcomes: an individual patient data meta-analysis of 9153 patients. *PLoS Med* 2012; 9: e1001300.

91. Ahmad N, Ahuja SD, Akkerman OW, *et al.* Treatment correlates of successful outcomes in pulmonary multidrug-resistant tuberculosis: an individual patient data meta-analysis. *Lancet* 2018; 392: 821–834.

92. Günther G, van Leth F, Alexandru S, *et al.* Clinical management of multidrug-resistant tuberculosis in 16 European countries. *Am J Respir Crit Care med* 2018; 198: 379–386.

93. Günther G, Lange C, Alexandru S, *et al.* Treatment outcomes in multidrug-resistant tuberculosis. *N Engl J Med* 2016; 375: 1103–1105.

94. World Health Organization. Rapid communication: key changes to treatment of multidrug- and rifampicin-resistant tuberculosis (MDR/RR-TB). Geneva, World Health Organization, 2018.

95. Hewison C, Bastar M, Khachatryan N, *et al.* Is 6 months of bedaquiline enough? Results from the compassionate use of bedaquiline in Armenia and Georgia. *Int J Tuberc Lung Dis* 2018; 22: 766–772.

96. World Health Organization. Global tuberculosis report 2017. Geneva, World Health Organization, 2017.

97. World Health Organization. Latent tuberculosis infection: updated and consolidated guidelines for programmatic management. Geneva, World Health Organization, 2018.

98. Andre E, Rusumba O, Evans CA, *et al.* Patient-led tuberculosis case-finding in the Democratic Republic of Congo. *Bull World Health Organ* 2018; 96: 522–530.

99. Zellweger JP, Sotgiu G, Block M, *et al.* Risk assessment of tuberculosis in contacts by IFNγ release assays: a Tuberculosis Network European Trials group study. *Am J Respir Crit care med* 2015; 191: 1176–1184.

100. Pai M, Zwerling A, Menzies D. Systematic review: T-cell-based assays for the diagnosis of latent tuberculosis infection: an update. *Ann Intern Med* 2008; 149: 177–184.

101. Bothamley GH, Ruhwald M, Goletti D. Omics and single molecule detection: the future of TB diagnostics. *In:* Lange C, Migliori GB, eds. Tuberculosis (ERS Monograph). Sheffield, European Respiratory Society, 2012; pp. 144–153.

102. Emilsson V, Ilkov M, Lamb JR, *et al.* Co-regulatory networks of human serum proteins link genetics to disease. *Science* 2018; 361: 769–763.

103. Chowdhury RR, Vallania F, Yang Q, *et al.* A multi-cohort study of the immune factors associated with *M. tuberculosis* infection outcomes. *Nature* 2018; 560: 644–648.

104. Bhattacharya A, Ranadive SN, Kale M, *et al.* Antibody-based enzyme-linked immunosorbent assay for determination of immune complexes in clinical tuberculosis. *Am Rev Respir Dis* 1986; 134: 205–209.

105. Jiang H, Luo TL, Kang J, *et al.* Expression of Rv2031c-Rv2626c fusion protein in *Mycobacterium smegmatis* enhances bacillary survival and modulates innate immunity in macrophages. *Mol Med Rep* 2018; 17: 7307–7312.

106. World Health Organization. Xpert MTB/RIF implementation manual: technical and operational "how-to"; practical considerations. Geneva, World Health Organization, 2014.

107. Theron G, Zijenah L, Chanda D, *et al.* Feasibility, accuracy and clinical effect of point-of-care Xpert MTB/RIF testing for tuberculosis in primary-care settings in Africa: a multicentre, randomised, controlled trial. *Lancet* 2014; 383: 424–435.

108. Lessells RJ, Cooke GS, McGrath N, *et al.* Impact of point-of-care Xpert MTB/RIF on tuberculosis treatment initiation. *Am J Respir Crit Care Med* 2017; 196: 901–910.

109. Vinuesa V, Borrás R, Briones ML, *et al.* Performance of a highly-sensitive *Mycobacterium tuberculosis*-complex real-time PCR assay for the diagnosis of pulmonary tuberculosis in a low prevalence setting: a prospective intervention study. *J Clin Microbiol* 2018; 56: e00116–8.

110. Vella V, broad A, Drobniewski F. Should all suspected tuberculosis cases in high income countries be tested with GeneXpert? *Tuberculosis* 2018; 110: 112–120.

111. Quan TQ, Bawa Z, Foster D, *et al.* Evaluation of whole-genome sequencing for mycobacterial species identification and drug susceptibility testing in a clinical setting: a large-scale prospective assessment of performance against line probe assays and phenotyping. *J Clin Microbiol* 2017; 56: e01480–17.

112. Yang Y, Niehaus KE, Walker TM, *et al.* Machine learning for classifying tuberculosis drug-resistance from DNA sequencing data. *Bioinformatics* 2018; 34: 1666–1671.

113. Xie YL, Chakravorty S, Armstrong DT, *et al.* Evaluation of a rapid molecular drug-susceptibility test for tuberculosis. *N Engl J Med* 2017; 377: 1043–1054.

114. Doyle RM, Burgess C, Williams R, *et al.* Direct whole genome sequencing of sputum accurately identifies drug resistant *Mycobacterium tuberculosis* faster than MGIT culture sequencing. *J Clin Microbiol* 2018: e00666–18.

115. Bothamley GH, Lange C TBNET. Infection control, genetic assessment of drug resistance and drug susceptibility testing in the current management of multidrug/extensively drug-resistant tuberculosis (M/XDR-TB) in Europe: a Tuberculosis Network European Trialsgroup (TBNET) study). *Respir Med* 2017; 132: 68–75.

116. Raviglione MC. Evolution of strategies for control and elimination. *In:* Migliori GB, Bothamley G, Duarte R, *et al.,* eds. Tuberculosis (ERS Monograph). Sheffield, European Respiratory Society, 2018; pp. 36–61.

117. Caminero JA, Scardigli A, van der Werf T, *et al.* Treatment of drug-susceptible and drug resistant TB. *In:* Migliori GB, Bothamley G, Duarte R, *et al.,* eds. Tuberculosis (ERS Monograph). Sheffield, European Respiratory Society, 2018; pp. 152–178.

118. Viney K, Wingfield T, Kuksa L, *et al.* Access and adherence to TB prevention and care for hard-to-reach groups. *In:* Migliori GB, Bothamley G, Duarte R, *et al.,* eds. Tuberculosis (ERS Monograph). Sheffield, European Respiratory Society, 2018; pp. 291–307.

119. Alipanah N, Jarlsberg L, Miller C, *et al.* Adherence interventions and outcomes of tuberculosis treatment: a systematic review and meta-analysis of trials and observational studies. *PLoS Med* 2018; 15: e1002595.

120. Wingfield T, Boccia D, Tover M, *et al.* Defining catastrophic costs and comparing their importance for adverse tuberculosis outcome with multi-drug resistance: a prospective cohort study, Peru. *PLoS Med* 2014; 11: e1001675.

121. World Health Organization. Protocol for survey to determine direct and indirect costs due to TB and to estimate proportion of TB-affected households experiencing catastrophic total costs due to TB. Geneva, World Health Organization, 2015.

122. Rudgard WE, Evans CA, Sweeney S, *et al.* Comparison of two cash transfer strategies to prevent catastrophic costs for poor tuberculosis-affected households in low- and middle-income countries: an economic modelling study. *PLoS Med* 2017; 14: e1002418.

123. Richterman A, Steer-Massaro J, Jarolimova J, *et al.* Cash interventions to improve clinical outcomes for pulmonary tuberculosis: a systematic review and meta-analysis. *Bull World Health Organ* 2018; 96: 471–483.

124. Wingfield T, Tovar MA, Datta S, *et al.* Addressing social determinants to end tuberculosis. *Lancet* 2018; 391: 1129–1132.

125. Valle AM. The Mexican experience in monitoring and evaluation of public policies addressing social determinants of health. *Glob Health Action* 2016; 9: 29030.

126. Knaul FM, González-Pier E, Gómez-Dantés O, *et al.* The quest for universal health coverage: achieving social protection for all in Mexico. *Lancet* 2012; 380: 1259–1279.

127. Nery JS, Rodrigues LC, Rasella D, *et al.* Effect of Brazil's conditional cash programme on tuberculosis incidence. *Int J Tuberc Lung Dis* 2017; 21: 790–796.

128. Anderson RM, May RM. Coevolution of hosts and parasites. *Parasitology* 1982; 85: 411–426.

129. Sreevatsan S, Pan X, Stockbauer KE, *et al.* Restricted structural gene polymorphism in the *Mycobacterium tuberculosis* complex indicates evolutionarily recent global dissemination. *Proc Natl Acad Sci USA* 1997; 94: 9869–9874.

130. Ribeiro SCM, Lima Gomes L, Amarai EP, *et al. Mycobacterium tuberculosis* strains of the modern sublineage of the Beijing family are more likely to display increased virulence than strains of the ancient sublineage. *J Clin Microbiol* 2014; 52: 2615–2624.

131. May RM, Anderson RM. Epidemiology and genetics in the coevolution of parasites and hosts. *Proc R Soc Lond, B, Biol Sci* 1983; 219: 281–313.

https://doi.org/10.1183/2312508X.10026118

132. Huffnagle GB, Dickson RP, Lukacs NW. The respiratory tract microbiome and lung inflammation: a two-way street. *Mucosal Immunol* 2017; 10: 299–306.

133. Kim D, Hofstaedter CE, Zhao C, *et al.* Optimizing methods and dodging pitfalls in microbiome research. *Microbiome* 2017; 5: 52.

134. Namasivayam S, Sher A, Glickman MS, *et al.* The microbiome and tuberculosis: early evidence for cross talk. *mBio* 2018; 9: e01420–18.

135. Von Mutius E, Pearce N, Beasley R, *et al.* International patterns of tuberculosis and the prevalence of symptoms of asthma, rhinitis and eczema. *Thorax* 2000; 55: 449–453.

136. Shirakawa T, Enomoto T, Shimazu S, *et al.* The inverse association between tuberculin responses and atopic disorder. *Science* 1997; 275: 77–79.

137. Alm JS, Lilja G, Pershagen G, *et al.* Early BCG vaccination and development of atopy. *Lancet* 1997; 350: 400–403.

138. Magis-Escurra C, Carvalho ACC, Kritski AL, *et al.* Comorbidities. *In:* Migliori GB, Bothamley G, Duarte R, *et al.*, eds. Tuberculosis (ERS Monograph). Sheffield, European Respiratory Society, 2018; pp. 276–290.

139. Bryant JM, Grogono DM, Greaves D, *et al.* Whole-genome sequencing to identify transmission of *Mycobacterium abscessus* between patients with cystic fibrosis: a retrospective cohort study. *Lancet* 2013; 381: 1551–1560.

140. Baker AW, Lewis SS, Alexander BD, *et al.* Two-phase hospital-associated outbreak of *Mycobacterium abscessus*: investigation and mitigation. *Clin Infect Dis* 2017; 64: 902–911.

141. Pasipanodya JG, Ogbonna D, Ferro BE, *et al.* Systematic review and meta-analyses of the effect of chemotherapy on pulmonary *Mycobacterium abscessus* outcomes and disease recurrence. *Antimicrob Agents Chemother* 2017; 61: e01206–17.

Disclosures: None declared.

Acknowledgements: With many thanks to the reviewers and members of the Dept of Immunology and Infection at the London School of Hygiene and Tropical Medicine (London, UK).

Chapter 25

Opportunities for training and learning

Caterina Casalini[1], Alberto Matteelli[2,3], Albert Komba[1], Lia D'Ambrosio[4] and Jan van den Hombergh[5]

This chapter discusses the key global learning platforms in TB, and describes findings from published studies about TB training and how such training has been evaluated. Key findings from our literature review show that training can be strengthened by: an understanding of the audience; conducting a needs assessment; designing an interactive course with specific learning objectives; including exercises and activities into the curriculum that allow trainees to practice their skills; performing onsite clinical mentoring and monitoring afterwards; and ensuring that healthcare providers and managers work collaboratively towards common outcomes. A favourable environment is also essential to motivate participants to transfer their knowledge to other colleagues at work and to apply their knowledge to service delivery. An evaluation of training provided is essential to understand the power of such investment and to guide future programming. However, evaluations need to be structured in a way that minimises bias and focuses on clinical outcomes.

Cite as: Casalini C, Matteelli A, Komba A, *et al.* Opportunities for training and learning. *In:* Migliori GB, Bothamley G, Duarte R, *et al.*, eds. Tuberculosis (ERS Monograph). Sheffield, European Respiratory Society, 2018; pp. 430–445 [https://doi.org/10.1183/2312508X.10022917].

🐦 @ERSpublications
The ingredients of effective training are: a participatory hands-on curriculum; long-term tutoring; regular supervision; a supportive working environment; and external evaluation that assesses fidelity to procedures and desirable clinical outcomes. http://ow.ly/cfVQ30lqCfE

O ver the years of development aid in TB control, resources have been allocated to ensure that: services are provided by competent healthcare workers, who are trained using robust task-oriented curricula implemented by highly-skilled facilitators; human resource plans are developed and coordinators are identified at government level; task shifting is included in the curricula and TB is addressed by pre-service education. For these reasons, the way in which training is delivered has also evolved, from formal classroom-based training, which was highly theoretical, to more hands-on curricula, which included practice sessions, and finally to the most recent distance learning platforms.

[1]Jhpiego Tanzania, Dar es Salaam, Tanzania. [2]WHO Collaborating Centre for TB/HIV and TB elimination. [3]Dept of Infectious and Tropical Diseases, University of Brescia, Brescia, Italy. [4]Public Health Consulting Group, Lugano, Switzerland. [5]AIDS Health Care Foundation, Los Angeles, CA, USA.

Correspondence: Caterina Casalini, Jhpiego Tanzania, Plot 72, Block 45B, Victoria Area, New Bagamoyo Road, PO Box 9170, Dar es Salaam, Tanzania. E-mail: caterina.casalini@jhpiego.org

Copyright ©ERS 2018. Print ISBN: 978-1-84984-099-6. Online ISBN: 978-1-84984-100-9. Print ISSN: 2312-508X. Online ISSN: 2312-5098.

This chapter aims to guide the reader through the variety of certified global training platforms that are currently available and discusses the lessons that can be learned from training implementation in the field (presented in text boxes), using currently published resources. The chapter focuses primarily on capacity-building amongst healthcare providers; education and training amongst patients, any cadre of educators and community workers, and pre-service training are only addressed in relation to the providers' training.

Search methods

We carried out a non-systematic review of the literature based on a PubMed search using specific keywords, including various combinations of the terms "TB", "training", "healthcare worker" or "healthcare provider" and "human resource" for the period 2011–2018 and from a variety of journals, including the *International Journal of Tuberculosis and Lung Diseases*. A reference list of the most important studies was also retrieved in order to improve the sensitivity of the research. Manuscripts written in English were selected. In addition, websites of the key TB training institutions were included; short clinical courses organised by international scientific societies were not considered, as they were out of the scope of this review.

Global training resources

This section provides an overview of the global distance learning platforms that have the most relevant training available and are supported by institutions with long-standing experience in TB.

Upcoming distance learning platforms represent an opportunity to reduce the time that frontline workers spend on travel to training, and offer (after having received a formal training) the option to enrol into long-term curricula with continuous mentoring and guidance on clinical management. However, despite the globalisation of distance education and learning, there remains an opportunity to rapidly scale up TB training at a fraction of the cost of classroom-based learning. Most countries in need do still face challenges, such as accessing reliable internet networks and using providers with basic computer skills. However, distance learning is not necessarily synonymous with internet-based learning; postal correspondence courses and narrow-cast radio and television media may be used to supplement onsite clinical training that aims to improve knowledge and skills for TB control [1, 2].

CDC has a readily accessible online resource for education and training (www.cdc.gov/tb/education/default.htm). It enables TB professionals to network, share resources, and build education and training skills. It also includes self-study modules on TB as well continuing-education activities. CDC's Division of Tuberculosis Elimination is funding four TB Centers of Excellence for Training, Education, and Medical Consultation during the period 2018–2022: the Curry International Tuberculosis Center (University of California, San Francisco, CA, USA); the Global Tuberculosis Institute (Rutgers, The State University of New Jersey, Newark, NJ, USA); Heartland National Tuberculosis Center (The University of Texas Health Science Center at Tyler, Tyler, TX, USA); and the Southeastern National Tuberculosis Center (Gainesville, FL, USA) [3]. The aim is to increase human resource development through education and training activities, and to increase the capacity for

Table 1. Main publications on training published by WHO

Title	WHO reference number	Objectives	Target audience
Checklist for the review of the human resource development component of national plans to control tuberculosis [4]	WHO/HTM/TB/ 2005.350	Conduct a systematic review of the human resource development component of the National Tuberculosis Programme	Anyone involved in a systematic review of the human resource development component of the National Tuberculosis Programme
Management of tuberculosis training for district TB coordinators. How to organize training for district TB coordinators [5]	WHO/HTM/TB/ 2005.353	Describe how to prepare for a full course, training or briefing facilitators, and directing a full course	National or provincial level staff responsible for training District TB Coordinators
Task analysis – the basis for the development of training in management of tuberculosis [6]	WHO/HTM/TB/ 2005.354	Conduct task analysis of the human resources engaged in TB control and clinical management, before developing a training course	Anyone involved in training curriculum development
Management of collaborative TB/HIV activities. Training for managers at the national and subnational levels [7]	WHO/HTM/TB/ 2005.359a,b, c; WHO/HIV/ 2005.10a	Assist countries in developing and organising country-specific TB/HIV courses for national and subnational TB and HIV/ AIDS managers	Managers at national and subnational levels
Strengthening the teaching of tuberculosis control in basic training programmes. A manual for instructors of nurses and other health care workers [8]	WHO/HTM/TB/ 2006.367	Provide information on the professional functions related to TB control based on the DOTS strategy Propose a standard curriculum for a training programme covering the professional functions related to TB control based on the DOTS strategy Provide information on educational methodology, planning and evaluation of the training programme	Heads of education programmes and instructors in basic training programmes responsible for education on TB control based on the DOTS strategy Authorities concerned with professional education and curriculum development Personnel responsible for human resource planning and development Administrators and supervisors of health services

Continued

https://doi.org/10.1183/2312508X.10022917

Table 1. Continued

Title	WHO reference number	Objectives	Target audience
ENGAGE-TB: Training of community health workers and community volunteers. Integrating community-based tuberculosis activities into the work of nongovernmental and other civil society organizations [9]	WHO/HTM/TB/ 2015.18	Assist facilitators in training community health workers and community volunteers in integrating community-based TB services into their work.	Facilitators of community worker training

appropriate medical evaluation and management of those with TB and LTBI through medical consultation.

Another equally important global resource is the WHO training course on "Implementing the WHO End TB strategy and on the new vision of TB elimination: skills for managers and consultants" (www.publichealthcg.com/training-courses.html). The course uses a fictitious country (Fictitia) in which all the activities take place. It is interactive and exercise-based, offering a mixture of presentations, exercises, workshops, site visits and role plays based on data from Fictitia. The course is aimed at individuals responsible for planning, organising, implementing and evaluating control activities for TB and MDR-TB, within the framework of the implementation of the End TB WHO Strategy, at a national and subnational level. The course's evaluation is based on: the participant's capacity to prepare high-quality mission reports for Fictitia; their problem-solving capacity; and the quality, feasibility and effectiveness of their recommendations about the Fictitia scenarios. Assessments are also subject-specific, including, for example: 1) evaluation of how the participants measure the air changes per hour immediately after the module on infection control; and 2) the participant's capacity to use the QuanTB Tool (created by Systems for Improved Access to Pharmaceutical and Services (SIAPS); http://siapsprogram.org/tools-and-guidance/quantb/), an electronic forecasting, quantification and early warning tool designed to improve procurement processes, ordering and planning for TB treatment. To date, such training has reached about half of the global workforce of the national TB programmes.

A number of publications are available on the WHO website (www.who.int/tb/publications). Table 1 lists all the publications and describes the key objective of each document [4–9].

The WHO End TB team has also developed a set of modules on "Management of TB training for health facility staff" [10]. This was coordinated by WHO and the following organisations contributed through the Tuberculosis Control Assistance Program (TB-CAP): the American Thoracic Society (ATS), Management Sciences for Health (MSH), the CDC and the KNCV Tuberculosis Foundation. The original versions of the training modules (published by WHO in 2003) were field-tested in Malawi with the support of the National Tuberculosis Control Programme of Malawi [11]. The updated version (2009) [10] was tested with the support of the Division of Tuberculosis Elimination of the CDC. The thirteen modules (table 2) were then rolled out globally by adapting the content to the local context, through national TB control programmes. Each module typically has: a closing section that provides a summary of the most important points; self-assessment questions and answers; exercises; and an annex of monitoring and evaluation tools that are relevant to the topic. The package is one of the first examples of a well-structured curriculum that is organised into modules, based on topics that can be taught separately at different times. Therefore, the facilitator can structure the teaching based on the knowledge and skills gap of the audience. The modules also combine theoretical aspects of TB control, along with activities that allow the participants to immediately apply their knowledge on clinical management and on the use of recording tools.

Adapting WHO training modules to the country context: an example from Ethiopia.
The modules on "Management of TB training for health facility staff" were adapted to a country-specific setting [10]. The WHO country team presented the package to the National Tuberculosis and Leprosy Control Programme, followed by consultations with other stakeholders and donors. Subsequently, a task analysis for each group of TB service providers was conducted and learning objectives were developed, using the WHO training package as a reference. Exercises were adapted to meet the local language and context, and modules were customised to comply with national guidelines, and monitoring and evaluation tools. The first draft of the modules was field tested and further adaptations were made prior to national roll out. As a spin-off of this activity, the Ministry of Education was approached to support the review of the TB module's pre-service curricula for nurses, clinical officers and medical doctors. Similarly, the in-service training package was used as a reference to develop the curriculum for a newly established group of health extension workers, who are dedicated to improving access to care in rural communities.

In 2008, WHO published an interesting handbook entitled *Planning the Development of Human Resources for Health for Implementation of the Stop TB Strategy* [12]. The handbook provides country-specific strategic and annual implementation plans for human resource development as part of a comprehensive TB control programme, and within overall human resource for health development.

The IUATLD offers training courses for a large variety of topics and competencies (www. unioncourses.org). The courses can be customised on request and are facilitated by medical doctors, researchers, clinicians and other public health professionals who specialise in TB, TB-HIV and MDR-TB. Participants are eligible for continuing education units and continuing medical education credits. The courses are accredited both by the International Association for Continuing Education and Training (IACET), and the European Board for Accreditation in Pneumology (EBAP). Some courses can be accessed online, while others are field-based (tables 3 and 4).

The WHO collaborating centre on prevention and control of TB in prisons in Azerbaijan [13], formally founded in 2012, offers a 16-module training course to medical and non-medical personnel in the penitentiary system. Amongst other areas, the curriculum includes: DR-TB management; laboratory quality management; the specifics of infection control measures in penitentiaries; and the application of new TB drugs in specialised treatment institutions. Training includes study tours to learn about TB control in penitentiary facilities.

The Curry International Tuberculosis Center (CITC) in California (USA) has a TB training and education toolbox that provides users with the tools and step-by-step guides required

https://doi.org/10.1183/2312508X.10022917

Table 2. Modules in WHO's *Management of Tuberculosis training for Health Facility Staff* [10]

Title	WHO reference number
Introduction	WHO/HTM/TB/2009.423a
Detect cases of TB	WHO/HTM/TB/2009.423b
Treat TB patients	WHO/HTM/TB/2009.423c
Inform patients about TB	WHO/HTM/TB/2009.423d
Identify and supervise community TB treatment supporters	WHO/HTM/TB/2009.423e
Manage drugs and supplies for TB	WHO/HTM/TB/2009.423f
Ensure continuation of TB treatment	WHO/HTM/TB/2009.423g
Monitor TB case detection and treatment	WHO/HTM/TB/2009.423h
TB infection control in your health facility	WHO/HTM/TB/2009.423i
Field exercise – observe TB management	WHO/HTM/TB/2009.423j
Management of tuberculosis – reference booklet	WHO/HTM/TB/2009.423k
Facilitator guide	WHO/HTM/TB/2009.423l
Answer sheets	WHO/HTM/TB/2009.423m

to develop and implement TB training for clinicians and other health workers [14]. CITC also offers a variety of courses on sexually transmitted infections/HIV/TB, TB case management and contact investigation, and TB in nursing. Under the leadership of the CITC, the University of California San Francisco and the ATS have been working to develop the implementation phases of the International Standards for Tuberculosis Care (ISTC) in five countries (Kenya, Tanzania, India, Indonesia and Mexico). The ISTC

Table 3. The field-based training courses offered by the IUATLD

Course	Objective	Key topics
International Management Development Programme (IMDP)	Train in the management competencies that are essential for the provision of quality healthcare	Developing budgets that meet governmental and/or donor requirements Organising and training healthcare staff at different levels Coordinating the procurement and management of medicines and supplies Handling human resources issues, such as motivating overworked staff Creating communication plans to disseminate important health messages Adhering to the practices required for monitoring and evaluating programme performance
TB and Lung Health	Train in clinical and programmatic aspects of TB, MDR-TB, TB-HIV and tobacco control	Contributing to the implementation of public health programmes that provide quality diagnosis, treatment and care for patients with TB Building the capacity of health professionals to record, report, monitor and evaluate the services that are provided Ensuring continuous quality assurance and strengthening consultation with patients and communities Responding to a country situation as necessary

Table 4. The online training courses offered by the IUATLD

Course	Content	Website
Childhood TB Learning Portal	Includes modules on: Childhood TB for Healthcare Workers; and Childhood MDR TB for Healthcare Workers	www.unioncourses.org/childhood-tb-learning-portal
Child TB Training Toolkit	Focuses on building the capacity of healthcare workers at the primary and secondary level to address and manage TB in children	www.unioncourses.org/child-tb-training-toolkit
TREAT TB E-tools	Develops the skills required to conduct high-quality operational research in high-burden countries	www.unioncourses.org/treat-tb-e-tools
Acid-Fast Direct Smear Microscopy: A Laboratory Training Programme	Complements laboratory manuals by demonstrating appropriate techniques, emphasising standard methods, and promoting consistent reading and reporting of smear results	www.unioncourses.org/acid-fast-direct-smear-microscopy-a-laboratory-training-programme
Structured Operational Research and Training Initiative (SORT IT)	Three 6-day modules spaced out over 9–12 months; the focus is on the development of the practical skills for conducting and publishing operational research	www.unioncourses.org/category/operational-research

https://doi.org/10.1183/2312508X.10022917

training materials provide educational tools that assist national TB programmes and other public and private TB providers to effectively adapt the standards to meet country-specific needs. Specialised webinars are available within the archive, on paediatric TB radiology, GeneXpert (Cepheid, Sunnyvale, CA, USA) field experiences, DILI, TB and diabetes.

The KNCV Tuberculosis Foundation to Eliminate TB in The Netherlands represents another valuable resource. Their Knowledge Center is a platform from which users can learn about the challenges in TB control in a vast range of countries (www.kncvtbc.org/en/knowledge-center/); its format offers a useful digest for both managers and healthcare workers. The Knowledge Center provides: expert training tools; a guide to the collection, analysis and use of TB data for healthcare workers; and country-specific training guides.

The Institute Pasteur in Paris (France) offers 2-week course (www.pasteur.fr/en/tuberculosis) to medical doctors, veterinarians, directors of clinical mycobacteriology laboratories, pharmacists and research scientists who wish to acquire up-to-date knowledge about TB and the practice of molecular methods for diagnosis, DST and epidemiology.

Clinical curricula for different categories of health staff

Landscaping training programmes

The development of efficient human resources is vital to facilitate TB control in developing countries; appropriate training of front-line staff is an important component of this process. With the resources that are available to improve TB control in countries in Africa and Central Asia, it is important to highlight context-specific training benchmarks and propose how deficiencies in human resources can be addressed, at least in part through the efficient (re-)training of frontline TB workers.

In most lower-middle income countries, when TB training is incorporated into the pre-service curriculum of physicians, nurses, community health officers and laboratory technicians, the quality of the training varies widely within and between countries. In many TB-endemic countries, the general education and health systems are not of optimal standard to support effective TB control and pre-training services. Moreover, systems for evaluating the quality of TB training need to be strengthened in these settings.

The effectiveness and sustainability of an integrated TB programme depends upon the extent to which training is of a uniformly high quality. Poor performance may be due to an insufficient number of health staff, or may be because care is not provided according to standards and/or is not responsive to the needs of the community and patients.

Assessment of the service outcome often recommends that providers should receive training. An example of this can be seen in a survey performed in Botswana, which recommended the roll out of additional TB training courses as result of variability in healthcare workers' knowledge about childhood TB [15]. Past investment in training courses may not always have impacted on the quality of service delivery and training evaluation often fails to describe an association with clinical outcome.

In addition to training, other factors can influence the productivity of TB control providers, including: personal and lifestyle-related factors; living circumstances; the adequacy of preparation for work during pre-service education; health system-related factors, such as the human resources policy and planning; job satisfaction-related factors, such as financial remuneration, infrastructure and working conditions, management capacity and styles, professional advancement and safety at work. These elements make up a "productivity mix"; TB training is an important component of this mix.

Even though there has been an increasing amount of funding healthcare provider training in TB, publications from robust evaluations that assess the impact on quality of care and behaviour change are limited. Such evaluations usually assess whether training objectives were achieved, and whether the accomplishment of those objectives resulted in enhanced performance on the job. In addition, evaluation results help ensure that training meets the needs of learners and organisations.

Training outcomes: country-specific examples

Findings from Kenya suggest that the increasing advocacy and involvement of specialised professional sectors with the National TB Programme, result in the development of more specific guidelines and training materials, and increases healthcare worker capacity in the implementation of TB prevention and cure [16].

FARLEY et al. [16] that healthcare providers with the highest level of clinical training have the greatest infection control knowledge, as well as a better attitude towards infection control practices; participation in facility-specific infection control training in the previous year was associated with a significantly higher knowledge score. However, an infection control plan and annual TB training was not associated with greater knowledge among participating healthcare providers [17]. Another study showed that greater knowledge was associated with in-service training by infection control nurses [18].

> A combination of robust pre-service training along with supervised clinical practice for a long period of time, might be the ingredient required for a long-term successful service outcome.

In Zambia and Botswana, longitudinal monitoring of TB infection control before and after the implementation of comprehensive training and an infection control-improvement intervention, resulted in significant improvements in infection control practices by healthcare workers at outpatient HIV facilities [19]. Other studies have shown that the presence of a trained TB infection control practitioner or focal person can result in reduced infection rates and improved outcomes [20].

In a descriptive, observational intervention study performed in the Philippines, a questionnaire was administered to X-ray facility radiology technologists before training. Chest radiographs were reviewed before and after technologists underwent the training course. The study's findings suggest that the training course had a positive impact on chest radiograph quality. The training course covered topics relating to chest radiograph quality in the context of the National Tuberculosis Programme, including lectures on the role of chest radiography in TB diagnosis, practices on the assessment sheet for chest radiograph imaging quality, developed by the Tuberculosis Coalition for Technical Assistance (TBCTA), and a field trip to X-ray facilities [21].

https://doi.org/10.1183/2312508X.10022917

This is another set of evidence that training, including practical exercises and field clinical experience, as well the identification of a trained focal person within the clinic, could play a key role in achieving a successful outcome.

An educational participatory theatre intervention that aimed to reduce the risk of occupational TB among healthcare workers in South Africa demonstrated that such an approach was acceptable to participants, met a defined demand, proved adaptable to the target group and was practical if performed during working hours or if integrated into existing training sessions [22]. The theatre approach, which is based on warm-up exercises, image theatre and role plays from the work of FREIRE [23] and BOAL [24], strengthened social cohesion *via* group work and reported a subsequent increase in vigilance regarding occupational TB; overall it was found to be a useful, culturally appropriate supplement to existing educational approaches to the prevention and management of occupational TB.

An assessment into the effect of participating in TB infection control training courses conducted at the Tuberculosis Infection Control Training Center in Machiton, Tajikistan, reported that participants were motivated to return to their work facility and engage with colleagues and facility leadership to share their knowledge about infection control principles and practices, and potential improvements that could be made within their facility. Training also appeared to have a positive impact on infection control practices in participants' workplaces [25].

In South African clinicians who regularly manage children with TB, an evaluation of training in the interpretation of chest radiographs in high TB-HIV settings showed that those with some paediatric or radiology training improved more than those with less training. Training also improved the participant's ability to correctly identify normal and unreadable chest radiographs but made only a minimal difference in their ability to correctly identify TB [26]. A cross-sectional and observational study performed in Manila (the Philipines), to evaluate the performance of radiology technicians 3 years after their participation in a training course that aimed to improve chest radiograph quality, showed that training had a positive and relatively long-term impact on maintaining quality, in terms of density, contrast, sharpness and artefacts. Two senior experts, blinded for dates and names of the facilities, evaluated the CXR films independently and the final scores were determined after free discussion between the two, to avoid systemic bias [27].

The more complex the competencies required for a particular task, the more crucial the background education of the provider in determining the outcome of the training. Therefore, training courses should be tailored to the baseline skills of the audiences, as well based on a specific set of competencies that the audience is expected to acquire as a result of the training. This approach would add more density to the work required for curriculum development and would require rolling out a larger volume of training to a variety of professionals based on their background and experience, layering different kind of skills.

When considering the outcome of training, stigma and discrimination, legal issues, peer-pressure and cultural factors should be considered. Findings from three service provision assessment surveys among healthcare workers in Kenya, Tanzania and Namibia, show that having received pre-service and on-the-job training in confidentiality was positively associated with the recognition of discriminatory behaviour [28]. Discrimination was more frequently observed in health facilities without regular supervision, as discrimination is usually fostered, and needs a permissive climate to persist; this also applies to healthcare settings with structural and organisational policies, which in practice are not always enforced.

It should be acknowledged that increased knowledge alone does not overcome all the barriers identified by the healthcare providers. Monitoring and supervisory field visits after training remain key to ensure sustained knowledge and adherence to standards by the providers. After training, supportive supervision is a critical tool to ensure that over time, providers are delivering the service according to the procedures and standards, and that staff turnover is addressed. If supervisors are available to answer questions from the providers, to identify and address incorrect practices, to recommend refresher training when necessary, and to assist providers in troubleshooting problems, the likelihood of achieving a successful clinical outcome will be higher.

The importance of offering client-centred services has recently been globally recognised, and training curricula have started addressing this as part of the learning objectives. For example, training developed by nurses with field expertise in Ethiopia used a best-practice, patient-centred approach and aimed to provide selected nurses with the skills required to train others on what is required to improve patient care [29]. In addition to lectures, problem-solving activities and negotiation skills, training involved a variety of participatory methods, including brainstorming, group work, discussion, and strengths, weaknesses, opportunities and threats (SWOT) analysis. Interview and assessment visits to observe clinical practice after training were conducted by the lead trainers without an external reviewer. Evaluation findings showed a behavioural change to reduce the risk of transmission of TB and MDR-TB, as most of the trained nurses showed a greater responsibility towards prevention and control of TB/MDR-TB in their healthcare facilities.

From a wide range of country-based evidence, we have learned that transforming attitudes, practice and outcomes requires several elements to come together: competency-based curricula with specific learning objectives, tailored to the participants' background and level of expertise. A curriculum that addresses issues related to accessing good-quality care at each stage of a patient's diagnosis and treatment, and that enables participants to identify and address barriers with their colleagues, is one of the key elements to a robust learning programme. Such training should be followed by long-term onsite mentoring activities. In addition, evidence shows that when training is conducted alongside other complementary activities (e.g. community awareness and village meetings with leaders and district health administrators, delivery of messages at schools, local associations, and meetings with community-based organisations and beneficiaries) the clinical outcome might improve further.

A cluster-randomised trial in which community awareness activities were held alongside healthcare worker training at microscopy centres in Bangladesh increased TB notification and treatment rates significantly more at intervention than control centres [30]. Similarly, a combination of community care worker training, structural adjustments, harmonisation of the scope of practice and stipend of community care workers, and enhanced supervision of community care workers to provide comprehensive TB-HIV prevention of mother-to-child transmission services in rural South African districts, showed a large increase in the uptake of services in the intervention arm compared to the control arm, particularly for TB and sexually transmitted infection screening, sputum collection and treatment adherence support, including adherence to dual therapy [31].

https://doi.org/10.1183/2312508X.10022917

In such complex scenarios, NGOs provide interim assistance to rapidly up-skill front-line workers in order to assist with the management of patients already in need of TB treatment. Task-shifting policies have been introduced that engage a variety of healthcare worker groups and aim to maximise human resource capabilities by striking a balance between quality, affordability and programme objectives.

A study in Bangladesh showed that training barely literate but motivated and supervised community healthcare workers in DOTS in rural areas produced similar cure and success rates to those seen with more qualified staff [32]. Malawi also moved towards a broad task-shifting approach and in this framework, offered one-day training on TB screening to community healthcare workers who were stationed at one ART clinic. Training involved an introduction to the TB screening questions as well as familiarisation with the flow of services to the client, until diagnosis. Those who were diagnosed with TB began treatment and, if a problem with adherence was identified, subjects were provided with adherence support by the community health worker at the facility or *via* home visits. The community healthcare worker case managers assisted with community tracing for anyone who was lost to follow-up, and linked with other community healthcare workers for combined home-based TB and HIV contact tracing. An evaluation of the effectiveness of the intervention (which was based on 16 months pre- and post-intervention data, extracted from registers and tools used by the community healthcare workers) showed a 20-fold increase in case detection, along with an immediate increase of 6.7 monthly diagnoses. The rate of increase of monthly TB diagnoses improved by 0.78 diagnoses per month in the post-intervention period compared with the pre-intervention period [33].

Another interesting example comes again from Malawi, where lay health workers received 2 weeks' training using didactic and interactive techniques, including case-based learning and role-playing to convey TB and adherence knowledge and counselling skills, and to allow for experiential learning through practice, using the point-of-care tool, critical reflection and the exchange of ideas [34]. This multicentre, pragmatic, cluster-RCT assessed the impact of a knowledge translation strategy of TB outcomes, by employing qualitative methods, such as interviews with lay healthcare workers and patients, document analysis of training logs, quarterly peer trainer meetings and mentorship meeting notes. The researchers found no significant treatment effect of the intervention.

Such findings highlight the complexity of the factors that influence compliance to procedures and standards, even after participatory training followed by onsite mentoring. Motivation, attitude, emotional intelligence, support from management and peers, environment, open-mindedness of trainees and mentors, job-related factors, self-efficacy and basic ability also affect training effectiveness and outcomes.

Training evaluation

A systematic review of publications evaluating training programmes for TB providers (*e.g.* doctors, nurses, paramedics and lay healthcare workers) was conducted *via* a search of the databases and websites of not-for-profit organisations [35]. The most common methods for assessing the outcomes of healthcare provider training were: 1) patient records to assess diagnostic and treatment outcomes after training; 2) post-training interviews with trainees; and 3) pre- and post-training tests to assess trainee knowledge gain after training. Approaches such as post-training focus group discussions with trainees and observations of the on-the-job performance of trainees were not commonly used; outcomes of the training in terms of improvement of service quality were rarely evaluated. Furthermore, in this specific review, most of the evaluations were conducted in Africa with very limited evidence about training program outcomes from Asia and America.

Post-training tests are limited as they only assess the factual knowledge of trainees and are often conducted right after training, thereby missing assessment of the long-term retention of such knowledge. Qualitative research is usually based on focus group discussions with a small number of trainees and focuses on their subjective feedback on the quality of the service. The actual external on-the-job performance of healthcare providers after training is often not assessed.

Furthermore, evaluations that are based on the trainees' perspective about their post-training practices, such as the assessment of TB infection control training at the Tuberculosis Infection Control Training Center in Machiton (Tajikistan) [25], have a key limitation in that participants' self-reported changes are subject to recall and social desirability bias. Similar concerns are seen in the Bangladesh study, which showed that training community healthcare workers in DOTS produced similar cure and success rates as training in healthcare workers [32], and in the Malawi training evaluation of TB screening in community healthcare workers who were stationed at one ART clinic [33].

Although such evaluations demonstrate interesting findings, their major limitations lay in their small sample size and the potential for selection bias; after training, community healthcare workers may select clients who are most likely to have TB.

Another training evaluation amongst lay healthcare workers from Malawi showed no significant treatment effect of the intervention [34]; however, it is possible that a significant effect was not found due to an implementation rather than a lack of effectiveness of the intervention itself.

Interestingly, this observation leads to the concept of "fidelity" of the implementation and to a wide array of reasons why knowledge does not always translate into the expected practice, despite the willingness and commitment of the service provider. However, fidelity to the expected procedures and standards along with other structural barriers are generally not included in the evaluation.

Multiple frameworks have been developed for the evaluation of training. The most frequently referenced training evaluation framework is the Kirkpatrick Model, which is based on reaction, learning, behaviour and results [36]. The Kirkpatrick-based evaluation has been combined with a novel approach to understanding how and why the outcomes occur through, for example, focus group discussions or in-depth interviews [37]. As existing evaluation models did not provide theoretical and practical resources that could be readily applied to training programs, the PEPFAR (President's Emergency Plan for AIDS Relief) Human Resources for Health Technical Working Group initiated a project to develop an outcome-focused training evaluation framework [38]. The purpose of the framework was to provide practical guidance to health training programmes in diverse international settings as they developed their approach to evaluation. The framework

https://doi.org/10.1183/2312508X.10022917

applies to HIV programmes but represents a useful reference platform for TB programmes in terms of standardising the evaluation approach; however, as it was based on qualitative inquiry (*e.g.* key informant interviews, feedback from stakeholders), the results were influenced by the experiences and perspectives of the researchers. Nevertheless, the framework guides users to consider and incorporate the influence of situational and contextual factors in determining training outcomes. It aims to help programmes target their outcome evaluation activities at a level that best meets their information needs, while recognising the practical limitations of resources, timeframes and the complexities of the systems in which international healthcare worker training programs are implemented.

Conclusion

Wide variations in training duration and structure are poorly correlated with programme performance. In order to demonstrate the outcome of substantial investment in healthcare worker training, WHO, TB associations, research and training institutes and international NGOs need to play an active role in working with national TB programmes to develop and implement standardised training curricula for front-line TB workers.

In order to practice, service providers need information, such as definitions of terms, rules and procedures, requirements, standards and principles. They need to practice skills until they can perform them competently, without assistance, and a mentor should provide opportunities for the trainees to practice skills, first in the classroom and then in the clinic. Use of examples, such as photos, illustrations, slides, audio or video recordings, as well practicing through classroom demonstration, role plays, observation in the field, or field exercise, are great techniques that allow a better understanding of the theoretical teachings. Participation is another essential element of successful training, as participants generally benefit from working directly with colleagues during the learning process.

Each training session must have a lesson plan, including the objective of the module, the duration, the material needed, a description of the preparatory activities, and a description of how to manage each subsection of the teaching module.

Increasing the availability and accessibility of educational materials is also an important aspect that supports and further strengthens capacity-building programmes. Within this framework, the development of a global network of training centres with exchange of knowledge through electronic conferences, discussions, consultations and educational materials, represents an important step towards improving training content and methodology.

Career advancement mechanisms should also be explored and created for all categories of healthcare providers, as well as motivational factors that encourage the continuation of learning and the application of knowledge following participation in a medical education programme.

At the same time, it is important to evaluate the contribution of training to improve healthcare workers' productivity and the quality of TB control programmes. Such evaluation should occur at three levels: 1) during training, through feedback from participants, quality of written and practical training-related assignments undertaken by participants, and pre-test/post-test evaluations; 2) within 12 months of training, through the use of questionnaires to facilitate participants' assessment of the impact of training on their performance, as well as site visits by trainers and external teams, to observe participants in clinical and field conditions; and 3) through assessment of the TB programme's outcomes, with particular attention to improvements in case detection and cure rates.

The skills and knowledge of service providers should be assessed at every opportunity, as they need continuous feedback on the extent of their learning, and the strengths and weaknesses of their attempts to perform skills.

To sum up, delivering effective training requires: a participatory hands-on curriculum that addresses the skills and competencies that trainees need to acquire or strengthen; competent trainers and long-term tutoring at the service delivery site; regular supportive supervision and a supportive working environment; robust external evaluation that assesses fidelity to procedures; and quantitative and qualitative assessment of the desirable clinical outcomes.

References

1. United Nations Educational, Social and Cultural Organization. Open and Distance Learning – Trends, Policy and Strategy Considerations. Paris, UNESCO, 2002. http://unesdoc.unesco.org/images/0012/001284/128463e.pdf

2. Zarocostas J. World Medical Association scales up training for multi-drug resistant tuberculosis to fight epidemic. *BMJ* 2008; 336: 1155.

3. Center for Disease Control and Prevention. Tuberculosis (TB). TB centers of excellence for training, education, and medical consultation. https://www.cdc.gov/tb/education/tb_coe/default.htm Date last accessed: May 29, 2018.

4. World Health Organization. Checklist for the Review of the Human Resource Development Component of National Plans to Control Tuberculosis. WHO/HTM/TB/2005.350. Geneva, World Health Organization, 2005. http://apps.who.int/iris/bitstream/handle/10665/69050/WHO_HTM_TB_2005.350.pdf; jsessionid=0F2009F52B306F1B73D02998913107F1?sequence=1

5. World Health Organization. Management of Tuberculosis Training for District TB Coordinators. How to Organize Training for District TB Coordinators. WHO/HTM/TB/2005.353. Geneva, World Health Organization, 2005. http://www.who.int/tb/publications/tb-training-management/en/

6. World Health Organization. Task Analysis - The Basis for Development of Training in Management of Tuberculosis. WHO/HTM/TB/2005.354. Geneva, World Health Organization, 2005. http://www.who.int/tb/publications/task-analysis-report/en/

7. World Health Organization. Management of Collaborative TB/HIV Activities. Training for Managers at the National and Subnational Levels. WHO/HTM/TB/2005.359a,b,c; WHO/HIV/2005.10a. Geneva, World Health Organization, 2005. http://www.who.int/tb/publications/who_htm_tb_2005_359/en/

8. World Health Organization. Strengthening the Teaching of Tuberculosis Control in Basic Training Programs. A Manual for Instructors of Nurses and other Health Care Workers. WHO/HTM/TB/2006.367. Geneva, World Health Organization, 2006. www.who.int/tb/publications/tb-training-manual/en/

9. World Health Organization. ENGAGE-TB: Training of Community Health Workers and Community Volunteers. Integrating Community-based Tuberculosis Activities into the Work of Nongovernmental and other Civil Society Organizations. WHO/HTM/TB/2015.18. Geneva, World Health Organization, 2015. www.who.int/tb/publications/2015/engage_tb_training/en/

10. World Health Organization. Management of Tuberculosis Training for Health Facility Staff. 2nd Edn. WHO/HTM/TB/2009.423a-m. Geneva, World Health Organization, 2010. www.who.int/tb/publications/2010/who_htm_tb_2009_423/en/

11. Tuberculosis Coalition for Technical Assistance. Task Force Training, World Health Organization. Management of tuberculosis: training for health facility staff. Geneva, World Health Organization, 2003.

12. World Health Organization. Planning the Development of Human Resources for Health for Implementation of the Stop TB Strategy: a Handbook. WHO/HTM/TB/2008.407. Geneva, World Health Organization, 2008. http://apps.who.int/iris/bitstream/handle/10665/44051/9789241597715_eng.pdf;jsessionid=D1491C90F13B7A9D5533F2E488127069?sequence=1

13. The WHO Collaborating Centre on prevention and control of tuberculosis in prisons in Azerbaijan. http://www.euro.who.int/en/countries/azerbaijan/news/news/2018/7/preventing-the-spread-of-tuberculosis-in-prisons-sharing-lessons-from-azerbaijan Date last accessed: May 29, 2018.

https://doi.org/10.1183/2312508X.10022917

14. The Curry International Tuberculosis Center, University of California, San Francisco. Developing and presenting TB control training courses toolbox. www.currytbcenter.ucsf.edu/products/view/developing-and-presenting-tb-control-training-courses-toolbox Date last accessed: May 29, 2018.

15. Arscott-Mills T, Masole L, Ncube R, et al. Survey of health care worker knowledge about childhood tuberculosis in high-burden centers in Botswana. *Int J Tuberc Lung Dis* 2017; 21: 586–591.

16. Maleche-Obimbo E, Wanjau W, Kathure I. The journey to improve the prevention and management of childhood tuberculosis: the Kenyan experience. *Int J Tuberc Lung Dis* 2015; 19: 39–42.

17. Farley E, Tudor C, Mphahlele M, et al. A national infection control evaluation of drug-resistant tuberculosis hospitals in South Africa. *Int J Tuberc Lung Dis* 2012; 16: 82–89.

18. Zoutman DE, Ford BD. The relationship between hospital infection surveillance and control activities and antibiotic resistant pathogen rates. *Am J Infect Control* 2005; 33: 1–5.

19. Emerson C, Lipke V, Kapata N, et al. Evaluation of a TB infection control implementation initiative in out-patient HIV clinics in Zambia and Botswana. *Int J Tuberc Lung Dis* 2016; 20: 941–947.

20. Haley RW, Quade D, Freeman HE, et al. The SENIC Project. Study on the efficacy of nosocomial infection control (SENIC Project). Summary of study design. *Am J Epidemiol* 1980; 111: 472–485.

21. Tuberculosis Coalition for Technical Assistance. Quality assessment of chest X-ray. Handbook for National TB Programs. The Hague, TBCTA, 2008.

22. Parent SN, Ehrlich R, Baxter V, et al. Participatory theatre and tuberculosis: a feasibility study with South African health care workers. *Int J Tuberc Lung Dis* 2017; 21: 140–148.

23. Freire P. Pedagogy of the oppressed. New York, Bloomsbury Publishing, 2000.

24. Boal A. The rainbow of desire: the Boal method of theatre and therapy. New York, Routledge, 1995.

25. Scott C, Mangan J, Tillova Z, et al. Evaluation of the Tuberculosis Infection Control Training Center, Tajikistan, 2014–2015. *Int J Tuberc Lung Dis* 2017; 21: 579–585.

26. Seddon JA, Padayachee T, Du Plessis AM, et al. Teaching chest X-ray reading for child tuberculosis suspects. *Int J Tuberc Lung Dis* 2014; 18: 763–769.

27. Ohkado A, Luna P, Querri A, et al. Impact of a training course on the quality of chest radiography to diagnose pulmonary tuberculosis. *Public Health Action* 2015; 5: 83–88.

28. Straetemans M, Bakker MI, Mitchell EMH. Correlates of observing and willingness to report stigma towards HIV clients by (TB) health workers in Africa. *Int J Tuberc Lung Dis* 2017; 21: 6–18.

29. Tadesse Y, Yesuf M, Williams V. Evaluating the output of transformational patient-centred nurse training in Ethiopia. *Int J Tuberc Lung Dis* 2013; 17: 9–14.

30. Talukder K, Salim MAH, Jerin I, et al. Intervention to increase detection of childhood tuberculosis in Bangladesh. *Int J Tuberc Lung Dis* 2012; 16: 70–75.

31. Uwimana J, Zarowsky C, Hausler H, et al. Community-based intervention to enhance provision of integrated TB-HIV and PMTCT services in South Africa. *Int J Tuberc Lung Dis* 2013; 17: Suppl. 1, 48–55.

32. Islam MA, Wakai S, Ishikawa N, et al. Cost-effectiveness of community health workers in tuberculosis control in Bangladesh. *Bull World Health Organ* 2002; 80: 445–450.

33. Flick R, Simon K, Munthali A, et al. Yield of community health worker-driven intensified case finding for tuberculosis among HIV-positive patients in rural Malawi. 21st International AIDS Conference, Durban, abstract WEAB0204, 2016. http://programme.aids2016.org/Abstract/Abstract/8970. Date last accessed: May 29, 2018.

34. Puchalski Ritchie LM, van Lettow M, Makwakwa A, et al. The impact of a knowledge translation intervention employing educational outreach and a point-of-care reminder tool vs standard lay health worker training on tuberculosis treatment completion rates: study protocol for a cluster randomized controlled trial. *Trials* 2016; 17: 439.

35. Wu S, Roychowdhury I, Khan M. Evaluating the impact of healthcare provider training to improve tuberculosis management: a systematic review of methods and outcome indicators used. *Int J Infect Dis* 2017; 56: 105–110.

36. Kirkpatrick D, Kirkpatrick J. Evaluating Training Programs. San Francisco, Berrett-Koehler Publishers, 2006.

37. Alvarez K, Salas E, Garofano C. An integrated model of training evaluation and effectiveness. *Hum Resour Dev Rev* 2004; 3: 385–416.

38. O'Malley G, Perdue T, Petracca F. A framework for outcome-level evaluation of in-service training of health care workers. *Hum Resour Health* 2013; 11: 50.

Disclosures: None declared.

![ERS logo] ERS | *monograph*

Clinical cases

Simon Tiberi[1,2], Marie Christine Payen[3], Katerina Manika[4], Inês Ladeira[5], Marta Gonzalez Sanz[6] and Marcela Muñoz-Torrico[7]

🐦 @ERSpublications
   Five clinical cases are described, showing some important and challenging presentations of TB
   http://ow.ly/cfVQ30lqCfE

The previous chapters of this *Monograph* have systematically presented various aspects of the presentation, diagnosis and management of TB. In this chapter, we embody these concepts and knowledge and apply them in a clinical context. TB can affect any organ of the body and any age group. The following selected five cases are real-world cases that present some important and challenging presentations, which we hope will be of interest to the reader and stimulate further learning, reflection and discussion.

A case of isoniazid-resistant extrapulmonary tuberculosis and pulmonary tuberculosis

Introduction

Isoniazid-monoresistant TB has been neglected for many years in the literature, despite being much more common than MDR-TB. In fact, the global average proportion of new TB cases resistant to isoniazid but without concurrent rifampicin resistance is 8.5% [1], which rises to 16% in the former Soviet Union countries [2]. Initial isoniazid monoresistance has been linked to poorer treatment outcomes [2, 3] and may lead to a greater risk of developing MDR-TB [4].

A 47-year-old woman of ex-Soviet-Union origin living in both Greece and Germany in the last 5 years presented with difficulty walking due to right ankle pain. She had a 3-month history of cough but no fever, night sweats or weight loss. A magnetic resonance imaging (MRI) scan of the ankle was performed, showing abnormal high signal intensity in the calcaneus and tarsal bones (figure 1a). Bone scintigraphy revealed hyperactive lesions in

[1]Division of Infection, Royal London Hospital, Barts Health NHS Trust, London, UK. [2]Blizard Institute, Barts and The London School of Medicine and Dentistry, Queen Mary University of London, London, UK. [3]Division of Infectious Diseases, CHU Saint-Pierre, Université Libre de Bruxelles (ULB), Brussels, Belgium. [4]Pulmonary Dept, "G. Papanikolaou" Hospital, Aristotle University, Thessaloniki, Greece. [5]Centro Hospitalar Vila Nova de Gaia, Vila Nova de Gaia, Portugal. [6]Division of Infection and Immunity, University College London Hospital, UCL Hospitals NHS Foundation Trust, London, UK. [7]Tuberculosis Clinic, Instituto Nacional de Enfermedades Respiratorias, Mexico City, Mexico.

Correspondence: Simon Tiberi, Division of Infection, Royal London Hospital, Barts Health NHS Trust, 80 Newark Street, London, E1 2ES, UK. E-mail: simon.tiberi@bartshealth.nhs.uk

Copyright ©ERS 2018. Print ISBN: 978-1-84984-099-6. Online ISBN: 978-1-84984-100-9. Print ISSN: 2312-508X. Online ISSN: 2312-5098.

https://doi.org/10.1183/2312508X.10023017

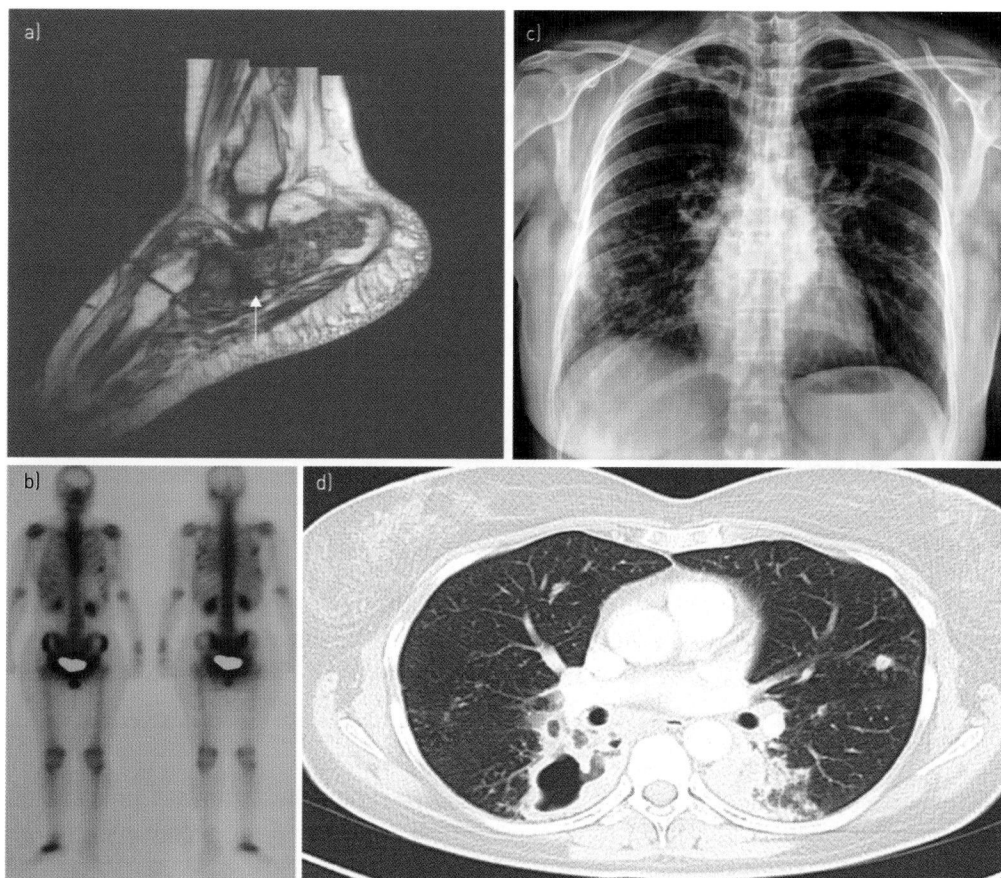

Figure 1. A case of isoniazid-resistant EPTB and PTB. a) Right ankle magnetic resonance imaging scan showing total destruction of the talcnavicular and calcaneocuboid (arrow) joints. b) Bone scintigraphy revealing hyperactive lesions in the sixth, seventh and eighth ribs and right ankle. c) Chest radiograph showing multiple infiltrations and a cavity at the level of the right hilum. d) Chest computed tomography scan showing a right lower lobe cavity along with infiltrations and nodule of the left lower lobe.

several ribs and the right ankle (figure 1b). Suspecting malignancy, a biopsy of the calcaneus was performed but was not diagnostic; no samples were sent for mycobacterial culture.

Pre-operatively, the patient underwent chest radiography, which revealed a cavity of the right lower lobe and infiltrations of the right upper lobe (figure 1c). A chest computed tomography (CT) scan revealed nodules bilaterally, tree-in-bud appearance, infiltrations of the lower lobes and presence of a large cavity in the right lower lobe (figure 1d). Sputum was positive for acid-fast bacilli and PCR positive for *Mycobacterium tuberculosis*, with no *rpoB*, *inhA* or *katG* gene mutations for rifampicin or isoniazid detected (MTBDRplus; Hain Lifescience GmbH, Nehren, Germany). The patient was transferred to the respiratory medicine department, where she was placed in respiratory isolation immediately after her biopsy, and standard quadruple anti-TB treatment was initiated.

The cause of the skeletal lesions was not established at this stage and concurrent metastatic disease was still considered possible. The patient was subjected to an abdomen CT scan, gastroscopy and colonoscopy, but no abnormal findings were detected.

3 weeks later, while the patient had clinically improved, she was still sputum smear positive and, surprisingly, phenotypic DST using the Mycobacteria Growth Indicator Tube revealed monoresistance to isoniazid. Levofloxacin was added to the regimen. The patient became smear negative after another 3 weeks of treatment, her erythrocyte sedimentation rate dropped from 86 to 14 mm·h^{-1} and she was discharged after obtaining three consecutive negative sputum smears. 8 weeks into treatment, she also converted to sputum culture negative.

On follow-up, after 6 months, the patient was no longer symptomatic apart from the pain in her right ankle, which had significantly subsided. Her chest radiography had improved. Her bone scintigraphy showed complete resolution of the rib lesions and improvement of the right ankle findings, retrospectively confirming the diagnosis of multifocal bone isoniazid-monoresistant TB. Continuation of treatment for another 6 months was decided, for a 12-month total course of treatment. A summary of the treatment regimen is shown in table 1. The patient was living with her sister, who was diagnosed with LTBI on contact screening and received treatment.

Discussion

Bone and joint TB is the third most common localisation of EPTB [5, 6] after pleural and lymphatic disease [7]. Rib and ankle joint involvements account for 2.8% and 10.3% of extra-spinal cases, respectively [5]. Concomitant pulmonary involvement is common, reported in 15–23% of cases [5, 8]. This reinforces the need to perform chest radiography on all patients with confirmed or possible TB.

In the present case, multiple skeletal involvement was initially attributed to metastatic disease, but pulmonary lesions led to diagnosis of TB and allowed for culture confirmation and DST. In the setting of isoniazid monoresistance, the discrepancy between molecular and phenotypic DST is not rare. Resistance-conferring mutations in *inhA* and *katG* genes, which are detected by line probe assays, account for ~90% of isoniazid resistance detected by phenotypic DST [9]. This is why conventional culture-based DST should be used in the follow-up evaluation of patients with a high risk for isoniazid resistance [9], as in the case presented here. Whole-genome sequencing was not available for this case but, in future, this may allow for more rapid detection of resistance as well as provide useful epidemiological information.

Table 1. Treatment regimen, duration and rationale for a case of isoniazid-resistant EPTB and PTB

Week	Treatment	Comment
0	RHZE	No resistance mutations detected
4	R(H)ZEL	Phenotypic H resistance; H not stopped because the single R tablets are not widely available in Greece
28	R(H)EL	Discontinuation of Z after 6 months of REZL; although there are no data supporting this decision, the main concern was hepatotoxicity; the patient significantly improved
52	R(H)EL	Discontinuation of treatment after 12 months; cavitating, multifocal TB

R: rifampicin; H: isoniazid; Z: pyrazinamide; E: ethambutol; L: levofloxacin.

https://doi.org/10.1183/2312508X.10023017

Although appropriate treatment of isoniazid-monoresistant TB is of crucial importance, different regimens have been proposed by WHO, American Thoracic Society and National Institute for Health and Care Excellence guidelines, reflecting a knowledge gap in this area. In 2018, the WHO published guidelines for treatment of isoniazid-monoresistant TB, recommending a 6-month regimen of rifampicin, ethambutol, pyrazinamide and levofloxacin in patients with rifampicin-susceptible and isoniazid-monoresistant TB. Addition of a fluoroquinolone to a regimen including rifampicin, ethambutol and pyrazinamide with or without isoniazid reduced the number of deaths and risk of amplification to MDR-TB [10] and was associated with better treatment success [11]. Unfortunately, no data were available for patients with EPTB but prolongation beyond 6 months may be considered in patients with extensive cavitary disease [10]. Based on a recent systematic review and meta-analysis [4], extending the duration of rifampicin and increasing the number of effective drugs for the first 4 months was linked to lower odds of unfavourable outcomes. Continuation of treatment to 12 months was decided in the present case, based on both the extent of pulmonary disease and multiple skeletal involvement.

A case of multidrug-resistant tuberculosis and cancer

Introduction

Concomitant cancer and TB is a major cause of morbidity and mortality and poses a challenge to diagnose and treat both conditions. TB and malignancy may interact in several ways: cancer and its treatment may lead to locally reduced infection barriers and generalised immunosuppression, rendering the cancer patient more susceptible to reactivation of TB [12, 13]; and shared risk factors for TB and cancer co-exist, such as smoking, alcoholism, COPD, immunosuppression and HIV [14–16]. Evidence of previous TB being an independent risk factor for the development of lung cancer has been inconsistent; however, in the large nationwide cohort study by Wu et al. [17], PTB was an independent risk factor for lung cancer. MDR-TB associated with cancer is an additional challenge due to treatment length, increased toxicity associated with chemotherapy and poorer outcomes.

Case presentation

A married man presented to his doctor with productive cough, fever and night sweats. Appetite and weight were stable. He was an ex-smoker (60 pack-years). He had a medical history of COPD, arterial hypertension and hypercholesterolaemia.

The patient was admitted for investigation and was found to be normotensive without tachycardia or tachypnoea; he had normal build (62 kg, body mass index 21 kg·m^{-2}) and no pallor, icterus, clubbing, cyanosis, oedema or peripheral lymphadenopathy. His breath sounds were vesicular and were diminished in the upper third of his left lung, without additional sounds. Examinations were otherwise normal.

Investigations

Initial plain chest radiography revealed a heterogeneous opacity in the upper third of the left lung, and CT scans confirmed the existence of a mass in the upper left lobe

https://doi.org/10.1183/2312508X.10023017

(30×30 mm) (figure 2) but also showed diffuse infiltrates in both lungs and mediastinal lymphadenopathy.

Fibreoptic bronchoscopy was performed and bronchoalveolar lavage showed neoplastic cells. Tests for acid-fast bacilli and PCR for TB were negative. Transbronchial biopsy confirmed a squamous lung carcinoma and the patient underwent further staging investigations. The stage was IIIB, T2aN3M0, for which chemotherapy was recommended. However, subsequently, the bronchoalveolar fluid sample was returned as culture positive for *M. tuberculosis* and, since there was a doubt about previous contact with a patient with MDR-TB (a nephew), rapid molecular tests for common mutations associated with drug resistance were performed and MDR-TB was identified (*rpoB* mutation for rifampicin and *inhA* mutation for isoniazid were detected). No resistance mutations were identified to aminoglycosides, quinolones or ethambutol. He tested negative for HIV.

Subsequently, phenotypic DST confirmed resistance to isoniazid, rifampicin, streptomycin and ethionamide, and susceptibility to pyrazinamide, ethambutol, amikacin, kanamycin, capreomycin, ofloxacin, cycloserine, PAS, moxifloxacin, levofloxacin and linezolid.

Treatment and follow-up

The patient started treatment with ethambutol, pyrazinamide, amikacin, moxifloxacin, cycloserine, PAS and linezolid (plus pyridoxine), with clinical and radiological improvement. At discharge, 8 weeks later, he had three sputum smears negative for acid-fast bacilli, all negative for mycobacterial culture. Ophthalmology and otorhinolaryngology specialists reviewed the patient during admission but made no further recommendations. Amikacin was dosed according to WHO recommendations. Audiometric testing, bloods, ECG and amikacin levels were monitored.

At 2-month follow-up following hospital discharge, the patient reported suicidal ideation and cycloserine was stopped. At 5-month follow-up he had developed acute renal failure and amikacin had to be withdrawn. 10 months after the start of treatment, pancytopaenia due to linezolid and gastric intolerance to PAS occurred; these two drugs were stopped and clinical improvement followed. The patient completed 20 months of treatment with significant clinical improvement: he gained ~5 kg and had resolution of cough; and dyspnoea (modified Medical Research Council score of 2) was similar to before TB and cancer diagnosis.

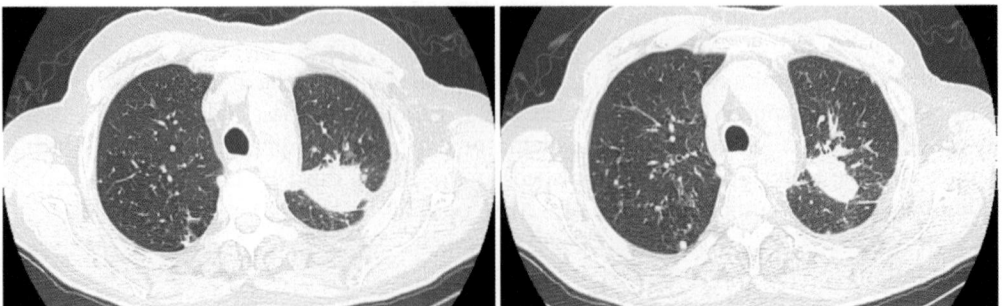

Figure 2. A case of MDR-TB and cancer: computed tomography scans presenting an upper left lobe mass (30×30 mm).

https://doi.org/10.1183/2312508X.10023017

Chemotherapy was postponed during all MDR-TB treatment, but the patient had radiotherapy during MDR treatment and initiated chemotherapy 1 month after ending TB treatment. At this point, the lung cancer was stage IIIC, T3N3M0 (figure 3).

Drug-resistant *Mycobacterium bovis* in a diabetic person living with HIV

A 37-year-old male was admitted with 2 months of fatigue, weakness, occasional low-grade fevers (37.5°C) and morning cough with scant greenish sputum. Chest radiography showed bilateral diffuse nodular opacities and a radiopaque area in the left hilar region (figure 4a). CT scans were also performed (figure 4b and c). Full blood count showed increased white cells with neutrophilia. The patient was diagnosed with community-acquired pneumonia and was hospitalised.

The patient had a 20-year history of DM type 1, and HIV infection since 2014, with an undetectable viral load and CD4 count of 160 cells·μL^{-1}. He was on abacavir/lamivudine and efavirenz treatment due to chronic kidney disease. The patient had *Mycobacterium bovis*, diagnosed in April 2014, and received 6 months of treatment (2HRZE/4HR: 2 months standard quadruple intensive phase/4 months isoniazid and rifampicin combination phase). He relapsed 1 month later with a positive sputum smear and a left psoas abscess, which had required drainage. Again, he cultured positive for *M. bovis*, on pulmonary and abscess samples; DST revealed resistance to isoniazid, rifampicin and pyrazinamide. The patient received treatment for 1 year with a regimen that included

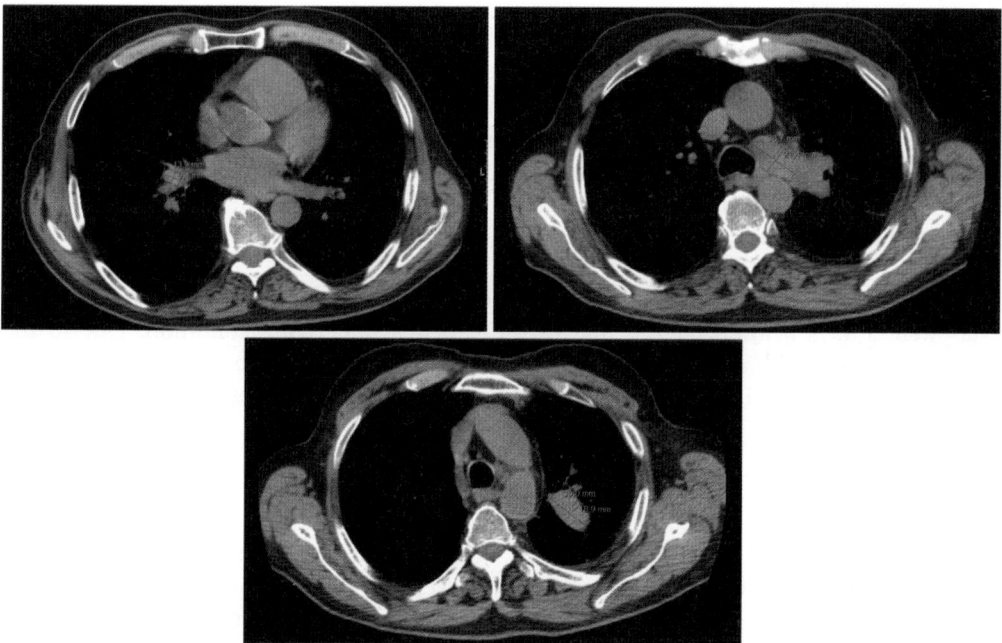

Figure 3. A case of MDR-TB and cancer: computed tomography scans at the end of MDR-TB treatment and after radiotherapy.

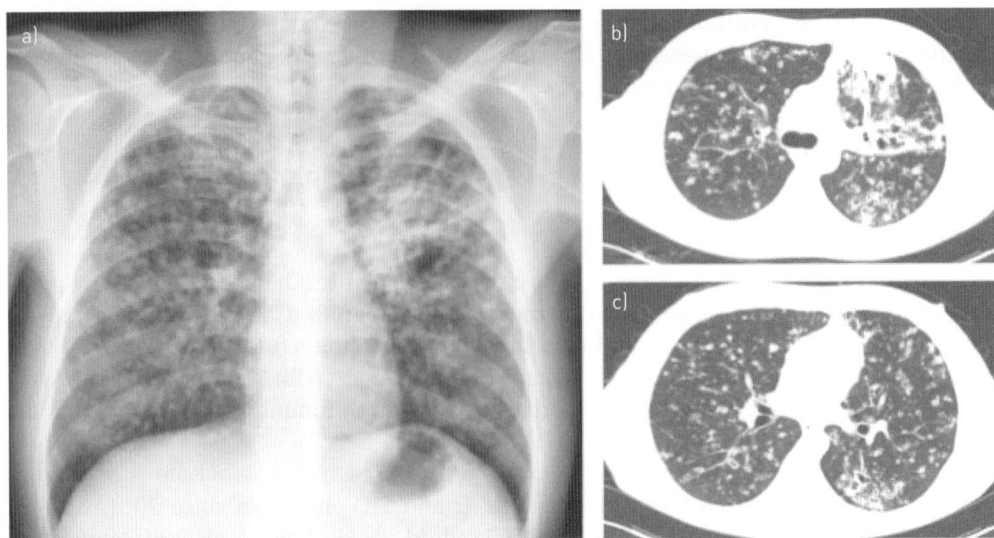

Figure 4. a) Chest radiograph, and b, c) computed tomography scans of the thorax at diagnosis, in a case of drug-resistant *Mycobacterium bovis*.

isoniazid, rifampicin, pyrazinamide and ethambutol, plus levofloxacin and clarithromycin, with clinical improvement as stated by his treating physician.

Due to the history of previous TB episodes, and the resultant risk of resistant TB, the patient was admitted directly to an isolation room and a sputum sample was taken and sent for molecular diagnosis with a GeneXpert system (Cepheid, Sunnyvale, CA, USA). This confirmed *M. bovis* infection and the *rpoB* gene mutation was detected.

The patient was considered as a high-risk pre-XDR-TB case, due to the long-term use of levofloxacin (XDR-TB would have resistance to a fluoroquinolone, such as levofloxacin). Laboratory results showed elevated blood urea nitrogen and serum creatinine (calculated glomerular filtration rate (GFR) 21 mL·min^{-1}), plus nephrotic-range proteinuria (5.96 g per 24 h); therefore, second-line injectable agents could not be used due to the high risk of progressive kidney failure.

The patient was considered a candidate for delamanid or bedaquiline; however, albumin levels were always below 2.8 g·L^{-1} due to the patient's underlying condition. Due to the current condition, with a high risk of death given the multiple comorbidities, treatment was started with moxifloxacin, linezolid, clofazimine, prothionamide, cycloserine, imipenem and amoxicillin/clavulanate.

On follow-up, although nephrotoxic drugs were avoided, the patient developed progressive renal dysfunction, azotaemia and hyperkalaemia with ECG changes that required medical management. Regimen doses were reduced according to the calculated GFR, and the patient was considered at a high risk of adverse events for bedaquiline or delamanid use. 20 days into admission, culture showed resistance to rifampicin, ethambutol, pyrazinamide and ofloxacin, and sensitivity to streptomycin, isoniazid (both 1 and 4 mg·L^{-1}), amikacin, kanamycin, capreomycin and moxifloxacin. The final regimen included moxifloxacin, linezolid, clofazimine, prothionamide, cycloserine and high-dose isoniazid.

 https://doi.org/10.1183/2312508X.10023017

The patient was culture negative after 1 month of treatment and remained negative after 10 months of follow-up. There was also important clinical improvement, with an increase in body weight of 20 kg and the absence of respiratory symptoms. Glucose levels remained in the normal range and glycated haemoglobin was 5.7%. Due to the better glucose control, renal function remained steady at GFR 70–75 mL·min^{-1}. To date, the patient continues on the same antiretroviral regimen and his viral load remains undetectable and CD4 count is 276 cells·mm^{-3}.

Discussion

TB due to *M. bovis* is a zoonosis that mainly infects cattle, and the disease is transmitted to humans through the consumption of unpasteurised and contaminated dairy products. Although the intake of contaminated food is the main route of infection, animal–human and human–human transmission is also possible by inhalation of contaminated particles, mainly in immunosuppressed patients [18].

According to the WHO Global Tuberculosis Report, in 2016 there were an estimated 147 000 new cases of zoonotic TB and 12 500 deaths due to this disease [1]. However, the real incidence of TB cases due to *M. bovis* is underestimated, due to the poor access to culture and identification methods in resource-limited setting [19].

TB due to *M. bovis* infection is clinically and radiologically indistinguishable from that caused by *M. tuberculosis*. The only possible way to differentiate them is through identification of the species on the basis of phenotypic and molecular tests; as a result, frequently *M. bovis* is reported as *M. tuberculosis* complex.

M. bovis should be considered if an isolate is monoresistant to pyrazinamide, as it lacks the enzyme pyrazinamidase, which transforms pyrazinamide into pyrazinoic acid, which is the active molecule against TB. DR-TB (including *M. bovis*) patients require management under programmatic conditions and *M. bovis* must be identified. In this case, all cultures were performed in another institution, and susceptibilities to second-line drugs were not performed.

Treatment of pyrazinamide-monoresistant *M. bovis* consists of 2 months of daily isoniazid, rifampicin and ethambutol, followed by 7 months of isoniazid and rifampicin [20]. Susceptibility testing and expert consultation should guide individualised therapy for polyresistant *M. bovis*.

The real impact of *M. bovis* infection on the outcome of the primary TB treatment and the risk of recurrence is unknown, as is the risk of developing acquired resistance to isoniazid and/or rifampicin, as in this case. There is some literature on the prognosis of *M. bovis* suggesting it is worse than for *M. tuberculosis* in both HIV-negative and HIV-positive patients [21].

HIV and DM are two powerful risk factors for the development of TB, but there is still a lack of information about whether DM should be considered by itself as a risk factor for the development of DR-TB. In the current case, the presence of advanced comorbidities and chronic complications limits the treatment options and increases the risk of development of adverse events; therefore, the regimen had to be individualised.

https://doi.org/10.1183/2312508X.10023017

Previously, it was considered that rifampicin-monoresistant cases could be treated just with the addition of a fluoroquinolone to the regimen; however, the risk of failure is great, and at present all rifampicin-monoresistant cases should be treated as MDR-TB cases. The present case was considered as an XDR-TB case from the beginning, since 1) there was a history of previous exposure to fluoroquinolones for a long time and 2) it was impossible to use a second-line injectable agent due to the great risk of renal failure.

According to the basic principles of DR-TB, a regimen should include at least four new drugs, never used before and likely to be effective. Two of them should be "core" drugs, at least one having a good bactericidal activity and one a good sterilising activity; the other two drugs are the so-called "companion" drugs, whose function is to protect the action of the core drugs [22]. In order to determine the selection of drugs, it is necessary to balance the benefit of a drug's ability to avoid resistance and the risks due to toxicity.

In the current case, taking into consideration pharmacological history and the current clinical state of the patient, empirical treatment included the use of moxifloxacin, linezolid, clofazimine, prothionamide, cycloserine, imipenem and amoxicillin/clavulanate. Once DST results were available, the regimen was individualised: imipenem and amoxicillin/clavulanate were stopped and high-dose isoniazid was added. To date, the clinical and microbiological evolution has been good and, most importantly, there has been improvement of renal function and the patient has not presented any serious adverse event that has required stopping any of the drugs that compose the regimen.

Pre-extensively drug-resistant tuberculosis with multiple limiting adverse reactions to second-line drugs

A 40-year-old man, of Central European origin and homeless since 2010, was admitted to hospital in October 2014 with suspected recurrent *Clostridium difficile* diarrhoea. His medical history was characterised by chronic alcohol abuse, seizures attributed to episodes of alcohol withdrawal and monoclonal gammopathy of unknown significance.

During hospitalisation, chest radiography revealed bilateral apical cavitating lesions. Sputum smear microscopy confirmed the presence of acid-fast bacilli. Anti-TB treatment with rifampicin, isoniazid, ethambutol and pyrazinamide was immediately started. The treatment was well tolerated, and the patient was discharged 6 weeks later with three consecutive negative sputum smears. His diarrhoea also improved and concomitant intestinal TB was suspected. GeneXpert was not performed systematically in 2015 and DST for first-line drugs was not available because of laboratory issues.

Complete DST was available after 6 weeks, a few days after the patient was discharged. The strain was phenotypically resistant to all first-line drugs as well as moxifloxacin. No genetic information was available. The MIC of the strain for moxifloxacin was $2.0\ \mu g\cdot mL^{-1}$. The patient was readmitted on January 23, 2015, to start an individualised second-line treatment for pre-XDR-TB consisting of amikacin, prothionamide, cycloserine and linezolid, plus pyrazinamide and high-dose moxifloxacin [23]. Note that the use of high-dose moxifloxacin was not ideal, as the drug should strictly not have been used. Monitoring of adverse drug reactions was routinely performed through monitoring of clinical symptoms and laboratory screening, according to recommendations [24].

https://doi.org/10.1183/2312508X.10023017

3 months after starting second-line treatment, the patient complained of tinnitus and dizziness associated with mild hearing loss. Amikacin was stopped and PAS started. Because of the lack of potentially active agents, bedaquiline was commenced on April 28, 2015, 3 months into second-line therapy.

During hospitalisation, the patient's mood changed. He developed a depressive effect and anxiety, as well as neuropsychiatric disorders (confusion and euphoria). Although these symptoms could be related to prolonged hospitalisation and alcohol withdrawal, we decided to stop cycloserine on April 30, 2015. Despite the interruption of cycloserine, depression increased. Psychological therapy was initiated, and escitalopram and trazodone were started on May 21, 2015. 3 days later, when the patient was found very sleepy, antidepressive drugs were stopped. The next day, the patient was found unconscious on the ground, with tonic clonic seizures. The episode lasted ~2 min before the patient regained consciousness but remained confused. A second episode occurred 30 min later. Diazepam 10 mg was slowly infused and the patient was transferred to the intensive care unit for observation and further management. As several second-line anti-TB drugs may cause neuropsychiatric disorders and seizures, TB treatment (pyrazinamide, linezolid, prothionamide, PAS, bedaquiline, moxifloxacin) was suspended and the seizures stopped. Brain imaging was reported to be normal. The patient slowly improved and was transferred back to the infectious diseases unit and the TB treatment was reintroduced stepwise every 3 days: PAS and pyrazinamide, then high-dose moxifloxacin then bedaquiline and finally linezolid. Prothionamide was not restarted due to its potential neurotoxicity and its weak effect. After complete review of the literature, the most probable cause of the sleepiness and subsequent fit was ascribed to the serotoninergic syndrome, related to the association of linezolid and antidepressive drugs (escitalopram and trazodone) in a patient with predisposition to seizures [25].

The TB treatment with pyrazinamide, high-dose moxifloxacin, bedaquiline, linezolid and PAS was reinforced by clofazimine in June 2015 and continued until the end of therapy. The patient underwent sputum smear conversion after 30 days and sputum culture conversion after 87 days. The patient was discharged on July 10, 2015, after confirmed sputum culture conversion, and was tolerating treatment.

Unfortunately, the patient was very independent and refused to attend different day centres for the homeless, and started drinking again as soon as he left the hospital. The patient stopped attending for directly observed therapy. The follow-up was characterised by treatment interruptions and readmissions until the end of the therapy.

In October 2016, after 16 months of effective treatment, the patient complained of visual disturbance. A bilateral optic neuritis was diagnosed, probably related to linezolid. At that time, sputum cultures had been negative since April 2015 and the patient had received about 13 months of cumulative treatment after culture conversion. Considering the severe adverse events and the difficulty of compliance of the patient, his TB treatment was withheld.

Unfortunately, the patient was found dead on the public highway a few weeks after his discharge from the hospital. No autopsy was performed.

In conclusion, this patient with pre-XDR-TB experienced several adverse events related to second-line TB treatment: vestibular and cochlear toxicity, neuropsychiatric disorders,

https://doi.org/10.1183/2312508X.10023017

Table 2. Adverse events related to the drugs used in a case of pre-XDR-TB

Drugs	Duration	Adverse event
Amikacin	3 months	Tinnitus, hearing loss
Cycloserine	3 months	Depression, cognitive disorders
Prothionamide	4 months	Depression, cognitive disorders, seizures?
Linezolid+SSRI	2 days	Seizures, serotoninergic syndrome?
Linezolid	17 months	Bilateral optic neuritis

SSRI: selective serotonin reuptake inhibitor (escitalopram and trazodone).

probable serotoninergic syndrome and bilateral optic neuritis (table 2). The treatment was nevertheless adapted to reach "treatment completion" (table 3). This case illustrates the importance of rapid genotypic identification of resistance mutations and the usefulness of systematic GeneXpert MTB/RIF testing. It also highlights the complex management of patients with difficult social contexts and alcohol addiction. Finally, one could consider avoiding drugs such as cycloserine and prothionamide in patients at risk for neuropsychiatric complications, like chronic alcohol users, and could introduce bedaquiline earlier.

A case of cheek tuberculosis: pan-sinusitis and osteomyelitis mimicking cancer

A 28-year-old man presented with severe right facial swelling, involving the zygomatic region. He complained of 5 months of right masseteric pain and bruxism, which were thought to be of dental origin. He had undergone an orthopantomogram, which was

Table 3. Treatment details for a case of pre-XDR-TB

Date[#]	H	R	E	Z	Mfx	Am	PAS	Cs	Pto	Lzd	Cfz	Bdq
06/11/2014	X	X	X	X								
26/01/2015				X	X	X		X	X	X		
23/04/2015				X	X		X	X	X	X		
28/04/2015				X	X		X		X	X		X
25/05/2015				X	X		X			X		X
13/06/2015				X	X		X			X	X	X
16/08/2015					Treatment interruption							
22/09/2015				X	X		X			X	X	X
10/12/2015					Treatment interruption							
22/12/2015				X	X		X			X	X	X
15/04/2016					Treatment interruption							
14/07/2016				X	X		X			X	X	X
15/10/2016					End of therapy							

H: isoniazid; R: rifampicin; E: ethambutol; Z: pyrazinamide; Mfx: moxifloxacin; Am: amikacin; Cs: cycloserine; Pto: prothionamide; Lzd: linezolid; Cfz: clofazimine; Bdq: bedaquiline. [#]: dates presented as day/month/year.

https://doi.org/10.1183/2312508X.10023017

reported to be normal. 2 weeks before his admission, he had an ultrasound scan of his parotid, showing a complex solid/cystic mass in the right parotid gland measuring 5 cm, suggestive of Warthin tumour and necessitating biopsy. The patient was referred to the ear, nose and throat (ENT) rapid diagnostic clinic, and a further ultrasound showed a larger lesion measuring 7 cm in diameter. A fine needle aspiration (FNA) obtained 10 mL of frank pus, demonstrating abundant neutrophils and a few macrophages. No necrosis, granulomas or malignant cells were seen.

The patient was admitted under ENT for further investigations. At that point, the swelling had progressed, and the patient had difficulty opening and closing his mouth. He was otherwise asymptomatic, never having had fevers, night sweats or any other systemic symptoms. On examination, the patient was afebrile and his observations were stable. His physical examination revealed severe facial oedema of the right side of his face, which was firm and non-tender, and which interfered with his right eye and jaw, with no other positive findings. His blood tests were unremarkable, including a negative HIV test. His chest radiograph was normal. The CT scan appearances suggested a sinonasal infective process with significant soft tissue involvement in the infratemporal fossa and complicated by central skull base osteomyelitis with a suggestion of bacterial and fungal (actinomycosis, mucormycosis) aetiologies. The CT was followed by an MRI scan (figure 5), which was reported as showing an abscess overlying the zygomatic arch measuring 5 cm (post FNA), involving the right temporomandibular joint (TMJ). Surrounding myositis was noted. Enhancing signal extending from the mandibular condyle along the cortex of the central skull base and invading the maxillary and ethmoid sinuses was present, with central skull base and right TMJ osteomyelitis suggesting the diagnosis of TB; however, a neoplastic process such as lymphoma or adenoid cystic carcinoma could not be excluded. Biopsies were performed, no acid-fast bacilli were seen, and the samples were sent for TB culture. The histopathology report showed mild chronic inflammatory infiltrate with necrosis. No malignancy was seen. Special stains did not reveal fungi or acid-fast bacilli.

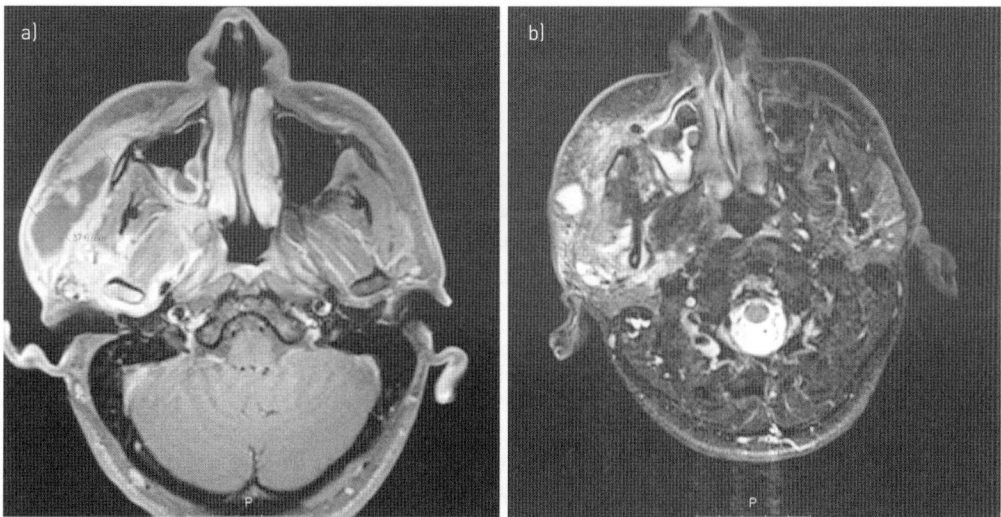

Figure 5. Magnetic resonance imaging scan images showing a) the abscess overlying the zygomatic arch and b) the enhancing soft tissue eroding the base of the skull, in a case of cheek TB.

At this point an infectious diseases consultation was requested. The infection team confirmed the lack of relevant past medical history, including no prior TB or TB contacts. The patient had entered the UK in 1996 and received prior BCG vaccination. He denied fevers, weight loss, night sweats, cough or any other systemic symptoms of TB. The patient had been assaulted 2.5 years before the current presentation, which had resulted in trauma to his right cheek. Anti-TB standard quadruple therapy was started with rifampicin, isoniazid, pyrazinamide and ethambutol. He also received vitamin B6 and vitamin D supplementation. The TB culture grew fully-sensitive *M. tuberculosis* after 18 days.

6 weeks into treatment, he developed high fevers, weakness, fatigue, progressive swelling of his right cheek and erythema nodosum on his shins, the latter erroneously treated in primary care as cellulitis with flucloxacillin. The patient was systemically unwell for the first time during his disease. These symptoms, given normal blood inflammatory markers and exclusion of other aetiologies, were thought to be a paradoxical TB reaction that would be improved with reassurance and ibuprofen. The symptoms did improve, and a new MRI scan performed 2 months into anti-TB therapy showed improvement. The patient was stepped down to continuation therapy with rifampicin and isoniazid. The patient completed 12 months of treatment, reporting good compliance and tolerability to therapy. The 12-month duration was considered necessary, given the localisation and extension of disease through the face and base of the skull. On completion of treatment, an MRI scan was performed, showing minimal residual post-treatment oedema within the right mandibular condyle with development of secondary osteoarthritis of the right TMJ. 6 months after this scan, he was seen again in clinic and he had no TMJ pain or dysfunction. He was asymptomatic, although some mild residual oedema was present on his right cheek. More than 1 year after he finished his treatment, he presented again with a 2-cm right laterocervical lymph node that caused him concern. He had no other TB signs or symptoms and he is currently being investigated for this new finding.

Discussion

TB has re-emerged in London in the last decades, with TB rates reaching above 100 per 100 000 in some boroughs, comparable with highly endemic countries and well above the national rate in the UK [26]. EPTB represents >50% of all TB cases and poses a diagnostic challenge translating into delays in diagnosis and treatment. A high index of suspicion, new diagnostic tests including biomarkers, better microbiological tests and appropriate imaging are needed [27, 28].

Cases of TB primarily affecting the face have been published in recent years, mainly from the Indian subcontinent, with most of the cases reported by dentists, maxillofacial or ENT surgeons [29–33]. TB and other conditions such as actinomycosis and some fungal infections have the capacity to cross tissue boundaries and fascial planes, commonly leading the clinicians to confuse them with malignancy. We demonstrate that TB can occur after trauma. This relationship between TB and trauma was initially suggested in 1975 by DuBrow and Landis [34], and other cases have subsequently been reported [35–37]. In the current case, neither Mantoux nor IGRA tests were performed; however, although these would have been useful to determine previous exposure to TB, they would probably not have helped clinicians to differentiate between BCG, past exposure and current infection. Given his paradoxical reaction, the patient may have demonstrated anergy or negative IGRA. Our case suffered a paradoxical reaction following initiation of therapy, which is less common in HIV-negative than HIV-positive patients with TB.

https://doi.org/10.1183/2312508X.10023017

In summary, the diagnosis of EPTB is often challenging, especially when unusual sites are affected. A higher index of suspicion together with improved diagnostic tools are required to avoid delays in treatment and help reduce morbidity.

References

1. World Health Organization. Global tuberculosis report 2017. WHO/HTM/TB/2017.23. Geneva, World Health Organization, 2017.
2. Stagg HR, Lipman MC, McHugh TD, *et al.* Isoniazid-resistant tuberculosis: a cause for concern? *Int J Tuberc Lung Dis* 2017; 21: 129–139.
3. Menzies D, Benedetti A, Paydar A, *et al.* Standardized treatment of active tuberculosis in patients with previous treatment and/or with mono-resistance to isoniazid: a systematic review and meta-analysis. *PLoS Med* 2009; 6: e1000150.
4. Stagg HR, Harris RJ, Hatherell HA, *et al.* What are the most efficacious treatment regimens for isoniazid-resistant tuberculosis? A systematic review and network meta-analysis. *Thorax* 2016; 71: 940–949.
5. Johansen IS, Nielsen SL, Hove M, *et al.* Characteristics and clinical outcome of bone and joint tuberculosis from 1994 to 2011: a retrospective register-based study in Denmark. *Clin Infect Dis* 2015; 61: 554–562.
6. Sandgren A, Hollo V, van der Werf MJ. Extrapulmonary tuberculosis in the European Union and European Economic Area, 2002 to 2011. *Euro Surveill* 2013; 18: 20431.
7. Leonard MK, Blumberg HM. Musculoskeletal tuberculosis. *Microbiol Spectr* 2017; 5: TNMI7-0046-2017.
8. Wibaux C, Moafo-Tiatsop M, Andrei I, *et al.* Changes in the incidence and management of spinal tuberculosis in a French university hospital rheumatology department from 1966 to 2010. *Joint Bone Spine* 2013; 80: 516–519.
9. World Health Organization. The use of molecular line probe assays for the detection of resistance to isoniazid and rifampicin: policy update. WHO/HTM/TB/2016.12. Geneva, World Health Organization, 2016.
10. World Health Organization. WHO treatment guidelines for isoniazid-resistant tuberculosis. Supplement to the WHO treatment guidelines for drug-resistant tuberculosis. WHO/CDS/TB/2018.7. Geneva, World Health Organization, 2018.
11. Fregonese F, Ahuja SD, Akkerman OW, *et al.* Comparison of different treatments for isoniazid-resistant tuberculosis: an individual patient data meta-analysis. *Lancet Respir Med* 2018; 6: 265–275.
12. Cha SI, Shin KM, Lee JW, *et al.* The clinical course of respiratory tuberculosis in lung cancer patients. *Int J Tuberc Lung Dis* 2009; 13: 1002–1007.
13. Vento S, Lanzafame M. Tuberculosis and cancer: a complex and dangerous liaison. *Lancet Oncol* 2011; 12: 520–522.
14. Engels EA, Shen M, Chapman RS, *et al.* Tuberculosis and subsequent risk of lung cancer in Xuanwei, China. *Int J Cancer* 2009; 124: 1183–1187.
15. Slama K, Chiang CY, Enarson DA, *et al.* Tobacco and tuberculosis: a qualitative systematic review and meta-analysis. *Int J Tuberc Lung Dis* 2007; 11: 1049–1061.
16. Çakar B, Çiledağ A. Evaluation of coexistence of cancer and active tuberculosis; 16 case series. *Respir Med Case Rep* 2017; 23: 33–37.
17. Wu CY, Hu HY, Pu CY, *et al.* Pulmonary tuberculosis increases the risk of lung cancer: a population-based cohort study. *Cancer* 2011; 117: 618–624.
18. de la Rua-Domenech R. Human *Mycobacterium bovis* infection in the United Kingdom: incidence, risks, control measures and review of the zoonotic aspects of bovine tuberculosis. *Tuberculosis* 2006; 86: 77–109.
19. de Kantor IN, LoBue PA, Thoen CO. Human tuberculosis caused by *Mycobacterium bovis* in the United States, Latin America and the Caribbean. *Int J Tuberc Lung Dis* 2010; 14: 1369–1373.
20. Nahid P, Dorman SE, Alipanah N, *et al.* Official American Thoracic Society/Centers for Disease Control and Prevention/Infectious Diseases Society of America clinical practice guidelines: treatment of drug-susceptible tuberculosis. *Clin Infect Dis* 2016; 63: e147–e195.
21. Lan Z, Bastos M, Menzies D. Treatment of human disease due to *Mycobacterium bovis*: a systematic review. *Eur Respir J* 2016; 48: 1500–1503.
22. Caminero JA, Piubello A, Scardigli A, *et al.* Proposal for a standardised treatment regimen to manage pre- and extensively drug-resistant tuberculosis cases. *Eur Respir J* 2017; 50: 1700648.
23. World Health Organization. Companion handbook to the WHO guidelines for programmatic management of drug-resistant tuberculosis. WHO/TB/2014.11. Geneva, World Health Organization, 2014.
24. Caminero JA, ed. Guidelines for Clinical and Operational Management of Drug-Resistant Tuberculosis. Paris, International Union Against Tuberculosis and Lung Disease, 2013.
25. Lawrence KR, Adra M, Gillman PK. Serotonin toxicity associated with the use of linezolid: a review of postmarketing data. *Clin Infect Dis* 2006; 42: 1578–1583.

26. Public Health England. Tuberculosis in London: annual review (2016 data). London, Public Health England, 2017.
27. Norbis L, Alagna R, Tortoli E, *et al*. Challenges and perspectives in the diagnosis of extrapulmonary tuberculosis. *Expert Rev Anti Infect Ther* 2014; 12: 633–647.
28. Gambhir S, Ravina M, Rangan K, *et al*. Imaging in extrapulmonary tuberculosis. *Int J Infect Dis* 2017; 56: 237–247.
29. Al-Hazmi WA. Tuberculosis of the malar and zygomatic bone: a case report. *Int J Health Sci* 2011; 5: 197–200.
30. Gupta R, Garg M, Gupta AK, *et al*. Tuberculous osteomyelitis of the maxilla: a rarest of rare case report. *Natl J Maxillofac Surg* 2014; 5: 188–191.
31. Kannaperuman J, Natarajarathinam G, Rao AV, *et al*. Primary tuberculous osteomyelitis of the mandible: a rare case report. *Dent Res J* 2013; 10: 283–286.
32. Dalmia D, Shah P, Pillai J. Primary tuberculous osteomyelitis of the mandible mimicking a parotid gland abscess. *Indian J Otolaryngol Head Neck Surg* 2016; 68: 257–260.
33. Bai S, Sun CF. Tuberculous osteomyelitis of the mandible with diffuse swelling of the floor of the mouth: a case report. *J Oral Maxillofac Surg* 2014; 72: 749.e1–749.e6.
34. DuBrow EL, Landis FB. Reactivation of pulmonary tuberculosis due to trauma. *Chest* 1975; 68: 596–598.
35. Perrone C, Altieri AM, D'Antonio S, *et al*. Breast tuberculosis after chest trauma – a case report and review of the literature. *Breast Care* 2016; 11: 200–203.
36. Sendi P, Friedl A, Graber P, *et al*. Reactivation of dormant microorganisms following a trauma. Pneumonia, sternal abscess and calcaneus osteomyelitis due to *Mycobacterium tuberculosis*. *Neth J Med* 2008; 66: 363–364.
37. Kim BS, Shin JH, Moon HS, *et al*. Post-traumatic back pain revealed as tuberculous spondylitis – a case report. *Korean J Pain* 2010; 23: 74–77.

Disclosures: M.C. Payen reports receiving a grant from Janssen Pharmaceutica, outside the submitted work, for work on an advisory board regarding bedaquiline in Belgium.

https://doi.org/10.1183/2312508X.10023017

Other titles in the series

ORDER INFORMATION

Monographs are individually priced.
Visit the European Respiratory Society bookshop
www.ersbookshop.com
For bulk purchases contact the Publications Office directly.
European Respiratory Society Publications Office,
442 Glossop Road, Sheffield, S10 2PX, UK.
Tel: 44 114 267 2860; Fax: 44 114 266 5064; E-mail: books@ersnet.org